Esra Meltem Koç
Hilal Aksoy
Editors

Common Diseases According to Family Medicine Practice Guidelines

nova
Medicine & Health
New York

DOI: https://doi.org/10.52305/MKYY8831

Library of Congress Cataloging-in-Publication Data

ISBN: 979-8-89530-302-3 (Hardcover)
ISBN: 979-8-89530-534-8 (eBook)

Published by Nova Science Publishers, Inc. † New York

Contents

Part 1

Musculoskeletal System Diseases

Chapter 1

Arthritis and Arthropathy

Ayşe Koçak*
Department of Medical Biochemistry, Kütahya Health Sciences University, Faculty of Medicine, Kütahya, Turkey

Abstract

Arthritis is caused by inflammation of the joints, also referred to as joint stress. Usually, it results in stiffness, edema, joint discomfort, and restricted mobility. There are more than 150 types of arthritis. Certain types of arthritis do not have a known cause, but other possible causes include illness, infection, genetic flaws, trauma, or overuse. In this chapter, guides to important developments in arthritis and arthropathies have been compiled.

Keywords: arthritis, arthropathy, guidelines

Introduction

Joint inflammation, often known as joint stress, is the cause of arthritis. Usually, it results in stiffness, edema, joint discomfort, and restricted mobility. More than 150 varieties of arthritis exist. Certain types of arthritis do not have a known cause, but other possible causes include illness, infection, genetic flaws, trauma, or overuse. Over 50 million individuals in the US suffer from arthritis, making it the most frequent cause of disability in the country. Although no recognized therapy is available, early intervention can help prevent irreversible joint injury. Joint symptoms associated with arthritis can include stiffness in the morning, particularly pain, inflammation, decreased mobility of the joint, warmth, and redness of the skin surrounding a joint. One kind of arthritic joint illness is called arthroscopy. Arthropathies may be related to an infection, such as Lyme disease, or a hematologic (blood) problem. This disease's signs and symptoms are stiffness and edema in the joints and a lower range of motion. Diagnosis: to identify the underlying cause of symptoms, a thorough clinical assessment is necessary. In this chapter, clinical guidelines for many types of arthritis that can be used in family medicine are listed.

* Corresponding Author's Email: kocak.ayse@gmail.com.

In: Common Diseases According to Family Medicine Practice Guidelines
Editors: Esra Meltem Koç and Hilal Aksoy
ISBN: 979-8-89530-302-3

Rheumatoid Arthritis

Recommendations for the use of disease-modifying antirheumatic medications (DMARDs) in the treatment of rheumatoid arthritis (RA) were created by the EULAR in 2010 (Smolen et al., 2010). Since then, as new information has become available and new definitions of remission, treatment approaches, categorization criteria, and medications have been developed, changes to these guidelines have been made every three years. The suggestions were last updated in 2019 (Neogi et al., 2010; Felson et al., 2011; Smolen et al., 2010; Smolen et al., 2020). Although recommendations are not required to be updated automatically, they do become necessary when new information becomes available, and their possible effects on guidance documents need to be taken into account. A line such as "With the current rate of development, we expect an update of these recommendations to be necessary for about 3–4 years" should be used to conclude the discussion portions of all prior publications on the EULAR RA treatment recommendations. It is necessary for the convenor of the Task Force, the methodologist, and the other members of the group to closely monitor any advancements in the area and determine if they warrant proposing an update to the EULAR Council. Many questions come to mind when analyzing the field's achievements, namely (Smolen et al., 2010) Which medications have recently received approval or successfully completed phase 3 trials? (Neogi et al., 2010)) Have real-world data analysis or clinical trials revealed any previously unidentified safety concerns? (Felson et al., 2011) What fresh data has emerged from strategic trials or from the patient's point of view? (Smolen et al., 2010) Has the level of evidence (LoE) for recommendations that were previously founded on a paucity of evidence increased? (Smolen et al., 2020) Have any fresh findings refuted any of the earlier recommendations? (6) Have fresh findings on topics covered in earlier research agendas been released?

It was especially wise to review the present proposals in light of two factors (US Food and Drug Administration, 2021). First, based on an analysis of a randomized trial, the US Food and Drug Administration (FDA) issued a statement and warning in 2021 regarding the cardiovascular and cancer risks of tofacitinib in comparison with TNF-inhibitors. The entire study was then published in the early months of 2022 (Ytterberg et al., 2022). Second, although it has a low to moderate evidence level, the American College of Rheumatology (ACR) updated its RA management guidelines recently and specifically discouraged the use of glucocorticoids (GCs), citing their greater toxicity than benefits (Fraenkel et al., 2021). Reexamining this matter proved necessary because EULAR has previously strongly supported the use of short-term GCs as a bridging therapy when beginning conventional synthetic (cs) DMARD therapy, with quick GC tapering to cessation afterward. Particularly in situations when a large number of medications are readily available, as is now the case with RA, management guidelines have to offer some direction on what specialists consider to be a reasonable, or perhaps even the most successful, strategy for treating a condition. How should one target the therapeutic objective, and what is it? When a patient receives a new diagnosis, which medications should they take? What steps should be taken in the event that a medicine, whether used initially or later, fails to achieve the intended therapeutic outcome because of ineffectiveness or side effects? In the framework of such guidelines, these and other concerns need to be addressed, and patient and knowledgeable input from many fields is crucial to their creation. Furthermore, expenses need to be taken into consideration not just in nations with lower incomes but also in those where the cost of medications is reasonable but the healthcare system mandates spending caps. All of this will be covered in the current update and is a component of the EULAR RA treatment recommendations.

Notably, no new medicine class has been authorized since the last update. Since then, the European Union and other regions have granted licenses for two more JAKi, upadacitinib, and filgotinib; however, the 2019 update has previously addressed them based on phase 3 studies. As a result, the task force concentrated on JAKi's safety features and the strategic usage of available agents in the sequence that was deemed most advantageous for GCs. It was crucial to restate these overarching principles as the cornerstone of all treatment approaches, even though the task force continued to use them in earlier iterations of these recommendations for information on general aspects of RA management that relate to common sense and do not require specific evidence levels.

A. The goal of treating patients with RA should be optimal treatment, determined by a joint agreement between the patient and the rheumatologist. The language of this concept and its designation as item A have been not altered. All participants agreed with the patient research partner's suggestion to explicitly state in the accompanying language that the "shared decision" entailed acknowledging patient preferences. If not, there was no more debate on this matter, and all participants (100%) agreed to maintain the current language. The level of agreement (LoA) was 10.0 ± 0.
B. Decisions on treatment are dependent on the state of the patient's illness, safety concerns, and other variables such as comorbidities and the rate at which structural damage develops. The task force determined that there was no need for a modification, although it was debated to emphasize the need of obtaining a complete history and information from the patient. All members of the task force voted in favor of maintaining this principle in its current form, with a LoA of 9.9 ± 0.4.
C. Patients suffering from RA should be treated primarily by rheumatologists. Similar to other task forces, this idea has generated discussion; it was proposed that the term "primarily" be removed. However, as previously stated, rheumatologists and/or rheumatology training are either completely unavailable in many nations, or the number of qualified rheumatologists is insufficient to care for all RA patients. In the end, 97.8% of the voters supported keeping the original phrasing and word arrangement, and the LoA was 9.8 ± 0.9.
D. To address the heterogeneity of RA, patients need access to a variety of medications with distinct mechanisms of action; they may need many subsequent treatments over the course of their lives. In 2019, this item was added to the principles, and in 2022, it received full endorsement. However, it was recommended to note in the context of the discussion that cycling should not happen too quickly because every agent may take a few weeks or months to show their full effects, and as a result, the effectiveness of any new therapy should not be determined too soon. In light of this, the EULAR guidance's general treat-to-target strategy centers on achieving the primary treatment target - remission in early and low disease activity in long-standing disease - at roughly 6 months, as well as at least a 50% improvement in disease activity within 3 months. Drug cycling should thus be avoided prior to these benchmarks and in the event of accidental or temporary flares, unless safety requires a different course of action. There was 100% agreement in the vote, and the LoA was 9.8 ± 0.6.

E. The treating rheumatologist should take these substantial human, medical, and social costs into account while managing RA. Once more, all task force members supported this item (100% of the votes), which also illustrates the overall cost-savings perspective of the EULAR Task Force: If two medications are equally suitable for a given patient, then the less expensive medication should be chosen. This proverb begins with oral vs. parenteral methotrexate (MTX), then it broadens to include the option between biologic originator (bo) and biosimilar (bs) DMARDs, and it concludes with a comparison between bDMARDs and tsDMARDs. However, prices must be seen broadly since they encompass not only the cost of a medication in the pharmacy, but also the expenses incurred by the hospital, the community, and individual patients. Remember that approximately ten years ago, EULAR approved the use of biosimilar (bs) DMARDs for this purpose, long before other organizations followed suit. The use of bsDMARDs has already significantly lowered medication costs, and a logical and evidence-based treatment prescription policy also contributes to cost savings: If two medications are equally safe and effective for a given patient, the less expensive one should be taken—a very common practice in all fields of medicine. It is noteworthy that healthcare systems in resource-poor nations, along with patients and rheumatologists within them, face significant financial and human resource constraints. This issue also affects certain high-income countries, particularly in the realm of rheumatology. While rheumatologists play a crucial role as patient advocates, it is equally important that payers and funders are aware of the wealth of data available to them and all other health professionals involved in managing RA. Without funding for advanced technologies, treatment success may be less likely to be achieved. Treatment for RA involves appropriate management from the beginning of the patient's journey as outlined in these suggestions, not only expensive treatment alternatives such as targeted DMARDs. At the meeting, every participant agreed with this premise, and the LoA was 9.7 ± 0.6.

Psoriatic Arthritis

Remarkable advances have been made in the treatment of psoriatic arthritis (PsA) in recent years. Ideas have changed over time, including the pre- and extremely early diagnosis of PsA, the identification of therapeutic targets, and the holistic management of comorbidities (Zabotti et al., 2023; Alharbi et al., 2020; Ferguson et al., 2019; Lubrano et al., 2023).

The following drugs are currently licensed for the treatment of PsA; conventional synthetic (cs) disease-modifying antirheumatic drugs (DMARDs), biologic DMARDs targeting tumor necrosis factor (TNF), interleukin (IL)-12/23 or IL-23 pathway, IL-17A and IL- Synthetic (ts) DMARDs that inhibit the 17A/F pathway and Janus kinases (JAKs) or phosphodiesterase 4 (PDE4) (Kerschbaumer et al., 2024). Following a large randomized controlled trial (RCT) of tofacitinib in rheumatoid arthritis (RA), new safety information regarding inflammatory arthritis has emerged, particularly a global warning against JAK inhibitors (JAKis) (Ytterberg et al., 2022; European League Against Rheumatism, 2024; Gossec et al., 2016). This field has undergone tremendous change since the 2019 EULAR. Guidelines for the pharmaceutical treatment of PsA have been published (Gossec et al., 2020; Coates et al., 2022; Coates & Gossec, 2023; Singh et al., 2019). Therefore, it was deemed appropriate to review the EULAR

PsA management guidelines in 2024 (FitzGerald et al., 2021). The steering group and 23 additional experts made up the task force. The members, who represented 19 different nations (of which 15 were EULAR countries), included 2 dermatologists, 1 infectious disease specialist, 2 rheumatology/epidemiology fellows/trainees, 3 HPRs, 2 affected individuals with PsA serving as patient research partners, and 27 rheumatology specialists. In total, 47% of the task force members did not participate in the 2019 update. The group convened in person in April 2023 to create the revised bullet points. Until an agreement was established, each topic was thoroughly addressed in both plenary sessions and smaller (breakout) groups. The task force first set the limit for acceptance of individual recommendations at ≥75% majority; later, (after discussions and possible reformulations) at ≥67% majority; and finally, if necessary, the last round of votes was accepted with >50% acceptance or else a proposal was rejected. Group approval was obtained through votes (with raised hands) for each bullet point (European League Against Rheumatism, 2024).

Of the seven overarching principles (OAPs), one has been added (overarching principle G), three have been reworded, and three have remained untouched. Please refer to the recommendation papers from 2015 and 2019 for further details on the methodology that resulted in the OAPs (either unchanged or significantly modified) (Zabotti et al., 2023; Gossec et al., 2016). The following highlights some of the main ideas from the OAPs discussion:

A. A comprehensive approach to the treatment of psoriatic arthritis may be necessary due to its diverse and possibly severe nature (unchanged). Not all patients with PsA will experience severe manifestations, despite the condition's potential for severity (FitzGerald et al., 2021; Kerola et al., 2022). Many patients benefit from interdisciplinary care when doctors from various disciplines work together with HPRs who possess the necessary knowledge (So & Tam, 2021; Wendling et al., 2022).
B. The goal of treating patients with psoriatic arthritis should be to provide the best treatment possible. This choice should be made jointly by the patient and the rheumatologist, taking into account costs, patient preferences, safety, and efficacy. This OAP was updated in 2019 to include patient preferences as a factor to be taken into account and to emphasize the value of shared decision-making to maximize treatment adherence and efficacy while minimizing complications caused by uncontrolled (active) disease and possible pharmaceutical side effects (Smolen et al., 2019; Caso et al., 2020)).
C. Rheumatologists are the experts who should handle psoriatic arthritis patients' musculoskeletal symptoms; when there is clinically significant skin involvement, they should work together to diagnose and treat the condition.
    a. Given their knowledge of the various medications used to treat PsA and other rheumatic and musculoskeletal illnesses (RMDs), including the crucial elements of safety and comorbidity, we believe that rheumatology specialists offer the best treatment for patients with PsA. In some clinical situations, seeing dermatologists and occasionally other experts may be beneficial (see also the overarching principles F and G). For better consistency with previous bullet points, very little rewording was done to characterize skin involvement as "clinically relevant" rather than "clinically significant." The role of HPRs, who are often not prescribers in EULAR nations, is not covered by this bullet point.

D. The main objective of treating psoriatic arthritis patients is to maximize their quality of life in terms of health by managing their symptoms, preventing structural damage, restoring normal function, and allowing them to participate in social activities. Reducing inflammation is a crucial step toward achieving these objectives (unchanged).
E. When treating patients with psoriatic arthritis, each musculoskeletal manifestation should be considered, and treatment decisions should be made (unchanged) accordingly.
F. Non-musculoskeletal symptoms (skin, eyes, and gastrointestinal system) and comorbidities (obesity, metabolic syndrome, cardiovascular disease, or depression) should be considered while managing individuals with psoriatic arthritis.
    a. The phrase "such as obesity" was included since it is common in PsA and has an impact on the results (Porta et al., 2021; (Leung et al., 2023). While metabolic syndrome is a group of risk factors that increase the possibility of developing type 2 diabetes and cardiovascular disease, obesity is the excess of body fat. A major factor in the development of metabolic syndrome is obesity. While the task force members debated whether other comorbidities ought to be included, they agreed that the phrase "such as" implied that comorbidities, in general, should be considered, negating the necessity to enumerate them. The decision about therapy may be influenced by depression and maybe other mental health conditions. In PsA, central sensitization to pain perception is common and affects results; this could make managing the condition more challenging (Trouvin et al., 2022; Ballegaard et al., 2021).
    b. Malignancies and bone health were also especially addressed. There are unique problems with managing comorbidities, especially in terms of assigning management responsibilities for different disease areas. Solutions must be implemented according to the unique needs of each patient, the unique environment of each nation, and the structure of the healthcare system.
G. To maximize the benefit-risk profile, the treatment option should consider safety concerns about specific modalities of action (new).
    a. The task force suggested this new OAP to underscore the need to consider safety factors for every patient in light of new information on the safety of various modalities of action (Ytterberg et al., 2022).

Osteoarthritis of the Hand, Hip, and Knee

The most prevalent kind of arthritis, osteoarthritis (OA), affects an estimated 302 million people globally (Cisternas et al., 2016; GBD 2015 DALYs and HALE Collaborators, 2016; Murphy et al., 2008; Murphy et al., 2010; Qin et al., 2017) and is the main cause of impairment in the elderly. The appendicular joints that are most frequently impacted are the hands, hips, and knees.

Osteophyte production, cartilage degradation, bone remodeling, and synovial inflammation are some of the joint-wide pathologies that define osteoarthritis (OA), which can cause pain, stiffness, swelling, and loss of normal joint function.

Patients with OA are likely to be treated with a variety of pharmacological and nonpharmaceutical therapies, frequently in combination, because the condition affects them for decades of their lives.

An all-encompassing strategy for the management of osteoarthritis (OA) in a particular patient can involve topical, oral, and intraarticular drugs in addition to behavioral, psychological, and educational treatments. The use of physical, psychological, and/or pharmaceutical therapy by a suitable practitioner is assumed in the recommendations. The objectives of management and the guidelines to achieve them are universally applicable to patients. However, a physical, psychological, mind-body, or pharmacological intervention may be sufficient to manage symptoms for certain people at certain times; for others, a series of therapies may be used sequentially or in combination. Patients will differ in what treatments they receive and in what order.

In addition to the patient's physical condition, treatment recommendations should consider their personal preferences and beliefs. Patients with OA who do not specifically contraindicate themselves from the suggested therapy are covered by this guideline. The presence of any medical conditions, such as hypertension, heart failure, cardiovascular disease, gastrointestinal bleeding risk, chronic kidney disease, or other comorbidities, should be evaluated for each patient, as it may affect the patient's risk of experiencing side effects from specific pharmaceutical agents. Additionally, the patient's history of surgery, disease severity, and injuries, as well as the availability and accessibility of services (such as transportation, distance, cost, insurance coverage, and ability to take time off work), may influence the patient's decision regarding physical, psychological, and mind-body approaches.

It is anticipated that this kind of evaluation will be carried out before a personalized treatment plan is finalized. The management should start with the pharmacologic medications that have the least toxicity or systemic exposure. Due to the pain and functional restrictions caused by OA and/or comorbidities, patients can suffer a wide range of extra symptoms. These include poor coping mechanisms, irregular sleep patterns, persistent, all-over discomfort, and mood disorders including anxiety and depression.

The Patient Panel stated that while selecting a course of therapy, it is important to consider the wider impact of OA on various comorbidities. This is best addressed by a multimodal treatment plan as opposed to one that is restricted to the prescription of a single medicine. The patient's general well-being and the effectiveness of their OA therapy can be enhanced by actions targeted at improving mood, reducing stress, treating sleeplessness, controlling weight, and increasing fitness. Indeed, even in cases where there is a paucity of evidence specifically pertaining to OA patients, therapies that have shown promise in the treatment of chronic pain may also prove helpful in OA (Skelly et al., 2018). Guidelines pertaining to physical, psychological, and mind-body approaches presume that the patient will be incorporating the intervention into their regular care unless otherwise noted. This guideline defines "usual care" as using over-the-counter oral nonsteroidal anti-inflammatory drugs (NSAIDs) and/or acetaminophen at maximally recommended or safely tolerated doses, as has typically been specifically approved in clinical trials of nonpharmacologic interventions.

In summary, a thorough, multimodal approach to treating patients with hand, hip, and/or knee OA must be provided in the framework of shared decision-making with patients in order to select the safest and most successful course of action. There is still a lot of research to be done, and there is a need for additional effective treatment choices for the millions of individuals who suffer from osteoarthritis globally.

Oligoarthritis, Temporomandibular Joint Arthritis, and Systemic Juvenile Idiopathic Arthritis

The American College of Rheumatology (ACR) reviews clinical practice recommendations every year and makes the necessary revisions in response to the evolving medical field. 2017 saw the start of an effort to update the juvenile idiopathic arthritis (JIA) recommendations (Beukelman et al., 2011; Ringold et al., 2013) from 2011 and 2013. To establish the recommendations' scope, a conference was held to identify important clinical themes. Due to the wide range of subjects covered, it was necessary to divide this clinical practice guideline into many sections to reflect advancements in JIA therapy and a deeper knowledge of pathophysiology. The first section was published in two pieces in 2019 (Ringold et al., 2019; Angeles-Han et al., 2019) and dealt with polyarthritis, sacroiliitis, enthesitis, and uveitis. We created clinically pertinent Patient/Population, Intervention, Comparison, and Outcomes (PICO) questions after the themes were chosen. The best available evidence was then used to produce recommendations using the Grading of Recommendations Assessment, Development, and Evaluation (GRADE) system for frequently encountered clinical situations.

Before the final vote, suggestions were solicited from pertinent parties, such as a panel of young adults with JIA and parents of JIA children, to consider their viewpoints and beliefs. The necessity for customized therapy while keeping an eye on the available data was emphasized by the patient/caregiver and guideline voting panels.

When starting treatment for active oligoarthritis, a planned nonsteroidal anti-inflammatory medication (NSAID) trial is cautiously advised. NSAIDs can reduce pain and have long been the mainstay of oligoarthritis therapy (Chhabra et al., 2020; Brik et al., 2005; Kvien et al., 1984). However, due to limited effectiveness (until the inactive illness is attained) and probable side effects (e.g., bruising, gastritis), the initial NSAID trial should be short. Because some voting panelists preferred that NSAID usage be avoided completely, the panelists could not agree on the proper period of first use prior to increasing the medication.

When treating active oligoarthritis, intraarticular glucocorticoids (IAGCs) are highly advised as part of the first treatment plan. The suggested preferable agent is triamcinolone hexacetonide, which is strongly advised. IAGCs are highly recommended despite the low quality of the evidence because of their high chance of sustained response and little possibility of side effects (Sato et al., 2014; Marti et al., 2008; Breit et al., 2000). Patients and caregivers expressed agreement over the usefulness of IAGC. Preferred over leflunomide, sulfasalazine, or hydroxychloroquine (in that order), methotrexate is conditionally advised. Given the overwhelming body of data demonstrating methotrexate's long-term safety and effectiveness in children, it is the recommended treatment even in the lack of comparative studies (Ravelli et al., 2017; Albarouni et al., 2014; Bava et al., 2019). There are other therapeutic choices available because methotrexate's tolerance varies (Franova et al., 2016; Imundo & Jacobs, 1996; Foeldvari & Wierk, 2005).

Conclusion

Arthritis encompasses over 150 types of joint inflammation diseases, causing significant disability and affecting over 50 million individuals in the US. While certain types have unknown causes, others may be the result of infections, genetic factors, trauma, or overuse. Common symptoms include joint stiffness, pain, swelling, and reduced mobility. Early diagnosis and intervention are crucial to prevent irreversible joint damage.

References

Albarouni, M., Becker, I., & Horneff, G. (2014). Predictors of response to methotrexate in juvenile idiopathic arthritis. *Pediatric Rheumatology Online Journal, 12*, 35. https://doi.org/10.1186/1546-0096-12-35.

Alharbi, S., Justine Y. Ye, Ker-Ai Lee et al., (2020). Remission in psoriatic arthritis: Definition and predictors. *Seminars in Arthritis and Rheumatism, 50*(6), 2020. https://doi.org/10.1016/j.semarthrit.2020.01.012.

Angeles-Han, S. T., Sarah Ringold, Timothy Beukelman, Daniel Lovell, Carlos A. Cuello, et al., (2019). 2019 American College of Rheumatology/Arthritis Foundation guideline for the screening, monitoring, and treatment of juvenile idiopathic arthritis-associated uveitis. *Arthritis Rheumatology, 71*, 864–877. https://doi.org/10.1002/art.40885.

Ballegaard, C., Marie Skougaard, Jørgen Guldberg-Møller, Christoffer V. Nissen et al., (2021). Comorbidities, pain and fatigue in psoriatic arthritis, psoriasis and healthy controls: A clinical cohort study. *Rheumatology, 60*(7), 3289–3300. https://doi.org/10.1093/rheumatology/keaa780.

Bava, C., Federica Mongelli, Angela Pistorio, Marta Bertamino, Giulia Bracciolini, Sara Dalprà, Sergio et al., (2019). A prediction rule for lack of achievement of inactive disease with methotrexate as the sole disease-modifying antirheumatic therapy in juvenile idiopathic arthritis. *Pediatric Rheumatology Online Journal, 17*, 50. https://doi.org/10.1186/s12969-019-0355-0.

Beukelman, T., Nivedita M. Patkar, Kenneth G. Saag, Sue Tolleson-Rinehart, Randy Q. Cron et al., (2011). American College of Rheumatology recommendations for the treatment of juvenile idiopathic arthritis: Initiation and safety monitoring of therapeutic agents for the treatment of arthritis and systemic features. *Arthritis Care Research (Hoboken), 63*, 465–482. https://doi.org/10.1002/acr.20460.

Breit, W., Frosch, M., Meyer, U., Heinecke, A., & Ganser, G. (2000). A subgroup-specific evaluation of the efficacy of intraarticular triamcinolone hexacetonide in juvenile chronic arthritis. *Journal of Rheumatology, 27*, 2696–2702.

Brik, R., Gepstein, V., & Berkovitz, D. (2005). Low-dose methotrexate treatment for oligoarticular juvenile idiopathic arthritis nonresponsive to intraarticular corticosteroids. *Clinical Rheumatology, 24*, 612–614. https://doi.org/10.1007/s10067-005-1116-7.

Caso, F., Maria Sole Chimenti, Luca Navarini, Piero Ruscitti, Rosario Peluso et al., (2020). Metabolic syndrome and psoriatic arthritis: Considerations for the clinician. *Expert Review of Clinical Immunology, 16*(4), 409–420. https://doi.org/10.1080/1744666X.2020.1740593.

Chhabra, A., Kiem Oen, Adam M. Huber, Natalie J. Shiff, Gilles Boire et al., (2020). Real-world effectiveness of common treatment strategies for juvenile idiopathic arthritis: Results from a Canadian cohort. *Arthritis Care Research (Hoboken), 72*, 897–906. https://doi.org/10.1002/acr.23922.

Cisternas, M. G., Murphy, L., Sacks, J. J., Solomon, D. H., Pasta, D. J., & Helmick, C. G. (2016). Alternative methods for defining osteoarthritis and the impact on estimating prevalence in a US population-based survey. *Arthritis Care Research (Hoboken), 68*, 574–580. https://doi.org/10.1002/acr.22721.

Coates, L. C., Enrique R. Soriano, Nadia Corp, Heidi Bertheussen, Kristina Callis Duffin et al., (2022). Group for Research and Assessment of Psoriasis and Psoriatic Arthritis (GRAPPA): Updated treatment recommendations for psoriatic arthritis 2021. *Nature Reviews Rheumatology, 18*(8), 465–479. https://doi.org/10.1038/s41584-022-00798-0.

Coates, L., & Gossec, L. (2023). The updated GRAPPA and EULAR recommendations for the management of psoriatic arthritis: Similarities and differences. *Joint Bone Spine, 90*(1), 105469. https://doi.org/10.1016/j.jbspin.2022.105469.

European League Against Rheumatism. (2024). *EULAR Recommendations.* https://www.eular.org/web/static/lib/pdfjs/web/viewer.html?file=https://www.eular.org/document/download/680/b9eb08d0-faca-4606-8ed9-d0539b3f312a/660.

Felson, D. T., Smolen, J. S., Wells, G., Zhang, B., van Tuyl, L. H., Funovits, J., Aletaha, D., Allaart, C. F., Bathon, J., Bombardieri, S., Brooks, P., Brown, A., Matucci-Cerinic, M., Choi, H., Combe, B., de Wit, M., Dougados, M., Emery, P., Furst, D., … Boers, M. (2011). American College of Rheumatology/European League Against Rheumatism provisional definition of remission in rheumatoid arthritis for clinical trials. *Arthritis & Rheumatism, 63*(3), 573–586. https://doi.org/10.1002/art.30129.

Ferguson, L. D., Stefan Siebert, Iain B. McInnes, Naveed Sattar (2019). Cardiometabolic comorbidities in RA and PsA: Lessons learned and future directions. *Nature Reviews Rheumatology, 15*(8), 461–474. https://doi.org/10.1038/s41584-019-0256-0.

FitzGerald, O., Alexis Ogdie, Vinod Chandran, Laura C. Coates, Arthur Kavanaugh et al., (2021). Psoriatic arthritis. *Nature Reviews Disease Primers, 7*(1), 59. https://doi.org/10.1038/s41572-021-00293-y.

Foeldvari, I., & Wierk, A. (2005). Effectiveness of leflunomide in patients with juvenile idiopathic arthritis in clinical practice. *Journal of Rheumatology, 37*, 1763–1767. https://doi.org/10.3899/jrheum.090874.

Fraenkel, L., Joan M. Bathon, Bryant R. England, E. William St Clair, Thurayya Arayssi et al., (2021). 2021 American College of Rheumatology guideline for the treatment of rheumatoid arthritis. *Arthritis & Rheumatology, 73*(7), 1108–1123. https://doi.org/10.1002/art.41752.

Franova, J., Š. Fingerhutová, K. Kobrová, R. Srp et al., (2016). Methotrexate efficacy, but not its intolerance, is associated with the dose and route of administration. *Pediatric Rheumatology Online Journal, 14*, 36. https://doi.org/10.1186/s12969-016-0099-z.

GBD 2015 DALYs and HALE Collaborators. (2016). Global, regional, and national disability-adjusted life-years (DALYs) for 315 diseases and injuries and healthy life expectancy (HALE), 1990–2015: A systematic analysis for the Global Burden of Disease Study 2015. *Lancet, 388*, P1603–1658.

Gossec, L., J. S. Smolen, S. Ramiro, M. de Wit, M. Cutolo, M. Dougados, P. Emery et al., (2016). European League Against Rheumatism (EULAR) recommendations for the management of psoriatic arthritis with pharmacological therapies: 2015 update. *Annals of the Rheumatic Diseases, 75*(3), 499–510. https://doi.org/10.1136/annrheumdis-2015-208337.

Gossec, L., Xenofon Baraliakos, Andreas Kerschbaumer, Maarten de Wit et al., (2020). EULAR recommendations for the management of psoriatic arthritis with pharmacological therapies: 2019 update. *Annals of the Rheumatic Diseases, 79*(6), 700–712. https://doi.org/10.1136/annrheumdis-2020-217159.

Imundo, L. F., & Jacobs, J. C. (1996). Sulfasalazine therapy for juvenile rheumatoid arthritis. *Journal of Rheumatology, 23*, 360–366.

Kerola, A. M., Amirhossein Kazemi, Silvia Rollefstad, Siri Lillegraven, Joseph Sexton et al., (2022). All-cause and cause-specific mortality in rheumatoid arthritis, psoriatic arthritis and axial spondyloarthritis: A nationwide registry study. *Rheumatology, 61*(12), 4656–4666. https://doi.org/10.1093/rheumatology/keac210.

Kerschbaumer, A., Josef S. Smolen, Ricardo J. O. Ferreira, Heidi Bertheussen et al., (2024). Efficacy and safety of pharmacological treatment of psoriatic arthritis: A systematic literature research informing the 2023 update of the EULAR recommendations for the management of psoriatic arthritis. *Annals of the Rheumatic Diseases*, 2024. https://doi.org/10.1136/ard-2024-225534.

Kvien, T. K., Hoyeraal, H. M., & Sandstad, B. (1984). Naproxen and acetylsalicylic acid in the treatment of pauciarticular and polyarticular juvenile rheumatoid arthritis: Assessment of tolerance and efficacy in a single-centre 24-week double-blind parallel study. *Scandinavian Journal of Rheumatology, 13*, 342–350. https://doi.org/10.3109/03009748409111307.

Leung, Y. Y., Lihi Eder, Ana-Maria Orbai, Laura C. Coates, Maarten de Wit et al., (2023). Association between obesity and likelihood of remission or low disease activity status in psoriatic arthritis applying index-based and patient-based definitions of remission: A cross-sectional study. *RMD Open, 9*(3), e003157. https://doi.org/10.1136/rmdopen-2023-003157.

Lubrano, E., Silvia Scriffignano, Kurt de Vlam, Mario Ronga, Fabio Massimo Perrotta et al., (2023). Triple jump for the optimal management of psoriatic arthritis: Diet, sleep and exercise–a review. *RMD Open, 9*(3), e003339. https://doi.org/10.1136/rmdopen-2023-003339.

Marti, P., Molinari, L., Bolt, I. B., Seger, R., & Saurenmann, R. K. (2008). Factors influencing the efficacy of intra-articular steroid injections in patients with juvenile idiopathic arthritis. *European Journal of Pediatrics, 167*, 425–430. https://doi.org/10.1007/s00431-007-0525-9.

Murphy, L. B., C. G. Helmick, T. A. Schwartz, J. B. Renner, G. Tudor, G. G. Koch, A. D. Dragomir et al., (2010). One in four people may develop symptomatic hip osteoarthritis in his or her lifetime. *Osteoarthritis Cartilage, 18*, 1372–1379. https://doi.org/10.1016/j.joca.2010.08.005.

Murphy, L., Todd A. Schwartz, Charles G. Helmick, Jordan B. Renner, Gail Tudor, Gary Koch et al., (2008). Lifetime risk of symptomatic knee osteoarthritis. *Arthritis Rheumatism, 59*, 1207–1213. https://doi.org/10.1002/art.24021.

Neogi, T., Aletaha, D., Silman, A. J., Naden, R. L., Felson, D. T., Aggarwal, R., Bingham, C. O., Birnbaum, N. S., Burmester, G. R., Bykerk, V. P., Cohen, M. D., Combe, B., Costenbader, K. H., Dougados, M., Emery, P., Ferraccioli, G., Hazes, J. M., Hobbs, K., Huizinga, T. W., … Hawker, G. (2010). The 2010 American College of Rheumatology/European League Against Rheumatism classification criteria for rheumatoid arthritis: Phase 2 methodological report. *Arthritis & Rheumatism, 62*(9), 2582–2591. https://doi.org/10.1002/art.27580.

Porta, S., Matilde Otero-Losada, Rodolfo A. Kölliker Frers, Vanesa Cosentino et al., (2021). Adipokines, cardiovascular risk, and therapeutic management in obesity and psoriatic arthritis. *Frontiers in Immunology, 11*, 590749. https://doi.org/10.3389/fimmu.2020.590749.

Qin, J., Kamil E. Barbour, Louise B. Murphy, Amanda E. Nelson, Todd A. Schwartz et al., (2017). Lifetime risk of symptomatic hand osteoarthritis: The Johnston County Osteoarthritis Project. *Arthritis Rheumatology, 69*, 1204–1212. https://doi.org/10.1002/art.40097.

Ravelli, A., Sergio Davì, Giulia Bracciolini, Angela Pistorio, Alessandro Consolaro et al., (2017). Intra-articular corticosteroids versus intraarticular corticosteroids plus methotrexate in oligoarticular juvenile idiopathic arthritis: A multicentre, prospective, randomised, open-label trial. *Lancet, 389*, 909–916. https://doi.org/10.1016/S0140-6736(17)30065-X.

Ringold, S., Angeles-Han, S. T., Beukelman, T., Lovell, D., Cuello, C. A., Becker, M. L., et al., (2019). 2019 American College of Rheumatology/Arthritis Foundation guideline for the treatment of juvenile idiopathic arthritis: Therapeutic approaches for non-systemic polyarthritis, sacroiliitis, and enthesitis. *Arthritis Rheumatology, 71*, 846–863. https://doi.org/10.1002/art.40884.

Ringold, S., Weiss, P. F., Beukelman, T., DeWitt, E. M., Ilowite, N. T., Kimura, Y., et al., (2013). 2013 update of the 2011 American College of Rheumatology recommendations for the treatment of juvenile idiopathic arthritis: Recommendations for the medical therapy of children with systemic juvenile idiopathic arthritis and tuberculosis screening among children receiving biologic medications. *Arthritis Rheumatism, 65*, 2499–2512. https://doi.org/10.1002/art.38092.

Sato, J. D., Fernandes, T. A., Nascimento, C. B., Corrente, J. E., & Saad-Magalhaes, C. (2014). Probability of remission of juvenile idiopathic arthritis following treatment with steroid joint injection. *Clinical Experimental Rheumatology, 32*, 291–296.

Singh, J. A., Gordon Guyatt, Alexis Ogdie, Dafna D. Gladman, Chad Deal et al., (2019). 2018 American College of Rheumatology/National Psoriasis Foundation guideline for the treatment of psoriatic arthritis. *Journal of Psoriasis and Psoriatic Arthritis, 4*(1), 31–58. https://doi.org/10.1177/2475530318812244.

Skelly, A. C., et al., (2018). Noninvasive nonpharmacological treatment for chronic pain: A systematic review. *Agency for Healthcare Research*. https://doi.org/10.23970/AHRQEPCCER209.

Smolen, J. S., Aletaha, D., Bijlsma, J. W., Breedveld, F. C., Boumpas, D., Burmester, G., Combe, B., Cutolo, M., de Wit, M., Dougados, M., Emery, P., Gibofsky, A., Gomez-Reino, J. J., Haraoui, B., Kalden, J., Keystone, E. C., Kvien, T. K., McInnes, I., Martin-Mola, E., … van der Heijde, D. (2010). Treating rheumatoid arthritis to target: Recommendations of an international task force. *Annals of the Rheumatic Diseases, 69*(4), 631–637. https://doi.org/10.1136/ard.2009.123919.

Smolen, J. S., Dafna Gladman, H. Patrick McNeil, Philip J. Mease, Joachim Sieper et al., (2019). Predicting adherence to therapy in rheumatoid arthritis, psoriatic arthritis or ankylosing spondylitis: A large cross-sectional study. *RMD Open, 5*(1), e000585. https://doi.org/10.1136/rmdopen-2017-000585.

Smolen, J. S., Landewé, R. B. M., Bijlsma, J. W. J., Burmester, G. R., Dougados, M., Kerschbaumer, A., McInnes, I. B., Sepriano, A., van Vollenhoven, R. F., de Wit, M., Aletaha, D., Aringer, M., Askling, J., Balsa, A., Boers, M., den Broeder, A. A., Buch, M. H., Buttgereit, F., Caporali, R., Cardiel, M. H., … van der Heijde, D. (2010). EULAR recommendations for the management of rheumatoid arthritis with synthetic and biological disease-modifying antirheumatic drugs. *Annals of the Rheumatic Diseases, 69*(6), 964–975. https://doi.org/10.1136/ard.2009.126532.

Smolen, J. S., Landewé, R. B. M., Bijlsma, J. W. J., Burmester, G. R., Dougados, M., Kerschbaumer, A., McInnes, I. B., Sepriano, A., van Vollenhoven, R. F., de Wit, M., Aletaha, D., Aringer, M., Askling, J., Balsa, A., Boers, M., den Broeder, A. A., Buch, M. H., Buttgereit, F., Caporali, R., … van der Heijde, D. (2020). EULAR recommendations for the management of rheumatoid arthritis with synthetic and biological disease-modifying antirheumatic drugs: 2019 update. *Annals of the Rheumatic Diseases, 79*(6), 685–699. https://doi.org/10.1136/annrheumdis-2019-216655.

So, H., & Tam, L. S. (2021). Cardiovascular disease and depression in psoriatic arthritis: Multidimensional comorbidities requiring multidisciplinary management. *Best Practice & Research Clinical Rheumatology, 35*(2), 101689. https://doi.org/10.1016/j.berh.2021.101689.

Trouvin, A. P., Attal, N., & Perrot, S. (2022). Assessing central sensitization with quantitative sensory testing in inflammatory rheumatic diseases: A systematic review. *Joint Bone Spine, 89*(5), 105399. https://doi.org/10.1016/j.jbspin.2022.105399.

US Food and Drug Administration. (2021). Initial safety trial results find increased risk of serious heart-related problems and cancer with arthritis and ulcerative colitis medicine Xeljanz, Xeljanz XR (tofacitinib). *FDA Report 2021.*

Wendling, D., Sophie Hecquet, Olivier Fogel, Jean-Guillaume Letarouilly et al., (2022). 2022 French Society for Rheumatology (SFR) recommendations on the everyday management of patients with spondyloarthritis, including psoriatic arthritis. *Joint Bone Spine, 89*(3), 105344. https://doi.org/10.1016/j.jbspin.2022.105344.

Ytterberg, S. R., Bhatt, D. L., Mikuls, T. R., Koch, G. G., Fleischmann, R., Rivas, J. L., Germino, R., Menon, S., Sun, Y., Wang, C., Shapiro, A. B., Kanik, K. S., & Connell, C. A. (2022). Cardiovascular and cancer risk with tofacitinib in rheumatoid arthritis. *New England Journal of Medicine, 386*(4), 316–326. https://doi.org/10.1056/NEJMoa2109927.

Zabotti, A., Gabriele De Marco, Laure Gossec, Xenofon Baraliakos et al., (2023). EULAR points to consider for the definition of clinical and imaging features suspicious for progression from psoriasis to psoriatic arthritis. *Annals of the Rheumatic Diseases, 82*(9), 1162–1170. https://doi.org/10.1136/ard-2023-224148.

Chapter 2

Neck Pain

Hüseyin Yetkin*, MD

Department of Orthopedics and Traumatology, Health Sciences University, Bursa, Turkey

Abstract

Neck pain can be attributed to various factors, including trauma, degeneration, inflammation, infection, tumors, and problems related to spinal cord compression. However, diagnosing non-traumatic neck pain can be challenging. To establish a diagnosis for individuals reporting neck pain, it is essential to consider their age and the characteristics of the pain. This process involves conducting diagnostic tests guided by a thorough medical history and a physical examination. The key is to determine whether the pain arises from musculoskeletal sources (muscles, ligaments, bones, and joints) or nervous system-related structures (myelopathy, radiculopathy, and spinal cord problems). In cases of acute neck pain without radicular or myelopathic symptoms, without trauma history, and without any association with fever, weight loss, malignancy, or inflammatory conditions, the condition is often benign. Conservative treatments are usually sufficient, and imaging may not be necessary. However, if there is a history of trauma, chronic neck pain, previous neck surgery, or malignancy, a 3-view cervical spine X-ray (AP, lateral, and open-mouth odontoid views) can help diagnose. If there is a known inflammatory disease history, assessing instability and the atlantoaxial joint is crucial, in addition to flexion and extension views. For patients with neurological symptoms, an MRI is recommended regardless of plain radiograph results. Furthermore, an MRI may be warranted in cases of instability, suspected infection, or when a malignancy needs to be ruled out. When MRI is not an option, a CT myelogram can serve as an alternative imaging approach.

Keywords: neck pain, cervical pain, cervicalgia, cervical radiculopathy, cervical myelopathy, neck pain management

Introduction

Neck pain is a common clinical complaint and can arise from a myriad of etiologies, including traumatic, degenerative, inflammatory, infectious, neoplastic, and conditions involving spinal cord compression (Deyo et al., 2006; Strine & Hootman, 2007; Martin et al., 2008). Nevertheless, there are instances of non-traumatic neck pain where determining the precise

* Corresponding Author's Email: hy.yetkin@gmail.com.

In: Common Diseases According to Family Medicine Practice Guidelines
Editors: Esra Meltem Koç and Hilal Aksoy
ISBN: 979-8-89530-302-3

cause can be challenging. The evaluation should be comprehensive, including a detailed medical history and a physical examination. The specific characteristics of pain, in addition to the age of the patient, play a vital role in reaching an accurate diagnosis and formulating an appropriate management plan. During the patient's medical history evaluation, it is imperative to inquire about the onset, duration, and specific location of the neck pain. Any history of recent or past traumatic events should be explored (Tsang, 2001). Certain red flags, such as periodic nocturnal pain and unexplained weight loss, can suggest malignancy, while the presence of fever and night sweats may indicate an underlying infection. In cases involving inflammatory conditions with stiffness in the morning and involvement of the atlantoaxial joint, atlantoaxial subluxation should be considered in the differential diagnosis (Levy, 2000). To effectively diagnose individuals with neck pain, a comprehensive medical history and thorough physical examination are imperative. It is vital to differentiate between pain originating from musculoskeletal components (e.g., muscles, ligaments, bones, and joints) and that arising from nervous system structures (e.g., myelopathy, radiculopathy, and spinal cord problems) (Kriss & Kriss, 2000; Tsang, 2001).

Mechanical neck pain attributed to musculoskeletal components is often described as deep and dull, frequently accompanied by stiffness. Patients may report the association of pain with atypical activities or poor posture before its onset. This type of pain tends to worsen with movement but improves with rest. Radiculopathy is characterized by a sharp, intense burning sensation that can radiate from the neck to the shoulder and down the arm. In the affected dermatome, patients may experience numbness, paresthesia, and motor weakness. Symptoms usually worsen with neck extension. Patients with myelopathic involvement may exhibit clumsiness, gait disturbances, and issues related to sexual or bladder dysfunction. Recognizing these specific characteristics is crucial during clinical assessment (Bennett, 2001; Freynhagen et al., 2006).

Diagnosis

Physical Examination Findings

A comprehensive clinical evaluation is paramount for diagnosing cervical spine disorders. Understanding the various types of pain associated with these disorders and recognizing specific clinical signs are essential to guide diagnosis and management. After an extensive physical examination, the evaluation of the active and passive neck movements of a patient's is crucial. The cervical spine consists of distinct joints that primarily contribute to flexion-extension, rotation, and lateral bending: the atlanto-occipital, atlantoaxial, and subaxial cervical spine joints, respectively. In cases of cervical disorders, especially mechanical neck pains, limited and painful neck movements are commonly observed.

Different types of pain characterize cervical spine disorders. Mechanical neck pain typically presents as restricted neck movements with dull and deep pain. In contrast, radicular pain is characterized by dysesthesia and paresthesia within the affected dermatome, accompanied by motor weakness in the respective muscle group. Myelopathic pain is associated with spasticity of the upper and lower extremities, hyperreflexia, clonus, positive Babinski sign, Hoffman sign, loss of fine motor skills in the hands, clumsiness, and gait disturbances (Levy, 2000). Radicular involvement suggests nerve root compression, whereas myelopathic involvement indicates signs of upper motor neurons due to spinal cord compression (Bennett, 2001; Freynhagen et al., 2006).

Several clinical signs assist in the diagnostic process. The Spurling sign, achieved by applying gentle pressure to the patient's head during extension and lateral rotation, can reproduce radicular pain with radiation to the ipsilateral upper extremity. The relief sign of abduction, where the patient places their affected upper extremity hand on their head, may suggest a soft disk protrusion causing radicular pain. A positive abduction relief sign helps differentiate the pain's origin from the shoulder (Fast et al., 1989).

The Lhermitte sign is a distinctive feature of cord compression, characterized by electric shock-like sensations radiating down the spine, especially with neck flexion. The Hoffman sign, an indicator of an upper motor neuron lesion, is observed by flicking the tip of the middle finger, eliciting a pinching motion response. Cervical sympathetic chain injuries can lead to Horner's syndrome, which manifests as partial ptosis, miosis (constricted pupil), and decreased sweating on the affected facial side (Alstadhaug, 2011).

The motor examination involves evaluating specific nerve root functions. For instance, assessing shoulder abduction and elbow flexion by examining the C5 nerve root, while evaluating elbow flexion is crucial for the C6 nerve root. For the C7 nerve root, it is essential to assess elbow extension, wrist flexion, and finger extension, and for the C8 nerve root, finger flexion should be examined. The evaluation of the T1 nerve root includes evaluating finger abduction and adduction (Tsang, 2001).

Sensory examination focuses on the detection of numbness, tingling, pain, paresthesia, and dysesthesia. Symptom locations can provide vital clues to the affected nerve root.

The reflex examination involves evaluating the reflexes associated with specific nerve roots. Weakness in the biceps reflex may suggest C5 and/or C6 nerve root compression, while a weakened brachioradial reflex may indicate C6 nerve root compression. Additionally, a weakened triceps reflex can suggest compression of the C7 nerve root (Tsang, 2001). Understanding pain characteristics, recognizing clinical signs, and performing a thorough examination of motor, sensory, and reflex functions enable an accurate diagnosis and facilitate appropriate treatment strategies.

Diagnostic Imaging

Neck pain is classified as acute (up to six weeks), subacute (around three months), or chronic (over three months). In cases where acute neck pain lacks radicular or myelopathic characteristics, is not associated with recent or past trauma, and does not present with symptoms such as fever, weight loss, malignancy, or a known inflammatory disease, the pain is likely benign. This type of pain often responds well to conservative treatment methods and may not necessitate immediate imaging (Levy, 2000).

In cases where there is a history of trauma, chronic neck pain, a prior history of neck surgery, or malignancy, obtaining a 3-view cervical spine X-ray (AP, lateral, and open-mouth odontoid views) may be beneficial for diagnosis. If there is a known history of an inflammatory disease, in addition to the views of flexion and extension, it is necessary to evaluate instability and the atlantoaxial joint (Tong & Barest, 2003). In patients with neurological symptoms, an MRI should be performed regardless of the findings on plain radiographs. Magnetic resonance imaging (MRI) is highly sensitive for detecting soft-tissue abnormalities such as disk problems. However, it often shows abnormalities in asymptomatic individuals. The prevalence of such abnormalities ranges from 60% in people in their 40s to over 80% in those older than 60 years old, with common findings being decreased signal intensity and disk protrusions (Lehto et al., 1994; Matsumoto et al., 1998). Additionally, an MRI may be considered in the presence of instability, infectious causes, and for the differential diagnosis of malignancy. When an MRI is not feasible, a CT myelogram can serve as an alternative imaging option. Electrodiagnostic testing can be useful in patients with unclear symptoms or inconclusive imaging results and to exclude peripheral neuropathy.

Mechanical Neck Pain

Mechanical neck pain encompasses a spectrum of causes, including strain, sprain, and hyperextension sprain. These etiologies often arise due to traumatic incidents such as acceleration-deceleration injuries, hyperextension-hyperflexion injuries, whiplash injuries, falls, sports-related injuries, and motor vehicle accidents.

In cases of severe blunt neck trauma or injury to the laryngeal region, symptoms such as dysphagia (difficulty swallowing) or hoarseness can manifest. It is crucial to recognize that these symptoms are indicative of more severe underlying issues, and therefore a detailed evaluation is warranted to ensure appropriate diagnosis and treatment.

Adult Cervical Spine Trauma

In the evaluation of trauma patients, the assumption of cervical spinal trauma is paramount. This requires the immediate application of a cervical collar at the incident scene. The primary survey focuses on addressing life-threatening issues, including Airway, Breathing, and Circulation (ABCs). Simultaneously, a comprehensive examination of the entire spine is performed, with particular attention to the cervical region, to identify potential injuries. After resolving immediate life-threatening concerns, the secondary survey involves a more detailed assessment of the cervical spine. This phase may require temporary removal of the cervical collar, accompanied by the application of manual inline traction to maintain spinal stability (Schouten et al., 2012).

The secondary survey includes an examination of the face and scalp for signs of direct trauma. Investigation of head positioning for angular or rotational deformities suggestive of severe cervical injuries. Palpation of the posterior cervical spine for tenderness in the midline or paraspinal tissues. Gentle rolling of the patient to facilitate the inspection and palpation of the entire spinal axis.

A critical component of the comprehensive evaluation is the neurological evaluation. This aims to identify sensory or motor deficits indicative of potential spinal cord injuries, ensuring a thorough understanding of the patient's condition.

The criteria of the National Emergency X-Radiography Utilization Study (NEXUS) are valuable in deciding which trauma patients require cervical spine imaging. In patients who are alert and stable, exhibit no focal neurological deficits, maintain unaltered consciousness, show no signs of intoxication, lack midline spinal tenderness, and have no distracting injuries, cervical spine imaging is unnecessary (Hoffman et al., 2000).

When cervical imaging is necessary, a series of radiographs are conducted, including views of cervical anteroposterior (AP), lateral, and open-mouth odontoid. Proper visualization of the lower endplate of C7 in the cervical lateral view is crucial. Abnormal findings or the presence of a fracture in conventional X-ray imaging prompt further evaluation with a cervical CT scan, with a focus on adequately visualizing the superior endplate of T1. For patients with neurological symptoms, an MRI should be performed (Como et al., 2009).

The need for a neurosurgical consultation should be determined based on the findings and clinical assessment. Ensuring a systematic approach to the evaluation of cervical spine trauma in the emergency setting is paramount to providing the best possible care to trauma patients.

Pediatric Cervical Spine Trauma

Pediatric trauma presents a significant public health concern, with trauma being the leading cause of death in children over the age of one. Among musculoskeletal injuries, spine fractures are the most common with the highest rates of morbidity and mortality. Cervical spine injuries, in particular, are more frequently observed in children under the age of eight (Jones et al., 2011).

When transporting pediatric patients under eight years of age, special considerations are essential to ensure their safety. One crucial measure is the use of an occipital cut in the spine boards during transportation. This adaptation is necessary because children in this age group possess larger heads in proportion to their bodies, which can lead to the flexion of an unstable cervical spine, thereby increasing the risk of injury during transport (Herzenberg et al., 1989).

The preponderance of cervical trauma in children under the age of eight occurs at levels C3 and above. This phenomenon can be attributed to several factors specific to the pediatric population. These factors include the relatively larger size of their heads compared to their bodies, the horizontal orientation of facet joints, increased ligamentous laxity, and relatively weaker neck muscles compared to adults (Dogan et al., 2006).

Conversely, individuals aged eight and older exhibit cervical traumas that more closely resemble those observed in adults. These injuries predominantly involve levels below C3. Understanding these age-related differences in cervical spine injuries is crucial for healthcare providers to provide appropriate care and take preventive measures in the management of pediatric trauma.

Pseudosubluxation of the Cervical Spine

Pseudosubluxation of the cervical spine is a radiographic occurrence primarily observed in children aged 8 years and under. This phenomenon is linked to the horizontal alignment of the facet joints in the cervical spine. The diagnosis is established by conducting lateral cervical X-ray views during flexion and extension. It is characterized by a relative anterior translation, frequently involving C2 on C3 or C3 on C4, with a range of up to 4 mm. Importantly, this translation self-corrects as the cervical spine extends, and there are no historical or physical findings that indicate significant trauma. The primary approach to managing this condition is observation, since pseudosubluxation of the cervical spine generally resolves spontaneously over time. It is of utmost importance to differentiate this radiographic variant from a genuine traumatic subluxation, which can occur due to a Hangman fracture (traumatic spondylolisthesis of C2), resulting from a fracture involving the bilateral pars interarticularis of the axis (Cattell & Filtzer, 1965; Swischuk, 1977; Adib et al., 2016).

Atlantoaxial Rotatory Displacement

Atlantoaxial rotatory displacement is a condition seen in pediatric patients that involves rotatory instability in the cervical spine, often stemming from C1-C2 subluxation or facet dislocation. This condition frequently occurs in young children and is associated with torticollis. The diagnosis is confirmed by dynamic CT scans of the cervical spine.

Cervical Spondylosis

Cervical spondylosis, a condition intrinsically associated with the natural aging process, primarily encompasses degenerative changes that unfold within the cervical spine. This age-related degeneration chiefly impacts the intervertebral disc, the facet joints, and the Luschka uncovertebral joints. It ushers in a diverse range of clinical manifestations, encompassing cervical neck pain, nerve root compression, and central cord compression. Notably, the cervical levels most frequently embroiled in this condition are C5-6 and C6-7. These segments are predisposed to degenerative alterations due to their significant role in flexion and extension movements within the subaxial spine. The approach to managing cervical spondylosis exhibits variability contingent on several factors. These factors encompass the severity and chronicity of pain, the presence of spinal instability, and the existence of neurological deficits. Treatment modalities span from vigilant observation to medical interventions, and, in select instances, surgical procedures performed to effectively address the condition. Recognizing cervical spondylosis, comprehending its clinical implications, and grasping the spectrum of management options are imperative facets of offering all-encompassing care to individuals grappling with this condition.

Cervical Radiculopathy

Cervical radiculopathy encompasses a constellation of symptoms, including occipital headaches, localized pain in the trapezial or interscapular regions, neck pain, radiating arm pain, numbness, tingling along specific dermatomes, and muscle weakness. This condition arises primarily from the compression of the spinal nerve roots.

Non-operative treatments have demonstrated efficacy in the majority of cases, aiming to alleviate symptoms and enhance the patient's overall condition. However, surgical intervention is considered in cases of persistent and incapacitating pain, despite a minimum of three months of conservative management. Additionally, surgical options are contemplated when there are significant neurologic deficits.

The management of cervical radiculopathy should be tailored to the individual patient, taking into account their specific symptoms, the progression of the condition, and the response to non-operative interventions. For those who do not attain adequate relief through conservative approaches, surgical decompression is a viable and effective alternative.

Cervical Myelopathy

Cervical myelopathy is a pathological condition marked by the compression of the cervical spinal cord. Its clinical presentation encompasses a spectrum of symptoms, including neck pain, stiffness, diffuse and bilateral paresthesias, non-dermatomal in nature, muscle weakness, clumsiness (often leading to object dropping), gait disturbances, and urinary retention.

While motor weakness constitutes a significant diagnostic indicator, it may pose challenges during a physical examination. More discernible is the weakness of the lower extremities. Noteworthy clinical signs include the "finger escape sign," where patients, extending and adducting their fingers, experience spontaneous abduction of the small finger, attributed to intrinsic muscle weakness. Another diagnostic test is the grip and release examination, involving a patient's ability to make and release a fist 20 times within 10 seconds, a task that may be problematic for those with myelopathy (Cook et al., 2007).

Sensory findings are a common feature of cervical myelopathy, with manifestations involving proprioception dysfunction and decreased pain sensation. Upper motor neuron signs, such as spasticity and hyperreflexia, are also prevalent. Clinical signs, notably the inverted radial reflex, Hoffmann's sign, sustained clonus, a positive Babinski test, and gait disturbances, further underscore the neurological implications of the condition.

Patients with cervical myelopathy frequently exhibit difficulties during the Romberg test and toe-to-heel walking. The preferred approach for treating cervical myelopathy typically involves surgical decompression and stabilization, with the aim of relieving spinal cord compression and addressing associated symptoms (Sadasivan et al., 1993; Matsumoto et al., 2001).

Inflammatory Diseases

Rheumatoid Cervical Spondylitis

Rheumatoid Cervical Spondylitis (RCS) represents a condition characterized by instability of the cervical spine, frequently found in individuals with rheumatoid arthritis. This instability is typically manifested as atlantoaxial subluxation, basilar invagination, and subaxial subluxation. Clinical manifestations and physical examination findings can closely resemble those observed in cervical myelopathy (Boden et al., 1993).

The diagnosis of RCS is established primarily through radiographic assessments, with a particular emphasis on cervical spine flexion-extension radiographs. Moreover, MRI studies are routinely employed to assess the degree of spinal cord compression, thus playing a pivotal role in both confirming the diagnosis and evaluating the condition's severity (Monsey, 1997).

Treatment strategies for RCS are contingent on various factors, including the patient's neurological status, the extent of mechanical instability, and the severity of spinal cord compression. These therapeutic options encompass a spectrum that ranges from conservative management strategies, including observation, to more aggressive approaches that incorporate decompression surgery and instrumentation. The formulation of a specific treatment plan is custom-tailored to each patient's unique clinical presentation and guided by the findings derived from diagnostic imaging (Kim & Hilibrand, 2005).

Ankylosing Spondylitis

Ankylosing Spondylitis (AS) is a chronic seronegative autoimmune spondyloarthropathy marked by the formation of bridging spinal osteophytes, enthesitis, sacroiliitis, and uveitis. The juvenile form, which occurs in individuals under 16 years of age, includes the presence of enthesitis (Azouz & Duffy, 1995). Its diagnostic criteria include bilateral sacroiliitis, uveitis, and HLA-B27 positivity (90% positive, but symptoms of AS are observed in fewer than 10% of HLA-B27 positive patients).

Radiographically, AS is characterized by squaring of the vertebrae along with the development of vertical or marginal syndesmophytes, leading to the distinctive "Bamboo spine" appearance. Other radiographic findings can include ossification of the disc space and osteopenia. Unlike Diffuse Idiopathic Skeletal Hyperostosis (DISH) syndrome, AS lacks an association with diabetes and is relatively more prevalent among younger age groups (Linden et al., 1984).

Patients with AS frequently present with lumbosacral pain and stiffness, which tend to be more pronounced in the morning. Neck pain typically emerges later in life. Notably, the occurrence of acute neck pain in a patient with AS should raise suspicion of a possible fracture (Taurog et al., 2016).

Treatment strategies for AS include the use of NSAIDs, COX-2 inhibitors, physical therapy, and TNF-alpha-blocking agents. These options are geared toward the management of symptoms and the improvement of the patient's quality of life.

Diffuse Idiopathic Skeletal Hyperostosis

Diffuse Idiopathic Skeletal Hyperostosis (DISH), commonly known as Forestier's disease, represents a prevalent disorder of uncertain etiology characterized by enthesopathy affecting the spine, often leading to symptoms of spinal pain and stiffness. The diagnosis of DISH can be confirmed by radiographic assessment of the cervical and thoracic spine. These images reveal the presence of non-marginal syndesmophytes that have been likened to the appearance of "Flowing candle wax." This phenomenon typically occurs at three successive levels, involving four contiguous vertebrae. DISH can manifest at various locations along the spine. Notably, the right thoracic spine is the most commonly affected, potentially due to the protective effect of the pulsatile aorta on the left side of the thoracic spine. It can also involve the cervical and lumbar regions. DISH differs from Ankylosing Spondylitis (AS) in several aspects. Unlike AS, DISH has been associated with diabetes. Radiographically, DISH typically exhibits preservation of disc space, does not display osteopenia, and is not linked with HLA-

B27, but rather with HLA-B8. Additionally, DISH does not involve sacroiliitis and is relatively more common in older age groups (Sarzi-Puttini & Atzeni, 2004; Le et al., 2021).

Management strategies for DISH often include activity modification, physical therapy, and bisphosphonate therapy. Surgery is considered for cases presenting with lumbar stenosis, cervical myelopathy, or significant spinal deformity, with the goal of improving the patient's quality of life and relieving symptoms.

Infectious Diseases

Adult Pyogenic Vertebral Osteomyelitis, also known as spondylodiskitis, encompasses a spectrum of spinal infections, including discitis, vertebral osteomyelitis, and epidural abscess. The causative agents are diverse, with approximately half of the cases are attributed to Staphylococcus aureus, making it the most prevalent pathogen. This is followed by Staphylococcus epidermidis. In the past decade, gram-negative infections have been on the rise, often associated with genitourinary and respiratory tract infections. Pseudomonas is observed in patients with a history of intravenous drug use, while Salmonella infections are common in individuals with sickle cell disease. Fungal and tuberculosis-related infections are also notable etiological factors (Tay et al., 2002; Cornett et al., 2016; Gentile et al., 2019).

The diagnostic approach predominantly relies on contrast-enhanced MRI studies. When it comes to therapeutic interventions, the choice between prolonged targeted antibiotic therapy as a standalone treatment or surgical intervention involving decompression and stabilization is based on several critical factors. These factors encompass the extent and chronicity of the infection, its location within the spinal column, as well as the identification and antimicrobial susceptibility of the causative pathogen. Opting for the most suitable treatment strategy requires a comprehensive assessment of these multifaceted considerations (Tay et al., 2002; Cornett et al., 2016; Gentile et al., 2019).

Spinal Cord Tumors

Spinal Cord Tumors are categorized as follows (Ciftdemir et al., 2016):

- Intradural Extramedullary Tumors: Schwannoma, Meningioma
- Intradural Intramedullary Tumors: Ependymoma, Astrocytoma
- Extradural Tumors: Metastasis (most commonly from the lung and breast), Lymphoma.

Congenital Diseases

Diastematomyelia

Diastematomyelia is a congenital spinal anomaly in which a fibrous, cartilaginous, or osseous septum divides the spinal cord longitudinally. Detection is commonly achieved by third-trimester prenatal ultrasound. Asymptomatic cases are typically observed. In contrast, symptomatic patients with neurological deficits often require surgical resection for optimal treatment.

Syringomyelia and Syringobulbia

Syringomyelia entails the formation of a fluid-filled cavity called a syrinx within the spinal cord. Over time, this syrinx expands, causing neurological impairments. In contrast, syringobulbia manifests as a syrinx within the brainstem, contributing to a range of neurological symptoms.

Congenital Muscular Torticollis

Congenital Muscular Torticollis results from abnormal sternocleidomastoid muscle contraction, typically observed in infants as a persistent head tilt toward the affected side. The clinical diagnosis relies on the identification of a palpable neck mass due to sternocleidomastoid muscle contraction, accompanied by chin rotation toward the opposite side. The primary treatment approach involves passive stretching, with resolution often occurring within a year. Surgical intervention to lengthen the sternocleidomastoid muscle is considered if significant improvement is not achieved after at least a year of stretching therapy (Do et al., 2006).

Klippel-Feil Syndrome

Klippel-Feil syndrome is an infrequent congenital condition attributed to the abnormal segmentation or formation of cervical somites during embryological development, resulting in cervical segment anomalies. While the classic triad of symptoms, seen in fewer than 50% of cases, includes a low posterior hairline, a short-webbed neck, and limited cervical range of motion, this syndrome is frequently associated with several other conditions. These include congenital scoliosis, Sprengel's deformity (characterized by high scapula) in approximately 1/3 of cases, renal aplasia in approximately 1/3 of cases, deafness in about 1/3 of cases, congenital heart disease, and atlantoaxial instability in roughly half of cases. The standard approach primarily involves observation with restrictions on participation in contact sports (Do et al., 2006; Tracy et al., 2004; Frikha, 2020; Öner et al., 2020).

Conclusion

Neck pain is a common musculoskeletal problem. The diagnosis of non-traumatic neck pain can be intricate and demands a comprehensive approach. The diagnostic process aims to determine whether the pain's origin is musculoskeletal or neurologically linked. In cases of acute neck pain without radicular or myelopathic signs, without trauma history, fever, weight loss, malignancy, or inflammation, the condition is typically benign. Non-operative treatments often suffice without extensive imaging. However, for those with a trauma history, chronic pain, previous neck surgery, or malignancy, a 3-view cervical spine X-ray can aid diagnosis. In cases of known inflammatory diseases, an evaluation of instability and the atlantoaxial joint is crucial, accompanied by views of flexion and extension. Patients with neurological symptoms should undergo an MRI, regardless of plain radiograph results. MRI may be necessary for instability, suspected infection, or ruling out malignancy. When MRI is not feasible, a CT myelogram serves as an alternative. This comprehensive approach ensures timely, tailored care for optimal patient outcomes. Understanding the causes and personalizing treatments are vital to managing this common but complex condition.

References

Adib, O., Berthier, E., Loisel, D., & Aubé, C. (2016). Pediatric cervical spine in emergency: radiographic features of normal anatomy, variants and pitfalls. *Skeletal Radiology, 45*(12), 1607–1617. https://doi.org/10.1007/s00256-016-2481-9.

Alstadhaug, K. B. (2011). Ervervet Horners syndrom [Acquired Horner's syndrome]. *Tidsskr Nor Laegeforen, 131*(9–10), 950–954. https://doi.org/10.4045/tidsskr.10.0935.

Azouz, E. M., & Duffy, C. M. (1995). Juvenile spondyloarthropathies: Clinical manifestations and medical imaging. *Skeletal Radiology, 24*(6), 399–408. https://doi.org/10.1007/BF00941234.

Bennett, M. (2001). The LANSS Pain Scale: The Leeds assessment of neuropathic symptoms and signs. *Pain, 92*(1–2), 147–157. https://doi.org/10.1016/s0304-3959(00)00482-6.

Boden, S. D., Dodge, L. D., Bohlman, H. H., & Rechtine, G. R. (1993). Rheumatoid arthritis of the cervical spine: A long-term analysis with predictors of paralysis and recovery. *The Journal of Bone and Joint Surgery. American Volume, 75*(9), 1282–1297. https://doi.org/10.2106/00004623-199309000-00004.

Cattell, H. S., & Filtzer, D. L. (1965). Pseudosubluxation and other normal variations in the cervical spine in children: A study of one hundred and sixty children. *The Journal of Bone and Joint Surgery. American Volume, 47*(7), 1295–1309.

Ciftdemir, M., Kaya, M., Selcuk, E., & Yalniz, E. (2016). Tumors of the spine. *World Journal of Orthopedics, 7*(2), 109–116. https://doi.org/10.5312/wjo.v7.i2.109.

Como, J. J., Diaz, J. J., Dunham, C. M., Chiu, W. C., Duane, T. M., Capella, J. M., Holevar, M. R., Khwaja, K. A., Mayglothling, J. A., Shapiro, M. B., & Winston, E. S. (2009). Practice management guidelines for identification of cervical spine injuries following trauma: Update from the Eastern Association for the Surgery of Trauma practice management guidelines committee. *The Journal of Trauma, 67*(3), 651–659. https://doi.org/10.1097/TA.0b013e3181ae583b.

Cook, C. E., Hegedus, E., Pietrobon, R., & Goode, A. (2007). A pragmatic neurological screen for patients with suspected cord compressive myelopathy. *Physical Therapy, 87*(9), 1233–1242. https://doi.org/10.2522/ptj.20060150.

Cornett, C. A., Vincent, S. A., Crow, J., & Hewlett, A. (2016). Bacterial spine infections in adults: Evaluation and management. *Journal of the American Academy of Orthopaedic Surgeons, 24*(1), 11–18. https://doi.org/10.5435/JAAOS-D-13-00102.

Deyo, R. A., Mirza, S. K., & Martin, B. I. (2006). Back pain prevalence and visit rates: Estimates from U.S. national surveys, 2002. *Spine (Philadelphia, PA 1976), 31*(23), 2724–2727. https://doi.org/10.1097/01.brs.0000244618.06877.cd.

Do, T. T. (2006). Congenital muscular torticollis: Current concepts and review of treatment. *Current Opinion in Pediatrics, 18*(1), 26–29. https://doi.org/10.1097/01.mop.0000192520.48411.fa.

Dogan, S., Safavi-Abbasi, S., Theodore, N., Horn, E., Rekate, H. L., & Sonntag, V. K. (2006). Pediatric subaxial cervical spine injuries: Origins, management, and outcome in 51 patients. *Neurosurgical Focus, 20*(2), E1. https://doi.org/10.3171/foc.2006.20.2.2.

Fast, A., Parikh, S., & Marin, E. L. (1989). The shoulder abduction relief sign in cervical radiculopathy. *Archives of Physical Medicine and Rehabilitation, 70*(5), 402–403. PMID: 2719545.

Freynhagen, R., Baron, R., Gockel, U., & Tölle, T. R. (2006). painDETECT: A new screening questionnaire to identify neuropathic components in patients with back pain. *Current Medical Research and Opinion, 22*(10), 1911–1920. https://doi.org/10.1185/030079906X132488.

Frikha, R. (2020). Klippel-Feil syndrome: A review of the literature. *Clinical Dysmorphology, 29*(1), 35–37. https://doi.org/10.1097/MCD.0000000000000301.

Gentile, L., Benazzo, F., De Rosa, F., Boriani, S., Dallagiacoma, G., Franceschetti, G., Gaeta, M., & Cuzzocrea, F. (2019). A systematic review: Characteristics, complications and treatment of spondylodiscitis. *European Review for Medical and Pharmacological Sciences, 23*(2 Suppl), 117–128. https://doi.org/10.26355/eurrev_201904_17481.

Herzenberg, J. E., Hensinger, R. N., Dedrick, D. K., & Phillips, W. A. (1989). Emergency transport and positioning of young children who have an injury of the cervical spine. The standard backboard may be hazardous. *The Journal of Bone and Joint Surgery. American Volume, 71*(1), 15–22. PMID: 2912996.

Hoffman, J. R., Mower, W. R., Wolfson, A. B., Todd, K. H., & Zucker, M. I. (2000). Validity of a set of clinical criteria to rule out injury to the cervical spine in patients with blunt trauma. *The New England Journal of Medicine, 343*(2), 94–99. https://doi.org/10.1056/NEJM200007133430203.

Jones, T. M., Anderson, P. A., & Noonan, K. J. (2011). Pediatric cervical spine trauma. *Journal of the American Academy of Orthopaedic Surgeons, 19*(10), 600–611. https://doi.org/10.5435/00124635-201110000-00004.

Kim, D. H., & Hilibrand, A. S. (2005). Rheumatoid arthritis in the cervical spine. *Journal of the American Academy of Orthopaedic Surgeons, 13*(7), 463–474. https://doi.org/10.5435/00124635-200511000-00006.

Kriss, T. C., & Kriss, V. M. (2000). Neck pain: Primary care work-up of acute and chronic symptoms. *Geriatrics, 55*(1), 47–57. PMID: 10659073.

Le, H. V., Wick, J. B., Van, B. W., & Klineberg, E. O. (2021). Diffuse idiopathic skeletal hyperostosis of the spine: Pathophysiology, diagnosis, and management. *Journal of the American Academy of Orthopaedic Surgeons, 29*(24), 1044–1051. https://doi.org/10.5435/JAAOS-D-20-01344.

Lehto, I. J., Tertti, M. O., Komu, M. E., Paajanen, H. E., Tuominen, J., & Kormano, M. J. (1994). Age-related MRI changes at 0.1 T in cervical discs in asymptomatic subjects. *Neuroradiology, 36*(1), 49–53. https://doi.org/10.1007/BF00599196.

Levy, H. I. (2000). Cervical pain syndromes: Primary care diagnosis and management. *Comprehensive Therapy, 26*(2), 82–88. https://doi.org/10.1007/s12019-000-0016-7.

Martin, B. I., Deyo, R. A., Mirza, S. K., Turner, J. A., Comstock, B. A., Hollingworth, W., & Sullivan, S. D. (2008). Expenditures and health status among adults with back and neck problems. *JAMA, 299*(6), 656–664. https://doi.org/10.1001/jama.299.6.656.

Matsumoto, M., Chiba, K., Ishikawa, M., Maruiwa, H., Fujimura, Y., & Toyama, Y. (2001). Relationships between outcomes of conservative treatment and magnetic resonance imaging findings in patients with mild cervical myelopathy caused by soft disc herniations. *Spine (Phila Pa 1976), 26*(14), 1592–1598. https://doi.org/10.1097/00007632-200107150-00021.

Matsumoto, M., Fujimura, Y., Suzuki, N., Nishi, Y., Nakamura, M., Yabe, Y., & Shiga, H. (1998). MRI of cervical intervertebral discs in asymptomatic subjects. *The Journal of Bone and Joint Surgery. British Volume, 80*(1), 19–24. https://doi.org/10.1302/0301-620X.80B1.7929.

Monsey, R. D. (1997). Rheumatoid arthritis of the cervical spine. *Journal of the American Academy of Orthopaedic Surgeons, 5*(5), 240–248. https://doi.org/10.5435/00124635-199709000-00002.

Öner, A., Aşansu, M. A., & Akman, Y. E. (2020). Sprengel deformity: Comprehensive evaluation of concomitant spinal and extraspinal anomalies in 90 patients. *Spine (Phila Pa 1976), 45*(18), E1150–E1157. https://doi.org/10.1097/BRS.0000000000003523.

Sadasivan, K. K., Reddy, R. P., & Albright, J. A. (1993). The natural history of cervical spondylotic myelopathy. *Yale Journal of Biology and Medicine, 66*(3), 235–242. https://pubmed.ncbi.nlm.nih.gov/8209559/.

Sarzi-Puttini, P., & Atzeni, F. (2004). New developments in our understanding of DISH (diffuse idiopathic skeletal hyperostosis). *Current Opinion in Rheumatology, 16*(3), 287–292. https://doi.org/10.1097/00002281-200405000-00021.

Schouten, R., Albert, T., & Kwon, B. K. (2012). The spine-injured patient: Initial assessment and emergency treatment. *Journal of the American Academy of Orthopaedic Surgeons, 20*(6), 336–346. https://doi.org/10.5435/JAAOS-20-06-336.

Strine, T. W., & Hootman, J. M. (2007). US national prevalence and correlates of low back and neck pain among adults. *Arthritis & Rheumatism, 57*(4), 656–665. https://doi.org/10.1002/art.22684.

Swischuk, L. E. (1977). Anterior displacement of C2 in children: Physiologic or pathologic. *Radiology, 122*(3), 759–763. https://doi.org/10.1148/122.3.759.

Taurog, J. D., Chhabra, A., & Colbert, R. A. (2016). Ankylosing spondylitis and axial spondyloarthritis. *The New England Journal of Medicine, 374*(26), 2563–2574. https://doi.org/10.1056/NEJMra1406182.

Tay, B. K., Deckey, J., & Hu, S. S. (2002). Spinal infections. *Journal of the American Academy of Orthopaedic Surgeons, 10*(3), 188–197. https://doi.org/10.5435/00124635-200205000-00005.

Tong, C., & Barest, G. (2003). Approach to imaging the patient with neck pain. *Journal of Neuroimaging, 13*(1), 5–16. https://pubmed.ncbi.nlm.nih.gov/12593126/.

Tracy, M. R., Dormans, J. P., & Kusumi, K. (2004). Klippel-Feil syndrome: Clinical features and current understanding of etiology. *Clinical Orthopaedics and Related Research, (424)*, 183–190. https://pubmed.ncbi.nlm.nih.gov/15241163/.

Tsang, I. (2001). Rheumatology: 12. Pain in the neck. *CMAJ, 164*(8), 1182–1187. https://pubmed.ncbi.nlm.nih.gov/11338807/.

van der Linden, S., Valkenburg, H. A., & Cats, A. (1984). Evaluation of diagnostic criteria for ankylosing spondylitis: A proposal for modification of the New York criteria. *Arthritis and Rheumatism, 27*(4), 361–368. https://doi.org/10.1002/art.1780270401.

Chapter 3

Lower Back Pain

Mehmet O. Bıyık[*], MD
Mehmet Aktoklu, MD
and Mehmet A. Demirci
Department of Neurosurgery, Karadeniz Technical University, Faculty of Medicine, Trabzon, Turkey

Abstract

According to recent data from the World Health Organization, 619 million people are affected by low back pain, which is described as pain between the lower edge of the ribs and the buttocks. It is one of the most common complaints from the past to the present and can cause chronic disability unless it is correctly diagnosed and treated. It can have many different causes, which range from small muscle or ligamentous damages and discopathy to metastases or other systemic disorders such as hematologic, infectious, or renal diseases. It may be treated with over-the-counter pain relievers to advanced pain treatments such as narcotic analgesics, nerve blocks, or even surgeries. In this section, it is aimed to provide awareness of the importance of causes, prognostic factors, and approaches to low back pain which is a very treatable situation, but if left untreated it can seriously affect quality of life.

Keywords: degenerative spinal cord diseases, low back pain, disease management, pain, radiculopathy, risk factors

Introduction

The World Health Organization (WHO) defines low back pain (LBP) as pain between the thoracic 12th vertebra and the hip. In 2020, 619 million people worldwide affected by LBP, and it is estimated that this number will be approximately 843 million by 2050 when it is evaluated together with population growth over the years (Ferreira et al., 2023). It is one of the factors contributing the most to the world's disability burden with 7.7% (Ferreira et al., 2023).

The general prevalence of low back pain is 28.8% and the gender distribution is 39% in men and 61% in women. It is also more prevalent in women in all age groups (Bento et al., 2020; de Souza et al., 2019; Ferreira et al., 2023). Associated factors for men include age over 36 years, smoking, having fewer years of formal education (0-4 years), and having a history of

[*] Corresponding Author's Email: mehmetorbaybyk@yahoo.com.

In: Common Diseases According to Family Medicine Practice Guidelines
Editors: Esra Meltem Koç and Hilal Aksoy
ISBN: 979-8-89530-302-3

hypertension. For women, factors associated with the complaint include lifting heavy loads, standing and sitting in a forward-bent position in daily and professional life, and sitting at the computer three or more days a week. Participants who were widowed or divorced were more likely to report low back pain in both sexes (Bento et al., 2020). The most recent assessment of the global prevalence of low back pain in all age groups shows that it is more common in older people and is characterized by longer attacks (de Souza et al., 2019). The prevalence of low back pain increases up to the age of 80 years and then decreases slightly, and it can be accepted that this complaint is mostly a continuation of pain from the past years and occurs as a part of aging. In other words, this complaint becomes less bothersome in old age and can simply be ignored (de Souza et al., 2019; Fejer & Ruhe, 2012; Sjøgren et al., 2009).

Pain can also be classified according to the type of damage, although not exclusively for low back pain. Basically, pain associated with tissue damage (bone, soft tissue, or organs) is called nociceptive pain, nerve damage is called neuropathic pain, and pain affected by psychological factors is called psychogenic pain. Nociceptive pain is often described as a sharp stabbing or throbbing pain. It can be relieved on its own but is often chronic; it can pass or be constant. Neuropathic pain is usually burning or tingling but can sometimes be described as an electric shock. It differs from nociceptive pain which occurs as a result of a specific stimulus in that it does not require such a stimulus, usually independent of nociceptor activation. Although psychogenic pain usually has a physical origin, psychogenic effects such as fear, depression, stress, or anxiety may cause pain to be more severe and/or longer lasting than it should be. These types of pain can sometimes be isolated and sometimes mixed in different proportions in a painful patient, and pain palliation can become quite complex in such cases (Manusov, 2012; Urits et al., 2019).

There are three types of low back pain: mechanical (muscle spasm, disc herniation, nerve root compression, degenerative facet joint disorders, spinal fracture, etc.), non-mechanical (tumors, inflammatory, or infectious conditions, etc.), and referred (gallbladder diseases, kidney stones, infections, and aortic aneurysm, etc.) (Manusov, 2012; Urits et al., 2019). Although the majority of cases are thought to be mechanical pain, a specific cause cannot be found in approximately 75% of cases and is thought to be related to muscle strain or ligament injury (Bailly et al., 2021; Huntoon & Huntoon, 2004; Manusov, 2012; Shokri et al., 2023).

Although there is no consensus, it is generally accepted that low back pain lasting up to 6 weeks is defined as acute, low back pain lasting between 6-12 weeks is defined as subacute, and low back pain lasting more than 12 weeks is defined as chronic low back pain (Musa POLAT Belgin KARAOĞLAN Gazi Üniversitesi Tıp Fakültesi FTR Ana Bilim Dalı & Üniversitesi Tıp Fakültesi FTR Ana Bilim Dalı ANKARA, n.d.; Urits et al., 2019). While the majority of non-chronic cases show self-limitation and improvement in 6 weeks or less, chronic symptoms can be seen in 10-40% of cases (Urits et al., 2019). Patients with acute and subacute low back pain should be treated in a different way from chronic cases (Bailly et al., 2021; Musa POLAT Belgin KARAOĞLAN Gazi Üniversitesi Tıp Fakültesi FTR Ana Bilim Dalı & Üniversitesi Tıp Fakültesi FTR Ana Bilim Dalı ANKARA, n.d.; Urits et al., 2019).

In many cases, the specific nociceptive source of lower back pain cannot be identified, and those affected are usually classified as "non-specific low back pain." In 90% to 95% of cases, non-specific low back pain is present. Although most patients with acute low back pain experience rapid improvement in pain and disability within 1 month, chronicity may occur in 4% to 25% of patients (Nieminen et al., 2021).

Chronic lower back pain can be caused by non-organic psychogenic factors or by a variety of causes such as degenerative, inflammatory, metabolic, infectious, neoplastic, traumatic, and congenital. The main goal of the treatment is to improve the symptoms and provide functionality by enabling mobilization and even exercise, thus improving the quality of life by helping to return to active life and work.

Etiopathogenesis

In terms of etiopathogenesis, any kind of innervated structure in the lumbar spine (such as muscles, zygapophyseal joints, ligaments, dura mater and nerve roots, ring fibrosis, vertebrae, and thoracolumbar fascia) may be the cause of low back pain. Additionally, the list of differential diagnoses is so wide, including non-spinal causes (Casato et al., 2019). It can be classified as congenital, degenerative, inflammatory, infectious, metabolic, neoplastic, traumatic, psychogenic, reflected pain, and post-surgical diseases (Figure 1).

Congenital causes include lumbolization, sacralization, scoliosis, spina bifida, and other developmental anomalies in the spine and related tissues during the growth and development period beginning from the neonatal period. Split cord malformations are associated with cutaneous lesions, spinal deformity, spina bifida, lipoma, and attached spinal cord. Patients are present with spinal deformity or neurological deficits, especially in the lower limbs, bowel, and bladder, or less frequently with a dysraphism discovered incidentally and may be completely asymptomatic (Karim Ahmed et al., 2020). The fusion of the five sacral vertebrae with the fifth lumbar vertebra is called sacralization, and the partial or complete separation of the first sacral segment from the rest of the sacrum to form a sixth lumbar vertebra is called lumbalization. This condition is caused by a defect in the segmentation of the lumbosacral spine during development and can result in a change in the structure of the lumbar and sacral vertebrae, leading to a change in the angle of the lumbosacral, increased stress on the L4-L5 motion segment, degenerative changes in the facet joint, disc degeneration, and anterior displacement of L4 over L5, and is responsible for low back pain due to altered biomechanics (Figure 1) (Sabnis & Nakhate, 2020).

In degenerative disc disease (DDD), due to the degeneration of the end plates, the nutrition of the disc decreases, followed by a decrease in disc heights, changing the biomechanics of the spine and leading to degenerative spinal stenosis, facet arthropathy, spondylosis and osteophytes, spondylolisthesis, and degenerative scoliosis and instability of the spine becomes inevitable (Deer et al., 2019; Harrop et al., n.d.). Lumbar spinal stenosis (LSS) is defined by the narrowing of the spinal canal, nerve root canals, and intervertebral foramen. Acquired LSS is generally associated with aging and progressive degenerative processes of the spine, and patients often have chronic pain (Figure 1) (Karim Ahmed et al., 2020).

Inflammatory joint diseases are chronic, progressive, inflammatory, autoimmune diseases affecting small joints, large joints such as the spine and sacroiliac joints, synovial fluid, often progressing in causing pain due to inflammation and mechanical causes, and the most common diseases are rheumatoid arthritis, ankylosing spondylitis, psoriatic arthritis, etc. Ankylosing spondylitis (AS) is a chronic, progressive, inflammation of the spine and sacroiliac joints and, in advanced cases, ossification of the vertebral ligaments, fusion of the vertebral bodies, and subsequent loss of spinal flexibility, generally between the ages of 20 and 40 with persistent, chronic low back pain and stiffness. RA is clinically characterized by joint swelling and pain, leading to progressive erosive joint destruction and causes functional disability, which is managed by rheumatologists based on the number of affected joints, serology, inflammatory markers, and duration of symptoms (Figure 1) (Aletaha et al., 2010; Fuchs et al., 2013; Kenar et al., 2023; Zamanpoor, 2019).

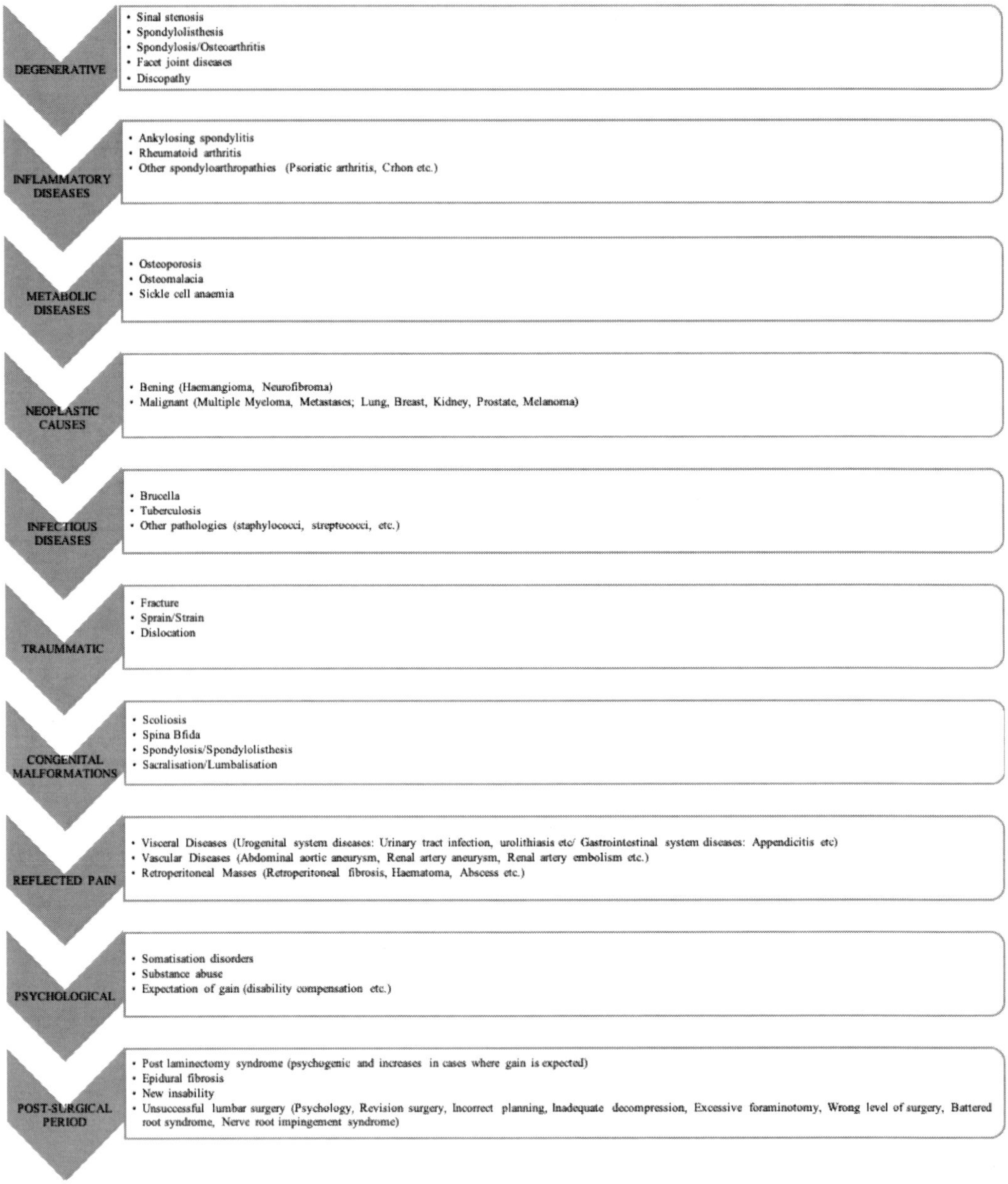

Figure 1. Summary of etiological factors.

Spondylodiscitis, osteomyelitis, subdural and epidural abscess, psoas, retroperitoneal, subphrenic, paravertebral, retropharyngeal, and mediastinal abscesses can develop as a result of hematogenous, neighborhood or direct (lumbar puncture) inflammatory diseases in which the vertebral body, intervertebral disc, facet joints are infected through spread (as a result of interventional procedures such as biopsy), usually causing nocturnal pain, fever, severe pain that increases with movement (Aljawadi et al., 2019; Babic & Simpfendorfer, 2017; Tsantes et al., 2020). Spondylodiscitis, which is a spinal infection, is most commonly seen in adults >50 years of age, but it should be considered that especially intravenous drug users or patients with diabetes mellitus, immunosuppressive diseases, the presence of intravascular foreign bodies (chemotherapy port, dialysis catheter, etc.) are highly susceptible to spinal infections. In general, the pain in these patients usually occurs at night and can wake them up from sleep. Pain can be triggered by movement. Although fever is a common symptom, half of the patients with pyogenic spinal infections and a high percentage of patients with fungal, mycobacterial, and brucella infections can be fever-free, which can delay the diagnosis. On physical examination, the presence of scars indicating previous surgery or trauma, and any infective findings on the skin (redness, swelling, fluctuations, etc.) should be evaluated. Paravertebral muscle spasm can be palpated, while marked tenderness on percussion is observed over the spinous processes of the infected spinal segment in 75% to 95% of cases. In patients with Charcot arthropathy and paraplegia, pain is minimal or absent. Neurological symptoms such as paresthesia and muscle weakness are present in approximately 30% of patients. Since the low specificity of symptoms and signs may result in delayed diagnosis, clinical suspicion is the first and the most important step for spinal infections (Figure 1) (Aljawadi et al., 2019; Babic & Simpfendorfer, 2017; Tsantes et al., 2020).

Osteoporosis is a systemic skeletal disease in which the balance between bone production and destruction cells is altered, resulting in loss of bone mass and microarchitectural bone structure, resulting in low fracture strength of bone, typically vertebral corpus, femoral neck, and distal fracture of the radius, with symptoms ranging from mild pain to neurological deficits (Fuchs et al., 2013). Sickle Cell Disease (SCD) is a genetic disorder caused by a single mutation in one of the hemoglobin chains, leading to structural changes in erythrocytes, resulting in shorter life expectancy, vascular occlusion, and organ damage. Height loss in the vertebral bodies, due to an infarction in the central part, can cause vertebral collapse, which can lead to significant pain (Figure 1) (Zanoni et al., 2021).

Primary and metastatic neoplasms of the spine and spinal cord are among the pathologies that can cause low back pain. Bone metastasis is the third most seen region of metastasis, followed by the lung and liver. Multiple myeloma, lung, breast, prostate, thyroid, colon, bladder, and renal cell are among the most common metastatic tumors to the bone. Having a history of cancer is the strongest risk factor for back pain due to bone metastases. The most prominent symptom of spinal metastases is back pain and can also be characterized as local pain, mechanical pain, or radicular pain (Macedo et al., 2017; Sutcliffe et al., 2013; Urits et al., 2019; Wewel & O'toole, 2020). Multiple myeloma is a neoplastic disease characterized by clonal proliferation of neoplastic plasma cells in the bone marrow, M protein in the body, and multiple organ damage, which can cause end-organ damage, often including hypercalcemia, renal dysfunction, anemia, lytic lesions in bone, osteolytic bone lesions, pathological fractures and various skeletal complications such as osteoporosis, and can progress from local pain to neurological deficit (Chen et al., 2021). The most prominent symptom found in 80% to 95% is pain. It may be characterized as local, mechanical, radicular, or nonspecific pain. 35% to 75%

may present with motor dysfunction. In patients without a known history of cancer, it should be suspected in the presence of weight loss, night sweating, pain that awakens from sleep at night, smoking, advanced age, and a family history of cancer despite efforts such as diet and sports (Chen et al., 2021; Macedo et al., 2017; Sutcliffe et al., 2013; Wewel & O'toole, 2020). Hemangiomas (HAs) are pathologically classified as capillary, cavernous, arteriovenous, or venous according to the type of vascular channel containing endothelial cells growing in the medulla of the vertebral body and rarely cause radicular and/or spinal cord compression due to invasion into the soft tissues of the spinal cord and epidural region. They are the most common benign tumors affecting the spine and can cause pain, paresthesia, and other neurological findings by causing enlargement of the bone matrix and compression of large vessels (Brindisino et al., 2022; Goldstein et al., 2015; Kunimoto et al., 2022). Spinal nerve sheath tumors (NSTs) are common types of spinal cord tumors, such as schwannomas or neurofibromas, and can occur both sporadically and in association with neurofibromatosis 1, an autosomal dominant disorder, and are essentially benign, grow slowly and have a low rate of local invasion or distant metastasis (Figure 1) (Mohamed & Ali, 2223).

Drug and opioid addiction, the expectation of disability compensation, and the presence of symptoms of depression may be indicators of psychosocial distress; similarly, patients with somatization and/or maladaptive coping disorders may have persistent, nonspecific low back pain and should be evaluated for social and psychological distress (Figure 1) (Urits et al., 2019).

The structural and functional organization of the somatic and visceral nociceptive systems is also found at the spinal level, where the somatic nociceptive afferents, which pass through the somatic nerves and have bodies in the corresponding ganglia of the dorsal roots of the spinal cord, transmit pain signals from different parts of the body to neurons in the posterior horn of specific parts of the spinal cord. In summary, stimuli of somatic and visceral origin in the spinal cord converge in common pathways toward the upper centers and produce reflected pain in areas where metameric innervation is shared, such as the urinary tract, colicky pain in urolithiasis, angina in myocardial infarction, biliary colic, abdominal aortic aneurysm, retroperitoneal abscess hematoma and masses (Figure 1) (Affaitati et al., 2020; Anagnostakos & Lal, 2021; Lyubashina et al., 2023; Pacheco-Carroza, 2021; Shokri et al., 2023).

Clinical Assessment

The evaluation of a patient with low back pain should begin with anamnesis, medical history, family history, general and complaint-oriented examination, as in almost every medical condition.

For example, acute onset of low back pain, history of trauma, osteoporosis, chronic kidney disease, multiple myeloma, dependent on dialysis, may indicate sprain and vertebral fracture; a burning rash along a dermatome may indicate herpes zoster. Additionally, intravenous substance abuse, being dialysis-dependent, catheterization, history of fever and injection in the lumbar region may indicate a possible infection; while dissatisfaction with work and family life, depression, somatization disorder, or having secondary gain such as the expectation of compensation from the workplace may indicate psychological reasons. Furthermore, unintentional weight loss, pain that wakes up from sleep at night, having a cancer diagnosis or a family history of malignancy can lead to spinal metastasis; while sedentary life, limited mobilization, edema in the feet, heat loss, varicose veins, and pulmonary embolism history can lead to the lower extremity or abdominal embolism. The pulsatile character of pain, and coldness sensation in the lower extremity can lead to an abdominal aortic aneurysm; while morning stiffness, relief during the day, decreased range of motion over time, swelling in small joints, and movement limitation may be indications of a rheumatic disease. Low back pain radiating to the leg and increasing with axial loading to disc hernias; advanced age, the gradual decrease in walking distance over the years, difficulty in going up and down slopes and sitting and getting up, the need to walk by leaning forward may be related to degenerative spine diseases. Anamnesis and physical examination, which are often sufficient on their own, are extremely critical in understanding the etiopathogenesis of low back pain.

The relationship between lower back pain and body position should be questioned. For example, a history of lumbar spinal stenosis, forward flexion while standing or walking, or pain relieved by sitting are typical. Most of the time, reflexes, including strength and sensation, are normal upon physical examination while sitting or lying down. There may also be a decrease in walking distance, which is called claudication. Neurogenic claudication arises as a result of ischemia (due to venous congestion and reduced arterial blood flow) but also as a result of mechanical compression of nerve roots and is characterized by pain or radiculopathy in the hips as well as in the lower limbs that increases with walking and is better with forward bending or stooping, but it should be noted that claudication can be of neurogenic or vascular origin. The differential diagnosis is briefly summarized in Table 1.

In addition to lumbar stenosis, spondylolisthesis also has a similar history and examination, as well as a more pronounced loss of strength in the roots affected by listhesis due to spinal movement, radicular pain, low back and leg pain triggered by sitting and standing on sloping floors, lifting loads, and although spinal stenosis is usually seen in advanced age, listhesis can be seen in any age group (Burton et al., 2023; Deer et al., 2019).

Physical examination should include examination, palpation, range of motion, strength testing, provocative maneuvers, and neurological assessments (limb strength, sensation, and deep tendon reflexes).

In Table 2, the etiologic factors are briefly summarized in terms of clinical and physical examination (Affaitati et al., 2020; Aljawadi et al., 2019; Anagnostakos & Lal, 2021; Burton et al., 2023; Casato et al., 2019; Deer et al., 2019; Harrop et al., n.d.; Karim Ahmed et al., 2020; Kenar et al., 2023; Lyubashina et al., 2023; Sabnis & Nakhate, 2020; Tsantes et al., 2020; Zamanpoor, 2019; Zanoni et al., 2021).

Prognosis

Although most patients with acute low back pain recover, 4 to 25% of them become chronic. The prognosis is also influenced by factors independent of the spine. Focusing only on pain, mechanics, and nominal diagnosis may lead to further disability (Nieminen et al., 2021). In terms of social or psychological distress, substance abuse and/or history of substance abuse, disability compensation, having symptoms of depression and accompanying psychiatric conditions, somatization, and/or maladaptive coping are associated with worse outcomes in patients with low back pain. It is found that those with a history of major depression are 5 times more likely, of anxiety 2.5 times more likely, and those with traumatic stress disorder 3 times more likely to become chronic pain (Mehling et al., 2015; Melloh et al., 2013; Shaw et al., n.d.; Urits et al., 2019). In another study, it was shown that smoking can cause decreased perfusion in the intervertebral discs through vasoconstriction, impaired blood flow in the spine through atherosclerosis in the long term, and degenerative lesions in the intervertebral discs. In the same study, it was found to be a risk factor for osteoporosis, to increase the level of proinflammatory cytokines in the circulation and cause increased pain, and the prevalence and incidence of low back pain were higher in both current and former smokers than in never smokers, and the prevalence was lower in former smokers than in current smokers (Shiri et al., 2010). In another study, those who exercised 1.0-1.9 hours a week had fewer pain complaints than those with a sedentary life (Nilsen et al., 2011). Another study showed a 10% to 60% reduction in the prevalence of low back pain and chronicity in people whose blood pressure increased slightly due to reduced baroreflex sensitivity (Hagen et al., n.d.). Therefore, when treating patients with low back pain, clinicians should consider all aspects of the disease. Conditions that worsen the prognosis, i.e., indicate chronicity, and those that indicate a good prognosis are summarized in the tables below to give an idea.

Tables 4 and 5 briefly summarize the prognostic factors that increase and decrease the chances of success in the treatment of low back pain (Hagen et al., n.d.; Mehling et al., 2015; Melloh et al., 2013; Nieminen et al., 2021; Nilsen et al., 2011; Shaw et al., n.d.; Shiri et al., 2010; Urits et al., 2019).

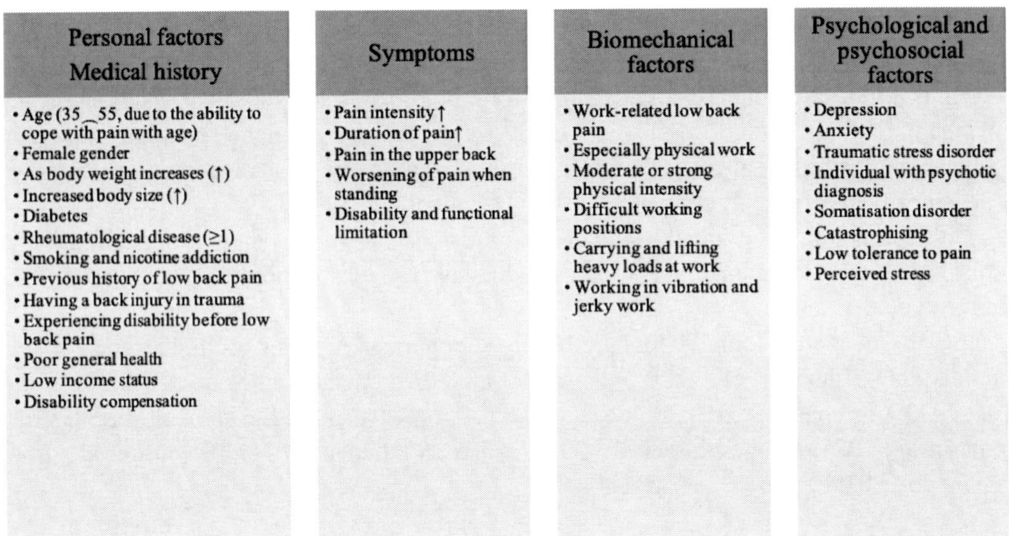

Figure 2. Negative prognostic factors.

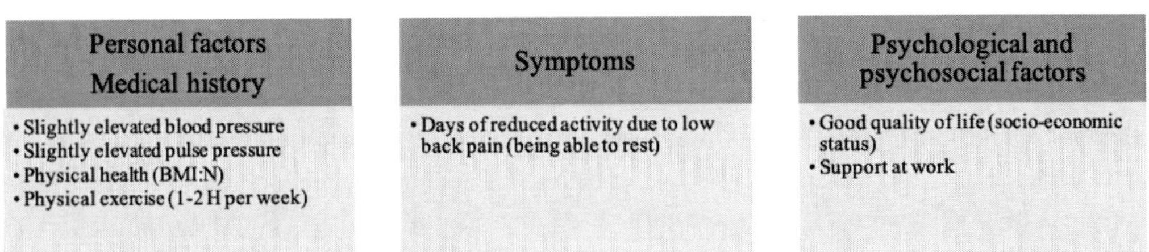

Figure 3. Positive prognostic factors (protective).

Table 1. Differential diagnosis of neurogenic and vascular claudication

	Pain location	Type of pain	Pain spread	Alleviation	Relief	Time to pass the complaint	Neurological finding	Pulsations
Neurogenic	Back, Hip Lower limb	Combustion Lethargy Numbness	Proximal to distal	Walking in extension and standing upright	Lumbar flexion Seating Rest	Minutes	+/-	Usually normal
Vascular	With calf-related vascular field	Cramp Printing Tension	Localized in the relevant vascular area	During walking and activity independent of lumbar position	At rest independent of lumbar position	Fast (seconds)	-	Decreased

Table 2. Summarized etiological factors in the differential diagnosis of clinical and physical examination

	Inguinal Pain	Back Pain	Hip Pain	Lower limb pain	Claudicasyo	Loss of Strength	Pain in Activity	Additional Features
Lumbar spinal stenosis		+	+	+/-	Neurogenic	+/-	↑	Anteflexion posture, Pain in felxion ↓
Spondylolisthesis		+	+/-	+/-	Neurogenic	+/-	↑	Single leg lift test + Straight leg lift +/-
Facet joint syndrome		+	+	+/-		-	↑	Pain on palpation of facets +
Degenerative disc	+/-	+	+/-	+/-			↑	Pain increases during sitting, bending forwards, standing ↑
Vertebral fracture		+	+/-	+/-	Neurogenic and Vascular	+/-	↑	Pain in the vertebrae on palpation + Claudication and neurological deficit may occur depending on the structure compressed by the fracture
Hip osteoarthritis	+	+	+	+/-			↑	Patrich and long-roll test+ Trandelenburg+
Piriformis syndrome		+	+	+/-			↑	Patrich test, + in rotation +/- in external rotation- Pain with walking and sitting Straight leg lift +
Ankylosing spondylitis and Other Spondyloarthropathies		+	+/-				↓	Morning stiffness+ Gaenslen test+ HLAB27+ (in AS) Pain at rest

Table 2. (Continued)

	Inguinal Pain	Back Pain	Hip Pain	Lower limb pain	Claudicasyo	Loss of Strength	Pain in Activity	Additional Features
Osteomyelitis Psoas abscess Empyema	+/-	+	+/-	+/-	+/-	+/-	↑	Neurological deficit, claudicasyo + depending on the presence of epidural, subdural empyema, etc. Tenderness with palpation + Acute phase reactants +, fever mostly+
Vascular (abdominal aortic aneurysm, renal artery embolism, etc.)	+	+		+	Vascular	+/-	↑	Pain at rest ↓ Lower limb cold Pulsations - (usually)
Cancer, Metastasis	+/-	+/-	+/-	+/-	+/-	+/-	+/-	Known history of cancer Involuntary weight loss Pain at night and rest

Management

When a patient with or without radicular pain presents, a detailed physical and neurological examination should be performed following anamnesis. This process should definitely include the evaluation of red flags, which are suspicion of serious or extraspinal pathology and conditions requiring urgent or specific treatment (Figure 4). If general symptoms of low back pain are present and no additional pathological condition is suspected, the patient should be informed about low back pain and radiculopathy, encouraged to participate in routine daily activities and work as much as possible, and informed that additional imaging is not required. If medical treatment is necessary for pain palliation and prevention of functional loss, NSAIDs are one of the first-line treatment options. However, patients should be re-evaluated after 2-4 weeks and if there is improvement, the treatment can be terminated by making the necessary recommendations for regular exercise and physical activity and protection. On the contrary, if improvement is not sufficient, red flags and yellow flags in terms of the risk of chronicity should be evaluated again and risk factors should be reviewed in terms of repeated work, rest leaves, long-term disability at work or barriers to return to work (Figure 4). Cases considered to have a strong risk of chronicity should be evaluated in a multidisciplinary manner (general practitioner, physiotherapist, rheumatologist, physical medicine and rehabilitation specialist, workplace physician) (Figure 4). At this time, home exercises and physiotherapy recommendations should be reviewed and the need for medical treatment should be re-evaluated. In all cases, patients should be encouraged to continue their daily activities and participate in physical activity. Spinal imaging is recommended for patients with persistent radicular complaints. At the end of all these processes, patients are re-evaluated after 6-12 weeks and if there is improvement in complaints, regular home exercises and physical exercises are recommended; if there is no improvement or if the multidisciplinary approach fails, necessary radiological imaging should be performed (Figure 4). Besides making an effort to diagnose a concrete cause, patients with chronic low back pain should also be psychologically evaluated. If necessary, SNRI, and tricyclic antidepressants, especially for neuropathic pain, can be added to the treatment. In case of detection of concrete unresponsive causes, the patient may be referred to other relevant specialists for further evaluation and treatments such as surgery or other pain interventions (Figure 4) (Bailly et al., 2021).

Conclusion

As mentioned in the section, low back pain is a multifactorial disorder with nonspecific causes. If it is chronic, it can cause loss of workforce, and mental health disorders, and is among the most common reasons for application to primary health-care centers. Anamnesis, medical history, family history, distribution and characteristics of pain, conditions that provoke pain, and the times when pain usually occurs, must be investigated. In order to determine the etiological factors such as trauma, infections, malignancies, etc., which should be diagnosed based only on anamnesis with a strong clinical suspicion, the best treatment can then be provided. At the same time, by identifying patients with neurological deficits in meticulous physical examination, a possible disability can be prevented.

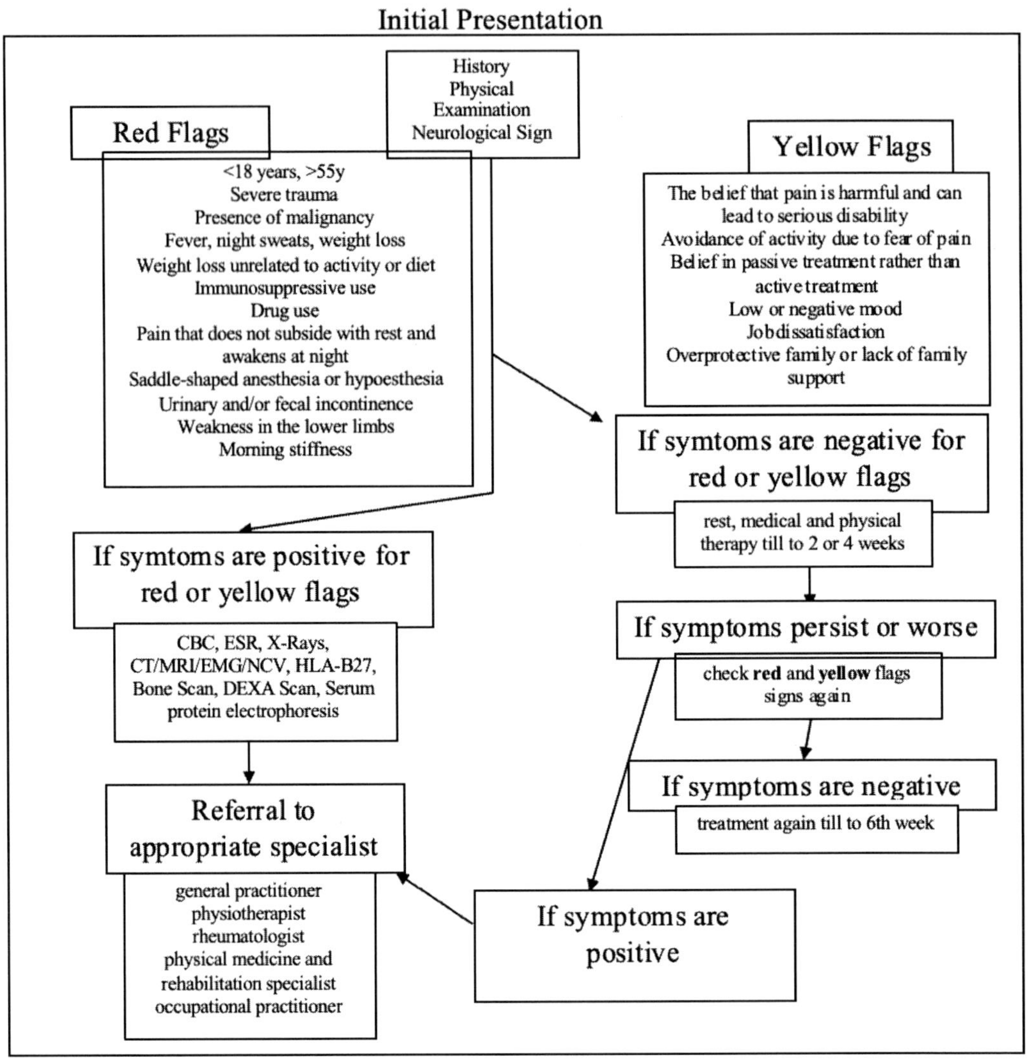

Figure 4. The management of low back pain.

Briefly, we should keep in mind:

1. Red and yellow flags should be well known, and, if necessary, specific treatments should be initiated by referring to the relevant specialists as soon as possible.
2. If there are no red or yellow flags, if necessary, treatment should be started and followed up.
3. The patient should be encouraged to return to daily activity and work by informing him/her that pain may last for a few weeks, providing reassurance that imaging will not be required in the first step.
4. If the pain persists during our follow-up, red and yellow flags should be re-evaluated, if necessary, initial examinations such as X-rays, and blood studies should be performed, and medical and physical therapy should be rearranged if there is no urgent condition such as red or yellow flags.

5. In case of any negative situation in follow-ups such as the occurrence of red or yellow flags, should be referred to the relevant specialists.
6. Or even if no alarming situation is encountered during follow-ups, one should insist on referring the patient to the relevant specialist for further examination and treatment concerning pain becomes chronic.

We should not forget that with proper diagnosis, treatment, and timely and correct referrals, 90% of low back pain can be treated by avoiding possible future chronicity, and psychological and physical disabilities. In this way, serious labor and financial loss can be prevented while the quality of life can also be improved significantly.

References

Affaitati, G., Costantini, R., Tana, C., Cipollone, F., & Giamberardino, M. A. (2020). Co-occurrence of pain syndromes. *Journal of Neural Transmission, 127*(4), 625–646. Springer. https://doi.org/10.1007/s00702-019-02107-8.

Aletaha, D., Neogi, T., Silman, A. J., Funovits, J., Felson, D. T., Bingham, C. O., Birnbaum, N. S., Burmester, G. R., Bykerk, V. P., Cohen, M. D., Combe, B., Costenbader, K. H., Dougados, M., Emery, P., Ferraccioli, G., Hazes, J. M. W., Hobbs, K., Huizinga, T. W. J., Kavanaugh, A., … Hawker, G. (2010). 2010 Rheumatoid arthritis classification criteria: An American College of Rheumatology/European League Against Rheumatism collaborative initiative. *Arthritis and Rheumatism, 62*(9), 2569–2581. John Wiley and Sons Inc. https://doi.org/10.1002/art.27584.

Aljawadi, A., Jahangir, N., Jeelani, A., Ferguson, Z., Niazi, N., Arnall, F., & Pillai, A. (2019). Management of pyogenic spinal infection: Review of literature. *Journal of Orthopaedics, 16*(6), 508–512. Reed Elsevier India Pvt. Ltd. https://doi.org/10.1016/j.jor.2019.08.014.

Anagnostakos, J., & Lal, B. K. (2021). Abdominal aortic aneurysms. *Progress in Cardiovascular Diseases, 65*, 34–43. W. B. Saunders. https://doi.org/10.1016/j.pcad.2021.03.009.

Babic, M., & Simpfendorfer, C. S. (2017). Infections of the spine. *Infectious Disease Clinics of North America, 31*(2). https://doi.org/10.1016/j.idc.2017.01.003.

Bailly, F., Trouvin, A. P., Bercier, S., Dadoun, S., Deneuville, J. P., Faguer, R., Fassier, J. B., Koleck, M., Lassalle, L., Le Vraux, T., Brigitte, L., Petitprez, K., Ramond-Roquin, A., Renard, J. F., Roren, A., Rozenberg, S., Sebire, C., Vuides, G., Rannou, F., & Audrey, P. (2021). Clinical guidelines and care pathway for management of low back pain with or without radicular pain. *Joint Bone Spine, 88*(6). https://doi.org/10.1016/j.jbspin.2021.105227.

Bento, T. P. F., Genebra, C. V. dos S., Maciel, N. M., Cornelio, G. P., Simeão, S. F. A. P., & Vitta, A. de. (2020). Low back pain and some associated factors: Is there any difference between genders? *Brazilian Journal of Physical Therapy, 24*(1), 79–87. https://doi.org/10.1016/j.bjpt.2019.01.012.

Brindisino, F., Scrimitore, A., Pennella, D., Bruno, F., Pellegrino, R., Maselli, F., Lena, F., & Giovannico, G. (2022). Aggressive vertebral hemangioma and spinal cord compression: A particular direct access case of low back pain to be managed - A case report. *International Journal of Environmental Research and Public Health, 19*(20). https://doi.org/10.3390/ijerph192013276.

Burton, M. R., Dowling, T. J., & Mesfin, F. B. (2023). Isthmic spondylolisthesis.

Casato, G., Stecco, C., & Busin, R. (2019). Fasciae and nonspecific low back pain: Role of fasciae in nonspecific low back pain. *Eur J Transl Myol, 29*(3). www.3bscientific.com.

Chen, B., Cai, L., & Zhou, F. (2021). Management of acute spinal cord compression in multiple myeloma. *Critical Reviews in Oncology/Hematology, 160*. Elsevier Ireland Ltd. https://doi.org/10.1016/j.critrevonc.2020.103205.

de Souza, I. M. B., Sakaguchi, T. F., Yuan, S. L. K., Matsutani, L. A., Do Espírito-Santo, A. de S., Pereira, C. A. de B., & Marques, A. P. (2019). Prevalence of low back pain in the elderly population: A systematic review. *Clinics, 74*. Universidade de Sao Paulo. https://doi.org/10.6061/clinics/2019/e789.

Deer, T., Sayed, D., Michels, J., Josephson, Y., Li, S., & Calodney, A. K. (2019). A review of lumbar spinal stenosis with intermittent neurogenic claudication: Disease and diagnosis. *Pain Medicine (United States, 20*, S32–S44). Oxford University Press. https://doi.org/10.1093/pm/pnz161.

Fejer, R., & Ruhe, A. (2012). What is the prevalence of musculoskeletal problems in the elderly population in developed countries? A systematic critical literature review. http://chiromt.com/content/20/1/31.

Ferreira, M. L., de Luca, K., Haile, L. M., Steinmetz, J. D., Culbreth, G. T., Cross, M., Kopec, J. A., Ferreira, P. H., Blyth, F. M., Buchbinder, R., Hartvigsen, J., Wu, A. M., Safiri, S., Woolf, A. D., Collins, G. S., Ong, K. L., Vollset, S. E., Smith, A. E., Cruz, J. A., … March, L. M. (2023). Global, regional, and national burden of low back pain, 1990–2020, its attributable risk factors, and projections to 2050: A systematic analysis of the global burden of disease study 2021. *The Lancet Rheumatology, 5*(6). https://doi.org/10.1016/S2665-9913(23)00098-X.

Fuchs, J., Rabenberg, M., & Scheidt-Nave, C. (2013). Prävalenz ausgewählter muskuloskelettaler Erkrankungen: Ergebnisse der Studie zur Gesundheit Erwachsener in Deutschland (DEGS1) [Prevalence of selected musculoskeletal diseases: Results from the study on adult health in Germany]. *Bundesgesundheitsblatt - Gesundheitsforschung - Gesundheitsschutz, 56*(5–6), 678–686. https://doi.org/10.1007/s00103-013-1687-4.

Goldstein, C. L., Varga, P. P., Gokaslan, Z. L., Boriani, S., Luzzati, A., Rhines, L., Fisher, C. G., Chou, D., Williams, R. P., Dekutoski, M. B., Quraishi, N. A., Bettegowda, C., Kawahara, N., & Fehlings, M. G. (2015). Spinal hemangiomas: Results of surgical management for local recurrence and mortality in a multicenter study. *Spine, 40*(9), 656–664. https://doi.org/10.1097/BRS.0000000000000840.

Hagen, K., Zwart, J.-A., Holmen, J., Svebak, S., Bovim, G., Lars, S., & Stovner, J. (n.d.). Does hypertension protect against chronic musculoskeletal complaints? *JAMA Network.* https://jamanetwork.com/.

Harrop, J. S., Youssef, J. A., Maltenfort, M., Vorwald, P., Jabbour, P., Bono, C. M., Goldfarb, N., Vaccaro, A. R., & Hilibrand, A. S. (n.d.). Lumbar adjacent segment degeneration and disease after arthrodesis and total disc arthroplasty. *SPINE, 33*(15). http://journals.lww.com/spinejournal.

Huntoon, E., & Huntoon, M. (2004). Differential diagnosis of low back pain. *Seminars in Pain Medicine, 2*(3), 138–144. https://doi.org/10.1016/j.spmd.2004.08.003.

Karim Ahmed, A., Howell, E. P., Harward, S., Sankey, E. W., Ehresman, J., Schilling, A., Wang, T., Pennington, Z., Gray, L., Sciubba, D. M., & Goodwin, C. R. (2020). Split cord malformation in adults: Literature review and classification. *Clinical Neurology and Neurosurgery, 193.* Elsevier B.V. https://doi.org/10.1016/j.clineuro.2020.105733.

Kenar, G., Yarkan-Tuğsal, H., Çetin-Özmen, P., Solmaz, D., Can, G., & Önen, F. (2023). A lower frequency of inflammatory back pain in male patients with ankylosing spondylitis compared with female patients. *Rheumatology International.* https://doi.org/10.1007/s00296-023-05449-5.

Kunimoto, K., Yamamoto, Y., & Jinnin, M. (2022). ISSVA classification of vascular anomalies and molecular biology. *International Journal of Molecular Sciences, 23*(4). MDPI. https://doi.org/10.3390/ijms 23042358.

Lyubashina, O. A., Sivachenko, I. B., & Busygina, I. I. (2023). Features of the neurophysiological mechanisms of visceral and somatic pain. *Neuroscience and Behavioral Physiology, 53*(2), 279–287. https://doi.org/10.1007/s11055-023-01418-4.

Macedo, F., Ladeira, K., Pinho, F., Saraiva, N., Bonito, N., Pinto, L., & Gonçalves, F. (2017). Bone metastases: An overview. *Oncology Reviews, 11*(1). https://doi.org/10.4081/oncol.2017.321.

Manusov, E. G. (2012). Evaluation and diagnosis of low back pain. *Primary Care - Clinics in Office Practice, 39*(3), 471–479. https://doi.org/10.1016/j.pop.2012.06.003.

Mehling, W. E., Ebell, M. H., Avins, A. L., & Hecht, F. M. (2015). Clinical decision rule for primary care patients with acute low back pain at risk of developing chronic pain. *Spine Journal, 15*(7), 1577–1586. https://doi.org/10.1016/j.spinee.2015.03.003.

Melloh, M., Elfering, A., Stanton, T. R., Käser, A., Salathé, C. R., Barz, T., Röder, C., & Theis, J. C. (2013). Who is likely to develop persistent low back pain? A longitudinal analysis of prognostic occupational factors. *Work, 46*(3), 297–311. https://doi.org/10.3233/WOR-131672.

Mohamed, A. A., & Ali, M. F. A. (2023). Surgical management of lumbar neurofibroma. *Cairo University, 88*(5). www.medicaljournalofcairouniversity.net.

Musa, P., Polat, B., & Karaoğlan, G. (n.d.). Derleme-Review approach to lumbar pain: Recognition treatment. *Klinik Tıp Dergisi.* www.kliniktipdergisi.com.

Nieminen, L. K., Pyysalo, L. M., & Kankaanpää, M. J. (2021). Prognostic factors for pain chronicity in low back pain: A systematic review. *Pain Reports, 6*(1). Lippincott Williams and Wilkins. https://doi.org/10.1097/PR9.0000000000000919.

Nilsen, T. I. L., Holtermann, A., & Mork, P. J. (2011). Physical exercise, body mass index, and risk of chronic pain in the low back and neck/shoulders: Longitudinal data from the Nord-Trøndelag Health Study. *American Journal of Epidemiology, 174*(3), 267–273. https://doi.org/10.1093/aje/kwr087.

Pacheco-Carroza, E. A. (2021). Visceral pain, mechanisms, and implications in musculoskeletal clinical practice. *Medical Hypotheses, 153.* https://doi.org/10.1016/j.mehy.2021.110624.

Sabnis, A., & Nakhate, M. (2020). A study of prevalence of sacralization of L5 vertebra. *International Journal of Anatomy and Research, 8*(1), 7399–7402. https://doi.org/10.16965/ijar.2020.112.

Shaw, W. S., Means-Christensen, A. J., Slater, M. A., Webster, J. S., Patterson, T. L., Grant, I., Garfin, S. R., Wahlgren, D. R., Patel, S., & Hampton Atkinson, J. (n.d.). Psychiatric disorders and risk of transition to chronicity in men with first-onset low back pain. *Pain Medicine.* https://academic.oup.com/painmedicine/article/11/9/1391/1859495.

Shiri, R., Karppinen, J., Leino-Arjas, P., Solovieva, S., & Viikari-Juntura, E. (2010). The association between smoking and low back pain: A meta-analysis. *American Journal of Medicine, 123*(1). https://doi.org/10.1016/j.amjmed.2009.05.028.

Shokri, P., Zahmatyar, M., Falah Tafti, M., Fathy, M., Rezaei Tolzali, M., Ghaffari Jolfayi, A., Nejadghaderi, S. A., Sullman, M. J. M., Kolahi, A. A., & Safiri, S. (2023). Non-spinal low back pain: Global epidemiology, trends, and risk factors. *Health Science Reports, 6*(9). John Wiley and Sons Inc. https://doi.org/10.1002/hsr2.1533.

Sjøgren, P., Ekholm, O., Peuckmann, V., & Grønbæk, M. (2009). Epidemiology of chronic pain in Denmark: An update. *European Journal of Pain, 13*(3), 287–292. https://doi.org/10.1016/j.ejpain.2008.04.007.

Sutcliffe, P., Connock, M., Shyangdan, D., Court, R., Kandala, N. B., & Clarke, A. (2013). A systematic review of evidence on malignant spinal metastases: Natural history and technologies for identifying patients at high risk of vertebral fracture and spinal cord compression. *Health Technology Assessment, 17*(42). https://doi.org/10.3310/hta17420.

Tsantes, A. G., Papadopoulos, D. V., Vrioni, G., Sioutis, S., Sapkas, G., Benzakour, A., Benzakour, T., Angelini, A., Ruggieri, P., & Mavrogenis, A. F. (2020). Spinal infections: An update. *Microorganisms, 8*(4). MDPI AG. https://doi.org/10.3390/microorganisms8040476.

Urits, I., Burshtein, A., Sharma, M., Testa, L., Gold, P. A., Orhurhu, V., Viswanath, O., Jones, M. R., Sidransky, M. A., Spektor, B., & Kaye, A. D. (2019). Low back pain, a comprehensive review: Pathophysiology, diagnosis, and treatment. *Current Pain and Headache Reports, 23*(3). Current Medicine Group LLC 1. https://doi.org/10.1007/s11916-019-0757-1.

Wewel, J. T., & O'Toole, J. E. (2020). Epidemiology of spinal cord and column tumors. *Neuro-Oncology Practice, 7*, I5–I9. https://doi.org/10.1093/nop/npaa046.

Zamanpoor, M. (2019). The genetic pathogenesis, diagnosis, and therapeutic insight of rheumatoid arthritis. *Clinical Genetics, 95*(5), 547–557. Blackwell Publishing Ltd. https://doi.org/10.1111/cge.13498.

Zanoni, C. T., Galvão, F., Maria, R. M., Zulli, R., Ricciardi, J. B., Cliquet, A., & Saad, S. T. O. (2021). Effectiveness of a home-based therapeutic exercise program on lower back pain and functionality in sickle cell disease (SCD) patients. *Hematology, Transfusion and Cell Therapy, 43*(3), 268–279. https://doi.org/10.1016/j.htct.2020.05.004.

Part 2

Endocrine System Diseases

Chapter 4

A Comprehensive Approach to Obesity Management in Family Medicine

Genco Görgü[1,*]
and Yasemin Özkaya[2]
[1]Bandırma 1St Family Health Center, Balıkesir, Turkey; Ministry of Health, Bandırma, Turkey
[2]Tepecik Training and Research Hospital, İzmir, Turkey

Abstract

The prevalence of obesity is rapidly increasing in societies due to the rapid industrialization of communities and the changing lifestyle habits of individuals, particularly in terms of diet and exercise. As a result, we are hearing the footsteps of a metabolic pandemic. Obesity, due to its association with numerous accompanying chronic diseases and organ damage in a cause-and-effect relationship, increases mortality and morbidity rates and exacerbates the burden of disease on the healthcare system. Family medicine will constitute the main component of the mechanism to combat the increasing threat of obesity. Such a widespread health issue can only be addressed through a patient-centered and community-oriented medical approach.

Keywords: obesity, family medicine, primary care, weight loss

Introduction

Obesity is considered one of the most important preventable causes of death due to its increasing prevalence in society, multifactorial, and complex nature. Diseases caused by obesity constitute the main burden of chronic diseases on populations (Who 1998). Diseases that are confirmed to be related to obesity, such as type 2 diabetes, hypertension (HT), hyperlipidemia (HL), cardiovascular diseases, cerebrovascular disease, obstructive sleep apnea syndrome, various cancers, non-alcoholic fatty liver disease, polycystic ovary syndrome, infertility, gastroesophageal reflux, biliary tract disease, osteoarthritis, and depression, lead to significant increases in healthcare expenditures. According to the World Health Organization's (WHO) statement in 1998, obesity is expected to be the most important health problem of the 21st century. Confirming the estimates of the Non-Communicable Diseases Risk Factor

---

* Corresponding Author's Email: ggorgu@gmail.com.

In: Common Diseases According to Family Medicine Practice Guidelines
Editors: Esra Meltem Koç and Hilal Aksoy
ISBN: 979-8-89530-302-3

Collaboration (NCD-RisC) Group, the prevalence of standardized obesity in the adult population worldwide has tripled in men and doubled in women from 1975 to 2014 (Who 1998, NCD-RisC 2016). According to the WHO, it is stated that there were 1.9 billion overweight and 650 million obese adults worldwide as of 2016 (Who 2021). Reversing this situation requires changes in individual behaviors and the elimination of social barriers to healthy lifestyle choices. This situation brings various responsibilities to the family physician. These responsibilities entail legal, ethical, and medical requirements. The duties of primary healthcare workers in the fight against obesity include the definition and detection of obesity, prevention with a preventive medicine approach, and ensuring its treatment through both lifestyle changes and medical approaches.

In this section, minimum qualifications and clinical approaches that will assist in combating obesity, which is increasingly prevalent in society and therefore frequently encountered in family medicine units, will be discussed. We hope that the relevant text will support our valuable colleagues by providing management for patients diagnosed with obesity in family health centers, where preventive health services are primarily provided, in solving this public health problem.

Definition

Obesity is a condition where excessive body fat can put a person at risk for health issues. Excessive body fat results from an imbalance between energy intake and energy expenditure (total energy expenditure includes energy used at rest, during physical activity, and for metabolism). Body mass index (BMI) is the most useful method used in the diagnosis of obesity. By looking at the BMI value, we can determine with high accuracy whether a person is obese or not. Generally, a BMI of 25-29 kg/m2 is considered overweight, while 30 kg/m2 and above are considered obese (U.S. Preventive Services Task Force 2003, Obezite, Lipid Metabolizması, Hipertansiyon Çalışma Grubu 2019). However, it is important to be aware of the special circumstances that can affect the sensitivity of BMI measurements in the assessment of obesity. For example, in older individuals, height decreases due to osteoporosis, muscle mass decreases, and fat percentage increases. Therefore, the body fat distribution changes, and more fat begins to accumulate around the waist. This raises questions about the validity of BMI cut-off points for diagnosing obesity in the elderly. Rapid changes in body size and composition during growth make the assessment of overweight and obesity in children and adolescents more complex compared to adults. The assessment generally involves comparing a child's BMI level with age- and gender-specific target values (Erlandson et al., 2016).

Obesity begins in individuals with a BMI > 33 kg/m2, which is different from other adults. Another special situation is that the BMI measurements of athletes with high muscle mass can be falsely high. Especially, the BMI values of some individuals who perform bodybuilding sports can be measured as 33-34 kg/m2; however, this does not necessarily mean that these individuals are obese (Romero-Corral 2008). In both athletes and in other individuals, waist circumference measurement is more sensitive to determining abdominal fat and detecting cardiovascular risk. Additionally, waist circumference measurement is not affected by confounding factors such as age, gender, and muscle mass. The cut-off points are determined separately for male and female genders. Knowledge of waist circumference values should be considered especially when diagnosing obesity in individuals with BMI values between 25-35 kg/m2. It is possible to consider everyone with a BMI > 35 kg/m2 as obese (Erlandson et al., 2016, Romero-Corral 2008, Expert Panel on Detection, Evaluation, and Treatment of High Blood Cholesterol in Adults 2001).

Obesity and Comorbid Conditions

Comorbid conditions and diseases are important factors to consider when determining the clinical approach to patients with obesity for primary care physicians, such as family doctors (Bays et al., 2013). After diagnosing obesity, it is essential to address medical conditions that may be related to obesity or may have an independent etiology but may affect the patient's clinical course. To understand the metabolic burden of obesity on the body, it is necessary to focus on metabolic syndrome and prediabetes. According to the NCEP-ATP III criteria, low high-density lipoprotein cholesterol (HDL cholesterol), high triglycerides, high blood pressure, and an increased waist circumference are interpreted to be in favor of metabolic syndrome. At least three of these criteria must be present for a diagnosis (Chalasani et al., 2012).

It has been reported that 80% of Type II Diabetes Mellitus cases are related to obesity (Obezite, Lipid Metabolizması, Hipertansiyon Çalışma Grubu 2019). Patients diagnosed with obesity must be evaluated for diabetes. Although glycemic targets for obese patients are similar to those of non-obese patients, treatment agents that prioritize weight loss are preferred in the selection of treatment approaches specific to obesity. Additionally, identifying overweight or obese individuals with diabetic symptoms or diagnoses creates an opportunity for weight loss through lifestyle changes.

As indicated by the diagnostic criteria for metabolic syndrome, dyslipidemic lipid profiles are also significant findings in obese patients. Lifestyle changes are the most effective tool in the hands of family doctors to combat this condition, which significantly increases cardiovascular risk. In overweight or obese patients with dyslipidemia, a lifestyle change should result in at least 5-10% weight loss. An average reduction of 15 mg/dL in triglyceride levels is observed with every 3 kg of weight loss, a decrease of approximately 5 mg/dL in LDL cholesterol levels with 5-8 kg, and an increase of 2-3 mg/dL in HDL cholesterol levels. When weight loss is less than 3 kg, the improvement in lipid profiles is less and more variable (Bays et al., 2013. Regular exercise also provides a decrease in VLDL cholesterol, an increase in HDL cholesterol, and, in some individuals, a decrease in LDL cholesterol. The recommended exercise should be moderate-intensity aerobic exercise that lasts at least 30 minutes, five days a week, burning at least 200 kcal per day. Resistance exercises to strengthen muscles should be recommended at least two days a week (Bays et al., 2013).

The relationship between obesity and the risk of cardiovascular disease has been studied for a long time. Studies have shown that obesity affects the development of atherosclerosis, symptomatic CAD, CHF, and atrial fibrillation. In one study, a 10 kg weight gain was shown to cause a 12% increase in coronary artery disease risk, a 3 mmHg increase in systolic blood pressure, and a 2.3 mmHg increase in diastolic blood pressure. Therefore, weight loss achieved by combating obesity has the secondary benefit of reducing blood pressure (Obezite, Lipid Metabolizması, Hipertansiyon Çalışma Grubu 2019).

The increasing prevalence of obesity leads us to indirectly compare it with symptoms or deteriorations seen in laboratory results that cause polyclinic referrals. For example, an individual with incidental liver function test abnormalities and anthropometric measurements in favor of obesity will be referred to an upper center for non-alcoholic fatty liver disease testing (Chalasani et al.2012). It would be appropriate to create a medical nutrition and exercise prescription for a patient with polycystic ovary syndrome, which is evaluated in terms of female infertility (Obezite, Lipid Metabolizması, Hipertansiyon Çalışma Grubu 2019). One of the services that family doctors provide in many healthcare systems is expert witness services, such as driver's license examinations. In this regard, obstructive sleep apnea syndrome (OSAS) should be ruled out in obese individuals being evaluated. In addition to the effects of adipokines on the lungs, obesity affects the collapsibility of the airways through either fat deposition in the airways or a decrease in lung volume. In contrast, OSAS leads to a decrease in leptin and an increase in ghrelin levels, resulting in increased hunger and weight gain. Obesity feeds into OSAS, and OSAS feeds into obesity, creating a dangerous cycle (Türk Toraks Derneği Obstrüktif Uyku Apne Sendromu Tanı ve Tedavi Uzlaşı Raporu 2024). If the condition is detected, treatment contributes to the well-being of the patient and the establishment of medico-legal obligations.

The patient-centered, community-oriented, and comprehensive clinical approach of family doctors also includes preventive services for patients and optimization of treatment in cases where clinical response is poor. For example, a significant proportion of individuals diagnosed with gastroesophageal reflux disease and asthma show resistance to treatment, and a significant proportion of these individuals have both of these diseases together and even with obesity (Obezite, Lipid Metabolizması, Hipertansiyon Çalışma Grubu 2019). Interventions targeting excess weight and obesity in these patients, including lifestyle changes and medical treatments, contribute to breaking the triple comorbid axis and achieving better treatment outcomes. The prevalence of disabilities, loss of workforce, and the occurrence of pathologies that can result in death increase in individuals living under the physical and metabolic burden caused by obesity. Osteoarthritis is a common joint disease that causes pain and limited mobility. Its prevalence has increased for two reasons: the aging population and the significant increase in obesity, which is a well-defined risk factor for the development of osteoarthritis in recent years. Excessive body weight leads to increased load on weight-bearing joints such as the knees, hips, and spine, causing wear and degeneration of the cartilage structure of the joints. The treatment of osteoarthritis, both in pharmacological and surgical aspects, imposes a burden on the healthcare system and individuals (Obezite, Lipid Metabolizması, Hipertansiyon Çalışma Grubu 2019).

One of the most notable aspects that makes the contribution of family doctors' fight against obesity to public health important is the relationship between obesity and cancer. In 2002, the International Agency for Research on Cancer stated that there is a relationship between obesity and many types of cancer. The most notable cancers are colon, postmenopausal breast, endometrial, kidney, and esophageal cancers. The mechanism behind the relationship between cancer and obesity is multifactorial. Increased insulin and IGF-1 levels lead to an increase in cancer cells, and adipokines are also thought to play a role in this mechanism. Leptin levels are positively correlated with colon, prostate, and breast cancer, while adiponectin levels are negatively correlated with endometrial, breast, colon, and prostate cancer. Additionally, hypoxia, genetic predisposition, and increased inflammation associated with obesity are also blamed factors in the obesity-cancer relationship (Obezite, Lipid Metabolizması, Hipertansiyon Çalışma Grubu 2019). Obese individuals should be monitored for cancer risk in addition to metabolic diseases and supported in their weight loss efforts.

Assessment

Family doctors should provide services to all individuals at risk of obesity, regardless of age, gender, or symptomatic organ system. Categorically, pregnant women, infants, children, adolescents, adults, and even the elderly are at risk for the consequences of obesity, making primary care the frontline in the fight against obesity. Primary care specialists should carefully address the underlying causes of weight gain by focusing on health behaviors and avoiding simplistic or stigmatizing explanations. Making body mass index (BMI) and waist circumference measurements, which are the most practical assessment criteria for obesity and overweight, a routine part of patient encounters in primary healthcare centers will increase awareness for both patients and healthcare professionals (Wharton et al., 2020).

Anyone with a body mass index (BMI) ≥25 kg/m2 needs weight control. Understanding the reasons and coping with the underlying causes of obesity based on personal life experiences, in collaboration with individuals, is important to develop personalized treatment plans. A detailed medical history should be obtained from obese patients, including personal and family history, medications, dietary behaviors, exercise habits, and emotional state (Wharton et al., 2020). It is recommended to take a comprehensive medical history to identify physical, mental, and psychosocial barriers that may prevent weight gain, in addition to addressing the underlying causes. During physical examination, possible secondary causes of obesity and complications of obesity should also be investigated. Laboratory measurements are not standard for every patient but are decided based on the clinical situation and do not need to be overly detailed (Wharton et al., 2020).

Treatment Options

When deciding on obesity treatment, the patient's expectations and motivation should be carefully assessed. In treatment, personalized treatment plans can be recommended by examining the causes of obesity in the patient and including behavior change (such as nutrition and physical activity) as well as psychological, pharmacological, and surgical interventions (Wharton et al., 2020).

A situation requiring weight control:

- Individuals with a BMI ≥ 25 kg/m2 who do not have additional cardiovascular risk factors (such as prediabetes, diabetes, hypertension, dyslipidemia, etc.) or obesity-related comorbid conditions (such as obstructive sleep apnea, osteoarthritis, etc.) should prevent further weight gain.
- Individuals with a BMI ≥ 25 kg/m2 who have additional cardiovascular disease risk or obesity-related comorbid conditions should have their weight loss needs evaluated and managed.
- Everyone with a BMI ≥ 30 kg/m2 needs weight control (Camhi et al., 2011).

For individuals with an increased Body Mass Index (BMI) (between 25 kg/m2 and 34.9 kg/m2), it is recommended to periodically measure waist circumference to identify increased visceral fat accumulation and adiposity that increases health risks (Obezite, Lipid Metabolizması, Hipertansiyon Çalışma Grubu 2019).

Obesity treatment contributes to reducing complications associated with obesity, maintaining overall health, and positively impacting life expectancy. Additionally, it provides economic benefits by reducing obesity-related healthcare expenses. Therefore, primary care physicians, who have a patient-centered, holistic, and comprehensive clinical approach, play an important role as natural health leaders managing multidisciplinary teams running weight loss programs. The primary goal of primary care physicians is to develop medical nutrition therapy and exercise plans and ensure their regular implementation. They should also assume the responsibility of providing education and counseling services to patients in the management of pharmacological and surgical treatment options for specific patient groups (Obezite, Lipid Metabolizması, Hipertansiyon Çalışma Grubu 2019).

When creating a treatment plan, the success criteria determined by both the primary care physician and the patient should be clearly understood, and realistic goals should be established. A weight loss of 5% to 10% is generally considered a successful outcome. If a weight loss of 10% to 15% is achieved, the patient is evaluated as highly successful. A weight loss >15% is considered an excellent outcome (Obezite, Lipid Metabolizması, Hipertansiyon Çalışma Grubu 2019).

Regular follow-up and control visits are of great importance to ensure that the treatment effectiveness is sustainable. Patients should be monitored by a healthcare professional every two weeks for the first two months after starting treatment, and then monthly for the next three months. Subsequent check-ups should be scheduled at intervals of no more than three months. All discussions with the patient should be recorded, including the amount of weight lost and the lifestyle changes made (Obezite, Lipid Metabolizması, Hipertansiyon Çalışma Grubu 2019).

Medical Nutrition Therapy

Medical nutrition therapy plays a fundamental role in the management of obesity. However, it should not be used alone in the management of obesity, as sustaining weight loss in the long term can be difficult (Obezite, Lipid Metabolizması, Hipertansiyon Çalışma Grubu 2019). Instead, medical nutrition therapy should be tailored to the individual's life in conjunction with other interventions (psychological, pharmacological, surgical) (Raynor, Champagne 2016).

It is valuable to gather information about the patient's habits, social environment, and economic situation in order to reduce barriers in the weight loss process. Especially for working individuals, choosing unhealthy fast food and high-energy ready-to-eat foods, constantly snacking when returning home in the evening and then eating another meal, eating quickly, taking large bites and not chewing the food enough, skipping meals and constantly snacking between meals, being preoccupied with other things during meals (chatting, watching TV, reading books, playing with the phone, etc.), staying at the table for a long time, overeating in times of distress, stress, and anger, frequently attending visits and events and not being able to refuse the offerings, constantly snacking before going to bed after dinner, waking up from sleep at night and eating, drinking little or no water and preferring high-calorie or sugary drinks instead. Therefore, it is valuable to gather information about the patient's habits, social environment, and economic situation to reduce the barriers in the weight loss process (Obezite, Lipid Metabolizması, Hipertansiyon Çalışma Grubu 2019).

The main goals of medical nutrition therapy in obesity are as follows:

- To meet the requirements of all nutrients in a sufficient and balanced manner according to the individual's age, gender, level of physical activity, lifestyle, and physiological condition.
- To reduce body weight to the targeted level (this level can be the individual's ideal weight or a weight above the ideal weight).
- To replace the individual's current unhealthy eating habits with correct and permanent eating habits, and to ensure the lifelong continuation of these correct habits.
- Once the targeted body weight is achieved, prevent weight regain, and maintain this weight consistently at the desired level.
- To maintain normal growth and development in children (Obezite, Lipid Metabolizması, Hipertansiyon Çalışma Grubu 2019).

An individual's daily energy intake should be reduced in a way that leads to a weight loss of 0.5-1.0 kg per week. This level can generally be achieved by reducing the daily energy requirement by approximately 500-1000 calories. An important point to consider here is that the recommended energy intake should not be below the basal metabolic rate and the weight loss should be long-term (Küçükerdönmez, 2014).

Protein: Approximately 12-15% of daily energy should come from protein, preferably focusing on high-quality (animal) protein sources.

Fat: Approximately 25-30% of the daily energy should come from fats. Fatty foods provide a feeling of satiety similar to that of protein-rich foods. Additionally, the proportion of energy from fats should not fall below 20% to support the availability of fat-soluble vitamins (A, D, E, K) in the body.

Carbohydrates: Approximately 55-60% of the daily energy should come from carbohydrates. It is recommended to reduce the consumption of simple carbohydrates such as refined sugar, honey, and jam, and increase the consumption of complex carbohydrates found in whole grains, legumes, etc.

Vitamins and Minerals: Generally, vitamin and mineral deficiencies are rare unless very low-energy diets are followed. However, in very low-energy diets, deficiencies in B vitamins, iron, and calcium can occur. Daily vitamin and mineral supplements may be necessary in diets providing less than 1500 kcal for men and 1200 kcal for women.

Fiber: A daily intake of 25-35 grams of fiber is sufficient for adults. It is recommended to consume natural sources of fiber such as vegetables, fruits, legumes, and whole grain products (such as unpeeled bulgur).

Alcohol: Alcohol consumption is not recommended in weight loss diets. If alcohol is consumed, the daily energy intake should be adjusted accordingly.

Fluids: It is important to consume at least 2 liters of fluids per day. It is recommended that 1-1.5 liters of this fluid be water. Avoid beverages with added sugar and carbonated drinks.

Salt: Salt intake should be reduced, especially in individuals with heart failure or other medical conditions such as edema and hypertension. Daily salt intake should not exceed 5-6 grams (1 teaspoon) (Obezite, Lipid Metabolizması, Hipertansiyon Çalışma Grubu 2019).

Various types of diets (low-calorie, low-fat/low-calorie, moderate-fat/low-calorie, or low-carbohydrate diets, as well as the Mediterranean diet) generally lead to weight loss. Regardless of the type of diet, adherence to the diet is considered a significant factor in weight loss (Dansinger et al., 2005). Therefore, it is recommended to adopt a diet that reduces energy intake below energy expenditure based on personal preferences, rather than focusing too much on the macronutrient composition of the diet. Diet counseling should be added, especially during the first year, to facilitate weight loss (Perreault, Apovian 2023).

Regardless of which diet or nutrition model is chosen, continuous monitoring and follow-up by both the physician and the patient are necessary for the success of the treatment. Clinicians should plan regular follow-up visits with a dietitian to assess barriers, discuss next steps, and provide encouragement. If weight loss is less than 5% in the first six months, alternative approaches should be considered (Perreault, Apovian 2023).

Exercise Therapy

The success of medical nutrition therapy cannot be achieved without following energy expenditure management following calorie restriction. Physical activity is a general term that describes all body movements that result in energy expenditure. While it is less effective in promoting weight loss compared to dietary restriction, increasing energy expenditure through physical activity is a strong indicator of maintaining weight loss. Exercise, on the other hand, is a planned and structured specific type of physical activity designed to improve an individual's fitness (Obezite, Lipid Metabolizması, Hipertansiyon Çalışma Grubu 2019).

Both weight loss and cardiovascular health require individuals to engage in structured exercises, and the knowledge and awareness of primary care physicians is important. Therefore, it would be beneficial to emphasize the following terms:

- Maximum heart rate is calculated by subtracting the age from 220.
- Exercises that target 40-50% of the maximum heart rate are classified as low-intensity exercises.
- Exercises that target 50-70% of the maximum heart rate are classified as moderate-intensity exercises.
- Exercises that target 70-90% of the maximum heart rate are classified as high-intensity exercises (Piercy et al., 2018).

Physical activity programs are cost-effective. When combined with a diet, physical activity has a synergistic effect on lipid levels and other cardiometabolic risk factors such as diabetes and hypertension. Additionally, physical activity can help mitigate the loss of lean mass (e.g., muscle) during active weight loss. Weight loss, particularly in overweight and obese individuals, leads to a more significant decrease in total cholesterol, LDL cholesterol, and triglyceride levels, while increasing HDL cholesterol levels (Reiner et al., 2011).

Even without a hypocaloric diet, moderate or high-intensity aerobic physical activity leads to the loss of visceral fat in overweight or obese individuals. Regardless of weight loss, physical activity has a positive impact on cardiovascular risk factors. The effect of moderate and high-intensity aerobic physical activity on visceral adipose tissue is greater than that of low-intensity physical activity or resistance exercises (Obezite, Lipid Metabolizması, Hipertansiyon Çalışma Grubu 2019).

When providing physical activity recommendations, factors such as age, gender, fitness level, preferences, lifestyle, and individual needs should be taken into account. The type, duration, frequency, and intensity of exercise should be determined on an individual basis.

- The choice of sport should be left to the patient's preference.
- As a general health recommendation, we suggest that all individuals, regardless of obesity, engage in 150 minutes of moderate-intensity aerobic physical activity per week, or 75 minutes of high-intensity aerobic physical activity per week, or an equivalent combination.
- We recommend performing resistance exercises two to three times a week as the main anaerobic strength training. Resistance exercises should target the major muscle groups such as shoulders, arms, back, abdomen, hips, and legs. Resistance exercises should be performed for at least one set of 8-15 repetitions.
- Resistance exercises are particularly recommended for overweight and obese patients starting weight loss treatment.
- The total duration of the exercise should be divided into three to five days within a week. Healthy individuals and athletes can exceed these values.
- Individuals who have achieved their weight loss goals and are in the weight maintenance phase are recommended to engage in at least 200 minutes of moderate-intensity exercise per week, or an equivalent (Piercy et al., 2018).

Psychological Interventions

Obesity is not only a physical problem but also a condition that can lead to psychosocial issues. Additionally, mental health problems can contribute to weight gain which leads to obesity. Eating disorders that may be present in obese individuals and should be questioned include binge eating disorder and night eating syndrome. Binge eating disorder is defined as eating a larger amount of food than most people would eat in a certain time period and feeling a lack of control overeating and the inability to stop. Night eating syndrome is associated with a disruption of the circadian eating pattern, where a person wakes up to eat (Obezite, Lipid Metabolizması, Hipertansiyon Çalışma Grubu 2019).

Cognitive Behavioral Therapy (CBT) is an effective method used in psychiatric approaches and can be applied at every stage of the treatment process. It can be implemented not only by psychiatrists but also by other healthcare professionals, primarily including family physicians. CBT is based on classical and operant conditioning principles. Before starting CBT, the patients are evaluated. The evaluation includes previous weight loss attempts, accompanying psychiatric and medical problems, motivation level, and a detailed understanding of eating habits. The most suitable patients for therapy are adults with a BMI between 30 and 50 kg/m2, who are willing to lose weight and do not have any additional psychiatric illnesses that would disrupt their adherence to therapy (Hilbert et al., 2012).

Behavior change or behavior therapy is one of the cornerstones of obesity treatment. The goal of behavioral therapy is to help patients make long-term changes in their eating behaviors by modifying and monitoring their food intake, changing their physical activities, and controlling the environmental cues and triggers that stimulate eating. The aim of behavior therapy is to create changes in the patient's eating and exercise behavior, and for this, the patient is asked to acquire certain skills.

Self-monitoring: This skill is among the basic principles of treatment. It involves keeping a daily record of food intake and exercise.

Goal setting: Patients are asked to set realistic goals at the beginning of therapy. Unrealistic goals can undermine motivation and adherence to therapy. The therapist serves as a guide in this regard.

Impulse control: The removal of stimuli that trigger unwanted behaviors, such as overeating, increasing positive stimuli, and encouraging the patient in this direction are targeted. The patient is informed about making some environmental arrangements, such as limiting the places where they eat, not making junk food at home, or keeping it easily accessible.

Behavioral substitution: Developing an alternative behavior to stimuli other than eating is necessary.

Positive reinforcement: The patient is encouraged to reward themselves with certain rewards as they achieve their goals. However, these rewards should not be related to eating (Obezite, Lipid Metabolizması, Hipertansiyon Çalışma Grubu 2019).

Pharmacological Treatment

The main duty of the family physician within the framework of primary healthcare is to screen the target population for obesity and implement a structured lifestyle intervention for identified cases. However, in cases where satisfactory results are not achieved and the medical condition contributed to this, a pharmacological approach may be considered. Medications that can achieve a weight loss of 5% within 3-6 months have been accepted as effective in treatment and approved for the management of chronic obesity. The expectations of an ideal obesity medication are as follows:

- Providing weight loss associated with dosage.
- Ensuring the continuity of the achieved target weight
- Being reliable for long-term use, without causing side effects, especially cardiac ones
- Not developing tolerance
- Not leading to misuse or addiction (Yumuk et al., 2015).

Pharmacological treatment indications for obesity:

1. Cases with BMI ≥30 kg/m2 that have failed to achieve weight control despite attempting diet, exercise, and behavioral modifications.

2. Patients with BMI levels between 27-29.9 kg/m2 who have comorbidities (such as Type 2 diabetes, coronary artery disease, cerebrovascular disease, hypertension, dyslipidemia, sleep apnea, etc.).

The efficacy of pharmacotherapy should be evaluated after the first three months. If the achieved weight loss is satisfactory (≥5% weight loss in non-diabetic individuals and ≥3% weight loss in diabetic patients), the treatment should be continued. Treatment should be discontinued in individuals who do not respond adequately to the treatment. A weight loss of 5-15% after six months is a realistic and appropriate target that can improve many comorbid conditions. Everyone involved, including patients, should be aware that obesity is a chronic disease, and weight management needs to be lifelong. Although there is no consensus, it is recommended to continue pharmacotherapy for at least 1 year and to continue treatment if there is a yearly weight loss of 10% in individual patients. A 15% weight loss over a two-year period is also considered an effective treatment. If weight loss can be maintained through lifestyle changes after two years, pharmacotherapy can be discontinued or treatment can be discontinued (Obezite, Lipid Metabolizması, Hipertansiyon Çalışma Grubu 2019).

Orlistat helps with weight loss when combined with diet and exercise. During its use:

The absorption of fat-soluble vitamins (A, D, E, and K) will be affected, so monitoring is necessary.

Multivitamin supplementation is recommended.

Patients should be warned about gastrointestinal side effects.

The impact on the absorption of co-administered drugs should be considered (Obezite, Lipid Metabolizması, Hipertansiyon Çalışma Grubu 2019).

During the use of another pharmacological agent, *Liraglutide:*

- Treatment is initiated with a daily dose of 0.6 mg and the dose is titrated weekly up to 3 mg/day based on side effects.
- It is generally well tolerated, with nausea and vomiting being the most common but usually transient side effects.
- It should not be used in individuals with a history of acute pancreatitis or medullary thyroid cancer, either individually or in their family (Obezite, Lipid Metabolizması, Hipertansiyon Çalışma Grubu 2019).

Surgical Treatment

The main treatment for obesity is lifestyle changes and diet, and pharmacotherapy is used in patients who cannot achieve the desired weight loss. Studies have shown that the average weight loss achieved with lifestyle changes, diet, and pharmacotherapy is about 10-15%. This rate contributes to the improvement of many obesity-related comorbid diseases. When a higher rate of weight loss is desired or when permanent weight loss cannot be achieved, bariatric surgery (BS) methods may be considered (Apovian et al., 2015, Sabuncu et al., 2017). The indications for bariatric surgery include:

- BMI should be ≥ 40 kg/m2 (without the condition of obesity being associated with any comorbidity; it should not increase the risk of surgical treatment)
- BMI should be ≥ 35 kg/m2 and should be accompanied by at least one comorbidity such as obesity-related type 2 DM, hypertension, dyslipidemia, sleep apnea syndrome, etc. (Sabuncu et al., 2017).

Although there are not sufficient randomized controlled studies, some studies have shown that bariatric surgery may be beneficial for patients with type 2 DM and BMI between 30-35 kg/m2 in terms of glycemic control. However, routine surgical treatment is not recommended for this group due to insufficient evidence (Obezite, Lipid Metabolizması, Hipertansiyon Çalışma Grubu 2019). However, bariatric surgery can be considered in selected cases where adequate glycemic control cannot be achieved despite effective and intensive antidiabetic treatment. Pregnancy, severe gastrointestinal diseases, active cancer, compensated heart and lung disease, advanced liver disease accompanied by portal hypertension, untreated sleep apnea syndrome accompanied by pulmonary hypertension, and severe hematological or autoimmune diseases are contraindications to bariatric surgery.

Conclusion

Obesity is a complex and multifactorial disease. It contributes to the development of many health problems such as type 2 diabetes, cardiovascular disease, hypertension, high cholesterol, cerebrovascular disease, various cancers, obstructive sleep apnea syndrome, fatty liver disease, gastroesophageal reflux, polycystic ovary syndrome, osteoarthritis, and depression, and places a significant burden on society's healthcare budgets. Obesity is increasing not only in adulthood but also in childhood and adolescence. Since it is known that obesity during childhood and adoloescence precedes obesity in adulthood, the goal of preventive medicine is to prevent weight gain during these periods. Decreased physical activity and changes in dietary intake in the elderly lead to "sarcopenic obesity." To prevent obesity, it is crucial to develop new intervention programs that include all segments of society, are easy to implement and cost-effective, and put them urgently into practice.

References

Apovian, C. M., Aronne, L. J., Bessesen, D. H., McDonnell, M. E., Murad, M. H., Pagotto, U., Ryan, D. H., Still, C. D., & Endocrine Society. (2015). Pharmacological management of obesity: An endocrine Society clinical practice guideline. *The Journal of Clinical Endocrinology and Metabolism, 100*(2), 342–362. https://doi.org/10.1210/jc.2014-3415.

Bays, H. E., Toth, P. P., Kris-Etherton, P. M., Abate, N., Aronne, L. J., Brown, W. V., Gonzalez-Campoy, J. M., Jones, S. R., Kumar, R., La Forge, R., & Samuel, V. T. (2013). Obesity, adiposity, and dyslipidemia: A consensus statement from the National Lipid Association. *Journal of Clinical Lipidology, 7*(4), 304–383. https://doi.org/10.1016/j.jacl.2013.04.001.

Camhi, S. M., Bray, G. A., Bouchard, C., Greenway, F. L., Johnson, W. D., Newton, R. L., Ravussin, E., Ryan, D. H., Smith, S. R., & Katzmarzyk, P. T. (2011). The relationship of waist circumference and BMI to visceral, subcutaneous, and total body fat: Sex and race differences. *Obesity (Silver Spring, Md.), 19*(2), 402–408. https://doi.org/10.1038/oby.2010.248.

Chalasani, N., Younossi, Z., Lavine, J. E., Diehl, A. M., Brunt, E. M., Cusi, K., Charlton, M., & Sanyal, A. J. (2012). The diagnosis and management of non-alcoholic fatty liver disease: Practice guideline by the American Association for the Study of Liver Diseases, American College of Gastroenterology, and the American Gastroenterological Association. *Hepatology (Baltimore, Md.), 55*(6), 2005–2023.

Dansinger, M. L., Gleason, J. A., Griffith, J. L., Selker, H. P., & Schaefer, E. J. (2005). Comparison of the Atkins, Ornish, Weight Watchers, and Zone diets for weight loss and heart disease risk reduction: A randomized trial. *JAMA, 293*(1), 43–53. https://doi.org/10.1001/jama.293.1.43.

Erlandson, M., Ivey, L. C., & Seikel, K. (2016). Update on office-based strategies for the management of obesity. *American Family Physician, 94*(5), 361–368.

Expert Panel on Detection, Evaluation, and Treatment of High Blood Cholesterol in Adults. (2001). Executive summary of the third report of the National Cholesterol Education Program (NCEP) expert panel on detection, evaluation, and treatment of high blood cholesterol in adults (Adult Treatment Panel III). *JAMA, 285*(19), 2486–2497. https://doi.org/10.1001/jama.285.19.2486.

Hilbert, A., Bishop, M. E., Stein, R. I., Tanofsky-Kraff, M., Swenson, A. K., Welch, R. R., & Wilfley, D. E. (2012). Long-term efficacy of psychological treatments for binge eating disorder. *The British Journal of Psychiatry: The Journal of Mental Science, 200*(3), 232–237. https://doi.org/10.1192/bjp.bp.110.089664.

Küçükerdönmez, Ö. (2014). *Obezite tedavisi [Obesity Treatment]* (Bölüm 5). *Obezite Tanı ve Tedavi Kılavuzu, Obezite, Dislipidemi, Hipertansiyon Çalışma Grubu*, Türkiye Endokrinoloji ve Metabolizma Derneği Yayını (1. Baskı, ss. 33-42). Ankara.

NCD Risk Factor Collaboration (NCD-RisC). (2016). Trends in adult body-mass index in 200 countries from 1975 to 2014: A pooled analysis of 1698 population-based measurement studies with 19.2 million participants. *The Lancet, 387*(10026), 1377–1396. https://doi.org/10.1016/s0140-6736(16)30054-x.

Obezite, Lipid Metabolizması, Hipertansiyon Çalışma Grubu. (2019). *Obezite tanı ve tedavi kılavuzu [Obesity Diagnosis and Treatment Guide].* https://file.temd.org.tr/Uploads/publications/guides/documents/20190506163904-2019tbl_kilavuz5ccdcb9e5d.pdf?a=1.

Perreault, L., & Apovian, C. (Accessed on October 15, 2023). *Obesity in adults: Overview of management.* In UpToDate, Pi-Sunyer FX, Seres D (Ed), Kunins L.

Piercy, K. L., Troiano, R. P., Ballard, R. M., Carlson, S. A., Fulton, J. E., Galuska, D. A., George, S. M., & Olson, R. D. (2018). The Physical Activity Guidelines for Americans. *JAMA, 320*(19), 2020. https://doi.org/10.1001/jama.2018.14854.

Raynor, H. A., & Champagne, C. M. (2016). Position of the Academy of Nutrition and Dietetics: Interventions for the treatment of overweight and obesity in adults. *Journal of the Academy of Nutrition and Dietetics, 116*(1), 129–147. https://doi.org/10.1016/j.jand.2015.10.031.

Reiner, Z., Catapano, A. L., G. De Backer, Graham, I., Taskinen, M.-R., Wiklund, O., Agewall, S., & Alegria, E. (2011). ESC/EAS guidelines for the management of dyslipidaemias: The Task Force for the management of dyslipidaemias of the European Society of Cardiology (ESC) and the European Atherosclerosis Society (EAS). *European Heart Journal, 32*(14), 1769–1818. https://doi.org/10.1093/eurheartj/ehr158.

Romero-Corral, A., Somers, V. K., Sierra-Johnson, J., Thomas, R. J., Collazo-Clavell, M. L., Korinek, J., Allison, T. G., Batsis, J. A., Sert-Kuniyoshi, F. H., & Lopez-Jimenez, F. (2008). Accuracy of body mass index in diagnosing obesity in the adult general population. *International Journal of Obesity (2005), 32*(6), 959–966.

Sabuncu, T., Kiyici, S., Eren, M., Sancak, S., Sönmez, A., Güldiken, S., Kutlutürk, F., Şahin, İ., Yilmaz, M., & Bayram, F. (2017). Summary of Bariatric Surgery Guideline of the Society of Endocrinology and Metabolism of Turkey. *Turkish Journal of Endocrinology and Metabolism, 21*(4), 140–147. https://doi.org/10.25179/tjem.2017-57388.

Türk Toraks Derneği Obstrüktif Uyku Apne Sendromu Tanı ve Tedavi Uzlaşı Raporu. (n.d.). *Official Journal of the Turkish Thoracic Society, Türk Toraks Derneği, Turkish Thoracic Society.* Retrieved March 24, 2024, from https://toraks.org.tr/site/sf/books/pre_migration/ad73ffecbc06107c01f3ffcfbf6b2ec10b56576e63fb970f57019fb497701d32.pdf.

U.S. Preventive Services Task Force. (2003). Screening for obesity in adults: Recommendations and rationale. *Annals of Internal Medicine, 139*(11), 930–932. https://doi.org/10.7326/0003-4819-139-11-200312020-00012.

Wharton, S., Lau, D. C. W., Vallis, M., Sharma, A. M., Biertho, L., Campbell-Scherer, D., Adamo, K., Alberga, A., Bell, R., Boulé, N., Boyling, E., Brown, J., Calam, B., Clarke, C., Crowshoe, L., Divalentino, D., Forhan, M., Freedhoff, Y., Gagner, M., Glazer, S., … Wicklum, S. (2020). Obesity in adults: A clinical practice guideline. *CMAJ: Canadian Medical Association Journal, 192*(31), E875–E891. https://doi.org/10.1503/cmaj.191707.

World Health Organization, Pan American Health Organization, & World Health Organization. (1998). *Obesity: Preventing and managing the global epidemic: Report of a WHO consultation on obesity.* https://iris.paho.org/handle/10665.2/43000.

World Health Organization. (2021, June 9). Obesity and overweight. *WHO.* http://www.who.int/mediacentre/factsheets/fs311/en/.

Yumuk, V., Tsigos, C., Fried, M., Schindler, K., Busetto, L., Micic, D., Toplak, H., & Obesity Management Task Force of the European Association for the Study of Obesity. (2015). European guidelines for obesity management in adults. *Obesity Facts, 8*(6), 402–424. https://doi.org/10.1159/000442721.

Chapter 5

Diabetes Mellitus

Filiz Mercantepe*, MD

Department of Endocrinology and Metabolism, Faculty of Medicine, Recep Tayyip Erdogan University, Rize, Turkey

Abstract

Diabetes mellitus (DM) is a chronic metabolic disorder that encompasses a wide range of symptoms and affects various metabolic processes. It is characterized by elevated blood glucose levels, resulting from either a lack of insulin or reduced insulin sensitivity in peripheral tissues, commonly termed "insulin resistance." This condition has widespread implications, affects multiple organs, and leads to systemic complications. Diabetes mellitus, an ancient ailment, holds the distinction of being the most widespread endocrine disorder. Establishing the classification of the illness is based on an understanding of its pathophysiology and serves as a crucial framework for informing appropriate treatment strategies. Failure to administer the proper treatment or adhere to the prescribed dietary regimen could result in the development of macrovascular and microvascular problems.
The effective management of diabetes mellitus requires the implementation of a comprehensive and interdisciplinary strategy. The ongoing education of patients, the community and healthcare professionals plays a vital role in the prevention of acute disease complications and the mitigation of long-term complication risks. The objective of this chapter is to present a thorough examination of diabetes, encompassing its pathophysiology, classification, clinical symptoms, diagnostic criteria, and management techniques for DM.

Keywords: diabetes mellitus, insulin deficiency, complications

Introduction

Diabetes Mellitus (DM) poses a substantial worldwide health challenge, resulting in reduced quality of life, elevated rates of mortality and morbidity, increased healthcare expenses, and mostly attributed to a rapid escalation in its prevalence. According to Saeedi et al., (2019), the estimated prevalence of DM currently is 463 million individuals, with a projected increase to 700 million by 2045. According to a study conducted by Cho et al., (2018), the global expenditure on DM healthcare is projected to reach $850 billion. The prevalence of this

* Corresponding Author's Email: filizmercantepe@hotmail.com.

In: Common Diseases According to Family Medicine Practice Guidelines
Editors: Esra Meltem Koç and Hilal Aksoy
ISBN: 979-8-89530-302-3

phenomenon has demonstrated a positive correlation with the rise in obesity rates, which can be attributed to the sedentary nature of modern urban living and the greater availability of unhealthy and obesogenic dietary options.

Etiology and Pathophysiology

Diabetes mellitus is a complex disease that is influenced by a combination of genetic predisposition, environmental variables, and lifestyle decisions. The main cause of type 1 diabetes is the autoimmune death of pancreatic beta cells, resulting in a complete lack of insulin. Individuals who possess genetic susceptibility may experience the activation of their immune system, leading to the destruction of pancreatic beta cells responsible for insulin production, upon exposure to specific environmental variables such as viruses or certain dietary components. In contrast, type 2 diabetes is characterized by the simultaneous presence of insulin resistance and impaired insulin production, both of which contribute to the development of the condition. Therefore, the release of insulin fails to adequately fulfill the increased demand caused by insulin resistance. Type 2 DM is a multifactorial disorder (Stumvoll et al., 2015) characterized by intricate interplays between genetic and environmental factors, potentially including a multitude of genetic components in its pathogenesis. The study conducted by Vujkovic et al., (2020) used large-scale genome research to identify more than 500 distinct genetic markers related to type 2 DM. This comprehensive multi-ancestry meta-analysis involved a substantial cohort of 1.4 million human participants. According to DeFronzo et al., (1991), obesity is associated with peripheral resistance to insulin-mediated glucose uptake and may also result in a decrease in the responsiveness of beta cells to glucose. Gestational diabetes manifests during pregnancy as a result of hormonal fluctuations and increased insulin resistance. The described hormonal changes are a result of the presence of diabetogenic hormones produced by the placenta, including growth hormone, corticotropin-releasing hormone, placental lactogen (also known as chorionic somatomammotropin), prolactin, and progesterone.

The Categorization of Diabetes Mellitus

Duchenne muscular dystrophy (DMD) can be classified into the four prevailing clinical classifications. The categories included in the field of diabetes include type 1 diabetes, and type 2 diabetes, as well as particular forms such as monogenic diabetes syndromes, exocrine pancreas disorders, drug-induced diabetes, and gestational diabetes mellitus (IDF Diabetes Atlas, 2017). Nevertheless, for certain individuals, the classification may not be definitively ascertained. Identifying the type of patient plays a crucial role in selecting the most suitable treatment strategy. Type 1 and type 2 DM are distinguished by their heterogeneity, which is evident in their distinct clinical manifestations and variations in the course of the disease. The classification at hand comprises all forms of diabetes characterized by the autoimmune destruction of β cells, which is referred to as type 1 DM. In 2019, the World Health Organization (WHO) released an alternative classification, as depicted in Table 1. Certain individuals cannot be easily classified as having either type 1 or type 2 diabetes at the time of initial diagnosis. The traditional insulin that type 2 DM mostly affects adults and type 1 DM predominantly affects children is no longer valid, as both conditions can now be observed in insulin demographics. The fundamental etiology of type 1 DM is the autoimmune death of beta cells, leading to a pronounced insulin insufficiency. This process encompasses latent autoimmune diabetes in adults as well. Type 2 DM arises as a result of a gradual decrease in insulin secretion from β-cells, which is not caused by an autoimmune response. This decrease in insulin secretion is accompanied by a partial deficit in insulin, often occurring along with insulin resistance and metabolic syndrome.

Diagnosis of Diabetes Mellitus

The diagnosis of diabetes can be made when a patient exhibits typical symptoms of diabetes together with a noticeably increased amount of glucose in the bloodstream. However, it is important to note that a significant number of people with diabetes may not exhibit any symptoms for prolonged periods, which highlights the need for blood tests to confirm the diagnosis. Both the WHO and the American Diabetes Association (ADA) follow the same diagnostic criteria for diabetes. These criteria are based on specific thresholds for fasting plasma glucose (FPG) levels, 2-hour post-load plasma glucose (PG) values obtained during an oral glucose tolerance test (2hPG), and glycated haemoglobin (HbA1c) levels. According to the ADA (2015), a diagnosis of diabetes is made when FPG levels are equal to or greater than 7.0 mmol/L (126 mg/dl), 2hPG values are equal to or greater than 11.1 mmol/L (200 mg/dl), or HbA1c levels are equal to or greater than 6.5% (48 mmol/mol). To validate the diagnosis, it is advisable to perform an iterative test on patients who do not exhibit symptoms.

Table 1. Classification of Diabetes Mellitus

Type 1 Diabetes Mellitus
Type 2 Diabetes Mellitus
Hybrid forms of Diabetes Mellitus
Other specific types Monogenic diabetes, exocrine pancreas diseases, drugs or chemical induced infections, immune diabetes,
Non-classified Diabetes Mellitus
Hyperglycemia First Detected During Pregnancy Diabetes During Pregnancy Gestational Diabetes

Table 2. Diagnostic Criteria for Diabetes Mellitus

FPG ≥126 mg/dL (7.0 mmol/L). Fasting is defined as no caloric intake for at least eight hours.
or
2-h PG ≥200 mg/dL (11.1mmol/L) during OGTT.
or
A1C ≥ 6.5% (48 mmol/mol)*
or
A patient presenting with a hyperglycaemic crisis or exhibiting typical symptoms of hyperglycaemia with a random PG≥200 mg/dL (11.1 mmol/L)

*with an NGSP-certified and standardized DCCT assay.

When there are suspicions or indications of diabetes, medical professionals employ various diagnostic procedures such as FPG, random (PG, 2nd hour PG levels during the 75 g oral glucose tolerance test (OGTT) and A1C testing. These tests aid in the diagnosis of DM. The next table, labelled Table 2, presents the relevant data.

The use of HbA1c as a diagnostic tool for diabetes has not been suggested for an extended period due to issues related to standardization and the ambiguity surrounding the diagnostic threshold. In recent years, due to global standardization efforts and mounting data on its predictive significance, the A1C test has gained acceptance as a diagnostic tool for diabetes. The A1C measurement methods used by laboratories in the United States have been certified by the National Glycohemoglobin Standardization Program (NGSP). These measurements are derived from the utilization of high-performance liquid chromatography (HPLC), which was used in the Diabetes Control and Complications Trial (DCCT) study and is widely acknowledged as the gold standard. Calibration according to the chromatographic method is necessary. The diagnostic threshold for diabetes mellitus was established at an A1C level of 6.5% (48 mmol/mol). Instances of discordance between A1C and PG outcomes could arise in certain circumstances, including the presence of haemoglobin variations (hemoglobinopathies), pregnancy, the postpartum period, haemodialysis, blood loss, or a history of transfusion. In instances such as these, it is advisable to employ a non-interfering A1C measuring technique to diagnose diabetes, or to take into account the diagnostic criteria of FPG. To establish a confirmed diagnosis in the absence of a conclusive clinical assessment, it is required to have two abnormal screening test results. These results can be obtained from either a single sample or two separate sample tests (Selvin et al., 2018). To examine gestational diabetes mellitus (GDM), screening and diagnostic assessments are typically conducted throughout the gestational period, between 24 and 28 weeks of pregnancy. Historically, a diagnostic methodology involving two stages has been widely used, utilizing glucose quantities of 50 grams and 100 grams, respectively. Alternatively, a diagnostic procedure known as the 'one-stage' method can be used, involving the administration of 75 grams of glucose.

Clinical Manifestations

The clinical manifestations observed in individuals are the result of elevated blood glucose levels and are also associated with the impact of hyperglycaemia on fluid and electrolyte equilibrium. In conjunction with conventional manifestations, such as polyuria, polydipsia, polyphagia or anorexia, weakness, fatigue, dry mouth, and nocturia, there are less prevalent symptoms, including impaired vision, unexplained weight loss, recurring fungal infections, and pruritus. Type 1 DM typically manifests before the age of 30. Three distinct peaks in development can be observed throughout the preschool years (often around the age of 6), the period of puberty (typically around the age of 13), and late adolescence (typically around the age of 20). Individuals diagnosed with type 1 diabetes may exhibit comorbid autoimmune conditions, such as Hashimoto's thyroiditis, Graves' disease, gluten enteropathy (Celiac disease), Addison's disease, vitiligo, and pernicious anaemia. Individuals diagnosed with type 1 diabetes are more susceptible to the development of diabetic ketoacidosis. Type 2 DM manifests predominantly in individuals over the age of 30 years. Nevertheless, the prevalence of type 2 diabetes in children and adolescents has seen a notable increase in recent years, primarily attributed to the increasing rates of obesity. This concerning trend has been particularly prominent over the past decade to fifteen years. Type 1 DM presents with an abrupt onset of symptoms and indications, but type 2 DM generally exhibits a more gradual and inconspicuous start.

Management

The management of diabetes mellitus requires the incorporation of lifestyle modifications and psychosocial support as essential components. The use of insulin therapy is recommended for people diagnosed with type 1 DM, GDM refractory to dietary management, and type 2 diabetic patients who have a reduced capacity for endogenous insulin production.

Insulin, a peptide hormone, plays a crucial role in the regulation of glucose metabolism in the human body. The injection of insulin into people who have either absolute or relative insulin deficiency serves not only to rectify hyperglycaemia but also to prevent or treat metabolic diseases and catabolic effects caused by insulin deficiency, such as hypertriglyceridemia and ketoacidosis. The primary mechanisms underlying the therapeutic effects of insulin involve the facilitation of glucose uptake into cells, augmentation of glycogen storage, suppression of hepatic glucose production, improvement of insulin sensitivity in peripheral and hepatic tissues, and inhibition of lipolysis and proteolysis. Type 1 DM is distinguished by a significant deficiency or complete absence of β-cell activity. Consequently, the administration of insulin is essential for those diagnosed with type 1 DM. Insulin replacement protocols commonly include the administration of basal insulin, short-acting insulin, and corrective insulin, as described by Holt et al., (2021). The available choices for basal insulin include NPH insulin, long-acting insulin analogues, and continuous administration of rapid-acting insulin via an insulin pump.

In individuals diagnosed with type 2 DM, it is imperative to promptly initiate insulin therapy in specific circumstances, including the presence of comorbidities that increase the need for insulin, severe insulin resistance, instances of acute metabolic decompensation such as diabetic ketoacidosis (DKA) or hyperosmolar hyperglycaemic state (HHS), surgical procedures, pregnancy, or the advancement of diabetes-related problems.

Hypoglycaemia is the prevailing adverse outcome associated with insulin therapy. Additional adverse effects include weight gain, lipohypertrophy, lipoatrophy, haemorrhaging, leakage, pain perception, significant hepatomegaly, and immunogenicity.

Glucose-Lowering Agents Other than Insulin

The selection of pharmacological therapy for type 2 DM should be approached on an individual basis, considering various factors. These factors include the severity of hyperglycaemia, duration of diabetes, specific attributes of the medications (such as their effectiveness, potency, adverse effects, cardiovascular safety, contraindications, risk of hypoglycaemia, and cost), the presence of diabetic complications, coexisting medical conditions, the patient's anticipated lifespan, and personal preferences. According to the consensus report titled "Managing Hyperglycaemia in Type 2 Diabetes" by Davies et al., (2022), a comprehensive and diverse strategy is recommended for the management of type 2 diabetes. This approach emphasizes the individual's needs and acknowledges the chronic character of the condition. Various individual factors play a significant role in shaping treatment decisions. These factors include personalized goals for glycaemic control and weight management, the impact on body weight, the prevention of hypoglycaemia and cardio-renal complications, underlying physiological considerations, the side effect profiles of medications, the complexity of the treatment regimen, the selection of the most appropriate regimen to optimize medication effectiveness and minimize treatment interruptions, as well as the consideration of factors such as medication accessibility, cost, and availability.

Given the current findings of many studies, it is imperative to acknowledge and address certain factors that must be considered in the management of type 2 DM. Metformin is considered the recommended first-line pharmacological intervention for the management of type 2 DM. It is considered suitable for administration in individuals with stable heart failure and an estimated glomerular filtration rate (eGFR) over 30 ml/min/1.73 m2. Nevertheless, metformin is contraindicated in instances of treatment-resistant severe congestive heart failure.

The use of pioglitazone is contraindicated in individuals with congestive heart failure or those suffering from significant coronary insufficiency. It is important for patients undergoing intense insulin therapy to be cognizant of the increased probability of oedema formation and exercise caution when administering the medicine. Dipeptidyl peptidase-4 (DPP-4) inhibitors are commonly considered pharmacological agents with a favourable cardiovascular safety profile. Nevertheless, they do not exhibit superior cardiovascular protective effects compared to conventional therapy modalities.

In individuals diagnosed with Type 2 diabetes who have a prior history of cardiovascular disease or are at increased risk for cardiovascular disease, and in cases where metformin monotherapy fails to achieve satisfactory glycaemic control, the addition of glucagon-like peptide-1 (GLP-1) receptor agonists or sodium-glucose cotransporter-2 (SGLT2) inhibitors is recommended. These medications have demonstrated cardiovascular safety and are therefore preferable treatment options.

The inclusion of a SGLT2 inhibitor in the therapeutic regimen for individuals with type 2 DM who are at increased risk of heart failure has been shown to potentially decrease the probability of hospitalization resulting from heart failure (Wiviott et al., 2019; Packer et al., 2021). The addition of an SGLT2 inhibitor to the treatment regimen in individuals with type 2 DM, a lower GFR, and proteinuria has been shown to potentially decelerate the course of nephropathy. Nevertheless, it is important to acknowledge that the decrease in GFR is associated with a reduction in the efficacy of SGLT2 inhibitor medications in controlling hyperglycaemia.

Complications of Diabetes Mellitus

Acute Complications

Despite the advancements in follow-up and treatment, diabetic emergencies can still result in mortality. The acute consequences most widely recognized in the context of diabetes are diabetic ketoacidosis, hyperosmolar hyperglycaemic condition, lactic acidosis, and hypoglycaemia.

Diabetic ketoacidosis (DKA) and hyperosmolar hyperglycaemic state (HHS) are two notable metabolic diseases that arise from insulin shortage and severe hyperglycaemia. These conditions have comparable pathophysiological and treatment approaches. The primary issue with DKA is a lack of insulin, while in an HHS, the main concern is dehydration. The mechanism of formation is almost the same. The suppression of lipolysis is not possible in DKA as a result of a complete absence of insulin, leading to the presence of ketonuria and ketonemia. In contrast to human hereditary hemochromatosis (HHD), the process of lipolysis is effectively inhibited by even a minimal concentration of insulin, thus preventing the production of ketone bodies. Lactic acidosis is a relatively infrequent clinical manifestation characterized by a notably elevated mortality rate, primarily attributed to the presence of concurrent severe comorbidities such as cardiac, renal, brain, and other health complications associated with diabetes.

Hypoglycaemia, a critical condition necessitating prompt attention in cases of diabetic emergencies, arises from the administration of excessive antidiabetic medications, including insulin and oral antidiabetic drugs (OAD), either in absolute or relative terms. From a clinical perspective, it is observed that hypoglycaemia can manifest in three distinct degrees, namely mild, moderate, and severe. Mild hypoglycaemia is characterized by the presence of only neurogenic symptoms, whereas moderate and severe hypoglycaemia exhibit both neurogenic and neuroglycopenic symptoms.

Chronic Complications of Diabetes Mellitus

Macrovascular Complications

The development of cardiovascular disease (CVD) is influenced by macrovascular problems, which can be alleviated through the successful control of blood glucose (BG) levels, hypertension, and dyslipidaemia. Atherosclerotic cardiovascular disease (ASCVD) encompasses various medical conditions including acute coronary syndrome (ACS), a history of myocardial infarction (MI), stable or unstable angina, coronary or other arterial revascularization, stroke, transient ischemic attack, or peripheral arterial disease. Individuals with diabetes have a much greater incidence of CVD compared to those without diabetes, with a risk magnitude ranging from two to four times higher (Mozaffarian et al., 2015). A significant proportion, ranging from 60% to 75% of individuals diagnosed with diabetes experience mortality as a result of macrovascular events. Atherosclerosis tends to manifest at a younger age and is more frequently observed in several segments among people diagnosed with diabetes. Moreover, the inclination toward risk-taking exhibits a positive trend as individuals age. The disparity is more pronounced between socioeconomically disadvantaged groups, especially those living in low- and middle-income countries, compared to their counterparts in high-income nations (IDF et al., 2017). To mitigate the potential for primary and secondary CVD, implementing certain lifestyle modifications such as maintaining a healthy weight, adhering to a nutritious diet, engaging in regular physical activity, and abstaining from smoking, along with achieving optimal blood pressure control, optimal glycaemic control, and administering statin treatment based on cardiovascular risk assessment, as well as considering the use of antiplatelet medications when appropriate, have been identified as beneficial strategies.

Microvascular Complications

There is a positive correlation between the prolonged duration of diabetes inadequate glycaemic management and the appearance of microvascular problems. One of the consequences that have a substantial impact on end-stage renal disease, morbidity, and mortality is diabetic kidney disease (DKD). The development of renal diseases in individuals with diabetes is believed to be influenced by the complex interaction of hemodynamic variables, particularly glomerular hypertension, and metabolic disorders such as hyperglycaemia and dyslipidaemia. To examine the early stages of nephropathy, it is necessary to do an estimation of the glomerular filtration rate (eGFR) in conjunction with the measurement of albuminuria.

Diabetic retinopathy (DR) is a significant microvascular problem that results in vision impairment in adults between the ages of 20 and 65. Approximately one-third of those diagnosed with diabetes are affected by this condition to variable degrees. Azad et al., (2016) have demonstrated that efficient cholesterol management can help decrease the course of DR. Similarly, Zhu et al., (2013) have found that intensive blood glucose control can reduce the severity of this condition. Engaging in regular exercise and increasing physical activity have been shown to have a beneficial effect on retinopathy. Nevertheless, it is important to consider that individuals with unstable proliferative retinopathy may experience vitreous haemorrhage as a consequence of engaging in activities that induce a Valsalva maneuver. Various therapeutic interventions, including laser photocoagulation, vitrectomy, and administration of anti-vascular endothelial growth factor (anti-VEGF) agents, have demonstrated efficacy in the management of proliferative retinopathy. The effectiveness of anti-VEGF medication in mitigating the advancement of retinal vascularization has been observed in cases with non-proliferative retinopathy. Nevertheless, empirical evidence has indicated that there is no discernible improvement in results on vision.

Diabetic neuropathy is a notable consequence of diabetes that contributes significantly to both morbidity and mortality rates. Diabetic peripheral neuropathy (DPN) is a frequently encountered neuropathic disease that can be attributed to metabolic and microvascular changes resulting from prolonged exposure to hyperglycaemia and increased cardiovascular risk (Tesfaye et al., 2010). Dysfunctions in autonomic control are commonly observed in people with long-term diabetes. The clinical manifestations of autonomic neuropathy encompass various physiological systems, including the cardiac system (such as sudden death, silent myocardial ischemia, and orthostatic hypotension), the gastrointestinal system (including gastroparesis, diarrhoea, and constipation), the urinary system (involving urinary incontinence or retention), sexual function (specifically erectile dysfunction), peripheral sweating (which may be reduced), and gustatory sweating. The use of tricyclic compounds, such as amitriptyline, serotonin-noradrenaline reuptake inhibitors (SNRI) such as duloxetine, and anticonvulsant medications such as pregabalin and gabapentin, is generally recommended by international consensus panels, including the National Institute for Health and Care Excellence (NICE), as the primary pharmacological agents to treat painful DPN (Centre for Clinical Practice at NICE, 2013).

Conclusion

It can be inferred that the aforementioned points lead to the logical conclusion that:

Diabetes Mellitus has emerged as a significant epidemic in contemporary times, requiring healthcare personnel to have a comprehensive understanding of its diagnosis in its incipient stages, thereby mitigating the risk of potential complications. By engaging in interdisciplinary collaboration, our objective is to create a future in which the burden of diabetes is mitigated, leading to an increased state of well-being and an improved quality of life for people affected by this condition.

References

American Diabetes Association. (2015). (2) Classification and diagnosis of diabetes. *Diabetes Care, 38*(Suppl), S8–S16. https://doi.org/10.2337/dc15-S005.

Azad, N., Bahn, G. D., Emanuele, N. V., Agrawal, L., Ge, L., Reda, D., Klein, R., Reaven, P. D., Hayward, R., & VADT Study Group. (2016). Association of blood glucose control and lipids with diabetic retinopathy in the Veterans Affairs Diabetes Trial (VADT). *Diabetes Care, 39*(5), 816–822. https://doi.org/10.2337/dc15-1897.

Centre for Clinical Practice at NICE (UK). (2013). *Neuropathic pain: The pharmacological management of neuropathic pain in adults in non-specialist settings*. National Institute for Health and Care Excellence (UK).

Cho, N. H., Shaw, J. E., Karuranga, S., Huang, Y., da Rocha Fernandes, J. D., Ohlrogge, A. W., & Malanda, B. (2018). IDF Diabetes Atlas: Global estimates of diabetes prevalence for 2017 and projections for 2045. *Diabetes Research and Clinical Practice, 138*, 271–281. https://doi.org/10.1016/j.diabres.2018.02.023.

Davies, M. J., Aroda, V. R., Collins, B. S., Gabbay, R. A., Green, J., Maruthur, N. M., Rosas, S. E., Del Prato, S., Mathieu, C., Mingrone, G., Rossing, P., Tankova, T., Tsapas, A., & Buse, J. B. (2022). Management of hyperglycemia in type 2 diabetes, 2022. A consensus report by the American Diabetes Association (ADA) and the European Association for the Study of Diabetes (EASD). *Diabetes Care, 45*(11), 2753–2786. https://doi.org/10.2337/dci22-0034.

DeFronzo, R. A., & Ferrannini, E. (1991). Insulin resistance: A multifaceted syndrome responsible for NIDDM, obesity, hypertension, dyslipidemia, and atherosclerotic cardiovascular disease. *Diabetes Care, 14*(3), 173–194. https://doi.org/10.2337/diacare.14.3.173.

Holt, R. I. G., DeVries, J. H., Hess-Fischl, A., Hirsch, I. B., Kirkman, M. S., Klupa, T., Ludwig, B., Nørgaard, K., Pettus, J., Renard, E., Skyler, J. S., Snoek, F. J., Weinstock, R. S., & Peters, A. L. (2021). The management of type 1 diabetes in adults. A consensus report by the American Diabetes Association (ADA) and the European Association for the Study of Diabetes (EASD). *Diabetes Care, 44*(11), 2589–2625. https://doi.org/10.2337/dci21-0043.

International Diabetes Federation. (2017). *IDF Diabetes Atlas* (8th ed.). Brussels: IDF.

Mozaffarian, D., Benjamin, E. J., Go, A. S., Arnett, D. K., Blaha, M. J., Cushman, M., de Ferranti, S., Després, J. P., Fullerton, H. J., Howard, V. J., Huffman, M. D., Judd, S. E., Kissela, B. M., Lackland, D. T., Lichtman, J. H., Lisabeth, L. D., Liu, S., Mackey, R. H., Matchar, D. B., McGuire, D. K., … American Heart Association Statistics Committee and Stroke Statistics Subcommittee. (2015). Heart disease and stroke statistics--2015 update: A report from the American Heart Association. *Circulation, 131*(4), e29–e322. https://doi.org/10.1161/CIR.0000000000000152.

Packer, M., Anker, S. D., Butler, J., Filippatos, G., Ferreira, J. P., Pocock, S. J., Carson, P., Anand, I., Doehner, W., Haass, M., Komajda, M., Miller, A., Pehrson, S., Teerlink, J. R., Brueckmann, M., Jamal, W., Zeller, C., Schnaidt, S., & Zannad, F. (2021). Effect of empagliflozin on the clinical stability of patients with heart failure and a reduced ejection fraction: The EMPEROR-Reduced Trial. *Circulation, 143*(4), 326–336. https://doi.org/10.1161/CIRCULATIONAHA.120.051783.

Saeedi, P., Petersohn, I., Salpea, P., Malanda, B., Karuranga, S., Unwin, N., Colagiuri, S., Guariguata, L., Motala, A. A., Ogurtsova, K., Shaw, J. E., Bright, D., Williams, R., & IDF Diabetes Atlas Committee. (2019). Global and regional diabetes prevalence estimates for 2019 and projections for 2030 and 2045: Results from the International Diabetes Federation Diabetes Atlas, 9th edition. *Diabetes Research and Clinical Practice, 157*, 107843. https://doi.org/10.1016/j.diabres.2019.107843.

Selvin, E., Wang, D., Matsushita, K., Grams, M. E., & Coresh, J. (2018). Prognostic implications of single-sample confirmatory testing for undiagnosed diabetes: A prospective cohort study. *Annals of Internal Medicine, 169*(3), 156–164. https://doi.org/10.7326/M18-0091.

Stumvoll, M., Goldstein, B. J., & van Haeften, T. W. (2005). Type 2 diabetes: Principles of pathogenesis and therapy. *Lancet (London, England), 365*(9467), 1333–1346. https://doi.org/10.1016/S0140-6736(05)61032-X.

Tesfaye, S., Boulton, A. J., Dyck, P. J., Freeman, R., Horowitz, M., Kempler, P., Lauria, G., Malik, R. A., Spallone, V., Vinik, A., Bernardi, L., Valensi, P., & Toronto Diabetic Neuropathy Expert Group. (2010). Diabetic neuropathies: Update on definitions, diagnostic criteria, estimation of severity, and treatments. *Diabetes Care, 33*(10), 2285–2293. https://doi.org/10.2337/dc10-1303.

Vujkovic, M., Keaton, J. M., Lynch, J. A., Miller, D. R., Zhou, J., Tcheandjieu, C., Huffman, J. E., Assimes, T. L., Lorenz, K., Zhu, X., Hilliard, A. T., Judy, R. L., Huang, J., Lee, K. M., Klarin, D., Pyarajan, S., Danesh, J., Melander, O., Rasheed, A., Mallick, N. H., … Saleheen, D. (2020). Discovery of 318 new risk loci for type 2 diabetes and related vascular outcomes among 1.4 million participants in a multi-ancestry meta-analysis. *Nature Genetics, 52*(7), 680–691. https://doi.org/10.1038/s41588-020-0637-y.

Wiviott, S. D., Raz, I., & Sabatine, M. S. (2019). Dapagliflozin and cardiovascular outcomes in type 2 diabetes. Reply. *The New England Journal of Medicine, 380*(19), 1881–1882. https://doi.org/10.1056/NEJMc1902837.

Zhu, C. H., Zhang, S. S., Kong, Y., Bi, Y. F., Wang, L., & Zhang, Q. (2013). Effects of intensive control of blood glucose and blood pressure on microvascular complications in patients with type II diabetes mellitus. *International Journal of Ophthalmology, 6*(2), 141–145. https://doi.org/10.3980/j.issn.2222-3959.2013.02.06.

Chapter 6

Thyroid Diseases

Mehmet Burak Öztop[1,*]
and Esra Meltem Koç[2]
[1]Department of General Surgery, Izmir Bakircay University, Faculty of Medicine, Izmir, Turkey
[2]Department of Family Medicine, Izmir Katip Celebi Univesity, Faculty of Medicine, Izmir, Turkey

Abstract

Thyroid diseases are common endocrine problems encountered in clinical practice and typically present with symptoms due to either excess or deficiency of hormonal activity. Additionally, pressure symptoms related to nodule formation, tumor development, or diffuse enlargement of the thyroid gland can also occur. An accurate diagnosis is essential for the appropriate treatment of thyroid diseases, and achieving this diagnosis requires a thorough history, physical examination, and well-planned laboratory investigations. Approaching thyroid problems in primary healthcare services is crucial to improve patients' quality of life and prevent serious complications. In this section, we will evaluate the approach to thyroid diseases commonly encountered in primary care.

Keywords: hypothyroidism, hyperthyroidism, thyroid nodules, thyroid diseases

Introduction

The thyroid gland is a midline structure located at the front of the neck. It functions as an endocrine gland and is responsible for producing thyroid hormone and calcitonin, thus contributing to the regulation of metabolism, growth, and serum concentrations of electrolytes such as calcium (Allen and Fingeret, 2023).

The thyroid gland is divided into two lobes connected by an isthmus that crosses the midline of the upper trachea at the second and third tracheal rings. In its anatomical position, the thyroid gland lies behind the sternothyroid and sternohyoid muscles and surrounds the cricoid cartilage and tracheal rings. It is located below the laryngeal thyroid cartilage and typically corresponds to the C5-T1 vertebral levels. The thyroid is attached to the trachea through a consolidation of connective tissue known as the lateral suspensory ligament or Berry's ligament. This ligament connects each lobe of the thyroid to the trachea. The thyroid

* Corresponding Author's Email: burakoztop@yahoo.com.

In: Common Diseases According to Family Medicine Practice Guidelines
Editors: Esra Meltem Koç and Hilal Aksoy
ISBN: 979-8-89530-302-3

gland, along with the esophagus, pharynx, and trachea, is located in the visceral compartment of the neck, bounded by the pretracheal fascia (Allen and Fingeret, 2023).

The thyroid gland is an endocrine gland that secretes hormones. It produces and secretes the hormones thyroxine (T4) and triiodothyronine (T3). These hormones are crucial in regulating the body's metabolic rate. The thyroid gland also produces and secretes the hormone calcitonin, which is effective in calcium metabolism. The hormones controlling the secretion of these hormones from the thyroid gland are thyroid-stimulating hormone (TSH) secreted from the anterior lobe of the pituitary gland and thyrotropin-releasing hormone (TRH) secreted by the hypothalamus (Hershman and Pittman, 1970). Thyroid hormone secretion is controlled by a negative feedback mechanism involving the hypothalamus-pituitary-thyroid (HPT) axis. A decrease in circulating T4 and T3 affects the secretion of TRH. TRH then increases the secretion of TSH through stimulation. TSH stimulates thyroid follicular cells through receptors, leading to the secretion of T3 and T4 hormones. When circulating T3 and T4 hormones increase, TRH and TSH secretion is inhibited, resulting in a decrease in T3 and T4 hormone secretion. This is a good example of a negative feedback mechanism (Goodman, 1996; Mandel et al., 1993). TSH and T3 are the main effective hormones in these control mechanisms (Scott et al., 1999).

The physiological effects of thyroid hormones are listed below:

- Increases the basal metabolic rate.
- Can induce lipolysis or lipid synthesis depending on the metabolic state.
- Stimulates carbohydrate metabolism.
- Plays a role in the anabolism of proteins and can induce protein catabolism in high doses.
- Has a permissive effect on catecholamines.
- In children, thyroid hormones act synergistically with growth hormone to stimulate bone growth.
- The effect of thyroid hormones on the central nervous system (CNS) is significant. They are necessary for brain maturation during the prenatal period. In adults, they can affect mood. Hyperthyroidism can lead to hyperexcitability and irritability, while hypothyroidism can cause memory impairment, slowed speech, and somnolence.
- Thyroid hormones also affect fertility, ovulation, and menstruation (Shadid MA).

Diagnostic Methods for Thyroid Diseases

A thyroid examination is very useful for identifying thyroid pathologies in primary care. A carefully conducted examination can detect enlargement of the thyroid gland, the presence of nodules, and increased blood flow to the thyroid gland. Additionally, a detailed history and systemic examination can identify many signs and symptoms related to thyroid diseases and facilitate the referral of the patient to secondary or tertiary care centers.

Which Test Should We Use?

In individuals without symptoms related to thyroid dysfunction, screening for thyroid disease using TSH is sufficient (Figure 1). In the absence of a systemic disease, a normal TSH concentration has a 99% negative predictive value in excluding primary hypothyroidism and hyperthyroidism (Turkish Society of Endocrinology and Metabolism, 2023). If TSH is normal in asymptomatic individuals, no further investigation is needed. If the TSH level is high, the sT4 level should be checked; if the TSH level is low, both the sT4 and sT3 levels should be assessed. In patients with symptoms and signs consistent with hypothyroidism, it is recommended to check both TSH and sT4 levels for diagnosis. In patients with symptoms and signs consistent with hyperthyroidism, it is recommended to check the levels of TSH, sT4, and T3/sT3 (Turkish Society of Endocrinology and Metabolism, 2023).

TSH and Thyroid Hormone Levels

TSH

TSH levels are higher in the early morning and decrease toward the evening. This circadian rhythm can cause a change in TSH levels that can affect treatment decisions, with variations between approximately 0.95 mIU/L and 2.0 mIU/L. Although the normal reference range for TSH is considered to be between 0.35 mIU/L and 4.50 mIU/L, the more frequently observed normal range is between 0.5 mIU/L and 2.50 mIU/L (Sheehan, 2016).

In regions without iodine deficiency, serum TSH concentrations increase with age in individuals without thyroid disease (Bremner et al., 2012). According to NHANES III data, the upper limit of TSH is 3.5 mIU/L in the 20-29 age range, 4.5 mIU/L in the 50-70 age range, and 7.5 mIU/L in individuals aged 80 and above (Sheehan, 2016). Therefore, the laboratory reference range for TSH and the threshold values for diagnosing hypothyroidism and initiating treatment are not the same (Turkish Society of Endocrinology and Metabolism, 2023). For pregnant women, the TSH reference ranges by trimester are 0.1–2.5 mIU/L in the first trimester, 0.2–3.0 mIU/L in the second trimester, and 0.3–3.0 mIU/L in the third trimester (Alexander Erik et al., 2017).

Total T4 and Total T3

Since TT3 and TT4 are heavily bound to proteins, slight changes in binding protein levels can make the interpretation of results challenging (Koulouri and Gurnell, 2013). Due to the effects of changes in binding proteins and their low sensitivity, total thyroid hormone tests are now used less frequently (Dufour, 2007). During pregnancy, the increase in T4-binding globulin can lead to lower measurements of ST4, making it unreliable. Instead of ST4 measurement, TT4 measurement is recommended. TT4 increases in the first trimester of pregnancy, and its reference range is 1.5 times that of non-pregnant individuals (Esfandiari and Papaleontiou, 2017). Any further increase is considered pathological (Turkish Society for Endocrinology and Metabolism, 2023).

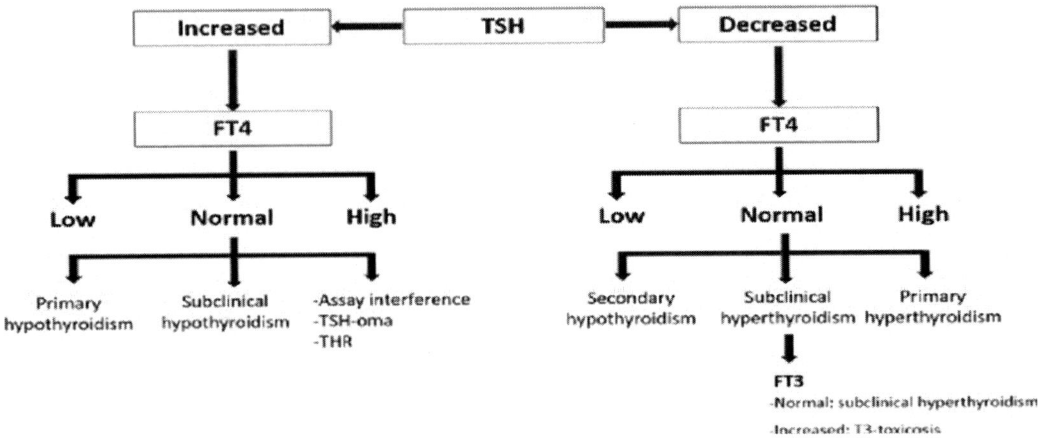

Figure 1. Differential diagnosis according to serum TSH Levels.

Free T4 (FT4)

The serum FT4 measurement has largely replaced total T4 for assessing thyroid status. It is used in conjunction with TSH to diagnose thyroid dysfunctions and adjust doses of medications in patients with secondary hypothyroidism (Esfandiari and Papaleontiou, 2017).

Free T3 (FT3)

The utility of serum T3 measurement in diagnosing hypothyroidism is limited. The FT3 level remains normal due to the excessive stimulation of the remaining healthy thyroid tissue by elevated TSH and the increase in type 2 iodothyronine deiodinase, which facilitates the conversion of T4 to T3 (Esfandiari and Papaleontiou, 2017). FT3 measurement is recommended in cases of drug use that blocks the conversion of T4 to T3, monitors patients using antithyroid medications, and distinguishes between hyperthyroidism and thyrotoxicosis (Koulouri et al., 2013).

Other Laboratory Tests

Thyroglobulin

Thyroglobulin is produced by thyroid follicular cells and secreted into the follicular lumen. Tg measurement has no role in the diagnostic process of thyroid cancer. However, Tg is used as a tumor marker in the follow-up of patients with operated thyroid cancer (Turkish Society of Endocrinology and Metabolism, 2023).

Calcitonin

Calcitonin is used as a tumor marker in medullary thyroid carcinoma (MTC). Therefore, calcitonin is used in the follow-up of all patients diagnosed with MTC after thyroidectomy (Turkish Society of Endocrinology and Metabolism, 2023).

Thyroid Autoantibodies

TSH Receptor Antibody (TRAb)

In approximately 98% of patients with Graves' disease, an antibody against the TSH receptor (TRAb) detected in the serum is pathognomonic for Graves' disease (Menconi et al., 2014). Evaluating TRAb concentration after antithyroid drug treatment in patients undergoing hyperthyroidism treatment is useful to predict the risk of disease recurrence after discontinuing treatment (Leo et al., 2016).

In pregnancy, if the mother has Graves' disease, fetal and neonatal thyrotoxicosis can occur due to the placental transfer of TRAb (Turkish Society of Endocrinology and Metabolism, 2023). It is recommended that serum TRAb levels be measured in all pregnant women with a history of Graves' disease at 20-24 weeks. Antibody titers greater than 300% of the upper limit of normal suggest that the fetus is at risk for hyperthyroidism (Pearce, 2015).

Anti-TPO and Anti-Thyroglobulin

In autoimmune thyroid disease, certain autoantibodies are present in the serum. Anti-TPO (thyroid peroxidase) and anti-Tg (thyroglobulin) are positive in 95-100% of cases of chronic thyroiditis (Hashimoto's thyroiditis) and 60-90% of cases of Graves' disease. Although the measurement of these antibodies is not recommended for evaluating thyroid function, they can be used to diagnose autoimmune thyroid disease (AITD). The most commonly used antibody for this purpose is anti-TPO. While valuable in diagnosing Hashimoto's thyroiditis, it is also detected in postpartum thyroiditis and Graves' disease, though it rarely contributes to the diagnosis of these diseases. Anti-thyroglobulin is an antibody against thyroglobulin. It can be elevated in healthy adults. Compared to anti-TPO, it is less sensitive and less specific (Caturegli et al., 2015). It is found in 10% of the normal population and 25% of patients with differentiated thyroid carcinoma (DTC) (Turkish Society of Endocrinology and Metabolism, 2023).

Other Methods

Thyroid Ultrasonography (US)

Thyroid ultrasonography is the most commonly used imaging tool in patients suspected of having thyroid disease (Caturegli et al., 2015). It is the most useful method for distinguishing normal thyroid parenchyma from diffuse or nodular thyroid disease by evaluating the size, echogenicity, border regularity, and vascularity of the gland (Alexander et al., 2020). Hypoechogenicity, irregular borders, microcalcifications, transverse length greater than width, solid structure, and increased vascularization are ultrasound features that carry a risk of malignancy. Purely cystic, spongiform, or comet-tail artifacts suggest a high likelihood of being benign (Wong et al., 2018).

Thyroid Scintigraphy

Thyroid scintigraphy should be performed when serum TSH is suppressed. 99 mTc is commonly used in routine practice due to its low cost and low radiation burden. It is useful to distinguish hypofunctioning nodules from hyperfunctioning nodules in patients with multinodular goiter to avoid unnecessary biopsies, and to evaluate suitability for radioactive iodine therapy (Durantem et al., 2023).

Thyroid Fine Needle Aspiration Biopsy (FNAB)

FNAB is an effective diagnostic method performed under ultrasound guidance in a clinical setting to distinguish between benign and malignant nodules. It is non-invasive, cost-effective, has a low risk of complications, and is effective (Turkish Society of Endocrinology and Metabolism, 2023).

Thyroid Function Disorders

Hypothyroidism

Hypothyroidism is one of the most common endocrine diseases. It is mostly caused by a decrease in thyroid hormone synthesis and secretion by the thyroid gland, leading to reduced thyroid hormone effects in peripheral tissues. Rarely, it is due to resistance to thyroid hormones in the periphery (Devdhar et al., 2007). If hypothyroidism is due to the thyroid gland, it is called primary hypothyroidism. If it develops due to insufficient TSH secretion, it is secondary hypothyroidism. If it develops due to insufficient synthesis and release of thyrotropin-releasing hormone (TRH) from the hypothalamus, it is called tertiary hypothyroidism. A condition where serum TSH is high and sT4 levels are normal is defined as subclinical hypothyroidism (Saglam and Cakir, 2012).

The most common cause of hypothyroidism worldwide is iodine deficiency (Vanderpump and Tunbridge, 2002). In areas where iodine deficiency is not seen, the most common cause of hypothyroidism is Hashimoto's thyroiditis (Almandoz and Gharib, 2012). Other causes include congenital conditions, goitrogens, medications, or iatrogenic causes due to the destructive treatment of thyrotoxicosis (Vanderpump and Tunbridge, 2002).

Clinical Features

In hypothyroidism, signs and symptoms arise due to the slowing of metabolic processes caused by thyroid hormone deficiency and the accumulation of glycosaminoglycans in the interstitial tissue. The observed symptoms vary widely depending on the degree of thyroid hormone deficiency and the speed with which the deficiency develops (Turkish Society of Endocrinology and Metabolism, 2023). The most common symptoms are dry skin, sensitivity to cold, fatigue, muscle cramps, changes in voice, and constipation (Garber et al., 2012) (Table 1).

Table 1. Symptoms of hypothyroidism and hyperthyroidism

Symptoms of Hypothyroidism	Symptoms of Hyperthyroidism
Weight gain	Palpitations/tachycardia/atrial fibrillation
Lethargy	Widened pulse pressure
Cold intolerance	Nervousness and tremor
Menstrual irregularities	Heat intolerance
Depression	Weight loss
Constipation	Muscular weakness
Dry skin	Usually, goiter is present

[1]Investıgatıon and Management of Primary Thyroid Dysfunction Clinical Practice Guideline, 2014.

Treatment

All patients with obvious hypothyroidism should be treated, regardless of whether they are symptomatic (Turkish Society of Endocrinology and Metabolism, 2023). There is a general consensus on treating all patients with a serum TSH level of 10 mU/L. The daily dose requirement of LT4 (Levothyroxine) varies according to age, gender, and body weight. In cases with partial thyroid function reserve, the initial average requirement is 1.2-1.6 µg/kg (approximately 75-100 µg/day). Patients without thyroid tissue and those with central hypothyroidism may require higher doses (100-250 µg/day). In young patients, treatment can start with the planned full dose. In elderly patients, especially those with coronary heart disease, the initial dose should be 12.5-25 µg/day, with dose increases of 12.5-25 µg/day. The goal of treatment is achieved by measuring TSH levels at 6-8 week intervals (Turkish Society of Endocrinology and Metabolism, 2023).

The target TSH values should be set at 0.4-2.5 mU/L for young, middle-aged, and pregnancy-planning patients; 3-6 mU/L for elderly patients (≥65-70 years); and ≤10 mU/L for very elderly patients (>80-85 years) (Turkish Society of Endocrinology and Metabolism, 2023). In patients receiving replacement therapy for central hypothyroidism, TSH is not used to determine replacement adequacy. Instead, the target is the middle and upper normal range of sT4 and sT3 levels measured before the daily T4 dose is taken (Devdhar et al., 2007).

Primary hypothyroidism is very common and can be treated by family physicians. However, consultation with an endocrinologist is necessary in the following situations:

- Suspected hypothyroidism in infants and children
- Cases where the treatment dose cannot be adjusted

- Pregnancy
- Those planning a pregnancy
- Patients with heart disease
- Presence of a nodule in the thyroid gland
- Endocrinological diseases such as pituitary disease or adrenal insufficiency
- Inconsistencies in thyroid tests
- Drug-induced hypothyroidism.

Hyperthyroidism and Thyrotoxicosis

Hypermetabolism and excessive exposure to thyroid hormones result in a state known as thyrotoxicosis. Hyperthyroidism is a form of thyrotoxicosis caused by the excessive synthesis of thyroid hormones by the thyroid gland. Graves' disease and nodular thyroid disease are the most common causes of endogenous hyperthyroidism.

Clinical Features

Hyperthyroidism can be categorized into an overt and subclinical based on its severity. Overt hyperthyroidism is defined by elevated serum levels of triiodothyronine (sT3) and/or serum thyroxine (sT4), along with subnormal (often undetectable) serum thyrotropin (TSH) levels. Subclinical hyperthyroidism is characterized by serum TSH levels that are low or undetectable, while T3 and free T4 levels remain within the normal reference range. Symptoms occur in both conditions but are milder in subclinical hyperthyroidism (Table 1). Thyroid hormones affect many tissues and organ systems, with the most significant impact on the cardiovascular system. The prevalence and severity of hyperthyroid symptoms are expected to be directly proportional to the elevation in sT3 and sT4 levels, but recent studies confirm the importance of age as a determinant (Ross et al., 2016).

When evaluating patients with clinically or incidentally diagnosed thyrotoxicosis, especially older patients, it is crucial to assess cardiovascular and neuromuscular complications and develop an appropriate treatment plan. All patients should undergo a thorough history and physical examination, including measurements of pulse rate, blood pressure, respiratory rate, and body weight. The evaluation should also include thyroid size, tenderness, symmetry, and nodularity, as well as pulmonary, cardiac, and neuromuscular function, and the presence or absence of peripheral edema, eye signs, or pretibial myxedema (Ross et al., 2016).

Graves' disease is a multisystem autoimmune disorder characterized by antibodies against the TSH receptor. It is more common in women and can occur at any age, with increased frequency in the fifth and sixth decades. Diagnosis is made based on clinical or biochemical evidence of thyrotoxicosis, positive serum TRAb, the presence of ophthalmopathy and/or dermopathy, and increased RAI uptake (Menconi et al., 2014). These findings are typically not present in toxic multinodular goiter and toxic adenoma (Saglam and Cakir, 2012).

Treatment

The primary treatment options for hyperthyroidism include antithyroid drugs, radioactive iodine therapy, and surgery. Methimazole (MMI) can be used once daily, whereas Propylthiouracil (PTU) requires administration three times daily due to its shorter half-life. A 100 mg dose of PTU is approximately equivalent to 5-6 mg of methimazole (15-20:1 ratio). Initial dosages are determined based on the severity of hyperthyroidism. For an sT4 level 1-1.5 times the upper limit of normal, 5-10 mg of methimazole are recommended; for 1.5-2 times, 10-20 mg; and for 2-3 times, 30-40 mg. The side effects of these medications include pruritus, skin rash, urticaria, elevated liver function tests, and agranulocytosis. The most common side effects are rash, itching, and urticaria, which can be managed with antihistamines without discontinuing the antithyroid drug in mild reactions. For moderate reactions, switching to another antithyroid drug or permanent treatment may be necessary, while severe reactions require complete avoidance of antithyroid drugs. Serious side effects necessitating drug discontinuation include agranulocytosis, toxic hepatitis, cholestasis, polyarthritis, and ANCA-positive vasculitis.

Depending on the severity of thyrotoxicosis, sT4 and total T3 should be reassessed in 2-6 weeks. TSH should not be used for monitoring, particularly in the early stages of treatment, as it can remain suppressed for an extended period. Once the patient is euthyroid, the antithyroid dose is reduced by 30-50%, and biochemical tests are repeated every 4-6 weeks. The optimal duration for antithyroid therapy is reported to be 12-18 months. Stopping the medication after just 6 months increases the risk of relapse. The achievement of biochemical euthyroidism for at least one year after stopping antithyroid therapy is defined as remission. Approximately half of the patients achieve remission after one year of antithyroid treatment. If relapse occurs after an adequate duration of antithyroid therapy, radioactive iodine (RAI) or surgery is recommended based on the patient's characteristics. A second round of antithyroid therapy can be considered, but the remission rates are lower. For toxic multinodular goiter or toxic adenoma, surgery or RAI is the preferred permanent treatment (Turkish Endocrinology and Metabolism Association, 2023).

The differential diagnosis, follow-up, and treatment of thyrotoxic conditions should ideally be managed by endocrinologists or internists. However, recognizing the symptoms of hyperthyroidism and monitoring for potential drug-related side effects are also responsibilities of primary care physicians.

Thyroid Nodules

Thyroid nodules are round or oval masses that form within the thyroid gland and do not resemble the normal tissue. These nodules can arise endemically due to iodine deficiency or sporadically. Thyroid nodules can be detected in 50-60% of healthy individuals, and these individuals often have euthyroid (normal thyroid function) status. Typically, nodules do not cause compressive symptoms or cosmetic concerns. However, when a thyroid nodule is detected, it is crucial to determine whether the nodule is benign (non-cancerous) or malignant (cancerous), whether it causes thyroid dysfunction, and whether it produces compressive symptoms.

Signs suggestive of malignancy include a family history of thyroid cancer, a history of neck radiation during childhood, firm and rapidly growing masses in the thyroid, sudden growth of an existing nodule, hoarseness, dysphagia (difficulty swallowing), stridor (a high-pitched wheezing sound), regional lymph node enlargement, and nodules larger than 4 cm. Ultrasonographic features that support malignancy include hypoechoic characteristics of the nodule, irregular margins, the presence of a thick and irregular halo, microcalcifications, and increased vascularity within the nodule on color Doppler imaging. Suspicious nodules should undergo a fine-needle aspiration biopsy (FNAB).

Evaluating a patient with a thyroid nodule involves four main components: clinical history and physical examination, serum thyroid-stimulating hormone (TSH) measurement, ultrasound, and FNAB if indicated. When taking a clinical history, the patient's age, gender, comorbidities, how the nodules were detected, their progression and associated complaints, history of medications and iodine intake, nodule history and previous tests and procedures, results of any previous thyroid surgery, symptoms of hypothyroidism and hyperthyroidism, compressive symptoms, history of radiation exposure to the neck, family history of thyroid nodules or thyroid cancer, and risk factors for thyroid cancer should be inquired about. During a physical examination, the size of the thyroid gland, signs of hyperthyroidism or hypothyroidism, nodule hardness, size, location, relation to surrounding tissues, presence of pain in the nodule or thyroid gland, signs of compression, and cervical lymph node examination should be assessed. The initial laboratory test is the TSH measurement. For incidentalomas and palpable thyroid nodules, thyroid ultrasonography is the first-line investigation, and routine screening ultrasound is not recommended (Gharib et al., 2016; Wong et al., 2018; Durante et al., 2018; Saglam and Cakir, 2012; Turkish Endocrinology and Metabolism Association, 2023).

When nodules are detected during physical examination by primary care physicians, patients should be referred to the appropriate center for further evaluation.

Thyroid Cancers

Thyroid cancer is the most frequently observed malignancy among endocrine malignancies, with differentiated thyroid cancers accounting for 95% of thyroid cancers. The main tumor types seen in thyroid cancers include papillary thyroid carcinoma, follicular thyroid carcinoma, Hurthle cell carcinoma, poorly differentiated thyroid carcinoma, anaplastic thyroid carcinoma, squamous cell carcinoma, medullary thyroid carcinoma, mixed medullary and follicular thyroid carcinoma, mucoepidermoid carcinoma, sclerosing mucoepidermoid carcinoma with eosinophilia, mucinous carcinoma, ectopic thymoma, spindle cell tumor with thymus-like differentiation, and intrathyroidal thymic carcinoma (current approaches to thyroid cancer). The most common type of differentiated thyroid cancer is papillary carcinoma, which originates from follicular epithelial cells (Cooper et al., 2009).

When primary thyroid carcinoma is a small, unifocal, intrathyroidal carcinoma without regional or distant metastasis, lobectomy is the recommended treatment. However, in general, two-thirds of patients undergo total thyroidectomy, while one-third undergo lobectomy. Therefore, comprehensive and accurate preoperative imaging to evaluate the primary tumor, multifocality, bilaterality, and central and lateral lymph node metastasis is crucial to determine the appropriate surgical approach. Ultrasound is the recommended initial imaging modality for patients with thyroid nodules, and suspected or known differentiated thyroid cancer (Turkish Endocrinology and Metabolism Association, 2023).

Conclusion

In primary healthcare, an accurate and effective approach to thyroid diseases is crucial for enhancing patients' quality of life and preventing serious complications. The diagnosis and treatment of thyroid diseases are based on a thorough history taking, a comprehensive physical examination, and well-planned laboratory tests. Early and precise intervention improves the patient's prognosis and prevents unnecessary treatments, thereby increasing the efficiency of healthcare services.

References

Alexander, L. F., Patel, N. J., Caserta, M. P., & Robbin, M. L. (2020). Thyroid ultrasound: Diffuse and nodular disease. *Radiologic Clinics of North America, 58*(6), 1041-1057.

Alexander, E. K., Pearce, E. N., Gregory, A. B., Brown, R. S., Grobman, W. A., Lazarus, J. H., Mandel, S. J., Peeters, R. P., & Sullivan, S. (2017). Guidelines of the American Thyroid Association for the diagnosis and management of thyroid disease during pregnancy and the postpartum. *Thyroid.*

Almandoz, J. P., & Gharib, H. (2012). Hypothyroidism: Etiology, diagnosis, and management. *Medical Clinics of North America, 96*(2), 203-221.

Bremner, A. P., Feddema, P., Leedman, P. J., Brown, S. J., Beilby, J. P., Lim, E. M., Wilson, S. G., O'Leary, P. C., & Walsh, J. P. (2012). Age-related changes in thyroid function: A longitudinal study of a community-based cohort. *The Journal of Clinical Endocrinology & Metabolism, 97*(5), 1554-1562. https://doi.org/10.1210/jc.2011-3020.

Caturegli, P., Remigis, A. D., & Rose, N. R. (2014). Hashimoto thyroiditis: Clinical and diagnostic criteria. *Autoimmunity Reviews, 13*, 391-397. https://doi.org/10.1016/j.autrev.2014.01.007.

Cooper, D. S., Doherty, G. M., Haugen, B. R., Kloos, R. T., Lee, S. L., Mandel, S. J., Mazzaferri, E. L., McIver, B., Pacini, F., Schlumberger, M., Sherman, S. I., Steward, D. L., & Tuttle, R. M. (2009). Revised American Thyroid Association management guidelines for patients with thyroid nodules and differentiated thyroid cancer: The American Thyroid Association (ATA) guidelines taskforce on thyroid nodules and differentiated thyroid cancer. *Thyroid, 19*(11), 1167-1214. https://doi.org/10.1089/thy.2009.0110.

Devdhar, M., Ousman, Y. H., & Burman, K. D. (2007). Hypothyroidism. *Endocrinology and Metabolism Clinics of North America, 36*, 595-615. https://doi.org/10.1016/j.ecl.2007.04.002.

Dufour, D. R. (2007). Laboratory tests of thyroid function: Uses and limitations. *Endocrinology and Metabolism Clinics of North America, 36*(3), 579-594. https://doi.org/10.1016/j.ecl.2007.04.008.

Durante, C., Grani, G., Lamartina, L., Filetti, S., Mandel, S. J., & Cooper, D. S. (2018). The diagnosis and management of thyroid nodules: A review. *JAMA, 319*(9), 914-924. https://doi.org/10.1001/jama.2018.0898.

Durante, C., Hegedüs, L., Czarniecka, A., Paschke, R., Russ, G., Schmitt, F., Soares, P., Solymosi, T., & Papini, E. (2023). European Thyroid Association clinical practice guidelines for thyroid nodule management. *European Thyroid Journal, 12*(5). https://doi.org/10.1530/ETJ-23-0025.

Esfandiari, N. H., & Papaleontiou, M. (2017). Biochemical testing in thyroid disorders. *Endocrinology and Metabolism Clinics of North America, 46*(3), 631-648. https://doi.org/10.1016/j.ecl.2017.04.006.

Garber, J. R., Cobin, R. H., Gharib, H., Hennessey, J. V., Klein, I., Mechanick, J. I., Pollack, R. C., Singer, P. A., & Woeber, K. A. (2012). Clinical practice guidelines for hypothyroidism in adults: Cosponsored by the American Association of Clinical Endocrinologists and the American Thyroid Association. *Thyroid, 22*(12), 1200-1235. https://doi.org/10.1089/thy.2012.0205.

Gharib, H., Papini, E., Garber, J. R., Duick, D. S., Harrell, R. M., Hegedus, L., Paschke, R., Valcavi, R., & Vitti, A. (2016). American Association of Clinical Endocrinologists, American College of Endocrinology, and Associazione Medici Endocrinologi medical guidelines for clinical practice for the diagnosis and management of thyroid nodules-2016 update appendix. *Endocrine Practice, 22*, 1-60. https://doi.org/10.4158/EP161208.GL.

Goodman, L. S. (1996). *Goodman and Gilman's the pharmacological basis of therapeutics* (Vol. 1549). McGraw-Hill New York.

Guyton, A. (1976). *Textbook of Medical Physiology* (5th ed.). WB Saunders. Philadelphia.

Hershman, J. M., & Pittman, J. A. Jr. (1970). Response to synthetic thyrotropin-releasing hormone in man. *The Journal of Clinical Endocrinology & Metabolism, 31*(4), 457-460. https://doi.org/10.1210/jcem-31-4-457.

Allen, E., & Fingeret, A. (2023). Anatomy, head and neck, thyroid. In *StatPearls* [Internet]. Treasure Island (FL): StatPearls Publishing. Available from: https://www.ncbi.nlm.nih.gov/books/NBK470452/.

Koulouri, O., & Gurnell, M. (2013). How to interpret thyroid function tests. *Clinical Medicine, 13*(3), 282. https://doi.org/10.7861/clinmedicine.13-3-282.

Koulouri, O., Moran, C., Halsall, D., Chatterjee, K., & Gurnell, M. (2013). Pitfalls in the measurement and interpretation of thyroid function tests. *Best Practice & Research Clinical Endocrinology & Metabolism, 27*(6), 745-762. https://doi.org/10.1016/j.beem.2013.10.003.

Leo, S. D., Lee, S. Y., & Braverman, L. E. (2016). Hyperthyroidism. *Lancet, 388*, 906–918. https://doi.org/10.1016/S0140-6736(16)00278-6.

Mandel, S. J., Brent, G. A., & Larsen, P. R. (1993). Levothyroxine therapy in patients with thyroid disease. *Annals of Internal Medicine, 119*(6), 492-502. https://doi.org/10.7326/0003-4819-119-6-199309150-00010.

Menconi, F., Marcocci, C., & Marinò, M. (2014). Diagnosis and classification of Graves' disease. *Autoimmunity Reviews, 13*(4-5), 398-402. https://doi.org/10.1016/j.autrev.2014.01.015.

Pearce, E. N. (2015). Thyroid disorders during pregnancy and postpartum. *Best Practice & Research Clinical Obstetrics & Gynaecology, 29*(5), 700-706. https://doi.org/10.1016/j.bpobgyn.2015.02.002.

Ross, D. S., Burch, H. B., Cooper, D. S., Greenlee, M. C., Laurberg, P., Maia, A. L., Rivkees, S. A., Samuels, M., Sosa, J. A., Stan, M. N., & Walter, M. A. (2016). American Thyroid Association guidelines for diagnosis and management of hyperthyroidism and other causes of thyrotoxicosis. *Thyroid, 26*(10), 1343-1421. https://doi.org/10.1089/thy.2016.0229.

Saglam, F., & Çakır, B. (2012). Clinical approach to thyroid diseases in primary health care. *Ankara Medical Journal, 12*(3), 136-139.

Scott, D., Wang, R., Kreman, T. M., Sheffield, V. C., & Karniski, L. P. (1999). The Pendred syndrome gene encodes a chloride-iodide transport protein. *Nature Genetics, 21*, 440-443. https://doi.org/10.1038/7785.

Shahid, M. A., Ashraf, M. A., & Sharma, S. (2023). Physiology, thyroid hormone. In *StatPearls* [Internet]. Treasure Island (FL): StatPearls Publishing. Available from: https://www.ncbi.nlm.nih.gov/books/NBK500006/.

Sheehan, M. T. (2016). Biochemical testing of the thyroid: TSH is the best and, oftentimes, only test needed–a review for primary care. *Clinical Medicine & Research, 14*(2), 83-92. https://doi.org/10.3121/cmr.2016.1309.

Türkiye Endokrinoloji ve Metabolizma Hastalıkları Derneği. (2023). *Tiroid Hastalıkları Tanı ve Tedavi Kılavuzu* [Diagnosis and Treatment Guide for Thyroid Diseases].

Wong, R., Farrell, S. G., & Grossmann, M. (2018). Thyroid nodules: Diagnosis and management. *Medical Journal of Australia, 209*(2), 92-98. https://doi.org/10.5694/mja17.00999.

Vanderpump, M. P., & Tunbridge, W. M. G. (2002). Epidemiology and prevention of clinical and subclinical hypothyroidism. *Thyroid, 12*(10), 839-847. https://doi.org/10.1089/105072502761016458.

Part 3

Dermatological Diseases

Chapter 7

Urticaria

Fatih M. Sari*, MD

Department of Emergency Medicine, Binali Yildirim University, School of Medicine, Erzincan, Turkey

Abstract

Urticaria is a condition characterized by the development of wheals (hives), angioedema, or both. Urticaria is classified as acute or chronic according to the duration of its occurrence. The most common symptoms are itching and wheals. The activity of the disease in spontaneous urticaria should be assessed both in clinical care and trials with the Urticaria Activity Score. The first goal of treatment should be the identification and elimination of the underlying causes. Although urticaria is one of the most common dermatoses, further research is required on the triggers and inflammatory processes that cause the disease.

Keywords: urticaria, allergy, angioedema

Introduction

Urticaria is a heterogeneous group of inflammatory diseases with a lifetime prevalence of up to 20% worldwide. It is one of the ten most common dermatoses. After activation of mast cells, plaques, angioedema, or both are observed. It begins acutely, and the lesion usually regresses within a few hours without leaving a scar (Charlesworth, 1996). Angioedema is diagnosed in the presence of edema in the subcutaneous tissue or mucosa. In cases of angioedema, pain is at the forefront of the lesions. Urticaria is usually self-limiting quickly, with eruptions rarely lasting a few days but may recur for weeks. If it lasts longer than 6 weeks, it is defined as chronic urticaria. The resolution of angioedema takes longer and may take up to 72 hours. While urticaria can occur anywhere in the body, angioedema is often seen in the uvula, tongue, lips, periorbital region, extremities, intestinal, and genital areas. The process of developing urticaria is usually an isolated event without a systemic reaction. Rarely, it may be the beginning of an anaphylactic reaction.

There are three characteristics of wheal in patients with urticaria:

* Corresponding Author's Email: drfmsari@gmail.com.

In: Common Diseases According to Family Medicine Practice Guidelines
Editors: Esra Meltem Koç and Hilal Aksoy
ISBN: 979-8-89530-302-3

1. a variable-sized central swelling that is almost always surrounded by reflex erytha;
2. an itching or occasionally burning sensation;
3. a transient nature, with the skin usually returning to its normal appearance between 30 minutes and 24 hours (Powell et al., 2015).

Epidemiology

Urticaria is one of the most common dermatological disorders, and its lifetime incidence reaches 20%. In general, it is more common in young adults than in the elderly and in women than in men. Physical urticaria and pressure urticaria are more common in men. Acute urticaria is more common in children than chronic urticaria. Although it affects all races, its incidence may vary between countries and races due to different allergens in different countries (Charlesworth, 1996). Differential diagnosis: Urticaria needs to be distinguished from other medical conditions such as anaphylaxis, urticarial vasculitis, auto-inflammatory syndromes or hereditary angioedema (HAE), and bradykinin-mediated angioedema, in which blisters, angioedema, or both may occur.

Classification

When angioedema, spontaneous wheals, or both occur for less than six weeks, it is referred to as acute spontaneous urticaria. If it lasts longer than 6 weeks, it is called chronic urticaria. When the etiology of acute urticaria is examined, no cause can be found in 50% of the patients, while it is thought to occur due to upper respiratory tract infections in 40% of the patients. In the remaining patients, the triggering agent was drugs in 9% and food in 1%. Chronic urticaria can be divided etiologically into two main classes (Table 1). The first of these is for the usual reason. These include auto-immune, idiopathic, pseudo-allergic, and infection-related chronic urticaria. The second class is inducible causes. These are; They can be listed as dermographism, delayed pressure urticaria, vibration angioedema, hot and cold urticaria, stress urticaria, solar urticaria, and aquagenic urticaria (Powell et al., 2015).

Table 1. Chronic Urticaria Subtypes

Chronic urticaria subtypes	
Chronic Spontaneous Urticaria (CSU)	*Inducible Urticaria (CIndU)*
Wheals, angioedema, or both appear on their own for longer than six weeks for reasons that are known or unclear.	Symptomatic dermographism
	Cold urticaria
	Delayed pressure urticaria
	Solar urticaria
	Heat urticaria
	Vibratory angioedema
	Cholinergic urticaria
	Contact urticaria
	Aquagenic urticaria

Table 2. Urticaria Activity Score

Score	Wheals	Pruritus
0	None	None
1	Mild (<20 wheals/24 h)	Mild (present but not annoying or troublesome)
2	Moderate (20-50 wheals/24 h)	Moderate (troublesome but does not interfere with normal daily activity or sleep)
3	Intense (>50 wheals/24 h or large confluent areas of wheals)	Intense (severe pruritus, which is sufficiently difficult to interfere with normal daily activity or sleep)

Pathophysiology

Urticaria is a disease that occurs after mast cell activation. The release of mediators such as histamine, platelet-activating factor (PAF), and cytokines causes vasodilation, activation of the sensory nerve, plasma extravasation, and cell recruitment to urticarial lesions. The signals that activate mast cells in the urticaria are not well defined. Histologically, edema in the upper and middle dermis causes blisters. This permeability increases as the upper dermis's lymphatic and postcapillary venules dilate, allowing the serum to seep into the tissue. Similar alterations mostly affect the lower dermis and subcutis in angioedema. Histopathological examination of skin biopsies performed on red and edematous urticarial plaques reveals an inflammatory infiltration consisting of active eosinophils and lymphocytes, with a predominance of neutrophils (Grattan, 2012).

Signs and Symptoms

Itching is by far the most common symptom. Wheals and flares of varying sizes are other distinctive symptoms. Wheals typically go away in a day or two without leaving behind hyperpigmentation. Angioedema, which usually affects the deep dermis and subcutaneous fat in areas such as the hands, lips, tongue, and periorbital tissues, can occasionally coexist with urticaria. Angioedema frequently has a burning sensation and/or mild pain, and it can last up to 72 hours. In cases of angioedema, itching is uncommon (Bernstein et al., 2014).

Diagnostic Methods in Acute Urticaria

Since acute urticaria is usually self-limiting, it does not require diagnostic investigation, except in susceptible patients.

Diagnostic Methods in Chronic Urticaria

The three primary goals of the CSU diagnostic workup are to (a) eliminate differential diagnoses; (b) examine disease activity, impact, and control; and (c) find exacerbation triggers or underlying causes where necessary. The detailed history of chronic spontaneous urticaria or angioedema should include its frequency, conditions of occurrence, triggers, timing, mode of occurrence, and duration of the attack. The history and examination should also include the nature of the lesion, the area of involvement, and whether the lesions are itchy or painful. It is important to take a history of patients with urticaria, as aggravating triggers are variable. In patients with long-standing and uncontrolled disease, further diagnostic procedures need to be carefully determined to reveal the underlying causes. Photographing the lesion may be helpful in monitoring the progression of the lesion. A detailed family and medication history is as important as the treatment of the disease (Zuberbier et al., 2022). In spontaneous urticaria, disease activity should be assessed for clinical care and follow-up purposes with the Urticaria Activity Score 7 (UAS7) (Table 2), a simple scoring system recommended and validated in the latest version of the guidelines. UAS7 refers to the main urticarial symptoms documented by the patient, and it is based on the evaluation of symptoms (blisters and itching). Because the activity of the urticaria constantly varies, patients are advised to document 24-hour self-assessment scores once daily for several days to best measure disease activity. In clinical practice, the total UAS7 score is used for 7 consecutive days. In clinical practice as well as during follow-up, it is crucial to assess the influence of the disease not only on disease activity but also on quality of life and disease control (Hollis et al., 2018).

Recommendations of the guidelines during the diagnosis process:

- Routine diagnostic measures are not recommended in acute spontaneous urticaria.
- It is recommended that basic tests, including blood count, CRP, and/or ESR, be used routinely in chronic spontaneous urticaria.
- Based on the patient's history and physical examination, additional diagnostic tests are advised at the CSU, particularly for patients whose disease is chronic or out-of-control.
- It is recommended to calculate the UAS7 score at each visit for all patients with chronic urticaria (Hollis et al., 2018).

Diagnosis in Children

Urticaria can occur in all age groups, including infants and young children. Recent studies show that the prevalence and underlying causes of CIndUs and CSU are very similar to the prevalence and causes in adults, with some minor differences. Therefore, the diagnostic approaches for children should be similar to those for adults (Muraro et al., 2007).

Management of Urticaria

1. To cure the disease completely is the aim of treatment.
2. The therapy of CU can involve
   a. Identifying the underlying causes and removing them,
   b. avoiding triggers,
   c. inducing tolerance,
   d. and/or use of medications to stop the production of mast cell mediators or to counteract their effects.

3. Following the fundamental guidelines of treating as little and as much as necessary should guide treatment. Depending on the progression of the disease, this can include adjusting the therapy protocol.

Identifying Underlying Causes and How to Avoid Them

An accurate diagnosis is a fundamental requirement before removing an underlying cause. In most circumstances, it can be challenging to pinpoint the exact cause of CU; for instance, infections may be the cause, an aggravating factor, or something completely unrelated. Urticaria can spontaneously clear up at any time, and it is also possible for a suspected cause or trigger to be accidentally removed (Zuberbier et al., 2022).

Drugs that cause non-allergic hypersensitivity reactions (NSAIDs are the prototypical examples of these) can both trigger and aggravate pre-existing CSU, such that their elimination in the latter scenario will only relieve symptoms in some patients (Doña et al., 2014).

For the therapy of CIndUs, avoiding physical stimulation is ideal but frequently very challenging to accomplish. The patient should be sufficiently informed about the physical characteristics of the relevant stimulus to be able to identify and manage exposure in regular daily life (Trevisonno et al., 2015).

Many patients have low thresholds for the relevant physical triggers, making complete symptom avoidance nearly impossible. For instance, severe symptomatic dermographism is occasionally mistaken for CSU due to the appearance of spontaneous hives in areas where even loose clothing rubs against the skin of the patient or where unintentional patient scratching results in the development of wheals (Trevisonno et al., 2015).

Unlike CIndU, CSU is frequently linked to a number of inflammatory or infectious diseases, according to reports. These infections, which need to be properly treated, include bacterial infections of the nasopharynx and H. pylori in the gastrointestinal tract (Chen et al., 2021).

There is some evidence that suggests a correlation between disease activity and severity and stress levels, even though the mechanisms of stress-induced exacerbation have not been thoroughly studied. This is true for both physical and emotional stress, which in some cases may be important for the emergence of symptoms such as cholinergic urticaria (Zuberbier et al., 2022).

Some CSU patients have shown evidence of pseudo-allergic reactions (non-IgE-mediated hypersensitivity reactions) to naturally occurring dietary constituents and, occasionally, to food additives. Numerous studies in different nations have shown encouraging results when it comes to low-histamine diets and pseudoallergen-free diets, which contain only trace levels of natural and synthetic dietary pseudoallergens (McNeil et al., 2015).

Inducing Tolerance

In some subtypes of urticaria, inducing tolerance may be helpful. Examples include cold urticaria, cholinergic urticaria, and solar urticaria, all of which can be treated quickly with UV-A within three days. It is necessary to consistently expose yourself to the stimulus at the threshold level every day because tolerance induction only lasts for a few days. Patients frequently object to the induction and maintenance of tolerance. Take cold urticaria, for instance, where daily cold baths or showers are required to treat the condition (Beissert et al., 2000).

Pharmacological Treatment

Reducing the impact of mast cell mediators on target organs, such as histamine, PAF, and others, is the main strategy in therapies intended to relieve symptoms.

Antihistamines were the first agents used in the treatment of urticaria. Although older, first-generation H1 antagonists (e.g., diphenhydramine, hydroxyzine) are effective in resolving lesions and itching, they can cause many side effects such as drowsiness, anti-cholinergic and cognitive effects that last until the next day. Therefore, it may be beneficial to take these agents before bed. According to the EAACI/GA²LEN/EuroGuiDerm/APAAACI treatment guidelines (Figure 1), first-generation antihistamines should no longer be used as the first treatment option, except when second-generation antihistamines are not available or when the benefits outweigh the risks. The guideline does not recommend the use of older, first-generation antihistamines with sedating effects in patients with urticaria unless there is a specific indication. If patients using first-generation antihistamines work in jobs that require attention, they should be warned in advance to be careful due to the sedative effects of these drugs. Most patients benefit from oral H1 antagonists alone. Modern second-generation H1 antagonists are the first choice. If treatment with the standard dose is not sufficient, the dose can be increased up to four times. For refractory cases, H1 and H2 antagonists can be used together (Zuberbier et al., 2022).

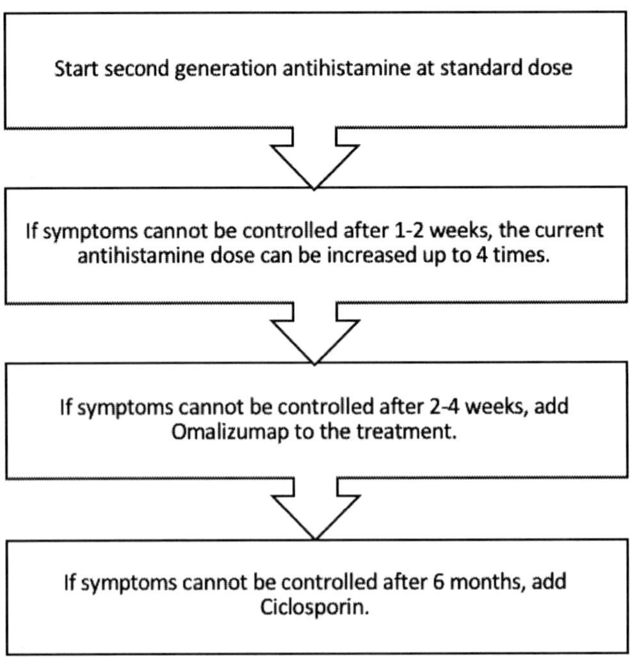

Figure 1. Recommended treatment algorithm for urticaria.

The newer second-generation antihistamines are not sedating in most patients. Side effects have been reported in a very small number of patients (cetirizine can cause drowsiness in up to 10% of patients). For this reason, many experts prefer to use these agents in patients with chronic urticaria while retaining first-generation agents for the treatment of acute or refractory urticaria. The most commonly used second-generation antihistamines are cetirizine, levocetirizine, desloratadine, loratadine, and fexofenadine. If necessary, it can be used four times a day in cases where symptom control is inadequate (Sharma et al., 2014).

Omalizumab (anti-IgE) treatment for CSU has been shown to be a very safe and effective treatment option. It has also been shown that omalizumab effectively treats CIndU, including cholinergic urticaria, cold urticaria, solar urticaria, heat urticaria, symptomatic dermographism, and delayed pressure urticaria. Omalizumab is safe for long-term treatment, efficiently treats recurrence after discontinuation in CSU patients, and greatly enhances quality of life. It also delays the onset of angioedema. In the CU, omalizumab is effective at doses ranging from 150 to 300 mg monthly. The total IgE in the serum does not have an effect on the dosage. In CSU, 300 mg are advised every four weeks. Different nations have different treatment durations and licensed doses (Zuberbier et al., 2022).

In terms of the release of mast cell mediators, Ciclosporin A also has a modest direct effect. In both placebo-controlled trials and open controlled trials in CSU, Ciclosporin A's efficacy in conjunction with a contemporary 2nd-generation H1-antihistamine was demonstrated. However, due to the higher incidence of side effects, this medication cannot be advised as standard care. The off-label use of closporin A for urticaria is only advised in cases where the condition is severe and has proven resistant to all doses of antihistamine and omalizumab combined. Contrasted with prolonged steroid use, ciclosporin A offers a much better risk/benefit ratio (Zuberbier et al., 2022).

Currently, topical corticosteroids are often and effectively used to treat a variety of allergic illnesses, although urticaria does not respond well to them. Prednisone doses between 20 and 50 mg/day are necessary if systemic corticosteroids are used, and long-term use of the drug inevitably results in side effects. It is strongly advised against using corticosteroids over an extended period of time outside of specialized clinics (Rutkowski & Grattan, 2017).

Conclusion

Although urticaria is one of the most common dermatoses, more research is required on the triggers and inflammatory processes that cause the disease and alternative medication options for the treatment of the disease.

References

Beissert, S., Stander, H., & Schwarz, T. (2000). UVA rush hardening for the treatment of solar urticaria. *Journal of the American Academy of Dermatology, 42*, 1030-1032. https://doi.org/10.1067/mjd.2000.104517.

Bernstein, J. A., Lang, D. M., Khan, D. A., Craig, T., Dreyfus, D., Hsieh, F., Sheikh, J., Weldon, D., Zuraw, B., Bernstein, D. I., Blessing-Moore, J., Cox, L., Nicklas, R. A., Oppenheimer, J., Portnoy, J. M., Randolph, C. R., Schuller, D. E., Spector, S. L., Tilles, S. A., & Wallace, D. (2014). The diagnosis and management of acute and chronic urticaria: 2014 update. *Journal of Allergy and Clinical Immunology, 133*(5), 1270-1277. https://doi.org/10.1016/j.jaci.2014.02.036.

Charlesworth, E. N. (1996). Urticaria and angioedema: A clinical spectrum. *Annals of Allergy, Asthma & Immunology, 76*(6), 484-495; quiz 495-499. https://doi.org/10.1016/S1081-1206(10)63267-X.

Chen, C. M., Huang, W. T., Chang, L. J., Hsu, C. C., & Hsu, Y. H. (2021). Peptic ulcer disease is associated with increased risk of chronic urticaria independent of *Helicobacter pylori* infection: A population-based cohort study. *American Journal of Clinical Dermatology, 22*, 129-137. https://doi.org/10.1007/s40257-020-00561-9.

Doña, I., Blanca-López, N., Torres, M. J., Gómez, F., Fernández, J., Zambonino, M. A., Monteseirín, F. J., Canto, G., Blanca, M., & Cornejo-García, J. A. (2014). NSAID-induced urticaria/angioedema does not evolve into chronic urticaria: A 12-year follow-up study. *Allergy, 69*, 438-444. https://doi.org/10.1111/all.12335.

Grattan, E. H. C. (2012). Urticaria and angioedema. In J. L. Bolognia (Ed.), *Dermatology* (pp. 291-306). Elsevier.

Hollis, K., Proctor, C., McBride, D., Balp, M. M., McLeod, L., Hunter, S., Tian, H., Khalil, S., & Maurer, M. (2018). Comparison of Urticaria Activity Score Over 7 Days (UAS7) values obtained from once-daily and twice-daily versions: Results from the ASSURE-CSU study. *American Journal of Clinical Dermatology, 19*(2), 267-274. https://doi.org/10.1007/s40257-017-0331-8.

McNeil, B. D., Pundir, P., Meeker, S., Han, L., Undem, B. J., Kulka, M., & Dong, X. (2015). Identification of a mast-cell-specific receptor crucial for pseudo-allergic drug reactions. *Nature, 519*, 237-241. https://doi.org/10.1038/nature14022.

Muraro, A., Roberts, G., Clark, A., Eigenmann, P. A., Halken, S., Lack, G., Moneret-Vautrin, A., Niggemann, B., & Rancé, F. (2007). The management of anaphylaxis in childhood: Position paper of the European academy of allergology and clinical immunology. *Allergy, 62*(8), 857-871. https://doi.org/10.1111/j.1398-9995.2007.01421.x.

Powell, R. J., Leech, S. C., Till, S., Huber, P. A., Nasser, S. M., & Clark, A. T. (2015). BSACI guideline for the management of chronic urticaria and angioedema. *Clinical & Experimental Allergy, 45*(3), 547-565. https://doi.org/10.1111/cea.12494.

Rutkowski, K., & Grattan, C. E. H. (2017). How to manage chronic urticaria 'beyond' guidelines: A practical algorithm. *Clinical & Experimental Allergy, 47*, 710-718. https://doi.org/10.1111/cea.12944.

Sharma, M., Bennett, C., Cohen, S. N., & Carter, B. (2014). H1-antihistamines for chronic spontaneous urticaria. *Cochrane Database of Systematic Reviews, 11*, Cd006137. https://doi.org/10.1002/14651858.CD006137.pub2.

Trevisonno, J., Balram, B., Netchiporouk, E., & Ben-Shoshan, M. (2015). Physical urticaria: Review on classification, triggers and management with special focus on prevalence including a meta-analysis. *Postgraduate Medicine, 127*, 565-570. https://doi.org/10.1080/00325481.2015.1045817.

Zuberbier, T., Abdul Latiff, A. H., Abuzakouk, M., Aquilina, S., Asero, R., Baker, D., Ballmer-Weber, B., Bangert, C., Ben-Shoshan, M., Bernstein, J. A., Bindslev-Jensen, C., Brockow, K., Brzoza, Z., Chong Neto, H. J., Church, M. K., Criado, P. R., Danilycheva, I. V., Dressler, C., Ensina, L. F., Fonacier, L., Gaskins, M., Gáspár, K., Gelincik, A., Giménez-Arnau, A., Godse, K., Gonçalo, M., Grattan, C., Grosber, M., Hamelmann, E., Hébert, J., Hide, M., Kaplan, A., Kapp, A., Kessel, A., Kocatürk, E., Kulthanan, K., Larenas-Linnemann, D., Lauerma, A., Leslie, T. A., Magerl, M., Makris, M., Meshkova, R. Y., Metz, M., Micallef, D., Mortz, C. G., Nast, A., Oude-Elberink, H., Pawankar, R., Pigatto, P. D., Ratti Sisa, H., Rojo Gutiérrez, M. I., Saini, S. S., Schmid-Grendelmeier, P., Sekerel, B. E., Siebenhaar, F., Siiskonen, H., Soria, A., Staubach-Renz, P., Stingeni, L., Sussman, G., Szegedi, A., Thomsen, S. F., Vadasz, Z., Vestergaard, C., Wedi, B., Zhao, Z., & Maurer, M. (2022). The international EAACI/GA²LEN/EuroGuiDerm/APAAACI guideline for the definition, classification, diagnosis, and management of urticaria. *Allergy, 77*, 734-766. https://doi.org/10.1111/all.15090.

Chapter 8

Eczema

Eda Türe*, MD

Department of Family Medicine, Samsun University Training and Research Hospital, Samsun, Turkey

Abstract

Eczema is a common skin disease worldwide that can affect individuals from infancy to adulthood. This skin reaction may show a chronic and recurrent clinical course due to endogenous and exogenous causes. Although the clinical course of eczema is defined as a temporary process, the patient can be diagnosed with mild and severe exacerbations from time to time. Skin irritation and loss of the protective barrier in patients may make them susceptible to infections. This skin condition may sometimes be accompanied by a food allergy. This may cause difficulty in diagnosis in infancy and early childhood. However, if the disease, whose very different etiological bases have been investigated, is sometimes an external cause, it can easily show a clinical recovery process with the removal of the causative agent. Therefore, in addition to an early and accurate diagnosis, different treatment strategies may need to be applied to patients.

Keywords: eczema, atopic dermatitis, prevention

Introduction

Skin tissue covers the entire body and serves as the first barrier in living things against external factors with its flora. Impaired skin barrier function, which may occur in patients for different reasons, may result in increased transepidermal water loss in the tissue. These changes in skin tissue may cause eczematous lesions to appear. While lesions can be seen in all age groups, the immune ability of the person and the persistence of the etiological cause may make the clinical picture chronic. The course of the disease is related to age and the chronic process. Eczema targets the epidermis as well as the dermis. It usually occurs in areas such as the face, hands, scalp, legs, elbows, back of the knees, and hips. Among the early findings, erythema, papules, and vesicles are frequently encountered in the affected skin area. However, cases diagnosed with serous exudate are also encountered. If there is a clinical process, the patient can be diagnosed with findings such as lesions, lichenification, and hyperpigmentation due to chronic

* Corresponding Author's Email: dr.edature@gmail.com.

In: Common Diseases According to Family Medicine Practice Guidelines
Editors: Esra Meltem Koç and Hilal Aksoy
ISBN: 979-8-89530-302-3

exposure to the agent (Raveendran, 2019; Lawton, 2009). Allergy-induced eczema can be seen together with different diseases such as allergic rhinitis and asthma based on immunological pathogenesis. Eczema, which is an inflammatory disease of the skin tissue, also has the potential to become chronic. This situation negatively affects the quality of life of individuals suffering from this disease. Additionally, in these patients, it is reported that the frequency of co-occurrence of anxiety and depression is increasing (Kouris et al., 2015).

Hand Eczema and Its Clinical Appearance

Hand eczema is an inflammatory skin reaction that can be seen throughout life. In this inflammatory reaction, the involvement of the hands and wrists, especially in the upper extremities, can accompany the clinical picture separately or together (Quaade et al., 2021). In fact, unless the endogenous and exogenous risk factors accompanying this disease, which are common in society, are eliminated, the patient's complaints continue. It is frequently emphasized in the literature that the most important underlying cause of the inflammatory reaction is atopic dermatitis. In particular, hand disinfectants, detergents, and surface cleaners that have the potential to irritate the skin may cause disruptions in treatment if the patient continues to use them. Irritation on the skin surface may cause changes in flora at different levels in the patient. There is an increase in wound infections, especially in these patients. In the results of the wound culture taken before treatment, S. aureus is isolated as the causative agent more frequently in patients (Agner & Elsner, 2020). To reduce contact allergy that develops due to exogenous factors, it is recommended to wash hands with soap, especially in healthcare units where frequent washing is required (Loh & Yew, 2022).

Eczema During Pregnancy

In light of different publications presented in the literature, it is suggested that atopic dermatitis or eczema may partially originate from the uterus. When we consider the issue for both the mother and the baby, genetic susceptibility and environmental interactions may affect the newly developing immune system. This may change the skin barrier, which has a protective function against the external environment, and cause damage. In this regard, it has been reported that daily 1000 IU cholecalciferol supplementation from the 14th week of pregnancy until birth may protect against infantile eczema in the first 12 months of life (El-Heis et al., 2022). Additionally, it makes recommendations for routine vitamin D supplementation during pregnancy, considering its effect on infantile eczema (Harvey et al., 2015).

Eczema in Infants

After birth, baby skin surface acidification, increased hydration in the first months, decreased hydration after months, and different levels of changes are observed in skin tissue cells (Fluhr et al., 2019). Eczema can occur in early infancy with skin irritation and deterioration of the skin barrier. Skin care is considered to be very effective in preventing infections, especially in premature newborns and babies with eczema. The main purpose here is to protect the immature skin barrier. In addition, the protective skin layer is defined as the stratum corneum. The maturation of this layer usually occurs in the third trimester, so stratum corneum hydration may not always be stable in premature newborns (Aksucu et al., 2022). These patients require attention in differential diagnosis in early childhood, as food allergy is added to the clinical picture (Kelleher et al., 2022). Inflammatory conditions such as seborrheic dermatitis, contact dermatitis, and nummular dermatitis seen during physical examination in infancy should be evaluated for eczema. If this patient group has a chronic course and is resistant to treatment, patients should be checked for the presence of immunodeficiency (Raveendran, 2019). In newborn skin care, personal experiences, individual training, as well as the developing socioeconomic environment become important. Due to the sensitive structure of newborn skin that needs protection, its anatomy and physiology need to be better understood. Natural products containing fewer additives may be preferred for individuals in the first years of life (Dyer, 2013).

Eczema in Elderly People

Today, as a result of new developments in the field of medicine, a significant increase is observed in the population of elderly individuals in society compared to the last century. One of the outpatient clinics that the elderly patient population frequently visits is undoubtedly the dermatology department. Eczema is also included in the differential diagnosis of many diseases that cause skin involvement, such as scabies, bullous pemphigoid, and mycosis fungoides. Additionally, antihypertensive drugs are frequently prescribed, especially when elderly patients apply to outpatient clinics. In different studies, antihypertensive drugs are preferred in this patient group. It is reported in the literature that eczema lesions may occur as a result of the use of effective drugs, especially calcium inhibitors and diuretics. Additionally, cases of de novo atopic dermatitis, which can be prevented by the use of locally effective skin softeners and steroid creams, have been described in these patients (Tétart & Joly, 2020).

Causes of Nummular Dermatitis

Nummular dermatitis is a skin condition of the type of eczematous dermatosis. Nummular eczema (NE) is a skin lesion that was first diagnosed by Marie Guillaume Alphonse Devergie in the 19th century (Iwahira et al., 2015). It can be diagnosed with numerous coin-shaped lesions during a general physical examination. Atopic dermatitis can appear as eczema. The avoidance of active ingredients and topical corticosteroids provides successful results in some cases. Although positive culture growth of Staphylococcus aureus, which causes a temporary change in the skin microflora, can also increase the severity of atopic dermatitis in cases (Kim et al., 2013). In the presence of infection, creams, and ointments containing topical antibiotics can be used (Robinson & Farci 2022). The use of tissue expanders and silicone implants has become very common today. In particular, these patients may develop nummular eczema during breast reconstruction. It is thought that skin lesions occur due to the disruption of the functioning of the sebaceous glands after surgical intervention (Iwhara et al., 2015). Although it has many side effects, isotretinoin preparations are frequently used in the treatment of cystic acne. However, this drug has some cutaneous or mucosal side effects and is frequently reported in the literature. Apart from common side effects such as xerosis and cheilitis, erythematous patches suggestive of nummular eczema have been reported to occur (Bettoli et al., 1987).

Eczema Treatment and Prevention

The aim of eczema treatment is to prevent transepidermal water loss in the skin tissue. Water loss appears to be a chronic problem, especially in eczema that enters the chronic process. In addition to the dermatological preparations used in these patients, daily skin care and warm water baths taken in the daily routine also contribute to the healing of the process. Another important issue is the choice of cosmetic products and soap. Soaps to be used by patients with eczema should be natural-based and mild, if possible. Additionally, preventing skin irritation should be the main goal when choosing soap. The use of products containing chemical additives and dyes should be avoided. Drying of the affected eczema skin area should be prevented in the working environment (Raveendran, 2019).

Conclusion

Eczema, a common inflammatory skin disorder, occurs as the result of a multifactorial etiology. Eczema, which can be seen in all age groups and genders, affects the patient's life in physical, financial, social, and psychological aspects. This effect paves the way for many different diseases in individuals whose quality of life is negatively affected. As a result, a multidisciplinary approach should be taken in the prevention and treatment of this common disease.

References

Agner, T., & Elsner, P. (2020). Hand eczema: epidemiology, prognosis and prevention. *Journal of the European Academy of Dermatology and Venereology: JEADV, 34 Suppl 1*, 4–12. https://doi.org/10.1111/jdv.16061.

Aksucu, G., Azak, M., & Çağlar, S. (2022). Effects of Topical Oils on Neonatal Skin: A Systematic Review. *Advances in skin & wound care, 35*(12), 1–9. https://doi.org/10.1097/01.ASW.0000891088.69828.2e.

Bettoli, V., Tosti, A., & Varotti, C. (1987). Nummular eczema during isotretinoin treatment. *Journal of the American Academy of Dermatology, 16*(3 Pt 1), 617. https://doi.org/10.1016/s0190-9622(87)80093-2.

Dyer, J. A. (2013). Newborn skin care. *Seminars in perinatology, 37*(1), 3–7. https://doi.org/10.1053/j.semperi.2012.11.008.

El-Heis, S., D'Angelo, S., Curtis, E. M., Healy, E., Moon, R. J., Crozier, S. R., Inskip, H., Cooper, C., Harvey, N. C., Godfrey, K. M., & MAVIDOS Trial Group. (2022). Maternal antenatal vitamin D supplementation and offspring risk of atopic eczema in the first 4 years of life: Evidence from a randomized controlled trial. *British Journal of Dermatology, 187*(5), 659-666. https://doi.org/10.1111/bjd.21721.

Fluhr, J. W., Bellemère, G., Ferrari, C., De Belilovsky, C., Boyer, G., Lachmann, N., McGuckin, C. P., Forraz, N., Darlenski, R., Chadoutaud, B., Msika, P., Baudouin, C., & Pellacani, G. (2019). Age-Dependent Transformation of Skin Biomechanical Properties and Micromorphology during Infancy and Childhood. *The Journal of investigative dermatology, 139*(2), 464–466. https://doi.org/10.1016/j.jid.2018.07.034.

Harvey, N. C., Holroyd, C., Ntani, G., Javaid, K., Cooper, P., Moon, R., Cole, Z., Tinati, T., Godfrey, K., Dennison, E., Bishop, N. J., Baird, J., & Cooper, C. (2014). Vitamin D supplementation in pregnancy: a systematic review. *Health technology assessment (Winchester, England)*, *18*(45), 1–190. https://doi.org/10.3310/hta18450.

Iwahira, Y., Nagasao, T., Shimizu, Y., Kuwata, K., & Tanaka, Y. (2015). Nummular Eczema of Breast: A Potential Dermatologic Complication after Mastectomy and Subsequent Breast Reconstruction. *Plastic surgery international*, *2015*, 209458. https://doi.org/10.1155/2015/209458.

Kelleher, M. M., Phillips, R., Brown, S. J., Cro, S., Cornelius, V., Carlsen, K. C. L., Skjerven, H. O., Rehbinder, E. M., Lowe, A. J., Dissanayake, E., Shimojo, N., Yonezawa, K., Ohya, Y., Yamamoto-Hanada, K., Morita, K., Axon, E., Cork, M., Cooke, A., Van Vogt, E., Schmitt, J., Weidinger, S., McClanahan, D., Simpson, E., Duley, L., Askie, L. M., Williams, H. C., & Boyle, R. J. (2022). Skin care interventions in infants for preventing eczema and food allergy. *The Cochrane database of systematic reviews*, *11*(11), CD013534. https://doi.org/10.1002/14651858.CD013534.pub3.

Kim, W. J., Ko, H. C., Kim, M. B., Kim, D. W., Kim, J. M., & Kim, B. S. (2013). Features of Staphylococcus aureus colonization in patients with nummular eczema. *The British journal of dermatology*, *168*(3), 658–660. https://doi.org/10.1111/j.1365-2133.2012.11072.x.

Kouris, A., Armyra, K., Christodoulou, C., Katoulis, A., Potouridou, I., Tsatovidou, R., Rigopoulos, D., & Kontochristopoulos, G. (2015). Quality of life, anxiety, depression and obsessive-compulsive tendencies in patients with chronic hand eczema. *Contact dermatitis*, *72*(6), 367–370. https://doi.org/10.1111/cod.12366.

Lawton, S. (2009). Assessing and treating adult patients with eczema. *Nursing standard (Royal College of Nursing (Great Britain) : 1987)*, *23*(43), 49–60. https://doi.org/10.7748/phc2010.05.20.4.32.c7770.

Loh, E. W., & Yew, Y. W. (2022). Hand hygiene and hand eczema: A systematic review and meta-analysis. *Contact dermatitis*, *87*(4), 303–314. https://doi.org/10.1111/cod.14133.

Quaade, A. S., Simonsen, A. B., Halling, A. S., Thyssen, J. P., & Johansen, J. D. (2021). Prevalence, incidence, and severity of hand eczema in the general population - A systematic review and meta-analysis. *Contact dermatitis*, *84*(6), 361–374. https://doi.org/10.1111/cod.13804.

Raveendran, R. (2019). Tips and Tricks for Controlling Eczema. *Immunology and allergy clinics of North America*, *39*(4), 521–533. https://doi.org/10.1016/j.iac.2019.07.006.

Robinson, C. A., Love, L. W., & Farci, F. (2022). Nummular Dermatitis. In *StatPearls*. StatPearls Publishing.

Tétart, F., & Joly, P. (2020). Eczema in elderly people. *European journal of dermatology: EJD*, *30*(6), 663–667. https://doi.org/10.1684/ejd.2020.3915.

Chapter 9

Scabies

Merve Alban[1,*], MD
and Mutlu Çoban[2], MD
[1]Department of Family Medicine, Izmir Katip Çelebi University, Atatürk Training and Research Hospital, Izmir, Turkey
[2]Department of Dermatology, Mutlu Çoban Dermatology Clinic, Aydın, Turkey

Abstract

Scabies is a contagious skin disease caused by Sarcoptes scabiei var hominis, a human ectoparasite, affecting approximately 300 million people worldwide each year (Hicks & Elston, 2009; Banerji, 2015). While it affects individuals of all races, genders, ages, and socioeconomic levels, it can cause outbreaks in densely populated areas where necessary hygiene conditions cannot be met (Cetin, 2017; Banerji, 2015; Akgöl & Köroğlu, 2022). It is transmitted through direct physical contact from person to person (Cetin, 2017). Itching, which intensifies at night, similar complaints in the immediate vicinity, and typically located lesions are indicative of diagnosis (Hicks & Elston, 2009; Cetin, 2017). The definitive diagnosis is based on the microscopic identification of mites, eggs, or feces from a skin scraping treated with 10% KOH (Cetin, 2017; Hicks & Elston, 2009). Treatment includes topical permethrin, benzyl benzoate, sulfur, and lindane, as well as oral ivermectin (Akgöl & Köroğlu, 2022; Cetin, 2017).

Keywords: scabies, sarcoptes scabies, scabies disease, permethrin, ivermectin

Introduction

The words "sarcopt" and "scabies" originate in Greek, derived from "sarx" (flesh), "coptein" (to cut), and "scabere" (to scratch) (Şimşek et al., 2019). The parasitic agent responsible for scabies was first discovered by the Italian physician Giovan Cosimo Bonomo and pharmacist Diacinto Cestoni in 1687. Although its etiology was not fully understood during Aristotle's time, it was first described as "akari" and has been referred to by different names in various sources since then. It is believed that Napoleon I suffered from scabies throughout most of his life due to the itching he experienced (Silva, 1998).

* Corresponding Author's Email: mervealban@gmail.com.

In: Common Diseases According to Family Medicine Practice Guidelines
Editors: Esra Meltem Koç and Hilal Aksoy
ISBN: 979-8-89530-302-3

Etiology

Scabies is a contagious parasitic skin infection caused by Sarcoptes scabiei var. hominis, an obligatory human parasite (Widaty et al., 2022; Yürekli, 2022; Sunderkötter et al., 2021; Cetin, 2017). The adult female sarcopt is approximately 0.3 × 0.4 mm in size, has eight legs and is about twice the size of the male sarcopt, making them invisible to the naked eye (Yürekli & Botsali, 2022; Sunderkötter et al., 2021). S. scabiei has an oval, single-segmented body and is dirty white in color. Humans are the only host for S. scabiei. It spends its entire life cycle in tunnels (burrows) within the stratum corneum layer of the human epidermis (Yücel & Yılmaz, 2021). Pregnant female mites burrow tunnels approximately 0.5-5 mm per day in the stratum corneum, the outermost layer of the skin, and typically remain in these tunnels for the rest of their 4-6 week lifespan, laying 2-3 eggs per day (Karimkhani et al., 2017; Sunderkötter et al., 2021). Some theories suggest that these parasites create tunnels close to the surface without penetrating deeper layers to meet their oxygen needs through diffusion from the skin (Yürekli, 2023).

Epidemiology

Scabies is a significant health problem in many developing countries; in 2009, the World Health Organization declared scabies a neglected skin disease (Anderson & Strowd, 2017). It is a widespread skin disease that can be seen not only in low socioeconomic groups, but also in developed countries and worldwide (Arora et al., 2020). Although it can occur at any age, it is more common in children and young adults (Karthikeyan, 2007). An average of 300 million cases are reported annually worldwide (Hengge et al., 2006). The prevalence globally ranges from 0.2% to 71%, with increases due to war and migration; during World War II, there were over 2 million cases, and regional outbreaks are known to occur in Turkey from time to time (Akgöl & Köroğlu, 2022). Transmission occurs most frequently through sexual contact but can also happen through close contact and the use of shared spaces and items (Yürekli, 2022). Common areas where transmission occurs frequently include communal living spaces such as hospitals, nursing homes, boarding schools, detention centers, and military barracks (Mounsey et al., 2013). It is estimated that scabies is responsible for 0.07% of diseases worldwide (Mumcuoğlu et al., 2023).

Diagnosis

Scabies diagnosis involves methods such as the "Ink Test" and "Topical Tetracycline Test" to identify tunnels, biopsy techniques like "Epidermal Shave Biopsy," and examination of skin scrapings to detect Sarcoptes adult larvae, nymphs, and/or eggs. The most commonly preferred and oldest method among these is the examination of skin scrapings (Yücel & Yılmaz, 2021). Sarcoptes can also be visualized by dermatologists using a device called a dermatoscope (Karimkhani et al., 2017; Yürekli & Botsali, 2022; Yücel & Yılmaz, 2021). Clinically inconspicuous scabies infection can be detected by a polymerase chain reaction (PCR) test through amplification of Sarcoptes DNA on the epidermal scale, and high IgE titers and eosinophilia can be observed (Bezold et al., 2001).

Differential Diagnosis

Scabies often mimics other pruritic skin conditions such as atopic or contact dermatitis, prurigo nodularis, folliculitis, impetigo, papular urticaria, dermatitis herpetiformis, and insect bites (Koç & Açıkel, 2023; Chouela et al., 2002).

Clinical Findings

Scabies can present in two forms: classic and crusted. Clinical symptoms appear approximately 2-6 weeks after infestation (Vasanwala et al., 2019; Sunderkötter et al., 2021; Cetin, 2017). The hands are the most common site of infestation (Yücel & Yılmaz, 2021). The most common type in humans, Sarcoptes scabiei var. hominis, typically resides in the finger web spaces, flexor surfaces of the wrists, feet, and ankles, nipples in women, and the penile shaft in men. The lesions present as classic burrows, erythematous itchy papules, pustules, vesicles, and/or inflammatory nodules (Mumcuoğlu et al., 2023; Zhao et al., 2023).

The skin lesions are slightly raised, brownish, pink-white colored burrows that extend 0.5-2 mm per day. At the end of the tunnel, there are vesicles the size of a pinhead, resembling pearls, containing female Sarcoptes mites. These tunnels and vesicles are areas where mites are densely located and are crucial for clinical diagnosis (Yücel & Yılmaz, 2021).

Nodular scabies, seen in about 7-10% of patients and more frequently in men, are characterized by inflamed, itchy, persistent, rough, hard, round nodules that are red, reddish-brown, or livid in color (Zhao et al., 2023). Antigens from the parasite cause an itchy hypersensitive reaction approximately 3-6 weeks after the initial infestation (Mumcuoğlu et al., 2023). Although not specific to scabies, itching that worsens at night and with high temperatures is typical (Sunderkötter et al., 2021).

Severe itching that intensifies at night, widespread maculopapular rash, the typical distribution of the lesions (palms, the finger web spaces, soles, around the navel, wrists, and the genital area), and the history of similar symptoms in close contacts (household members with a history of scabies or similar rash and itching) suggest scabies (Cetin, 2017; Şimşek et al., 2019).

In the extremely contagious form known as Norwegian scabies, typically seen in disabled or immunosuppressed individuals, itching is less pronounced. Hyperkeratosis in the nails, hyperkeratotic papules and plaques in the body, and especially lesions located on the head and neck are typical (Koç & Açıkel, 2023).

Treatment

Before treatment, factors such as the patient's age, clinical condition, immunity, pregnancy-lactation status in women of reproductive age, the presence of additional dermatological conditions, potential harms of medications, cost-effectiveness, availability of the drug, and previous treatment resistance history are important. The most crucial aspect of treatment is patient compliance (Akgöl & Köroğlu, 2022).

There are various treatments for scabies. Topical permethrin 5% is widely used and is the most effective agent, with pregnancy category B (Cetin, 2017). However, resistance to this treatment, challenges in patient compliance, and allergic reactions should not be overlooked. Some studies have shown that 1% permethrin cream is more effective than lindane in the treatment of lice and is safer due to lower systemic absorption. In scabies treatment, a single application of 5% permethrin is expected to achieve a response of over 90%, and a second course can increase treatment success (Cox, 2000). Before topical treatment, the skin should be cool and dry, and the treatment should cover all skin areas, including the scalp, external genital organs, groin, navel, between the fingers and toes, and nail edges. The treatment should be applied at night and washed off after 8-12 hours. A second course should be applied 7-14 days later. All individuals in close contact with the patient must undergo the same treatment simultaneously (Cetin, 2017).

Underwear, towels, and bed sheets should be washed in a machine (at ≥ 50°C), dry cleaned, or stored in a sealed plastic bag for a week (Cetin, 2017).

Other treatment options include topical lindane, 5% precipitated sulfur, malathion, and topical and oral ivermectin. However, lindane, also known as gamma benzene hexachloride, is no longer used due to potential neurotoxic effects (Cetin, 2017). Factors such as resistance to S. scabiei, cost, availability, and potential toxicity, especially in children and pregnant women, limit the use of these treatments (Anderson & Strowd, 2017).

Benzyl benzoate, a component of Peru balsam, was first used against scabies in 1932, and its mechanism of action is unknown (Holst et al., 2000). Benzyl benzoate can be used alone (10% and 25% lotions) or with sulfur, and different application protocols exist. It can be applied once or twice on the same day, 10 minutes apart; or once every 24 hours or once a week (Buffet & Dupin, 2003). It is contraindicated in pregnant and breastfeeding women and children under 2 years old. It can cause skin irritation and burning sensation, leading to eczematous skin reactions (Akgöl & Köroğlu, 2022).

Sulfur preparations, although malodorous, are preferred agents due to cost-effectiveness. In our country, they are the first-choice alternative to permethrin. For adults, precipitated sulfur is applied in 10% Vaseline and 5% ointment for children. There is also Wilkinson ointment, containing cade oil and sulfur (Akgöl & Köroğlu, 2022).

One of the topical treatments, crotamiton, is less effective than permethrin and lindane, and resistance has been reported after a single application of 8-12 hours (Chouela et al., 2002).

Oral ivermectin, a safe and well-tolerated anthelmintic, is frequently used in scabies treatment (Koç & Açıkel, 2023; Chouela et al., 2002). A second course of ivermectin is recommended between the second and third days of egg hatching and between the seventh and fifteenth days when fertilized female mites start laying new eggs (Koç & Açıkel, 2023). Levy et al., found that ivermectin was more effective than lindane and benzyl benzoate when used as a single dose but less effective than permethrin. However, when a second dose of ivermectin was administered, it had a comparable efficacy to permethrin. In many countries, oral ivermectin for scabies treatment is approved by the US Food and Drug Administration (FDA) and is recommended at 200 micrograms/kg, with two doses one week apart (Levy et al., 2019; Maghrabi et al., 2014; Salavastru et al., 2017). However, its use is not approved for infants and children weighing less than 15 kg (Levy et al., 2019). A study by Maghrabi and colleagues indicated that surgical debridement is a complementary treatment that enhances the success of topical and systemic treatments in Norwegian crusted scabies (Maghrabi et al., 2014).

Conclusion

Scabies is a highly contagious disease that affects individuals of all socioeconomic backgrounds, particularly in impoverished and densely populated areas, spreading through close contact. The risk of scabies is significantly higher in young children, the elderly, and immunocompromised individuals. It is a disease that can lead to depression, insomnia, secondary infections, and associated complications, as well as financial burdens, and can cause social stigma (Yazar et al., 2012; Banerji, 2015). Occasionally, scabies cases with atypical presentations are misdiagnosed, prolonging the condition. Incorrect treatments with topical corticosteroids can suppress symptoms, making the condition more atypical and complicating the diagnosis (Şen et al., 2013). Delays in diagnosis and treatment significantly negatively impact the quality of life (Turan & Metin, 2021). Early diagnosis, treatment, and adherence to hygiene rules are crucial in preventing transmission and outbreaks (Sofuoğlu, 2023).

References

Akgöl, J., & Köroğlu, A. (2022). Scabies, scabies treatment and plants used in the treatment of scabies. *Ankara Ecz. Fak. Derg./J. Fac. Pharm. Ankara, 46*(2), 600-618. https://doi.org/10.33483/jfpau.1085681.

Anderson, K. L., & Strowd, L. C. (2017). Epidemiology, diagnosis, and treatment of scabies in a dermatology office. *JABFM, 30*(1). https://doi.org/10.3122/jabfm.2017.01.160190.

Arora, P., Rudnicka, L., Sar-Pomian, M., Wollina, U., Jafferany, M., Lotti, T., Sadoughifar, R., Sitkowska, Z., & Goldust, M. (2020). Scabies: A comprehensive review and current perspectives. *Dermatologic Therapy, 33*(4), e13746. https://doi.org/10.1111/dth.13746.

Arslan, H., & Gündüz, Ö. (2023). Bullous scabies, the light shed on etiopathogenesis and treatment: Report of five paediatric cases. *Postepy Dermatol Alergol, 40*(3), 432-436. https://doi.org/10.5114/ada.2023.128976.

Banerji, A. (2015). Scabies. *Paediatrics & Child Health, 20*(7), 395-402. https://doi.org/10.1093/pch/20.7.395.

Bezold, G., Lange, M., Schiener, R., Palmedo, G., Sander, C. A., Kerscher, M., & Peter, R. U. (2001). Hidden scabies: Diagnosis by polymerase chain reaction. *British Journal of Dermatology, 144*(3), 614-618. https://doi.org/10.1046/j.1365-2133.2001.04096.x.

Buffet, M., & Dupin, N. (2003). Current treatments for scabies. *Fundamental & Clinical Pharmacology, 17*, 217-225. https://doi.org/10.1046/j.1472-8206.2003.00173.x.

Cetin, B. S. (2017). Uyuz Hastalığına Yaklaşım (Güncel Kılavuz Değerlendirmesi). *J Pediatr Inf, 11*(2), 107-109. https://doi.org/10.5578/ced.201727.

Chouela, E., Abeldaño, A., Pellerano, G., & Hernández, M. I. (2002). Diagnosis and treatment of scabies: A practical guide. *American Journal of Clinical Dermatology, 3*(1), 9-18. https://doi.org/10.2165/00128071-200203010-00002.

Cox, N. H. (2000). Permethrin treatment in scabies infestation: Importance of the correct formulation. *BMJ, 320*(7226), 37-38. https://doi.org/10.1136/bmj.320.7226.37.

Feng, S., Shi, M., Yin, Z., Di, W., Guillot, J., & Fang, F. (2023). Can ivermectin kill Sarcoptes scabiei during the molting process? *PLoS Neglected Tropical Diseases, 17*(5), e0011337. https://doi.org/10.1371/journal.pntd.0011337.

Hengge, U. R., Currie, B. J., Jäger, G., Lupi, O., & Schwartz, R. A. (2006). Scabies: A ubiquitous neglected skin disease. *Lancet Infectious Diseases, 6*(12), 769-779. https://doi.org/10.1016/S1473-3099(06)70654-5.

Hicks, M. I., & Elston, D. M. (2009). Scabies. *Dermatologic Therapy, 22*(4), 279-292. https://doi.org/10.1111/j.1529-8019.2009.01243.x.

Holst, R. F., Rufli, T., & Christophers, E. (2000). Die Skabiestherapie unter besonderer Berücksichtigung des frühen Kindesalters, der Schwangerschaft und Stillzeit. *Hautarzt, 51*(7), 7-13. https://doi.org/10.1007/s001050050003.

Karimkhani, C., Colombara, D. V., Drucker, A. M., et al., (2017). The global burden of scabies: A cross-sectional analysis from the Global Burden of Disease Study 2015. *Lancet Infectious Diseases, 17*, 1247-1254. https://doi.org/10.1016/S1473-3099(17)30483-8.

Karthikeyan, K. (2007). Scabies in children. *Archives of Disease in Childhood - Education & Practice Edition, 92*(3), ep65-69. https://doi.org/10.1136/adc.2005.073825.

Koç, H. A., & Açıkel, S. Ü. (2023). Scabies: Clinical signs, diagnosis and current treatment. *Archives of Current Medical Research, 4*(2), 62-69. https://doi.org/10.47482/acmr.1244299.

Levy, M., Martin, L., Bursztejn, A. C., Chiaverini, C., Miquel, J., Mahé, E., Maruani, A., & Boralevi, F. (2020). Ivermectin safety in infants and children under 15 kg treated for scabies: A multicentric observational study. *British Journal of Dermatology, 182*(4), 1003-1006. https://doi.org/10.1111/bjd.18369.

Mounsey, K. E., McCarthy, J. S., & Walton, S. F. (2013). Scratching the itch: New tools to advance understanding of scabies. *Trends in Parasitology, 29*(1), 35-42. https://doi.org/10.1016/j.pt.2012.09.006.

Maghrabi, M. M., Lum, S., Joba, A. T., Meier, M. J., Holmbeck, R. J., & Kennedy, K. (2014). Norwegian crusted scabies: An unusual case presentation. *Journal of Foot & Ankle Surgery, 53*, 62-66. https://doi.org/10.1053/j.jfas.2013.09.002.

Mumcuoğlu, K. Y., Şenel, E., & Özkan, A. T. (2023). Scientometric evaluation of the itch mite, Sarcoptes scabiei (Acari: Sarcoptidae): The last four decades of global academic output on scabies. *Turkiye Parazitol Derg, 47*(3), 171-178. https://doi.org/10.4274/tpd.galenos.2023.51423.

Salavastru, C. M., Chosidow, O., Boffa, M. J., Janier, M., & Tiplica, G. S. (2017). European guideline for the management of scabies. *Journal of the European Academy of Dermatology and Venereology, 31*(8), 1248-1253. https://doi.org/10.1111/jdv.14351.

Silva, M. R. (1998). Giovan Cosimo Bonomo (1663–1696): Discoverer of the etiology of scabies. *International Journal of Dermatology, 37*, 625-630. https://doi.org/10.1046/j.1365-4362.1998.00323.x.

Sofuoğlu, K., Atış, T. H., Yıldız, İ., Uraz, M., Ertabaklar, H., & Okyay, P. (2023). Uyuz Hastalığı Korkusu Ölçeğinin Türkçe Formunun Geçerlik Güvenirlik Çalışması. *Halk Sağlığı Araştırma ve Uygulamaları Dergisi, 1*(1), 71-80. https://doi.org/10.5281/zenodo.10433342.

Sunderkötter, C., Wohlrab, J., & Hamm, H. (2021). Scabies: Epidemiology, diagnosis, and treatment. *Deutsches Ärzteblatt International, 118*(41), 695-704. https://doi.org/10.3238/arztebl.m2021.0296.

Şen, B. B., Rifaioğlu, E. N., Ekiz, Ö., Aksakal, M., Gökçe, H., & Doğramacı, A. Ç. (2013). Mastositozu taklit eden skabiyez inkognito. *Med J SDU Tıp Fak Derg: Çocuk Özel Sayısı,* 1-4. https://dergipark.org.tr/tr/pub/sdutfd/issue/24701/261248.

Şimşek, E., Keskin, A., & Dağcıoğlu, B. F. (2019). Common and frequently overlooked disease scabies: Case report. *Ankara Medical Journal,* (1), 205-209. https://doi.org/10.17098/amj.542208.

Turan, Ç., & Metin, N. (2021). Pandeminin Skabiyez Sıklığı Üzerindeki Etkisi: COVID-19 Sonrasında Olası Skabiyez Salgını Senaryosu. *Turkiye Parazitol Derg, 45*(3), 190-194. https://doi.org/10.4274/tpd.galenos.2021.7236.

Vasanwala, F. F., Ong, C. Y., Aw, C. W. D., & How, C. H. (2019). Management of scabies. *Singapore Medical Journal, 60*(6), 281-285. https://doi.org/10.11622/smedj.2019058.

Veraldi, S., Schianchi, R., Silvio, M., & Aromolo, I. F. (2023). Pseudoresistance to permethrin in scabies. *Journal of Infection in Developing Countries, 17*(5), 713-715. https://doi.org/10.3855/jidc.17750.

Widaty, S., Miranda, E., Cornain, E. F., & Rizky, L. A. (2022). Scabies: Update on treatment and efforts for prevention and control in highly endemic settings. *Journal of Infection in Developing Countries, 16*(2), 244-251. https://doi.org/10.3855/jidc.15222.

Yücel, A., & Yılmaz, M. (2021). Prevalence of Sarcoptes scabiei in patients with suspected scabies. *Turkiye Parazitol Derg, 45*(2), 133-136. https://doi.org/10.4274/tpd.galenos.2021.6874.

Yürekli, A. (2022). Is there really resistance to scabies treatment with permethrin? In vitro killing activity of permethrin on Sarcoptes scabiei from patients with resistant scabies. *Dermatologic Therapy, 35*, e15260. https://doi.org/10.1111/dth.15260.

Yürekli, A. (2023). How does Sarcoptes scabiei var. hominis meet its oxygen needs? *Journal of the American Academy of Dermatology, 89*(4), e161-e162. https://doi.org/10.1016/j.jaad.2023.05.055.

Yürekli, A., & Botsali, A. (2022). Can we increase the success of scabies treatment? The effect of removing tunnels from patients in the success of scabies treatment. *Dermatologic Therapy,* e15701. https://doi.org/10.1111/dth.15701.

Yürekli, A., Can, İ., & Oğuz, M. (2023). Using ultraviolet light in diagnosing scabies: Scabies' Sign via Wood's Lamp. *Journal of the American Academy of Dermatology, 89*(5), e195-e196. https://doi.org/10.1016/j.jaad.2023.07.006.

Zhao, Y. K., Lu, J. F., Liu, J. H., Wu, H. H., Song, L. L., Wan, C. L., & Luo, D. Q. (2023). Recalcitrant nodular scabies showing excellent response to tofacitinib: Five case reports. *Therapeutic Advances in Chronic Disease, 14*, 1-7. https://doi.org/10.1177/20406223231195632.

Yazar, S., Kuk, S., Çetinkaya, Ü., Gözgenç, N., & Şahin, İ. (2012). Uyuz ön tanılı hastalarda Sarcoptes scabiei araştırılması. *Kafkas Üniversitesi Veteriner Fakültesi Dergisi, 18*(Suppl-A), A85-A87. https://doi.org/10.9775/kvfd.2011.6059.

Chapter 10

Fungal Infections

Volkan Atasoy*, MD

Department of Family Medicine, University of Health Sciences,
Trabzon Faculty of Medicine, Trabzon, Turkey

Abstract

More than 400 species of fungi can cause disease in humans. Changes in climate, migration and an increasing number of people with weakened immune systems have accelerated the incidence of fungal infections. In the United States alone, there are nearly 9 million outpatient visits annually for fungal infections. New fungal species that can develop antifungal resistance, such as Candida auris, raise concerns about treatment. Thus, it is important that primary care physicians understand the dermatological signs of fungal infections so they know how to identify them. Dermatophytoses is a common clinic manifestation among fungal infections affecting individuals of all ages around the world. These infections can easily be diagnosed by tests conducted in primary care settings. A delay in diagnosis results can cause complications and increase a patient's economic burden. Nevertheless, oral antifungal therapy should not be prescribed until the pathogen fungal organism has been identified, except in certain circumstances. Referral to a specialist is required for systemic forms or resistance to initial therapy. Family physicians should warn their patients about predisposing factors of fungal infections such as wearing tight clothing, walking barefoot, and traveling to endemic regions.

Keywords: dermatophytoses, fungal infection, mycoses, primary healthcare

Introduction

In clinical dermatology practice, fungal infections are often identified by the depth of the infected skin area. Classification based on the route of acquisition categorizes mycoses according to the entry source into the host's body: exogenous when transmitted via airborne, cutaneous, or subcutaneous routes, and endogenous when resulting from the colonization or reactivation of normal flora. Classification based on virulence categorizes mycoses into primary pathogens, which can infect normal hosts, and opportunistic pathogens, which cause disease when there is a deficiency in the host's defenses. The organization of mycosis infections

* Corresponding Author's Email: drvova@hotmail.com.

In: Common Diseases According to Family Medicine Practice Guidelines
Editors: Esra Meltem Koç and Hilal Aksoy
ISBN: 979-8-89530-302-3

consists of superficial, cutaneous, subcutaneous, and deep (systemic) fungal infections. Fungal skin infections are among the common causes of skin illnesses (Nigat et al., 2023). Approximately two billion people worldwide are affected by fungal infections of the skin, hair, and nails, while millions suffer from Candida infections and systemic forms (Howell, 2023). Fungi have a worldwide domain and can affect people of all ages. Indeed, fungal infections are often associated with certain host factors such as occupation, living geographic area, use of systemic anti-bacterial drugs, and immunosuppressive conditions that can facilitate the occurrence. Direct contact with infected material or traumatic inoculation into the dermis are potential routes for initiating infection. Chronic diseases and medications that causes immunodeficiency may be underlying factors resulting in treatment resistance or recurrence.

Fungal infections are easy to diagnose and treat but, if not managed properly, they can spread and become permanent, leading to dangerous complications, reducing quality of life and disrupting social relationships (Bewley, 2017). Diagnosis is typically based on a visual examination of relevant clinical signs, supported by patient history. Microscopic evaluation of skin scrapings, dermoscopy, and fungal culture are also commonly used diagnostic procedures, especially for cutaneous forms. Systemic fungal infections may require skin biopsy, blood tests for serology, or image-based approaches. Histological studies constitute the gold standard in the diagnosis of fungal infections (Howell, 2023). Treatment includes topical antifungal creams and gels, oral antifungal agents, and many other medications. Meanwhile, increasing antifungal resistance deserves a global attention. Fungi are now developing resistance to commonly used agents through novel mutations in their genes, and dermatophytes and non-dermatophyte molds and/or yeasts can cause mixed infections, leading to a growing problem in the treatment of superficial mycoses (Gupta et al., 2021). To overcome treatment failures and prevent fungal infections, early detection of clinical signs and implementation of evidence-based treatment in accordance with current guidelines is essential. Public Health England's guidance for the management offungal skin and nail infections provides a quick reference tool for primary care professionals to diagnose and treat uncomplicated cases based on clinical signs (Public Health England, 2009).

Main Body

Superficial Fungal Infections

These infections take place in the non-living superficial layer of the skin and do not trigger a host cellular response. They are limited to the stratum corneum of the epidermis and targets skin, hair and nail tissues. They originate from human, animal, or soil sources. They are mostlycurable. Clinical patterns include Pityriasis versicolor, Tinea nigra, White piedra, and Black piedra.

Pityriasis Versicolor

Pityriasis versicolor occurs when the pathogenic mycelial form of Malassezia yeast invades the stratum corneum. It presents with macules, patches, and thin plaques with areas of hypopigmented or hyperpigmented skin on the neck, shoulders, chest, and back (Leung et al., 2022). This distribution is consistent with the lipid-dependent nature of the causative organism, which requires rich sebum production. The prevalence is higher in tropical regions of the earth, suggesting that heat, humidity, and hyperhidrosis are risk factors. Diagnosis depends on clinical features, but a potassium hydroxide (KOH) preparation from scraped skin under a light microscope shows the diagnostic 'spaghetti and meatballs' pattern. Initial topical antifungal therapy includesketoconazole (2% shampoo, 2% cream), ciclopirox olamine (1.5% shampoo), miconazole (cream), clotrimazole (cream), terbinafine (cream, jel), and miscellaneous products of selenium sulfide (2.5% shampoo), zinc pyrithione (1% shampoo), propylene glycol (50% in water). If topical agents are ineffective or cannot be applied, oral antifungal drugs flucanazole and itraconazole are primarily recommended (Hald et al., 2015). In case of treatment failure, it is rational to reevaluate the diagnosis. Even after successful treatment, skin discoloration may persist for weeks to several months. Maintenance therapy may be required in patients with recurrence, which is common in Pityriasis versicolor. In this situation, applying selenium sulfide 2.25% shampoo or ketoconazole 2% shampoo once a month may be preferred.

Tinea Nigra

Tinea Nigra is a rare disease mostly caused by the pigmented yeast-like fungus Hortaeawerneckii, which accounts for less than 1% of superficial fungal infections. Although it is common in children and young adults, individuals of all ages, regardless of gender, can suffer from this condition. The clinical picture is usually an asymptomatic, unilateral hyper pigmented patch on the palm (Lee & Schwartz, 2022). Less popular areas are the fingers, between the toes, and the soles of the feet. The typical lesion is brown to grey-green in colour, has sharp edges, and is velvety or slightly scaly. The aquatic environment of tropical climates plays a role in the formation of hyperhidrosis that provides a suitable media for the reproduction of the organism (Bonifaz et al., 2010). Physical examination and history of predisposing factors support the diagnosis. Dermoscopy, KOH preparation, culture, and Wood's lamp examination are useful diagnostic procedures. Skin biopsy is required for the differential diagnosis of melanoma, palmar lichen planus, phytophotodermatitis and drug eruptions. In the absence of randomized studies, treatment of tinea nigra is based on evidence from clinical experience and small case series. Cream forms of imidazole's (ketoconazole 2%, bifonazole 1%, terbinafine 1% cream) and keratolytics (Whitfield's ointment; contains salicylic acid 3% and benzoic acid 6%) are used effectively (Bonifaz et al., 2008).

Piedra

Piedra is a fungal infection of the hair shaft with nodular concretions. There are two subtypes: white piedra, caused by pathogenic Trichosporon species, and black piedra, caused by Piedraiahortae. White piedra is characterized by white-brown nodules and predominantly affects facial, axillary, and genital hair. Black piedra has a resemblance to scalp hair, appearing with stone-like brown concretions, especially on the frontal scalp (Schwartz, 2004). Diagnosis is made by microscopic examination of the KOH preparation, but fungal culture provides a confirmed diagnosis. The best treatment for both White and Black piedra is to shave the infected hair, which is almost curable, and use a 1/1000 sublimate solution in 60% alcohol after trichotomy. Ketoconazole shampoo and systemic antifungals may be preferred in patients who avoid epilation and to prevent recurrence (Dias et al., 2013).

Cutaneous Fungal Infections

These infections affect the superficial keratinized layer of non-living tissues in the skin, creating a pathological response in the host by the metabolic products of the infectious agent. Dermatophytoses, dermatomycosis, and candidiasis are prominent members. The diseases under this heading primarily consist of fungal infections that family physicians can manage within the scope of primary care practice.

Tinea Capitis

Tinea capitis (TC) is a dermatophyte infection of the scalp and hair that is particularly common in prepubertal children aged 3-7 years (Fuller et al., 2014). Its incidence in infants is low and its occurrence may be related to immune deficiency. Although numerous organisms associated with different clinical types have been identified, the generaMicrosporum and Trichophytonpre dominate. M.Microsporum canis is a widespread organism throughout Europe, and T.tonsurans has superseded it in the United States (Mayser et al., 2020). The clinical appearance of TC varies depending on etiological factors, such as a gray patch, black dot, and favus appearance. Itching is a common symptom across species. Scaly and crusty patches several centimeters in size, along with alopecic areas and erythema, are visible features. Generalized scaling of the scalp may also occur without hair loss. Kerion is a progressive form of TC due to the host's hypersensitivity reaction to infection. Boggy, inflammatory plaques with pustules that can lead to pain, posterior lymphadenopathy, and fever are characteristic. Another unusual form, favus, develops mainly after T.Trichophyton schoenleinii infection and is characterized by yellow, cup-shaped lesions. If not treated appropriately it can result in cicatricial alopecia. The differential diagnosis of TC includes seborrheic dermatitis, alopecia areata, atopic dermatitis, psoriasis capitis, and bacterial folliculitis.

Typical features onphysical examination usually determine the diagnosis. Wood's light examination, dermoscopy, culture, and molecular methods are thefore most diagnostic aids. Fungal cultures are more sensitive than microscopy and the KOH preparation, but should be stored on agar for 3 to 4 weeks and observed at weekly intervals. An easy sampling technique is to moisten a cotton applicator or toothbrush with water and rub it to the lesion. Sabouraud agar or dermatophyte test medium is preferred for the application of samples. Wood lamp examination is useful for M. canis, which reflects green fluorescence, but is not for T. tonsurans, which does not reflect fluorescence. To achieve clinical and mycological improvement, oral antifungal treatment is recommended instead of topical treatment, which cannot penetrate the hair shaft (Higgins et al., 2000). Griseofulvin, terbinafine, fluconazole, and itraconazole are options. Griseofulvin is more effective in Microsporum infections, while terbinafine is more effective in T. tonsurans infection. They have accepted and safe drug efficacy in children (Chan et al., 2016). International recommendations for the treatment of pediatric TC include one or two single doses of 20 mg/kg griseofulvin ultra-micronized 6-8 weeks for Tricophyton spp. and 8-12 weeks for Microsporum/Nannizzia spp, once daily terbinafine 62.5 mg for cases <20 kg, 125 mg for cases 21-40 kg, 250 mg for cases >40 kg 4 weeks for Tricophyton spp. and 8-12 weeks for Microsporum spp. (Mayser et al., 2020). With the start of treatment, patients can return to their social or school lives within the scope of head-to-head contact precautions for 14 days. Use of sporicidal shampoo containing 2.5% selenium sulphide or 2% ketoconazole for 2 to 4 weeks may benefit the patient and household in reducing spread and reinfection (Kelly, 2012). Clinical follow-up is prudent to recognize persistent erythema, crusting, and drainage, which usually occur due to inconsistent or incorrect application of treatment or insensitivity of the organism.

Tinea Pedis

Tinea pedis (TP) is a dermatophytosis of the feet, also called "athlete's foot." It has a prevalence that increases with age. The most common etiological genera are T.rubrum, T.mentagrophytes, and E.floccosum. Clinical findings vary among different types. In the interdigital form, scaling and itchy erosion are observed, especially on the lateral three toes. The hyperkeratotic form is usually bilateral and is characterized by diffuse scaling and plantar erythema on the medial and lateral surfaces of the feet, which called the moccasin-pattern. The vesiculobullous or inflammatory form is seen with vesicles or bullae that can be itchy and painful, especially in the medial side of the foot (Kovitwanichkanont & Chong, 2019). The ulcerative form associated with bacterial co-infection is less common and presents with erosions and ulcers on the plantar surface. The diagnosis of TP is made based on clinical appearance. In case of atypical findings, KOH preparation or culture can be performed. Topical creams containing terbinafine and butenafine applied once or twice daily for four weeks are effective. Systemic antifungal therapy should be reserved for patients who have failed topical therapy, have disseminated disease, or are immunocompromised.

Tinea corporis

Tinea corporis (TC), also known as "ringworm of the body," is a dermatophyte infection of hairless skin areas other than the palms, soles, face, and groin. Trichophytan and Microsporiumspecies are common pathogens, of which T.rubrum is the predominant organism. The etiology of M. canis suggests cat or dog contact. It is prevalent in children and young adults. The typical clinical appearance is a red, circular or oval, scaly patch with clear, central areaswith an erythematous border. Lesions may be single or multiple, generally 1 to 5 cm in size and may merge. Differential diagnoses of TC include discoid eczema, annular psoriasis, erythema annulare centrifugum, and subacute cutaneous lupus erythematosus. The findings in the KOH preparation confirm the diagnosis. It is well treated with the topical antifungal creams discussed in treatment of TP above. In large lesions, oral antifungal treatment with terbinafine, itraconazole, fluconazole, and griseofulvin is reasonable (Sahoo & Mahajan, 2016).

Tinea Cruris

Tinea cruris, also known as "jock itch," is a dermatophyte infection of the groin fold. T.rubrum is the common causative organism. It is prevalent in adolescents and young adult males. Concomitant fungal infections, especially TP, may be the source. It is characterized by an erythematous, well-emarginated patch on the medial upper thigh. Itching and pain may occur as symptoms. The genitalia is usually preserved, scrotal involvement point out Candida etiology. Psoriasis, seborrheic dermatitis, candidiasis, and erythrasma are the most likely differential diagnosis. KOH preparation is usually feasible and the presence of hyphae supports a fungal etiology. Treatment is similar to TC.

Other Clinical Dermatophytoses

Tinea manuum, Tinea faciei, Tinea barbae, Tinea incognita, Tinea imbricate, and Tinea gladiatorum are other diagnoses encountered in clinical practice. There are peer diagnostic approaches and treatment methodsfor the more common tinea infections described above. Tinea manuum is a hand infection that mimics features of TC. It is usually synchronous with TP. The condition that affects the patient's one hand (tinea manuum) and bilateral feet (TP) is called "two feet-one hand syndrome." Tinea faciei is the infection of the facial skin. Tinea barbae involved in the unilateral beard area and requires oral antifungal treatment. Tinea incognitaoccurs when a fungal infection is poorlytreated with topical steroids. With the local immunosuppressive effect of steroids, erythema and sharp emarginated border may fade, makingaccurate diagnosis difficult. If the hair follicle and dermis are invadedby infection, it is called Majocchi's granuloma and systemic antifungal treatment is required. Tinea imbricate is characterized by concentric, erythematous plaques caused by T.concentricum. Tinea gladiatorum is a different type of TCseen in athletes who play contact sports, especially wrestlers.

Tinea Unguium (Onychomycosis)

Tinea unguium is a fungal infection of the toenails or fingernails caused by dermatophytes, yeasts, and non-dermatophyte molds. It is more common in adults than in children and account half of all nail disorders (Sigurgeirsson& Baran, 2014). There are five main clinical subtypes (Ameen et al., 2014). Distal and lateral subungual onychomycosis, which is more common, is manifestedbythickening and discoloration of the distal edge of the nail along with subungual hyperkeratosis leading to nail dystrophy. T. rubrum is the major responsible organism (Foster at al., 2004). Proximal subungual onychomycosis is a rare condition and its possible relationship with immune deficiency is important. T. rubrum, C. albicans, Fusarium and Aspergillus species have been reported to be the causative organisms (Hay &Baran, 2011). Superficial white onychomycosis is characterized by white spots and lines on the surface of the nail plate, which is common in children. It is usually caused by T. mentagrophytes (Piraccini&Tosti, 2004). In endonyxonychomycosis, the fungus penetrates the nail plate keratin, causing nail whitening in the absence of subungual hyperkeratosis. T. soudanence is most commonly associated with endonyxonychomycosis (Hay &Baran, 2011). Total dystrophic onychomycosis is a condition in which the nail plate is completely destroyed and covered withkerototic debris. It is often theend-stage form of other patterns or is caused by Candida species in immunocom promised patients. Chronic trauma and psoriasis should be rule out in Tinea unguium, where little toe involvement is less common. In addition, continuous participation in shared moist places such as pools, gyms, or baths should be questioned in terms of predisposing factors.

The diagnosis of onychomycosis is based on physical appearance. Since the treatment is long-term, expensive, and non-fungal mimics are common, it is recommended to confirm it with KOH preparation, fungal cultures, PAS stain, or histopathologic examination. Accordingly, the Australasian College of Dermatologists and the American Academy of Dermatology do not recommend the use of topical or antifungal medications for thickened, distorted toenails unless dermatophyte infection is mycologically confirmed. Terbinafine and fluconazole for oral treatment, although do not yet have United States Food and Drug Administration approval, and ciclopirox for topical use are the treatment options. The efficacy of terbinafine is superior to fluconazole with short-term treatment. Ciclopirox nail polish can be used in conjunction with oral therapy in patient resistant to systemic therapy. Terbinafine treatment in children is similar to the TC treatment mentioned above, and 250 mg oral tablets are available for adults. The duration of terbinafine treatment is six weeks for fingernails and 12 weeks for toenails daily, and baseline liver function test monitoring is advised. In case of treatment failure, presence of comorbidities or involvement of the nail matrix required specialist referral (Piraccini et al., 2022).

Candidiasis

Candida species are a broad family that can cause local mucocutaneous infections as well as systemic forms, especially in immunocompromised and hospitalized individuals. Although there are over 160 species in nature, the most common pathogens that cause disease in humans are C. albicans, C. glabrata, C. tropicalis, C. parapsilosisand C. crusei (Turner & Butler, 2014). C. albicans is the main organism responsible for Candidiasis in adults and pediatric patients (Macias-Paz et al., 2022). There are various factors that predispose to candida infections; some of these are obesity, diabetes, pregnancy, medications and the nutritional status of the host. Moist body areas may facilitate cutaneous candidiasis. Lesions appear as erythematous, macerated patches in the involved tissue.

Oropharyngeal candidiasis or "thrush" is common in infants. It also occurs in adults who wear dentures or immunodeficient. White pseudomembranous patches resembling milk clots on the tongue, buccal mucosa, gums, and palate are typical. Patients who have denture stomatitis, edema and erythema can be seen at the contact sides. Although it is usually asymptomatic, symptoms such as loss of taste, pain, and cottony feeling are observed. Microscopic examination of the scraped lesion prepared with KOH confirms the diagnosis by seeing budding yeasts with hyphae or pseudohyphae. In the treatment of mild oropharyngeal candidiasis, clotrimazole troches, 10 mg 5 times daily or miconazole mucoadhesive buccal 50 mg tablet once daily for 7-14 days have high-quality evidence. For denture-associated candidiasis, disinfection of the denture is recommended in addition to antifungal therapy. Oral azoles and nystatin are alternative agents (Pappas et. al., 2016). C. albicans is one of the causative factors of angular cheilitis, also known as “perleche,” which presents itself with fissuring, maceration, and erythema in the corners of the mouth. It is usually bilateral and sore. Cutaneous candidiasis includes forms of intertrigo, miliaria, and paronychia. Intertrigo refers to erythematous, eroded plaques with satellite pustular lesions that generally involve the scrotum and inguinal area, perianal and perigenital skin in infants, and interdigital areas between the fingers. Candida miliaria often affects bedridden patients or patients wearing occlusive clothing. Candidal paronychia usually occurs in patients whose hands frequently come into contact with wet conditions. Redness, swelling and tenderness in the nail folds are common. Topical antifungal creams are the initial treatment for cutaneous forms. Candida infections may be responsible for mastitis in breastfeeding women with painful, shiny nipples that are often accompanied by infant thrush or diaper candidal dermatitis. Mammary candidiasis is diagnosed clinically and treated primarily with topical azoles. Chronic mucocutaneous candidiasis is superficial candidal infections of the skin, nails, and oropharynx caused by a genetic defect in the immune system. Various autoimmune manifestations, mostly endocrinopathies, may be associated with the disease. Sharp-edged, massive, scaly lesions on the skin are usually chronic and difficult to treat. Genetic tests are available for definitive diagnosis.

Balanitis is a candidal infection of male genitalia characterized by itchy, red, small papules with whitish exudates on the glans and shaft. Vaginal intercourse with an infected sexual partner within three months is a common predisposing factor. In addition to hygiene measures, empirical regimens with topical antifungals are used in the treatment. Vulvovaginal candidiasis (VVC) is vulvitis and vulvovaginitis of the non-keratinized genital mucosa, usually caused by C.albicans in combination with other Candida species or yeasts. Approximately three-quarters of women will experience an episode of VVC in their lifetime (Workowski et al., 2021). Oral contraceptive use, pregnancy, diabetes, HIV infection, and immunosuppressive therapy are risk factors. Pruritus and white, curd vaginal discharges are typical findings. Patients also experience dysuria, dyspareunia, vulvar burning and pain. Diagnostic considerations include wet preparation and culture or other test results. In a patient with suspected VVC, examination of a wet mount with KOH preparation should be performed, and test positivity should be treated. Vaginal cultures for candida should be obtained in patients with VVC symptoms but negative test results. As initial treatment, a short-term topical antifungal medication with azoles in 1-3 days, without superiority to each other, or a single 150-mg oral dose of fluconazole is recommended (Workowski et al., 2021). Nevertheless, recurrent VVC, defined as three or more episodes of infection per year, is estimated to affect 158 million women each year by 2030, leading to more than 20 million additional visits (Denning et al., 2018). Longer-term treatment is required to maintain mycological remission in these patients. Except for men with balanitis, there are no data to support treatment of sex partners of VVC patients.

Subcutaneous Fungal Infections

These uncommon fungal skin lesions are usually chronic, sporadic and localized to the skin and subcutaneous tissue. Sporotrichosis, chromoblastomycosis, phaeohyphomycosis, lobomycosis, mycetoma, mucormycosis, and entomophthoromycosis are some known clinical forms. Their mainlands are the tropical and sub-tropical regions of the earth. They may be the cause of opportunistic infections in immunocompromised patients with HIV and patients with malignancy. Skin involvement is common, but they can disseminate to inner organs. Histopathological examinations create the gold standard diagnostic approaches except Sporotrichosis, which is best diagnosed with cultures. Spontaneous resolution is rare, so oral antifungal regimens is required in most cases. Treatment can easily resolve cutaneous involvement, although disseminated forms are difficult to manage.

Sporotrichosis is caused by the dimorphic fungus S. schenckii. It is usually penetrated to people from a small break on the skin with the fungal spores in contaminated plants. Hands and arms are mostly affected. It presents with reddish, small, and ulcerated dermal nodule in the acquisition site from 1 to 12 weeks after exposure. A swollen draining lymphatic can be seen under the skin. Treatment with itraconazole 200 mg oral daily for 2 to 4 weeks is recommended which is usually extended for a total of 3 to 6 months (Kauffman et al., 2007). Chromoblastomycosis is caused by a various pigmented fungi leading a chronic infection of the skin. Lesions may be nodular, verrucous, plaque-like, tumoral, and cicatricial (Brito & Bittencourt, 2018). It is an occupational disease which mostly affects agricultural workers. Treatment requires a long time of duration which includes physical treatments and immunotherapy along with antifungal medications.

Mycetoma is a chronic, destructive inflammatory disease that usually occurs in the foot. Since it was first reported in the town of Madura in India, it is so called "Madura foot." While various types of fungi called eumycetoma may play a role in its etiology, there are also bacteria called actinomycetoma. It affects more often young adult males living in poor regions of developing countries. It is characterized by painless subcutaneous mass, discharging sinuses and grains that contains causative organism (Verma & Jha, 2019). A long-term antifungal treatment is required yet surgical amputation may be performed in ineffective cases. Mucormycos is can involve cutaneous and soft tissues which is the most common form, when causative fungi which are named mucormycetes penetrate to skin via a cut. Clinical presentation includes abscesses, skin swelling, necrosis, ulcers, and eschars (Cornely et al., 2019). The other less frequent types may occur by inhaling spores in patients having comorbidities such as diabetes or underlying malignancy that lower their immunity against fungi. The infection can spread and affect muscle and bones so early detection is important.

Deep (Systemic) Fungal Infections

Deep fungal infectionstend to affect internal organs such as lungs, gastrointestinal tract, and central nervous system but may manifest with skin involvement. They are common over 60 years and men (Wen et al., 2022). Primer lesion of the skin or hematogenous dissemination of systemic infections may cause cutaneous inoculation. This group of infections includes endemic mycoses such as Histoplasmosis, Blastomycosis, Coccidioidomycosis, and Paracoccidioidomycosis, and opportunistic mycoses such as Systemic Candidiasis, Cryptococcosis, Aspergillosis and Fusarium species. Skin involvement is closely associated with immunodeficient status of host. A rare presentation, it composes opportunity for diagnosis by allowing biopsy from visible lesion. Cutaneous manifestations of deep fungal infections include ulcerated nodules with lymphadenopathy, areas of indurated skin, erythematous papules, and plaques that develop several weeks after inoculation. Necrotic lesions may be seen in Aspergillus and Fusarium species. Obtaining information from medical history about the endemic regions visited, exposure to certain animal droppings, and the underlying diseases sheds light on physicians. In patients with community-acquired pneumonia, there are clinical testing algorithms for Coccidioidomycosis, Histoplasmosis, and Blastomycosis that provide useful guidance in primary care (Smith et al., 2023). It would be appropriate to refer patients who are suspected of having these infections in primary care to a specialist, as they may progress to a life-threatening clinical condition and parenteral therapy and advanced laboratory tests for diagnosis may be needed. Intravenous amphotericin B and oral azoles are used to treat systemic fungal infections, with proven efficacy (Wheat et al., 2007; Chapman et al., 2008; Perfect et al., 2010; Galgiani et al., 2016; Patterson et al., 2016).

Conclusion

Fungal infections are a common clinical entity that imposes a large workload and economic burden on healthcare systems. Diagnosis of cutaneous forms, especially, in primary health care is possible and necessary. Primary care providers should be familiar with fungi-specific clinical findings and medical history inquiries in accordance with up-to-date guidelines for optimal management.

References

Bewley, A. (2017). The neglected psychological aspects of skin disease. *BMJ (Clinical Research Ed.)*, 358, j3208. https://doi.org/10.1136/bmj.j3208.

Bonifaz, A., Badali, H., de Hoog, G. S., Cruz, M., Araiza, J., Cruz, M. A., Fierro, L., & Ponce, R. M. (2008). Tinea nigra by *Hortaea werneckii*: A report of 22 cases from Mexico. *Studies in Mycology*, 61, 77–82. https://doi.org/10.3114/sim.2008.61.07.

Bonifaz, A., Gómez-Daza, F., Paredes, V., & Ponce, R. M. (2010). Tinea versicolor, tinea nigra, white piedra, and black piedra. *Clinics in Dermatology*, 28(2), 140–145. https://doi.org/10.1016/j.clindermatol.2009.12.004.

Brito, A. C., & Bittencourt, M. J. S. (2018). Chromoblastomycosis: An etiological, epidemiological, clinical, diagnostic, and treatment update. *Anais Brasileiros de Dermatologia*, 93(4), 495–506. https://doi.org/10.1590/abd1806-4841.20187321.

Chapman, S. W., Dismukes, W. E., Proia, L. A., Bradsher, R. W., Pappas, P. G., Threlkeld, M. G., Kauffman, C. A., & Infectious Diseases Society of America. (2008). Clinical practice guidelines for the management of blastomycosis: 2008 update by the Infectious Diseases Society of America. *Clinical Infectious Diseases*, 46(12), 1801–1812. https://doi.org/10.1086/588300.

Chen, X., Jiang, X., Yang, M., González, U., Lin, X., Hua, X., Xue, S., Zhang, M., & Bennett, C. (2016). Systemic antifungal therapy for tinea capitis in children. *The Cochrane Database of Systematic Reviews*, 2016(5), CD004685. https://doi.org/10.1002/14651858.CD004685.pub3.

Cornely, O. A., Alastruey-Izquierdo, A., Arenz, D., Chen, S. C. A., Dannaoui, E., Hochhegger, B., Hoenigl, M., Jensen, H. E., Lagrou, K., Lewis, R. E., Mellinghoff, S. C., Mer, M., Pana, Z. D., Seidel, D., Sheppard, D. C., Wahba, R., Akova, M., Alanio, A., Al-Hatmi, A. M. S., ... Mucormycosis ECMM MSG Global Guideline Writing Group. (2019). Global guideline for the diagnosis and management of mucormycosis: An initiative of the European Confederation of Medical Mycology in cooperation with the Mycoses Study Group Education and Research Consortium. *The Lancet. Infectious Diseases*, 19(12), e405–e421. https://doi.org/10.1016/S1473-3099(19)30312-3.

Denning, D. W., Kneale, M., Sobel, J. D., & Rautemaa-Richardson, R. (2018). Global burden of recurrent vulvovaginal candidiasis: A systematic review. *The Lancet. Infectious Diseases*, 18(11), e339–e347. https://doi.org/10.1016/S1473-3099(18)30103-8.

Dias, M. F., Quaresma-Santos, M. V., Bernardes-Filho, F., Amorim, A. G., Schechtman, R. C., & Azulay, D. R. (2013). Update on therapy for superficial mycoses: Review article part I. *Anais Brasileiros de Dermatologia*, 88(5), 764–774. https://doi.org/10.1590/abd1806-4841.20131996.

Foster, K. W., Ghannoum, M. A., & Elewski, B. E. (2004). Epidemiologic surveillance of cutaneous fungal infection in the United States from 1999 to 2002. *Journal of the American Academy of Dermatology*, 50(5), 748–752. https://doi.org/10.1016/s0190-9622(03)02117-0.

Fuller, L. C., Barton, R. C., Mohd Mustapa, M. F., Proudfoot, L. E., Punjabi, S. P., & Higgins, E. M. (2014). British Association of Dermatologists' guidelines for the management of tinea capitis 2014. *The British Journal of Dermatology*, 171(3), 454–463. https://doi.org/10.1111/bjd.13196.

Fungal skin and nail infections: Diagnosis and laboratory investigation Quick reference guide for primary care: For consultation and local adaptation. (2017). *Public Health England website*. https://assets.publishing.service.gov.uk/media/5a82d72c40f0b6230269cfbd/Fungal_skin_and_nail_infections_guidance.pdf.

Galgiani, J. N., Ampel, N. M., Blair, J. E., Catanzaro, A., Geertsma, F., Hoover, S. E., Johnson, R. H., Kusne, S., Lisse, J., MacDonald, J. D., Meyerson, S. L., Raksin, P. B., Siever, J., Stevens, D. A., Sunenshine, R., & Theodore, N. (2016). 2016 Infectious Diseases Society of America (IDSA) clinical practice guideline for the treatment of coccidioidomycosis. *Clinical Infectious Diseases*, 63(6), e112–e146. https://doi.org/10.1093/cid/ciw360.

Gupta, A. K., Renaud, H. J., Quinlan, E. M., Shear, N. H., & Piguet, V. (2021). The growing problem of antifungal resistance in onychomycosis and other superficial mycoses. *American Journal of Clinical Dermatology*, 22(2), 149–157. https://doi.org/10.1007/s40257-020-00580-6.

Hald, M., Arendrup, M. C., Svejgaard, E. L., Lindskov, R., Foged, E. K., Saunte, D. M., & Danish Society of Dermatology. (2015). Evidence-based Danish guidelines for the treatment of Malassezia-related skin diseases. *Acta Dermato-Venereologica*, 95(1), 12–19. https://doi.org/10.2340/00015555-1825.

Hay, R. J., & Baran, R. (2011). Onychomycosis: A proposed revision of the clinical classification. *Journal of the American Academy of Dermatology*, 65(6), 1219–1227. https://doi.org/10.1016/j.jaad.2010.09.730.

Higgins, E. M., Fuller, L. C., & Smith, C. H. (2000). Guidelines for the management of tinea capitis. *British Journal of Dermatology*, 143, 53–58. https://doi.org/10.1046/j.1365-2133.2000.03530.x.

Howell, S. A. (2023). Dermatopathology and the diagnosis of fungal infections. *British Journal of Biomedical Science*, 80, 11314. https://doi.org/10.3389/bjbs.2023.11314.

Kauffman, C. A., Bustamante, B., Chapman, S. W., Pappas, P. G., & Infectious Diseases Society of America. (2007). Clinical practice guidelines for the management of sporotrichosis: 2007 update by the Infectious Diseases Society of America. *Clinical Infectious Diseases*, 45(10), 1255–1265. https://doi.org/10.1086/522765.

Kelly, B. P. (2012). Superficial fungal infections. *Pediatrics in Review*, 33(4), e22–e37. https://doi.org/10.1542/pir.33-4-e22.

Kovitwanichkanont, T., & Chong, A. H. (2019). Superficial fungal infections. *Australian Journal of General Practice*, 48(10), 706–711. https://doi.org/10.31128/AJGP-05-19-4930.

Lee, J. B., & Schwartz, Z. (2022). Tinea nigra. *The New England Journal of Medicine*, 387(16), 1501. https://doi.org/10.1056/NEJMicm2204411.

Leung, A. K., Barankin, B., Lam, J. M., Leong, K. F., & Hon, K. L. (2022). Tinea versicolor: An updated review. *Drugs in Context*, 11, 2022-9-2. https://doi.org/10.7573/dic.2022-9-2.

Ameen, M., Lear, J. T., Madan, V., Mohd Mustapa, M. F., Richardson, M., Hughes, J. R., Sahota, A., Griffiths, M., McDonagh, A. J., Punjabi, S., Buckley, D. A., Nasr, I., Swale, V. J., Duarte-Williamson, C. E., McHenry, P. M., Levell, N. J., Leslie, T., Mallon, E., Towers, K., ... Exton, L. S. (2014). British Association of Dermatologists' guidelines for the management of onychomycosis. *British Journal of Dermatology*, 171(5), 937–958. https://doi.org/10.1111/bjd.13358.

Macias-Paz, I. U., Pérez-Hernández, S., Tavera-Tapia, A., Luna-Arias, J. P., Guerra-Cárdenas, J. E., & Reyna-Beltrán, E. (2023). *Candida albicans*: The main opportunistic pathogenic fungus in humans. *Revista Argentina de Microbiologia*, 55(2), 189–198. https://doi.org/10.1016/j.ram.2022.08.003.

Mayser, P., Nenoff, P., Reinel, D., Abeck, D., Brasch, J., Daeschlein, G., Effendy, I., Ginter-Hanselmayer, G., Gräser, Y., Hipler, U. C., Höger, P., Kolb-Mäurer, A., Ott, H., Schaller, M., & Zidane, M. (2020). S1 guidelines: Tinea capitis. *Journal der Deutschen Dermatologischen Gesellschaft = Journal of the German Society of Dermatology: JDDG*, 18(2), 161–179. https://doi.org/10.1111/ddg.14026.

McNulty, Cliodna. (2009). Fungal skin and nail infections: Diagnosis and laboratory investigation. Quick reference guide for primary care: For consultation and local adaptation. *Public Health England.* Reformatted June 2017 for British Infection Association, Royal College of General Practitioners. https://assets.publishing.service.gov.uk/media/5a82d72c40f0b6230269cfbd/Fungal_skin_and_nail_infections_guidance.pdf.

Nigat, T. D., Sitote, T. M., & Gedefaw, B. M. (2023). Fungal skin disease classification using the convolutional neural network. *Journal of Healthcare Engineering*, 2023, 6370416. https://doi.org/10.1155/2023/6370416.

Pappas, P. G., Kauffman, C. A., Andes, D. R., Clancy, C. J., Marr, K. A., Ostrosky-Zeichner, L., Reboli, A. C., Schuster, M. G., Vazquez, J. A., Walsh, T. J., Zaoutis, T. E., & Sobel, J. D. (2016). Clinical practice guideline for the management of candidiasis: 2016 update by the Infectious Diseases Society of America. *Clinical Infectious Diseases*, 62(4), e1–e50. https://doi.org/10.1093/cid/civ933.

Patterson, T. F., Thompson, G. R., III, Denning, D. W., Fishman, J. A., Hadley, S., Herbrecht, R., Kontoyiannis, D. P., Marr, K. A., Morrison, V. A., Nguyen, M. H., Segal, B. H., Steinbach, W. J., Stevens, D. A., Walsh, T. J., Wingard, J. R., Young, J. A., & Bennett, J. E. (2016). Practice guidelines for the diagnosis and management of aspergillosis: 2016 update by the Infectious Diseases Society of America. *Clinical Infectious Diseases*, 63(4), e1–e60. https://doi.org/10.1093/cid/ciw326.

Perfect, J. R., Dismukes, W. E., Dromer, F., Goldman, D. L., Graybill, J. R., Hamill, R. J., Harrison, T. S., Larsen, R. A., Lortholary, O., Nguyen, M. H., Pappas, P. G., Powderly, W. G., Singh, N., Sobel, J. D., & Sorrell, T. C. (2010). Clinical practice guidelines for the management of cryptococcal disease: 2010 update by the Infectious Diseases Society of America. *Clinical Infectious Diseases*, 50(3), 291–322. https://doi.org/10.1086/649858.

Piraccini, B. M., & Tosti, A. (2004). White superficial onychomycosis: Epidemiological, clinical, and pathological study of 79 patients. *Archives of Dermatology*, 140(6), 696–701. https://doi.org/10.1001/archderm.140.6.696.

Piraccini, B. M., Starace, M., Rubin, A. I., Di Chiacchio, N. G., Iorizzo, M., Rigopoulos, D., & A working group of the European Nail Society. (2022). Onychomycosis: Recommendations for diagnosis, assessment of treatment efficacy, and specialist referral. The CONSONANCE Consensus Project. *Dermatology and Therapy*, 12(4), 885–898. https://doi.org/10.1007/s13555-022-00698-x.

Sahoo, A. K., & Mahajan, R. (2016). Management of tinea corporis, tinea cruris, and tinea pedis: A comprehensive review. *Indian Dermatology Online Journal*, 7(2), 77–86. https://doi.org/10.4103/2229-5178.178099.

Schwartz, R. A. (2004). Superficial fungal infections. *The Lancet*, 364(9440), 1173–1182. https://doi.org/10.1016/S0140-6736(04)17107-9.

Sigurgeirsson, B., & Baran, R. (2014). The prevalence of onychomycosis in the global population: A literature study. *Journal of the European Academy of Dermatology and Venereology: JEADV*, 28(11), 1480–1491. https://doi.org/10.1111/jdv.12323.

Smith, D. J., Free, R. J., Thompson, G. R., III, Baddley, J. W., Pappas, P. G., Benedict, K., Gold, J. A. W., Endemic Mycoses Diagnostic Algorithm Subject Matter Expert Group, Tushla, L. A., Chiller, T., Jackson, B. R., & Toda, M. (2023). Clinical testing guidance for coccidioidomycosis, histoplasmosis, and blastomycosis in patients with community-acquired pneumonia for primary and urgent care providers. *Clinical Infectious Diseases*, ciad619. https://doi.org/10.1093/cid/ciad619.

Turner, S. A., & Butler, G. (2014). The *Candida* pathogenic species complex. *Cold Spring Harbor Perspectives in Medicine*, 4(9), a019778. https://doi.org/10.1101/cshperspect.a019778.

Verma, P., & Jha, A. (2019). Mycetoma: Reviewing a neglected disease. *Clinical and Experimental Dermatology*, 44(2), 123–129. https://doi.org/10.1111/ced.13642.

Wen, S. R., Yang, Z. H., Dong, T. X., Li, Y. Y., Cao, Y. K., Kuang, Y. Q., & Li, H. B. (2022). Deep fungal infections among general hospital inpatients in southwestern China: A 5-year retrospective study. *Frontiers in Public Health*, 10, 842434. https://doi.org/10.3389/fpubh.2022.842434.

Wheat, L. J., Freifeld, A. G., Kleiman, M. B., Baddley, J. W., McKinsey, D. S., Loyd, J. E., Kauffman, C. A., & Infectious Diseases Society of America. (2007). Clinical practice guidelines for the management of patients with histoplasmosis: 2007 update by the Infectious Diseases Society of America. *Clinical Infectious Diseases*, 45(7), 807–825. https://doi.org/10.1086/521259.

Workowski, K. A., Bachmann, L. H., Chan, P. A., Johnston, C. M., Muzny, C. A., Park, I., Reno, H., Zenilman, J. M., & Bolan, G. A. (2021). Sexually transmitted infections treatment guidelines, 2021. *MMWR Recommendations and Reports*, 70(4), 1–187. https://doi.org/10.15585/mmwr.rr7004a1.

Part 4

Psychiatric Disorders

Chapter 11

Personality Disorders

Gulin Ozdamar Unal*, MD
Department of Psychiatry, Suleyman Demirel University, Isparta, Turkey

Abstract

Personality disorders are intricate psychiatric conditions that impact cognitive processes, emotional experiences, and behavioral patterns. They exhibit a diverse range of enduring internal emotions and behaviors that result in difficulty and impairment throughout multiple domains of life. Various personality disorders have unique characteristics. Typically, these problems emerge throughout adolescence or early adulthood. These diseases can result in considerable anguish and hinder relationships, jobs, and daily functioning, making it challenging to cope with life. Specific treatments do not exist for personality disorders. Dialectical behavior therapy, cognitive-behavioral therapy, and psychodynamic therapy could enhance the ability of patients to manage stress, interact effectively with others, and address factors directly related to their disease. A significant number of individuals diagnosed with personality disorders also experience comorbid mental conditions, such as anxiety or depression, which can be effectively managed with pharmacological interventions. By employing suitable therapeutic interventions, individuals can acquire the skills to effectively control their symptoms, enhance their overall state of being, and cultivate more robust interpersonal connections. To provide compassionate care and support to those facing these difficult conditions, it is essential to promote greater awareness, reduce social stigma, and foster a deeper knowledge of personality disorders.

Keywords: personality disorders, paranoid personality disorder, borderline personality disorder, narcissistic personality disorder, obsessive-compulsive disorder

Introduction

Personality disorders are prevalent throughout all medical settings, thus necessitating frequent encounters with such conditions by all medical practitioners. In clinical settings, there is a significant population of people with personality problems who do not receive adequate attention, which can lead to ineffective or inadequate treatments being administered. The co-

---

* Corresponding Author's Email: gülin_ozdamar@hotmail.com.

In: Common Diseases According to Family Medicine Practice Guidelines
Editors: Esra Meltem Koç and Hilal Aksoy
ISBN: 979-8-89530-302-3

occurrence of comorbidity with other mental disorders is an often-documented phenomenon, and the presence of a personality disorder often has a negative influence on the course and outcome of treatment. The presence of personality disorders has been found to have a significant association with premature mortality and suicide, highlighting the need for a greater focus on their detection and management within clinical interventions, surpassing the present approaches in place (McClelland et al., 2023).

Personality characteristics refer to enduring and distinct perceptions that individuals have about themselves and their surroundings, as well as their constant patterns of interpersonal relationships and cognitive processes. Personality disorders are characterized by enduring patterns of rigid and maladaptive personality traits that typically manifest throughout adolescence or early adulthood. These patterns result in significant functional impairment and distress for individuals, and they differ markedly from the cultural norms and expectations of their society. Personality disorders present with persistent challenges in a minimum of two domains, including cognition, affect, interpersonal functioning, and impulse control. This pattern cannot be better explained as a manifestation or because of another psychiatric condition. It does not manifest because of the influence of a substance, such as a substance of abuse, a pharmaceutical drug, or poison, nor does it arise from the influence of any pathological disease.

Prevalence of Personality Disorder

The prevalence of personality disorders differs between various populations and can be impacted by other factors, such as demography, cultural disparities, and the research methods used. Based on recent studies and estimations from multiple sources as of 2020, the approximate prevalence of personality disorders in the general population is approximately 10% (Winsper et al., 2020).

Prevalence percentages may vary between certain forms of personality disorders. Borderline personality disorder (BPD) is estimated to affect approximately 0.7% to 2.7% of the general population, indicating that it is frequently identified among individuals with personality problems (Leichsenring et al., 2023). On the contrary, schizotypal, antisocial, or narcissistic personality disorders may have lower prevalence rates.

It is crucial to acknowledge that these statistics may differ based on the diagnostic criteria, the population under study, and the assessment methodologies used. Moreover, certain persons afflicted with personality disorders may choose not to pursue professional assistance or go untreated, resulting in potential underestimations of the true frequency.

Continuous advances are being made in the study and diagnosis of personality disorders, with continued research focused on improving the accuracy of prevalence estimates and expanding the treatment and support available to those affected by these problems.

Evaluation of Personality Disorder

To ascertain the presence of a personality disorder, it is imperative to assess the individual's enduring behavioral patterns and level of functioning over an extended period. Personality disorders are diagnosed in clinical practice only very infrequently. The evaluation of whether personality traits undergo changes over time and the identification of patterns that indicate lasting qualities are subjects that warrant investigation. A solitary interview may not suffice for the purpose of establishing a diagnosis. The evaluation of personality features has significance when several sources of information are considered, such as conducting interviews at various time points, gathering data from patient relatives, and using psychometric test methods.

The assessment of personality disorder can be conducted using several methods, such as self-report questionnaires, checklists, and structured clinical interviews. Structured interviews offer several advantages due to their ability to provide in-depth and comprehensive information. Nevertheless, the clinician must dedicate more time to effectively conducting these interviews. In contrast, self-report scales offer more practicality, efficiency, and reduced time requirements for clinicians compared to structured interviews. Nevertheless, the appropriate use of the data acquired from these scales requires the application of clinical expertise and discernment. There are a variety of instruments at the disposal of physicians to help in the process of diagnosing personality disorders, each possessing its distinct limits in terms of both validity and reliability. However, it is important to note that there is currently no universally recognized gold-standard assessment instrument for personality disorders. Commonly used self-rated questionnaires are Personality Assessment Inventory (Morey & Hopwood, 2004), Minnesota Multiphasic Personality Inventory–II (Butcher et al., 1989), Millon Clinical Multiaxial Inventory–III (Sellbom et al., 2022), Eysenck Inventory Questionnaire (Sato, 2005), NEO Five-Factor Inventory (McCrae et al., 1998).

Cluster A Personality Disorders

Paranoid Personality Disorder

Individuals diagnosed with paranoid personality disorder exhibit a pervasive and unwarranted distrust of others, harboring persistent fears that they may be subjected to harm, exploitation, deception, or betrayal, although lacking substantiating proof. They exhibit a reluctance to engage in interpersonal relationships or establish emotional proximity with others due to the apprehension that their expressed thoughts or statements may be used in a manner that is detrimental to their well-being. Individuals derive feelings of embarrassment or fear from commonplace language or occurrences. They consistently exhibit this personality trait and tend to harbor long-standing resentments and display a reluctance to offer forgiveness for perceived instances of humiliation, disrespect, or harm inflicted upon them. Individuals exhibit a pronounced response when they perceive themselves to be subjected to acts of humiliation. Individuals may encounter baseless uncertainties over their partners' faithfulness, and in certain cases, they may encounter feelings of insecurity that escalate to the point of exhibiting pathological jealousy. Those in the issue consistently inquire about the location of their partners, their activities, their ambitions, and their level of dedication. Individuals with a propensity for severe skepticism, unfriendly attitudes, and argumentative and grumbling tendencies often encounter challenges when it comes to establishing and maintaining personal relationships (Triebwasser et al., 2013).

Research has demonstrated a correlation between experiences of emotional neglect, physical neglect, supervisory neglect, and physical abuse throughout childhood and the occurrence of PPD (Lee, 2017). Additionally, studies have shown a correlation between brain trauma and hearing impairments with the manifestation of paranoid tendencies (Koponen et al., 2002). There is a prevailing assumption that the personality disorders classified under cluster A share a connection with schizophrenia (Webb & Levinson, 1993). Patients diagnosed with PPD have been shown to exhibit anomalies in the dopaminergic system that are comparable to those observed in those with schizophrenia. The prevalence of PPD is higher among relatives of individuals diagnosed with delusional disorder compared to relatives of individuals diagnosed with schizophrenia (Lee, 2017).

Individuals diagnosed with PPD often have a formal or serious manner and consistently maintain a posture characterized by tension. They tend to maintain emotional and social distance from individuals, displaying a lack of warmth and friendliness in their attitudes. Due to their inclination to avoid acknowledging personal errors, individuals strive to preserve their self-esteem by attributing their deficiencies to external sources. Individuals who are unable to confront their shortcomings may engage in the construction of a self-perception that portrays an elevated sense of personal value. They respond to perceived intimidation originating from their surroundings. Although they may face legal issues, they often resort to initiating legal proceedings by exhibiting behavior aimed at asserting their rights.

Individuals afflicted with this disease may have transient episodes of psychosis, particularly in times of increased stress. The co-occurrence of recurrent depression, agoraphobia, and obsessive-compulsive disorder might be regarded as comorbid conditions. The most common personality disorders are schizotypal, schizoid, narcissistic, withdrawn, and borderline personality disorders (Lee, 2017).

Schizoid Personality Disorder

The primary characteristic of schizoid personality disorder entails a pervasive tendency towards social detachment and limited affective expression. It appears that they lack the inclination to establish intimate connections. Individuals exhibit a preference for solitude over social interaction. They do not derive pleasure from their membership in a community. They prefer to participate in solitary pursuits that do not require interpersonal engagement. They demonstrate minimal inclination toward participating in sexual activity. Individuals with this condition experience reduced levels of enjoyment in sensory, physical, or interpersonal interactions compared to individuals without the condition (Triebwasser et al., 2012).

They appear to disregard both positive and negative feedback from others. The individuals exhibit a lack of discernible emotional response. They have a cold appearance. Infrequently, they encounter intense emotional states, such as anger or excitement. Individuals exhibit a subdued demeanor when confronted with unfavorable circumstances. Individuals can encounter challenges in effectively expressing their anger. The efficacy of their performance is diminished in professional environments that require the establishment of interpersonal connections. Individuals tend to thrive in situations where they are separated from the broader social context (Fariba et al., 2023).

Individuals may potentially encounter brief episodes of psychosis when faced with mentally demanding circumstances. Schizoid personality disorder may be considered a potential precursor to the development of schizophrenia and delusional disorder during their initial phases (Kotlicka-Antczak et al., 2019). Recurrent depression can be seen as a comorbid condition. It may also be observed in conjunction with schizotypal, paranoid, and avoidant personality disorders.

Schizotypal Personality Disorder

A schizotypal personality disorder is characterized by an aversion to intimate connections, cognitive and perceptual abnormalities, and disorganized behavior. Individuals exhibiting this personality pattern may display cognitive-perceptual abnormalities such as magical thinking, peculiar perceptual experiences, and the tendency to attribute personal significance to unrelated events, as well as paranoid beliefs. The absence of intimate friendships, restricted emotional expression, excessive social anxiety, and paranoid ideation may manifest in interpersonal interactions. Within the disorganization dimension, patients can exhibit aberrant speech and strange behavior (Kwapil & Barrantes-Vidal, 2022).

Many individuals diagnosed with schizotypal personality disorder have a proclivity for misconstruing commonplace occurrences and external stimuli as possessing a distinct and exceptional significance, particularly tailored to their own experiences. These individuals may hold superstitious and mystical notions. They hold the belief that they possess premonitory abilities, the capacity to perceive the thoughts and intentions of others, and the ability to exert supernatural control over others. Their speech and conduct may involve ritualistic, odd, and unique phrases and actions. Their speech is disorganized and unintelligible.

These individuals exhibit unsuitable, disheveled, and untidy clothing. Due to their distinctive appearance, peculiar speech, and unconventional behavior, they are seen as peculiar by society and are categorized as eccentric individuals. They engage in inappropriate, inflexible, and limited interactions with others. These individuals may harbor dubious or mistrustful sentiments. Their circle of friends is extremely small. Individuals express dissatisfaction with their inability to form connections with others and experience discomfort when they manage to create relationships (Rosell et al., 2014). When they must interact with other people for a long time, their anxiety does not calm down over time; on the contrary, their doubts increase, and they may become even more nervous.

Depression and anxiety disorders often occur together as comorbid illnesses in patients diagnosed with schizotypal personality disorder. They may experience temporary periods of psychosis, especially when they are under significant stress (Kotlicka-Antczak et al., 2019). It is feasible to conduct an additional diagnosis of schizoid, paranoid, and avoidant personality disorders.

Cluster B Personality Disorders

Antisocial Personality Disorder

Antisocial Personality Disorder (ASPD) is a psychiatric disorder distinguished by a variety of behavioral presentations. These presentations encompass enduring patterns of indifference and transgressions against the rights of others, lack of responsibility, impulsive tendencies, aggressive behavior, disregard for personal and collective safety, and nonadherence to legal obligations. These behavioral patterns commonly manifest in the early stages of development and tend to intensify as individuals transition into adulthood. Individuals diagnosed with ASPD, colloquially known as sociopathy, demonstrate a conspicuous lack of concern for the emotions and rights of others. Individuals with such characteristics demonstrate a tendency to deliberately incite, cause anguish, and assert dominance over others. The observable indicators include the recurrence of conflicts, the engagement in deceitful actions for personal benefit, the display of hostility, aggression, violence, or threats against others, the absence of regret for causing harm, the inability to fulfill employment and financial responsibilities, and the repeated involvement in legal processes (Rodrigo et al., 2010).

The development of ASPD has been underscored by numerous causes. The issue that receives the greatest emphasis is the interplay between genetic and environmental influences (van de Groep et al., 2023). Several research methods have been used, including twin and family studies, genome studies, gene-environment interaction analysis, and genome-wide association studies, to investigate the underlying mechanisms of ASPD. Research has revealed that the etiology is influenced by irregularities in various biological factors, including the serotonergic and dopaminergic neurotransmitter pathways, the hypothalamo-hypopitutory adrenal axis, as well as the production, release, transport, and interaction with receptors for steroid hormones and thyroid hormones (Fairchild et al., 2018). The genesis of ASPD cannot be fully explained by genetic factors in isolation. The formation of ASPD is influenced by the interplay between genetic genes and environmental influences. Environmental factors encompass a range of circumstances that might influence an individual's development. These factors may include being raised by a parent diagnosed with ASPD, having a single parent, exposure to criminal behavior within the home, experiences of emotional neglect and abuse, instances of sexual harassment, occurrences of brain trauma, and involvement in criminal peer connections.

During the childhood of individuals diagnosed with ASPD, there is a notable presence of deleterious behaviors, including aggression towards both humans and animals, dishonesty or theft, destruction of property or goods, and non-compliance with established rules. These behaviors manifest themselves in diverse settings and contexts. They exhibit a significant lack of tolerance for the concepts of discipline and authority. Instances of maladjustment in various contexts, such as military service and professional settings characterized by hierarchical structures, can manifest themselves in a range of behaviors. These include evading assigned responsibilities, neglecting to fulfill duties, engaging in deceit, embellishing facts, abandoning obligations, expressing intentions to cause harm to oneself or others, displaying attitudes indicative of self-harm, and engaging in acts of self-mutilation (Fisher & Hany, 2023).

ASPD exhibits a substantial prevalence of comorbidity (Esposito et al., 2023). Mood disorders, including alcohol and substance use disorders, anxiety disorders, psychotic disorders, somatoform disorders, conduct disorders, and attention deficit and hyperactivity disorder, are commonly observed as comorbid psychiatric conditions. Furthermore, it is related to those diagnosed with borderline personality disorder and narcissistic personality disorder. The differential diagnosis of ASPD has considerable significance due to the presence of behavioral patterns that are similar to other mental disorders. These patterns include emotional instability, inconsistencies in social interactions, impulsive tendencies, proclivity toward violence, and a propensity for alcohol and substance abuse.

Borderline Personality Disorder

Borderline personality disorder exhibits a significant prevalence in both the general population and clinical practice settings. Currently, it is widely accepted in the academic community that borderline personality disorder emerges from a multifaceted interplay between genetic and environmental influences, which impact brain development through many mechanisms, including phenotypes, hormones, and neuropeptides (Lazzari & Rabottini, 2023). The etiopathogenesis of borderline personality disorder is attributed to epigenetic modifications that arise from issues within the baby-caregiver interaction, as well as trauma, including childhood psychological, physical, and sexual abuse (Bradley et al., 2005).

The primary clinical characteristics of this condition encompass volatility in interpersonal connections, self-perception, and emotional states, as well as pronounced impulsiveness. Splitting is an often-seen defense mechanism in individuals diagnosed with borderline personality disorder (Fertuck et al., 2018). They tend to perceive others or the situations they encounter in a dichotomous manner, categorizing them as either positive or negative. Idealization and revalidation are observed within interpersonal relationships. An individual can perceive someone who they previously held in high regard as an adversary within a short period of time.

They exhibit a limited capacity to endure solitude and consistently encounter a persistent sensation of emptiness. Within the context of interpersonal relationships, individuals experience a profound internal conflict from their fear of abandonment and rejection, and their simultaneous need for deep commitment and dependency. They may demonstrate episodes of anger and engage in behaviors that are harmful to themselves as a result of the confusion they encounter within their interpersonal connections. In this case, it causes deterioration in their relationships (Luyten et al., 2020).

Patients may potentially participate in impulsive and high-risk sexual activities to alleviate their sense of emptiness and alleviate the emotional strain resulting from emotions of abandonment or rejection. Emotional crises are a common occurrence. During these crises, patients commonly encounter a variety of emotional experiences, including anxiety, fear, threat, doubt, hopelessness, rage, and shame (Kernberg & Yeomans, 2013). When patients are under stress, they may have disorganized thoughts that tend to lead to suspicion and brief psychotic episodes. They may engage in self-harming behaviors, suicide behaviors, regressive behaviors, and dissociative behaviors as a means to alleviate the stress they are directly or indirectly experiencing, thus eliciting a response from individuals in their immediate environment. Patients may have identity confusion. The phenomenon of frequent and abrupt shifts in aims, beliefs, and discrepancies is commonly observed.

It is imperative to maintain awareness of and scrutinize the diagnosis of borderline personality disorder starting from the initial interview in individuals with enduring mental difficulties who present with pervasive symptoms in various domains and exhibit insufficient response to treatment. Psychiatric comorbidities are quite common in borderline personality disorder, and these comorbidities tend to recur. The most common comorbidities are major depression, bipolar disorder, anxiety disorders, alcohol and substance use disorders, trauma and stressor-related disorders, and eating disorders. Studies are reporting that it is frequently seen as a comorbidity of avoidant, dependent, paranoid, and antisocial personality disorders (Shah & Zanarini, 2018).

It is important to evaluate whether life safety is ensured when the clinician encounters patients with borderline personality disorder (Pape et al., 2023). Suicidal tendencies, self-harming behaviors, and risky sexual behaviors should be evaluated during the examination. In circumstances involving potential hazards, patients should be referred to a psychiatrist for follow-up and treatment.

Histrionic Personality Disorder

Histrionic Personality Disorder (HPD) is characterized primarily by affecting relationships and interactions, and inappropriate interpersonal behavior is recognized as the central feature of these disorders. Individuals diagnosed with HPD exhibit behavioral patterns that are marked by self-dramatization, suggestibility, and a propensity to seek attention (Yalch et al., 2023). Patients exhibiting HPD can also be characterized by traits such as theatricality, superficiality, self-centeredness, and susceptibility to emotional distress. Moreover, persons who are classified inside this specific diagnostic category frequently exhibit a proclivity to engage in sexually provocative behavior. Individuals diagnosed with HPD may engage in disruptive behaviors to elicit attention from their social counterparts (French & Shrestha, 2023). Nevertheless, over time, this conduct has the potential to result in the disengagement and eventual dissolution of the relationship by the individual with whom one is interacting.

Individuals with HPD can openly express their feelings in a manner that is amplified or exaggerated, such as the act of greeting people insincerely with excessive enthusiasm, shedding tears in response to a small emotional occurrence, displaying sudden bursts of rage, and exhibiting quick fluctuations. Their perspectives and emotions are susceptible to external influences and transient interests. They often tend to rely on their intuition and readily assimilate the viewpoints of others. They tend to see their interpersonal relationships as more intimate and emotionally connected than they objectively are. They exhibit enthusiasm for the initiation of novel interpersonal connections. They anticipate a consistent level of attention within their interpersonal relationships (Lengel, 2020).

HPD is frequently co-occurring with somatoform disorder, conversion disorder, and depression. It has been observed that individuals often have an association with other personality disorders such as borderline, narcissistic, antisocial, and dependent personality disorders (Smith & Lilienfeld, 2012).

Narcissistic Personality Disorder

Narcissistic Personality Disorder (NPD) is characterized by a pervasive pattern of grandiosity, a constant need for admiration, a lack of empathy, a strong desire for approval, and a notable deficiency in empathetic abilities. They anticipate amplifying their capabilities, enhancing their achievements, making an impression on others, garnering their admiration, and obtaining preferential treatment. Individuals exhibiting this personality pattern perceive themselves as possessing a sense of superiority, uniqueness, and exceptionalism. There is a belief among certain individuals that their thoughts and ideas can only be comprehended by a select group of individuals who hold esteemed positions, leading them to exclusively form connections with such individuals. These individuals require admiration and care from their peers. Individuals who perceive a lack of preferential treatment, which they believe they are entitled to, may experience emotional distress and exhibit signs of anger (Mitra & Fluyau, 2023).

People with narcissistic personality disorder often cannot empathize and have difficulties comprehending the wishes, subjective experiences, and feelings of others. They expect one's expectations to be met in inappropriate, exaggerated ways while ignoring the needs and desires of others. They discuss it in great depth. When others express their demands, they can accuse them of incompetence and humiliate them. They imagine that other people are jealous of them. When they encounter people who are considered successful and admired, they insult them, criticize them aggressively, and humiliate them (Caligor et al., 2015).

The self-esteem of individuals with NPD is fragile. They are hypersensitive to criticism and defeat. They do not forget the criticism directed at them, they feel belittled and humiliated. They experience serious difficulties in interpersonal relationships due to their constant need to be liked and appreciated, their disregard for others' demands and feelings, and their belief that they deserve everything.

Individuals diagnosed with NPD can exhibit symptoms such as recurring episodes of depression, dysthymia, anorexia nervosa, and substance use disorder (Richter et al., 2023). Additionally, histrionic, borderline, paranoid, and antisocial personality disorders may also be listed as additional diagnoses (Eaton et al., 2017).

Cluster C Personality Disorders

Avoidant Personality Disorder

Avoidant personality disorder involves the avoidance of social interactions due to a fear of criticism, disapproval, or exclusion. Due to their emotions of inadequacy, individuals lack certainty regarding acceptance and affection. Forming intimate interpersonal connections with these individuals proves to be challenging. They have social anxiety and a reluctance to engage in social gatherings due to concerns about potential embarrassment. They perceive themselves as being of lower status compared to others and label themselves as lacking skill and unattractive (Fariba & Sapra, 2023).

Introverted, timid, quiet, and unobtrusive actions are typical of individuals who suffer from avoidant personality disorder. These behaviors are often displayed within the context of social situations. Individuals are reluctant to take personal initiatives in social circumstances that are foreign to them because they are afraid of being misunderstood or embarrassed (Lampe & Malhi, 2018). They have an excessive concentration on the emotional and behavioral responses of other people when they interact with them. They are susceptible to experiencing considerable emotional pain because of receiving rejection or criticism from an individual or group.

Psychiatric diseases that are frequently diagnosed along with avoidant personality disorder are depression and social phobia (Reich & Schatzberg, 2021). Additionally, a diagnosis of dependent personality disorder is made along with avoidant personality disorder. Because these individuals have a limited number of relatives with whom they interact, they become attached to and dependent on them.

Dependent Personality Disorder

Individuals diagnosed with dependent personality disorder exhibit a pronounced and exaggerated dependency on others to fulfill their caregiving needs. Consequently, they might exhibit dependent and obedient conduct. They believe that they are incapable of functioning well without assistance from others. They rely on the perspectives and counsel of others, even while making mundane choices in their everyday lives, such as selecting attire, deciding on meals, determining social companions, and choosing meeting locations. They require others to assume responsibility. They hesitate to express their dissent to their dependents, apprehensive that it may result in the withdrawal of support or rejection. They lack self-assurance. They anticipate encountering challenges in the beginning and sustaining of a business. They can generate satisfactory work when they possess the assurance of someone else's presence and experience a sense of validation. Due to their reliance on others to address problems, individuals frequently fail to develop self-sufficiency abilities, thereby intensifying their dependence (Watson, 2008).

Individuals diagnosed with dependent personality disorder may willingly undertake disagreeable tasks that they may not personally endorse, to preserve the care and assistance of others. They can submit acquiescing to the desires of others, regardless of the irrationality or detriment it may cause to themselves. The need to maintain the relationship can often lead to distorted and unbalanced relationships. They exhibit a high degree of selflessness and are willing to make significant sacrifices. They may occasionally experience financial, physical, verbal, and sexual exploitation. Due to their fear of being alone, they endure behaviors that they disapprove of (Disney, 2013).

Individuals diagnosed with dependent personality disorder exhibit a pattern of seeking new partnerships promptly after terminating previous close relationships to fulfill their need for care and support. They rapidly form emotional bonds with others, without discrimination, due to the dread of being abandoned. They tend to underestimate their abilities and attributes. They desire others to guard them and exert control over them. They avoid jobs that require autonomous action and accountability. Individuals with this personality condition frequently experience depression, anxiety disorder, and adjustment problems (Bornstein, 1995). It is commonly associated with avoidant, histrionic, and borderline personality disorders.

Obsessive Compulsive Personality Disorder

Individuals with obsessive-compulsive personality disorder are characterized by perfectionism, need for control, and cognitive rigidity. They may express their emotions in a very controlled manner and feel uncomfortable around people who are very emotionally expressive. Their daily relationships are formal and serious. They hold themselves back until what they say/do is perfect. They may have difficulty with competence, flexibility, openness to order, perfectionism, and mental and interpersonal control (Rizvi & Torrico, 2023).

Individuals affected by obsessive-compulsive personality disorder exhibit an excessive preoccupation with rules, details, processes, lists, and timetables, to the extent that they become oblivious to the primary objectives of the task at hand. These individuals exhibit a high degree of caution and are inclined toward repetition, displaying meticulousness by attentively scrutinizing details, and repeatedly verifying for potential errors. They could exhibit poor time management skills, resulting in crucial chores being postponed till the last minute. The self-imposition of high standards and perfectionism can result in notable dysfunctions and distress for individuals. Their excessive preoccupation with achieving perfection in every aspect of a job or endeavor may impede its completion.

These individuals, characterized by a need for control and inflexible thinking, tend to take on a dominant position in their relationships and may display excessive reliance or defiance towards authority. They exhibit emotional restraint and experience discomfort in the presence of those who display high levels of emotional expressiveness (Villemarette-Pittman et al., 2004). Their daily relationships are formal and serious. They restrain themselves until their words or actions reach a state of perfection. The individual exhibits a lack of flexibility when it comes to moral and ethical principles, an unwillingness to dispose of obsolete or valueless possessions, a hesitancy to delegate work to others, a tendency to be miserliness with oneself and others, and a fixed and obstinate mindset. Individuals with this personality characteristic may demonstrate a proclivity to excessively elaborate or qualify remarks, engage in repetitive error-checking, experience bouts of wrath when their sense of control is jeopardized, and engage in procrastination. They frequently encounter interpersonal conflicts due to their excessively demanding expectations of others' behavior, inflexibility, and reluctance to consider alternative perspectives. Additionally, their dependence on strict rules and expectations for both their conduct and that of others in relationships contributes to these conflicts (Pinto et al., 2022).

Obsessive-compulsive personality disorder can have comorbidities with various psychiatric conditions. While distinct from an obsessive-compulsive personality disorder, obsessive-compulsive disorder shares similarities in terms of obsessive thoughts and compulsive behaviors. People with obsessive-compulsive personality disorder could also have obsessive-compulsive disorder or exhibit obsessive-compulsive disorder-like symptoms (Pollak, 1987). Also, some of the common comorbid conditions include anxiety disorders such as generalized anxiety disorder, social anxiety disorder, or specific phobias, major depressive disorder or persistent depressive disorder, paranoid, schizotypal, avoidant, or dependent personality disorders, eating disorders such as anorexia nervosa, bulimia nervosa, or binge eating disorder, substance use disorders.

Treating Personality Disorders

Treating personality disorders often entails employing a combination of several therapeutic approaches (Bateman et al., 2015). It is crucial to recognize that treatment strategies may differ depending on the condition, its level of severity, and the unique requirements of each individual. Below are some prevalent therapy techniques used for personality disorders:

Psychotherapy: Psychotherapy is the main therapeutic approach used to address personality disorders. Various therapeutic modalities, including cognitive-behavioral therapy, dialectical behavior therapy, psychodynamic therapy, and schema-focused therapy, are frequently used. These therapies have the objective of assisting individuals in comprehending their ideas, feelings, and actions, as well as cultivating more beneficial coping mechanisms and relational abilities.

Family Therapy: In certain instances, incorporating family members into therapy can be beneficial. The primary objective of family therapy is to strengthen communication, resolve problems, and foster understanding among family members, thereby promoting the individual's recovery.

Group Therapy or Support Groups: Engaging in group therapy or support groups can yield advantageous outcomes. Engaging with individuals encountering comparable difficulties can foster a feeling of inclusion, assistance, and the opportunity to gain insight from mutual encounters.

Pharmacotherapy: Medication is not the main treatment for personality disorders, but it can be used to address symptoms commonly associated with these illnesses. Antidepressants or anti-anxiety drugs can be used to mitigate the symptoms of depression or anxiety frequently observed in patients with personality disorders.

Skills Training: Certain programs may provide specialized sessions aimed at enhancing social, communication, and emotional regulation abilities. These programs facilitate the acquisition of adaptive strategies to deal with stressors and effectively manage interpersonal interactions.

Hospitalization or Intensive Treatment Programs: In severe cases or when safety is at risk due to self-harm or suicidality, hospitalization or intensive treatment programs may be required to offer a more organized and intensive form of therapy.

Self-help and self-care strategies: These approaches involve participating in activities that encourage self-care, stress reduction, mindfulness, and making healthy lifestyle choices. These strategies can be used alongside professional therapy procedures to enhance their effectiveness.

The management of personality disorders typically involves a protracted course of treatment that requires perseverance and dedication from both the individual and mental health practitioners. The objective is to enhance overall functioning, optimize quality of life, and empower individuals to properly manage their symptoms. Collaborating with proficient mental health practitioners who can customize the treatment regimen to accommodate specific requirements and track advancement over time is of utmost importance.

Conclusion

To summarize, personality disorders are intricate psychiatric conditions that have a profound effect on individuals' cognition, emotions, and actions. There are multiple discrete personality disorders, each characterized by its unique array of symptoms and difficulties. Recurring tendencies in behaviors related to personality patterns often lead to discomfort, setbacks, and underperformance in relationships, employment, and general performance. While the exact incidence of personality disorders is difficult to determine, it appears that a significant portion of the population is affected by them. Nevertheless, the actual prevalence of the condition may surpass the reported percentages due to possible cases that go undiagnosed and people who opt not to seek assistance. To ensure that those impacted by personality disorders receive the necessary empathetic treatment and assistance, it is imperative to enlighten the general public, diminish social prejudice, and enhance comprehension of these conditions. The ongoing research, new diagnostic criteria, and growing therapy options provide encouragement for the improved identification, treatment, and empowerment of individuals with personality disorders. This will facilitate their progress towards enhanced mental health and well-being.

References

Aldrete, J. A. (1995). The post-anesthesia recovery score revisited. *Journal of Clinical Anesthesia, 7*(1), 89-91. https://doi.org/10.1016/0952-8180(94)00001-k.

Bateman, A. W., Gunderson, J., & Mulder, R. (2015). Treatment of personality disorder. *Lancet, 385*(9969), 735-743. https://doi.org/10.1016/S0140-6736(14)61394-5.

Bornstein, R. F. (1995). Comorbidity of dependent personality disorder and other psychological disorders: An integrative review. *Journal of Personality Disorders, 9*(4), 286-303. https://doi.org/10.1521/pedi.1995.9.4.286.

Bradley, R., Jenei, J., & Westen, D. (2005). Etiology of borderline personality disorder: disentangling the contributions of intercorrelated antecedents. *Journal of Nervous and Mental Disease, 193*(1), 24-31. https://doi.org/10.1097/01.nmd.0000149215.88020.7c.

Butcher, J. N., Graham, J. R., Ben-Porath, Y. S., Tellegen, A., Dahlstrom, W., & Kaemmer, B. (1989). *MMPI-2: Manual for administration, scoring, and interpretation*. University of Minnesota Press.

Caligor, E., Levy, K. N., & Yeomans, F. E. (2015). Narcissistic personality disorder: diagnostic and clinical challenges. *American Journal of Psychiatry, 172*(5), 415-422. https://doi.org/10.1176/appi.ajp.2014.14060723.

Disney, K. L. (2013). Dependent personality disorder: A critical review. *Clinical Psychology Review, 33*(8), 1184-1196. https://doi.org/10.1016/j.cpr.2013.10.001.

Eaton, N. R., Rodriguez-Seijas, C., Krueger, R. F., Campbell, W. K., Grant, B. F., & Hasin, D. S. (2017). Narcissistic personality disorder and the structure of common mental disorders. *Journal of Personality Disorders, 31*(4), 449-461. https://doi.org/10.1521/pedi_2016_30_260.

Esposito, C. M., Ceresa, A., Auxilia, A. M., Zanelli Quarantini, F., Caldiroli, A., Capuzzi, E., ... Buoli, M. (2023). Which clinical and demographic factors are related to incarceration in male patients with antisocial personality disorder? *International Journal of Offender Therapy and Comparative Criminology, 67*(16), 1630-1641. https://doi.org/10.1177/0306624X221139073.

Fairchild, G., Baker, E., & Eaton, S. (2018). Hypothalamic-pituitary-adrenal axis function in children and adults with severe antisocial behavior and the impact of early adversity. *Current Psychiatry Reports, 20*(10), 84. https://doi.org/10.1007/s11920-018-0952-5.

Fariba, K. A., & Sapra, A. (2023). Avoidant personality disorder. In *StatPearls*. https://www.ncbi.nlm.nih.gov/pubmed/32644751.

Fariba, K. A., Madhanagopal, N., & Gupta, V. (2023). Schizoid personality disorder. In *StatPearls*. https://www.ncbi.nlm.nih.gov/pubmed/32644660.

Fertuck, E. A., Fischer, S., & Beeney, J. (2018). Social cognition and borderline personality disorder: Splitting and trust impairment findings. *Psychiatric Clinics of North America, 41*(4), 613-632. https://doi.org/10.1016/j.psc.2018.07.003.

Fisher, K. A., & Hany, M. (2023). Antisocial personality disorder. In *StatPearls*. https://www.ncbi.nlm.nih.gov/pubmed/31536279.

French, J. H., & Shrestha, S. (2023). Histrionic personality disorder. In *StatPearls*. https://www.ncbi.nlm.nih.gov/pubmed/31194465.

Jackson, L. M. (2019). *The psychology of prejudice: From attitudes to social action* (2nd ed.). American Psychological Association. https://doi.org/10.1037/0000168-000.

Kernberg, O. F., & Yeomans, F. E. (2013). Borderline personality disorder, bipolar disorder, depression, attention deficit/hyperactivity disorder, and narcissistic personality disorder: Practical differential diagnosis. *Bulletin of the Menninger Clinic, 77*(1), 1-22. https://doi.org/10.1521/bumc.2013.77.1.1.

Kim, Y. M., Kang, C., Joo, Y. B., & Lee, S. H. (2019). The role of ultrasound-guided single-shot femoral and sciatic nerve blocks on pain management after total knee arthroplasty. *Knee, 26*(4), 881-888. https://doi.org/10.1016/j.knee.2019.05.002.

Koponen, S., Taiminen, T., Portin, R., Himanen, L., Isoniemi, H., Heinonen, H., ... Tenovuo, O. (2002). Axis I and II psychiatric disorders after traumatic brain injury: A 30-year follow-up study. *American Journal of Psychiatry, 159*(8), 1315-1321. https://doi.org/10.1176/appi.ajp.159.8.1315.

Kotlicka-Antczak, M., Karbownik, M. S., Pawelczyk, A., Zurner, N., Pawelczyk, T., Strzelecki, D., & Urban-Kowalczyk, M. (2019). A developmentally-stable pattern of premorbid schizoid-schizotypal features predicts psychotic transition from the clinical high-risk for psychosis state. *Comprehensive Psychiatry, 90*, 95-101. https://doi.org/10.1016/j.comppsych.2019.02.003.

Kwapil, T. R., & Barrantes-Vidal, N. (2022). Schizotypal personality disorder in the alternative model for personality disorders. *Personality Disorders, 13*(4), 392-396. https://doi.org/10.1037/per0000538.

Lampe, L., & Malhi, G. S. (2018). Avoidant personality disorder: Current insights. *Psychology Research and Behavior Management, 11*, 55-66. https://doi.org/10.2147/PRBM.S121073.

Lazzari, C., & Rabottini, M. (2023). Biopsychosocial theories of borderline personality disorder: A meta-synthesis and psychopathological network model from a systematic review. *Rivista di Psichiatria, 58*(6), 258-270. https://doi.org/10.1708/4143.41406.

Lee, R. (2017). Mistrustful and misunderstood: A review of paranoid personality disorder. *Current Behavioral Neuroscience Reports, 4*(2), 151-165. https://doi.org/10.1007/s40473-017-0116-7.

Leichsenring, F., Heim, N., Leweke, F., Spitzer, C., Steinert, C., & Kernberg, O. F. (2023). Borderline personality disorder: A review. *JAMA, 329*(8), 670-679. https://doi.org/10.1001/jama.2023.0589.

Lengel, G. (2020). Histrionic personality disorder. In *The Wiley Encyclopedia of Personality and Individual Differences: Clinical, Applied, Cross-Cultural Research* (pp. 187-191).

Luyten, P., Campbell, C., & Fonagy, P. (2020). Borderline personality disorder, complex trauma, and problems with self and identity: A social-communicative approach. *Journal of Personality, 88*(1), 88-105. https://doi.org/10.1111/jopy.12483.

McClelland, H., Cleare, S., & O'Connor, R. C. (2023). Suicide risk in personality disorders: A systematic review. *Current Psychiatry Reports, 25*(9), 405-417. https://doi.org/10.1007/s11920-023-01440-w.

McCrae, R. R., Costa, P. T., Jr., Del Pilar, G. H., Rolland, J.-P., & Parker, W. D. (1998). Cross-cultural assessment of the five-factor model: The Revised NEO Personality Inventory. *Journal of Cross-Cultural Psychology, 29*(1), 171-188.

Mitra, P., & Fluyau, D. (2023). Narcissistic personality disorder. In *StatPearls*. https://www.ncbi.nlm.nih.gov/pubmed/32310461.

Morey, L. C., & Hopwood, C. J. (2004). Efficiency of a strategy for detecting back random responding on the Personality Assessment Inventory. *Psychological Assessment, 16*(2), 197-200. https://doi.org/10.1037/1040-3590.16.2.197.

Pape, V. R., Braun, S., Peters, S., Stingl, M., Tucha, O., & Sammer, G. (2023). The riddle of deliberate self-harm: Physiological and subjective effects of self-cutting cues in patients with borderline personality disorder and healthy controls. *Personality and Mental Health, 17*(4), 328-351. https://doi.org/10.1002/pmh.1583.

Pinto, A., Teller, J., & Wheaton, M. G. (2022). Obsessive-compulsive personality disorder: A review of symptomatology, impact on functioning, and treatment. *Focus (American Psychiatric Publishing), 20*(4), 389-396. https://doi.org/10.1176/appi.focus.20220058.

Pollak, J. (1987). Relationship of obsessive-compulsive personality to obsessive-compulsive disorder: A review of the literature. *Journal of Psychology, 121*(2), 137-148. https://doi.org/10.1080/00223980.1987.9712651.

Rattan, A. (2019). How lay theories (or mindsets) shape the confrontation of prejudice. In R. K. Mallett & M. J. Monteith (Eds.), *Confronting prejudice and discrimination: The science of changing minds and behaviors* (pp. 121-140). Academic Press. https://doi.org/10.1016/B978-0-12-814715-3.00008-4.

Reich, J., & Schatzberg, A. (2021). Prevalence, factor structure, and heritability of avoidant personality disorder. *Journal of Nervous and Mental Disease, 209*(10), 764-772. https://doi.org/10.1097/NMD.0000000000001378.

Richter, M., Mota, S., Hater, L., Bratek, R., Goltermann, J., Barkhau, C., ... Opel, N. (2023). Narcissistic dimensions and depressive symptoms in patients across mental disorders in cognitive behavioral therapy and in psychoanalytic interactional therapy in Germany: A prospective cohort study. *The Lancet Psychiatry, 10*(12), 955-965. https://doi.org/10.1016/S2215-0366(23)00293-6.

Rizvi, A., & Torrico, T. J. (2023). Obsessive-compulsive personality disorder. In *StatPearls*. https://www.ncbi.nlm.nih.gov/pubmed/37983323.

Rodrigo, C., Rajapakse, S., & Jayananda, G. (2010). The 'antisocial' person: An insight into biology, classification, and current evidence on treatment. *Annals of General Psychiatry, 9*, 31. https://doi.org/10.1186/1744-859X-9-31.

Rosell, D. R., Futterman, S. E., McMaster, A., & Siever, L. J. (2014). Schizotypal personality disorder: A current review. *Current Psychiatry Reports, 16*(7), 452. https://doi.org/10.1007/s11920-014-0452-1.

Sato, T. (2005). The Eysenck personality questionnaire brief version: Factor structure and reliability. *The Journal of Psychology, 139*(6), 545-552.

Sellbom, M., Flens, J., Gould, J., Ramnath, R., Tringone, R., & Grossman, S. (2022). The Millon Clinical Multiaxial Inventory-IV (MCMI-IV) and Millon Adolescent Clinical Inventory-II (MACI-II) in legal settings. *Journal of Personality Assessment, 104*(2), 203-220. https://doi.org/10.1080/00223891.2021.2013248.

Shah, R., & Zanarini, M. C. (2018). Comorbidity of borderline personality disorder: Current status and future directions. *Psychiatric Clinics of North America, 41*(4), 583-593. https://doi.org/10.1016/j.psc.2018.07.009.

Smith, S. F., & Lilienfeld, S. O. (2012). Histrionic personality disorder. In *Encyclopedia of Human Behavior* (pp. 312-315).

Triebwasser, J., Chemerinski, E., Roussos, P., & Siever, L. J. (2012). Schizoid personality disorder. *Journal of Personality Disorders, 26*(6), 919-926. https://doi.org/10.1521/pedi.2012.26.6.919.

Triebwasser, J., Chemerinski, E., Roussos, P., & Siever, L. J. (2013). Paranoid personality disorder. *Journal of Personality Disorders, 27*(6), 795-805. https://doi.org/10.1521/pedi_2012_26_055.

van de Groep, I. H., Bos, M. G. N., Popma, A., Crone, E. A., & Jansen, L. M. C. (2023). A neurocognitive model of early onset persistent and desistant antisocial behavior in early adulthood. *Frontiers in Human Neuroscience, 17*, 1100277. https://doi.org/10.3389/fnhum.2023.1100277.

Villemarette-Pittman, N. R., Stanford, M. S., Greve, K. W., Houston, R. J., & Mathias, C. W. (2004). Obsessive-compulsive personality disorder and behavioral disinhibition. *Journal of Psychology, 138*(1), 5-22. https://doi.org/10.3200/JRLP.138.1.5-22.

Watson, C. (2008). Dependent personality disorder. *Australian and New Zealand Journal of Psychiatry, 42*, A118-A118.

Webb, C. T., & Levinson, D. F. (1993). Schizotypal and paranoid personality disorder in the relatives of patients with schizophrenia and affective disorders: A review. *Schizophrenia Research, 11*(1), 81-92. https://doi.org/10.1016/0920-9964(93)90041-g.

Winsper, C., Bilgin, A., Thompson, A., Marwaha, S., Chanen, A. M., Singh, S. P., ... Furtado, V. (2020). The prevalence of personality disorders in the community: A global systematic review and meta-analysis. *British Journal of Psychiatry, 216*(2), 69-78. https://doi.org/10.1192/bjp.2019.166.

Yalch, M. M., Ceroni, D. B., & Dehart, R. M. (2023). Influence of child abuse and neglect on histrionic personality pathology. *Journal of Trauma & Dissociation, 24*(1), 111-124. https://doi.org/10.1080/15299732.2022.2119458.

Chapter 12

Depression

Ceyhun Yurtsever[*], MD

Department of Family Medicine, Kanuni Training and Research Hospital, Trabzon, Turkey

Abstract

Depression, a pervasive and escalating global health concern, significantly contributes to morbidity and mortality. Many national and international guidelines have been published on the management of this disease. Considering that symptoms may not always be obvious or patients may not express them, screening recommendations become important, although there may be variability between them. According to the "Diagnostic and Statistical Manual of Mental Disorders - Fifth Edition," the presence of depressive mood or dysphoria is an essential criterion for the diagnosis of Major Depressive Disorder, which is the leading condition among depressive disorders. Antidepressants, psychological interventions, complementary and alternative medicine practices, and exercise are viable treatment options, and an individualized approach must be taken. Effective depression management in primary care will contribute to improving the outcomes of the disease.

Keywords: antidepressive agents, depression, diagnostic and statistical manual of mental disorders, practice guideline, primary care

Introduction

Depression, which can be defined as a depressed mood that includes feelings such as sadness, hopelessness, anxiety, emptiness, discouragement, loss of interest or pleasure in activities, is an important health problem that brings great costs to society and healthcare systems (GBD 2019 Diseases and Injuries Collaborators, 2020; Greenberg et al., 2015). The rate of admission for depression is more than 10% in both outpatient clinics and emergency departments (Santo & Kang, 2023).

Primary care physicians have the potential to play an important role in the management of depression because they are always accessible, can ensure continuity of care, can develop long-term relationships with the patient and have empathetic listening and motivational interviewing skills (United States Department of Veterans Affairs (VA), 2020). In this article, depression

[*] Corresponding Author's Email: ceyhunyurtsever@hotmail.com.

In: Common Diseases According to Family Medicine Practice Guidelines
Editors: Esra Meltem Koç and Hilal Aksoy
ISBN: 979-8-89530-302-3

management will be discussed in accordance with the recommendations of international guidelines.

Main Body

Epidemiology

The World Health Organization (WHO) reports a global prevalence of adult depression of 5%, affecting approximately 300 million individuals (WHO, 2023). A 2017 multi-country study on the 12-month prevalence of depression in 21 countries aligns with this statistic (Thornicroft et al., 2017). The lifetime prevalence is 12%, with a twofold increase in developed countries compared to developing ones (Kessler et al., 2011). The variability in depression risk factor profiles between nations, coupled with sociocultural nuances, and disparities in health perception and awareness, likely contributes to this observed difference (Weissman et al., 1996). Additionally, it should not be forgotten that the frequency of depression may vary depending on the diagnostic method used (Sjöberg et al., 2017).

Childhood onset of depression is a recognized phenomenon, with the Centers for Disease Control and Prevention (CDC) reporting a diagnosis rate of 4.4% among children aged 3-17 years in the USA between 2016-2019 (CDC, 2023). Adolescents, however, face an even more alarming scenario, with an estimated 1 in 5 individuals between the ages of 12 and 17 experiencing depression (National Institute of Mental Health [NIMH], 2023). Recent findings suggest a concerning uptrend in depression prevalence among adolescents (Shorey et al., 2022).

Within the adult population, the highest incidence of depression is observed among individuals aged 18-29 years, with a prevalence rate that jumped to 20% (NIMH, 2023; Villarroel & Terlizzi, 2020). Studies indicate that the average onset age for depressive disorders is around 29 years (Falk et al., 2008; Hasin et al., 2018; Kessler et al., 2005). Gender differences reveal a higher prevalence among adolescent and adult females, with both annual and lifetime rates approximately twice as high as in males (Hasin et al., 2018; NIMH, 2023; Weinberger et al., 2018). Etiological distinctions between genders are speculated to contribute to this observed variance (Kendler & Gardner, 2014).

Depression is approximately 3 times more common in patients with general medical disorders, with a reported prevalence of 27% (VA, 2020; Wang et al., 2017). Additionally, depression negatively impacts various aspects of healthy living, including lifestyle behaviors, compliance with medication and diet, glycemic control, and personal self-care, thus exacerbating the morbidity and mortality associated with certain diseases.

Depression is more common in those with lower income, in those who are unmarried, especially in those who are divorced, separated, or widowed, and in physically inactive individuals (Hasin et al., 2018; Pearce et al., 2022).

The ramifications of depression extend beyond individual well-being, significantly affecting the quality of life for both patients and their families (Ferenchick et al., 2019). It also significantly limits activities of daily living and contributes greatly to non-fatal health loss. Depressive disorders are a major cause of disability and rank third worldwide in terms of years lived with disability (GBD 2017 Disease and Injury Incidence and Prevalence Collaborators, 2018). Moreover, depression imposes a substantial financial burden, increasing through medical and pharmaceutical costs, suicide-related expenses, and loss of productivity due to presenteeism (Greenberg et al., 2021). In the United States, the economic burden of depression increased from 2010 to 2018, reaching a staggering 326 billion dollars.

Screening

Patients avoid sharing depressive symptoms with their family physicians for reasons such as fear of stigmatization and privacy concerns. At the same time, the thought that this service is outside the scope of primary health care, the desire to avoid antidepressants, or the belief that they can cure their problems with their own efforts contribute to this behavior (Bell et al., 2011). Furthermore, while emotional symptoms can be attributed to stress of daily life (work, relationship, etc.), the reason for admission can be more somatic symptoms such as headache, fatigue, and chronic pain (Lam et al., 2016; Simon et al., 1999; Tylee & Gandhi, 2005). This situation is even more evident in elderly patients, and usually only physical complaints or cognitive impairment are at the forefront (Ferenchick et al., 2019). That is why symptoms of depression are often overlooked when not asked directly.

When screening is not done in primary care, half of the patients with depression are missed, and only one-third receive treatment within a year (Mitchell et al., 2009; Strakowski et al., 2003). Conversely, research supports that routine screening for depression increases the detection rate, can reduce disparities in care, improves disease outcomes such as the prevalence of symptoms, response to treatment, and remission, and is cost-effective (Barry et al., 2023; Garcia et al., 2022; Gilbody et al., 2008; O'Connor et al., 2023; Pyne et al., 2003; Valenstein et al., 2001). Ultimately, depression screening can be considered an important component of diagnosis and treatment (Maurer et al., 2018). Unfortunately, despite all the recommendations of the authorities regarding screening, it has been reported that only 5% of adults are screened for depression in primary care (Akincigil & Matthews, 2017).

The U.S. Preventive Services Task Force (USPSTF), the American Academy of Family Physicians (AAFP), and the VA recommend depression screening for all adults over 18 years of age, including pregnant and postpartum individuals and older adults, regardless of risk factors (Barry et al., 2023; Maurer et al., 2018; VA, 2022). The United Kingdom's National Institute for Health and Care Excellence (NICE) and the Canadian Network for Mood and Anxiety Treatments (CANMAT) advise against screening the general population (Lam et al., 2016; NICE, 2022). NICE considers it appropriate to screen individuals with a previous history of depression or significant physical illness, and CANMAT to screen individuals with risk factors.

There is insufficient evidence on the timing of the screening and the appropriate screening interval (Ferenchick et al., 2019). This situation led the USPSTF to propose a pragmatic approach (Barry et al., 2023). It is considered reasonable to screen previously unscreened adults and evaluate the need for additional screening in patients at increased risk using clinical judgment. AAFP reports that screening during routine health visits will facilitate implementation (Maurer et al., 2018). The VA recommends annual screening (VA, 2022).

The diagnosis of depression is often an ongoing process that relies on building trust rather than a single visit. However, the use of validated scales is valuable in detecting and monitoring depressed patients in primary care (Ferenchick et al., 2019). There is not enough evidence on the superiority of screening tools over each other (Maurer et al., 2018). AAFP and VA recommend using the Patient Health Questionnaire-2 (PHQ-2) for initial testing and, if the test is positive, a more detailed evaluation of the PHQ-9, symptoms, and risk level (Maurer et al., 2018; VA, 2022). The PHQ-2 consists of two statements: "Little interest or pleasure in doing things" and "Feeling down, depressed, or hopeless." A positive test result is indicated when a total of 3 or more points are obtained from the statements, scored between 0-3. CANMAT and NICE recommend a rapid 2-question screening (Lam et al., 2016; NICE, 2022). Accordingly, if the answer to either of the questions " During the last month, have they often been bothered by feeling down, depressed, or hopeless?" and " During the last month, have they often been bothered by having little interest or pleasure in doing things?" is yes, the patient should be reviewed with further evaluations. Other screening tools that the USPSTF states can be used for adults are the Center for Epidemiologic Studies Depression Scale and the Geriatric Depression Scale in older adults (Barry et al., 2023).

While the USPSTF does not recommend screening for depression in those aged 11 and under, it concluded that screening of adolescents aged 12-18 would be beneficial in cases where accurate diagnosis, effective treatment, and appropriate follow-up can be provided (Mangione et al., 2022). It is stated that repetitive screening can be productive in adolescents at risk, and opportunistic screening can be effective in those who do not receive health care frequently. The American Academy of Pediatrics (AAP) similarly expresses the opinion that adolescents should be screened and states that an annual screening would be appropriate (AAP, 2023). The PHQ for adolescents and the primary care version of the Beck Depression Inventory are the most used screening tools for depression in adolescents (Maurer et al., 2018).

Pregnant and postpartum women are at high risk for depression. When left untreated, postpartum depression can negatively affect the bond between mother and baby and cause cognitive, emotional, and behavioral consequences in children (VA, 2022). It has been reported that postpartum depression screening is effective, and the prevalence is lower in those who are screened (O'Connor et al., 2016). The USPSTF, AAFP, VA, AAP, and the American College of Obstetricians and Gynecologists (ACOG) recommend that all women be tested for depression after birth (AAP, 2023; ACOG, 2018; Barry et al., 2023; Maurer et al., 2018; VA, 2022). Screening should be performed at least once during pregnancy and repeated 4-8 weeks after birth. The Edinburgh Postpartum Depression Scale (EPDS) and PHQ-2 are suitable for this purpose (Cox et al., 2014). The most used tool, EPDS, is available in more than 50 languages and is easy to score. It has been reported to be superior to the PHQ-9 or the Postpartum Depression Screening Scale in detecting postpartum depression.

The USPSTF concluded that the evidence is insufficient for the benefits of screening for suicide risk in children, adolescents, and adults, including pregnant and postpartum persons and older adults (Barry et al., 2023; Mangione et al., 2022). Additionally, NICE recommends that people with depression should always be asked directly about suicidal thoughts and intentions (NICE, 2022).

Diagnosis

Although Major Depressive Disorder (MDD) classically comes to mind when depression is mentioned, the "Diagnostic and Statistical Manual of Mental Disorders Fifth Edition Text Revision (DSM-5)" categorized depressive disorders into 8 different diagnoses (American Psychiatric Association [APA], 2013). These diagnoses differ in terms of duration, timing, or etiology. However, in all of them, the individual's functionality is affected and is accompanied by a sad, empty, or irritable mood. Diagnostic criteria for MDD are shown in Figure 1. Other diagnoses of depressive disorder are summarized in Figure 2.

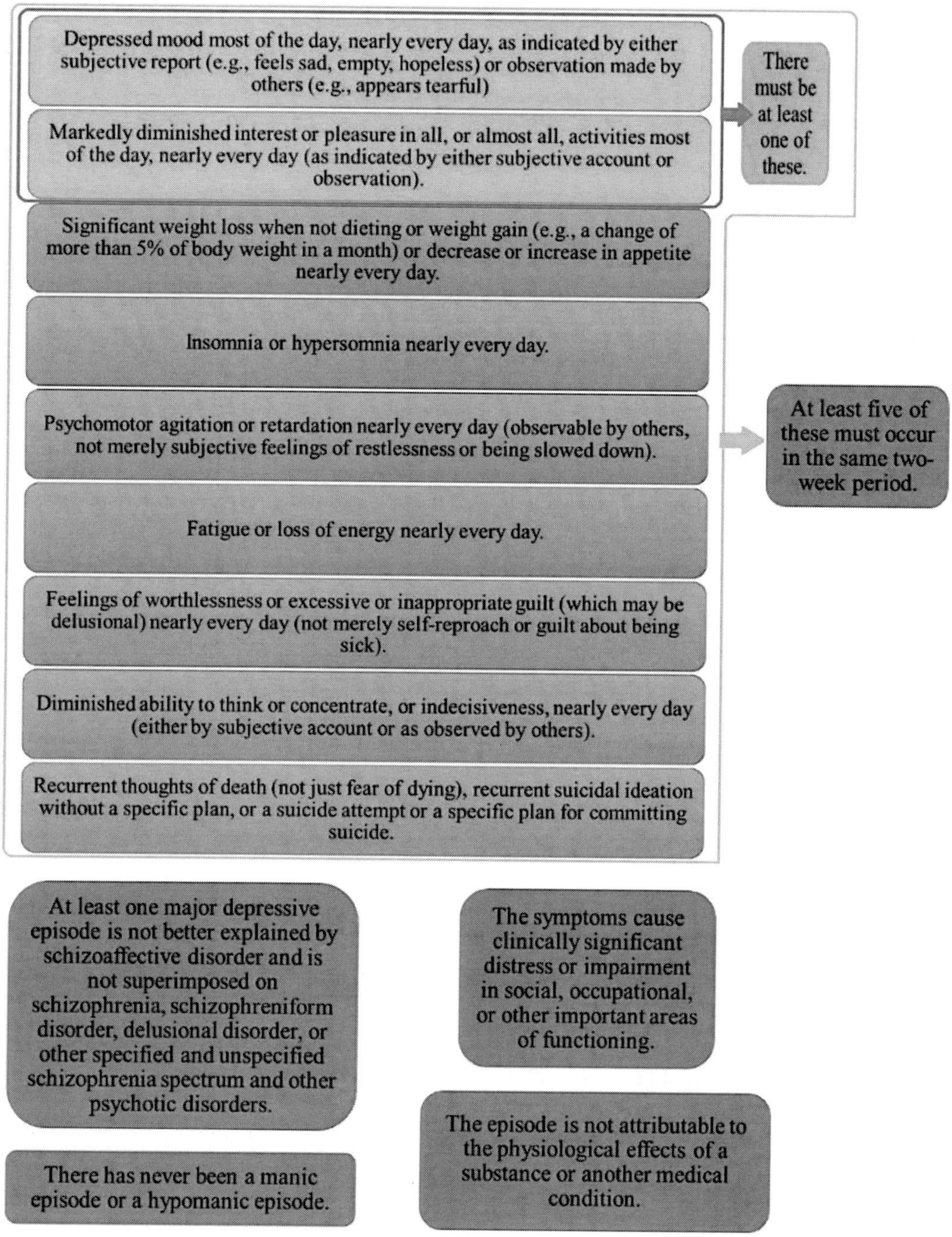

Figure 1. DSM-5 Diagnostic Criteria for Major Depressive Disorder (APA, 2013).

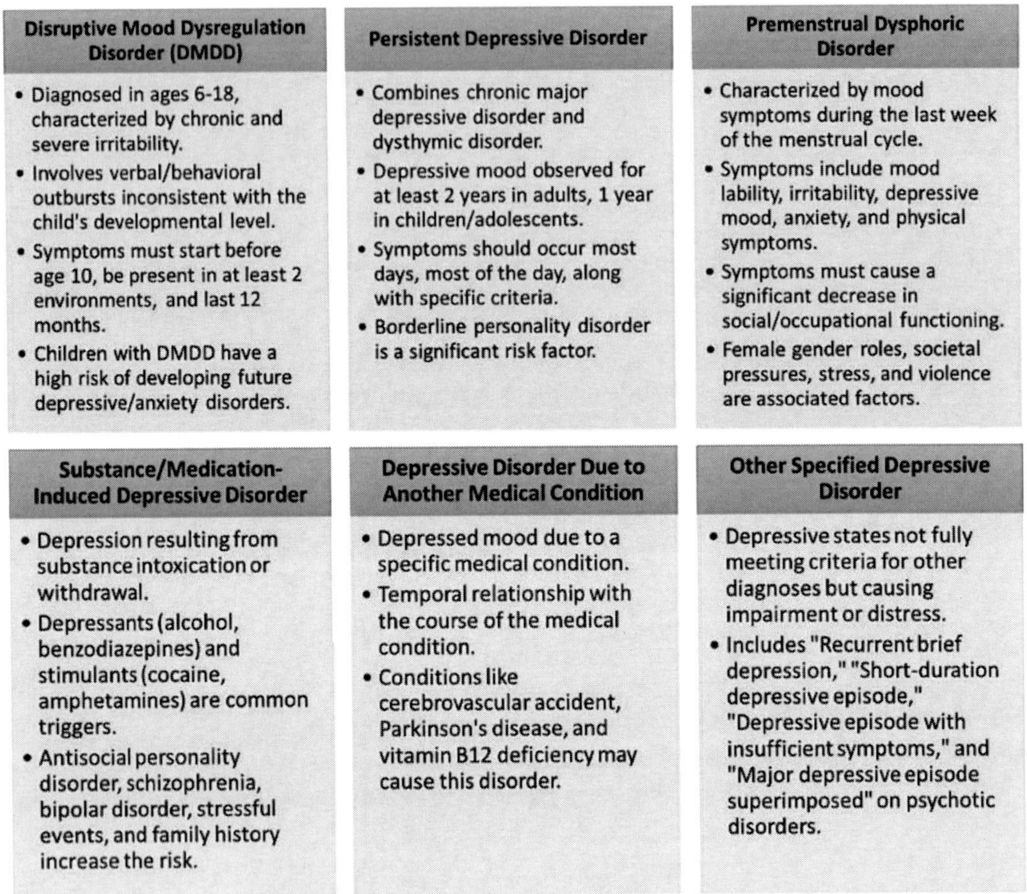

Figure 2. Depression diagnoses other than Major Depressive Disorder (APA, 2013).

Treatment

Treatment options including second-generation antidepressants, psychological interventions, complementary and alternative medicine practices, and exercise can be used alone or in combination for depression. All guidelines generally indicate initial treatment with psychotherapy or pharmacotherapy (Buelt & McQuaid, 2023). VA guidelines recommend combination therapy only in patients with severe, persistent, or recurrent depression (VA, 2022). The APA considers it appropriate that if combined treatment is to be applied, the choice of psychotherapy should be cognitive behavior therapy or interpersonal psychotherapy (American Psychological Association, 2019). The VA, American College of Physicians, and the American Psychological Association recommend exercise or St. John's Wort when participation in pharmacotherapy or psychotherapy is unwilling or unavailable (American Psychological Association, 2019; Qaseem et al., 2023; VA, 2022). Recommendations of the NICE and VA guidelines are shown in Figures 3 and 4.

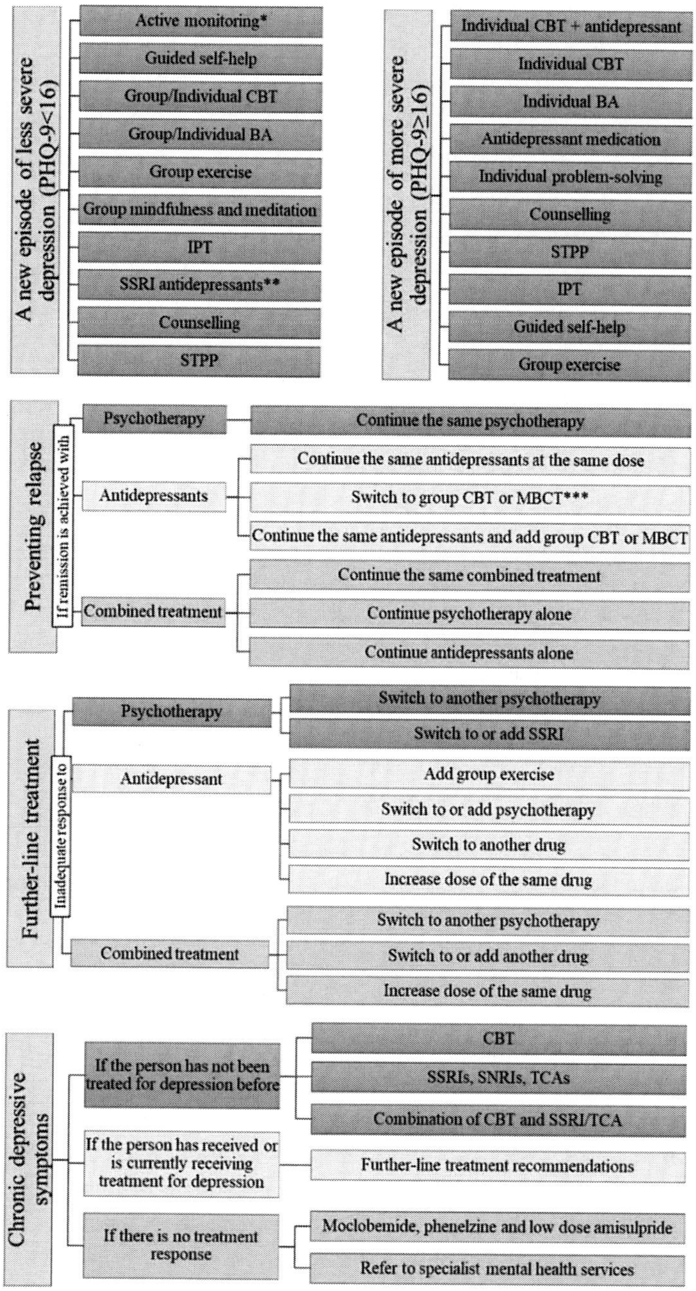

***If the person does not want treatment; inform and evaluate after 2-4 weeks.**

**Do not recommend antidepressants as initial treatment unless this is the person's preference.

***If the person wants to stop the antidepressants.

CBT: Cognitive behavioral therapy. BA: Behavioral activation, IPT: Interpersonal psychotherapy. SSRI: Selective serotonin reuptake inhibitors. STPP: Short-term psychodynamic psychotherapy. MBCT: Mindfulness-based cognitive therapy. SNRI: Serotonin–norepinephrine reuptake inhibitor. TCA: Tricyclic antidepressant.

Figure 3. National Institute for Health and Care Excellence depression treatment algorithm (NICE, 2022).

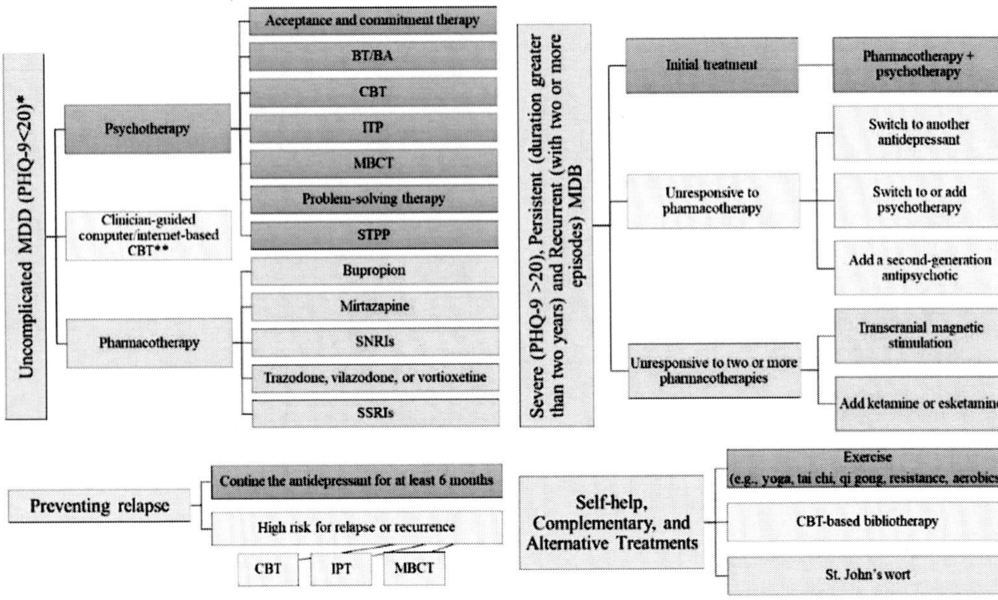

*Psychotherapy in breastfeeding or pregnant women and older adults (≥65 years). Couple-focused therapy for patients with significant relationship distress. Light therapy for those with or without a seasonal pattern (previous seasonal affective disorder).

**Alone or as an adjunct to pharmacotherapy.

CBT: Cognitive behavioral therapy. BA: Behavioral activation, IPT: Interpersonal psychotherapy. SSRI: Selective serotonin reuptake inhibitors. STPP: Short-term psychodynamic psychotherapy. MBCT: Mindfulness-based cognitive therapy. SNRI: Serotonin–norepinephrine reuptake inhibitor. TCA: Tricyclic antidepressant.

Figure 4. United States Department of Veterans Affairs depression treatment algorithm (VA, 2022).

Basic Principles

AAFP and VA report that collaborative care models (including multi-professional care, structured management, planned follow-up, and interprofessional communication) and psychiatrist involvement in the process have a positive impact on patient management. (Buelt, 2023; VA, 2022). It is also stated that telemedicine applications are effective.

A joint decision should be made with the patient about treatment (Kovich et al., 2023; NICE, 2022). Sufficient time should be allocated to discuss with the patient their ideas about starting treatment, their preferences, previous treatment experiences, and what they hope from treatment. If necessary and if the patient agrees, other individuals related to the patient should also be included in the process. Patients should be explained in detail what the guidelines' recommendations are. When choosing treatment, a feasible and individualized approach should be taken, considering needs, preferences, and additional physical or mental illnesses, and prioritizing treatments that have previously shown benefit should be given priority (Gartlehner et al., 2023; NICE, 2022).

The patient should be evaluated 2-4 weeks after starting treatment and whether the treatment is working or not. The patient's compliance with treatment, possible side effects, and suicidal ideation should be reviewed throughout treatment, especially in the first weeks of treatment. There will be additional benefits to monitoring the success of treatment with quantitative and validated scales such as the PHQ-9 (NICE, 2022; VA, 2022).

They should be told that regular physical activity, especially outdoors, and healthy lifestyle behaviors such as healthy eating, avoiding alcohol, and getting enough sleep will make them feel better (NICE, 2022; VA, 2020).

It should be noted that the likelihood of relapse is high in cases of a history of recurrent episodes of depression, inadequate response to previous treatments, avoidance behavior, a history of severe depression, additional physical or mental health problems, and the presence of personal or environmental factors contributing to depression (NICE, 2022).

Pharmacotherapy

Selective serotonin reuptake inhibitors (SSRI; escitalopram, paroxetine, etc.), serotonin-norepinephrine reuptake inhibitors (SRNI; duloxetine, venlafaxine, etc.), serotonin modulators (nefazodone, trazodone, etc.), and atypical antidepressants (bupropion, mirtazapine, etc.) are first-line drugs used in the treatment of depression (Kovich et al., 2023; Park & Zarate, 2019). Drug selection should be individualized, but it should be considered that escitalopram, mirtazapine, paroxetine, venlafaxine, and amitriptyline are the most effective drugs in reducing depressive symptoms (Cipriani et al., 2018).

If antidepressant medication is prescribed, the patient should be informed at the beginning of the treatment that it may be affected, that these effects may last up to 4 weeks, the need to come for a check-up after 2 weeks or in some cases (18-25 years of age or concern about suicide risk), 1 week later, how and at what time to take the medication, the importance of using the medication regularly, the treatment should continue for at least 6 months and about possible side effects (NICE, 2022). When prescribing antidepressants to the elderly, attention should be paid to possible interactions with other medications used and comorbidities. Dosage adjustments should be made every 2 weeks, starting with low doses (Park & Zarate, 2019). Recovery can be observed in 2 weeks or may take up to 3 months. In such cases, it would be appropriate to switch to another antidepressant.

Gastrointestinal bleeding	• SSRIs, SNRIs
Hepatotoxicity	• Nefazodone, bupropion, duloxetine, trazodone
Hyponatremia	• SSRIs, SNRIs, mirtazapine, TCAs
Osteoporosis and fractures	• SSRIs, SNRIs
QT prolongation	• Citalopram, escitalopram, amitriptyline
Sexual adverse effects	• Escitalopram and paroxetine
Suicidality	• Duloxetine, fluoxetine, paroxetine, sertraline, venlafaxine
Weight gain	• SSRIs, SNRIs, TCAs

SSRI: Selective serotonin reuptake inhibitor; SNRI: Serotonin-norepinephrine reuptake inhibitor; TCA: Tricyclic antidepressant.

Figure 5. Side effects due to antidepressants and related drug groups (Kovich et al., 2023).

Nausea and vomiting, which are especially common with SNRIs, are the side effects that most often lead to discontinuation of the antidepressant (Gartlehner et al., 2008). Additionally, sexual side effects and weight gain may also occur (Alonso-Pedrero et al., 2019; Gartlehner et al., 2008). While QT prolongation may occur with the use of SSRI and TCA, the risk of ventricular arrhythmia or sudden cardiac death has been shown to be low (Prasitlumkum et al., 2021). Sertraline may be preferred in patients with ischemic heart disease, considering its side effect profile and potential for beneficial antiplatelet activity (Teply et al., 2016). Some evidence suggests that SSRI use increases the risk of falls, fractures, and all-cause death (Coupland et al., 2018). Side effects related to antidepressants and related drug groups are shown in Figure 3.

The US guidelines do not specify the duration of treatment for antidepressants. Canadian guidelines recommend treatment for two years or longer for those with a high risk of disease recurrence for at least six months (Kovich et al., 2023). Because each episode of depression increases the patient's risk of future attacks, indefinite maintenance treatment is often recommended for patients who have experienced three or more episodes of depression.

The dose of antidepressant medication should gradually be reduced and discontinued. The patient should be informed that withdrawal symptoms (FINISH; flulike symptoms, insomnia, nausea, imbalance, sensory disturbances, hyperarousal) may occur when stopped suddenly (Kovich et al., 2023; NICE, 2022). While these symptoms usually disappear within 1-2 weeks, in some cases they may last longer. Withdrawal symptoms may also occur when the dose of the drug is gradually reduced. It should be borne in mind that paroxetine and venlafaxine are likely to cause withdrawal symptoms (NICE, 2022). Cognitive behavioral therapy may help prevent relapse and recurrence of depressive symptoms when discontinuing antidepressants (Maund et al., 2019). Reducing the dose by approximately 25% every four weeks or 12.5% every two weeks are reasonable strategies (Kovich et al., 2023).

When starting medication, especially in people at risk of suicide, it should be considered that the risk of suicide can increase at the beginning of treatment, and this should be reviewed after 1 week (NICE, 2022).

Paroxetine and sertraline are recommended as the first choice for breastfeeding mothers. Fluoxetine, which has a higher risk of agitation and overstimulation, and paroxetine, which has more anticholinergic effects, should be avoided in elderly patients. Recommended alternatives include duloxetine, sertraline, and escitalopram (Kovich et al., 2023).

Psychotherapy

Psychotherapy is defined as the whole of clinical methods and interpersonal attitudes that are applied informedly and deliberately, aiming to change people's behaviors, cognitions, or emotions in a desired way and based on ongoing psychological principles (Campbell et al., 2013). These interventions are treatments that have been used and accepted for many years in depression, the variety (individual-group, short-term-long-term, etc.) of which has been increasing in recent years (Cuijpers et al., 2019; Ramanuj et al., 2019). Although many primary care physicians tend to prescribe antidepressant medications for depression, patients often prefer psychological treatments (McHugh et al., 2013; Olfson & Marcus, 2010).

Electroconvulsive Therapy (ECT)

NICE recommends ECT in cases of depression if there is no response to other treatments, if rapid intervention is desired, or if the person prefers it based on previous experience (NICE, 2022). VA adds catatonia, psychotic depression, and severe suicidality to this list (VA, 2022).

Conclusion

The management of depression in primary care is a multifaceted endeavor that requires a comprehensive understanding of its epidemiology, screening challenges, diverse diagnostic categories, and evidence-based treatment options. By prioritizing early detection, patient-centered care, and collaborative approaches, primary care practitioners can significantly contribute to alleviating the individual and societal burdens imposed by depression.

References

ACOG Committee on Gynecologic Practice. (2018). Screening for perinatal depression. *Obstetrics & Gynecology, 132*(5), e208–e212. https://doi.org/10.1097/aog.0000000000002927.

Akincigil, A., & Matthews, E. B. (2017). National rates and patterns of depression screening in primary care: Results from 2012 and 2013. *Psychiatric Services, 68*(7), 660-666. https://doi.org/10.1176/appi.ps.201600096.

Alonso-Pedrero, L., Bes-Rastrollo, M., & Marti, A. (2019). Effects of antidepressant and antipsychotic use on weight gain: A systematic review. *Obesity Reviews, 20*(12), 1680-1690. https://doi.org/10.1111/obr.12934.

American Academy of Pediatrics. (2023). *Recommendations for Preventive Pediatric Health Care*. https://downloads.aap.org/AAP/PDF/periodicity_schedule.pdf.

American Psychiatric Association. (2013). *Diagnostic and statistical manual of mental disorders* (5th ed.). Washington, DC: American Psychiatric Association.

American Psychological Association. (2019). *Clinical practice guideline for the treatment of depression across three age cohorts*. https://www.apa.org/depression-guideline.

Barry, M. J., Nicholson, W. K., Silverstein, M., Chelmow, D., Coker, T. R., Davidson, K. W., Davis, E. M., Donahue, K. E., Jaén, C. R., Li, L., Ogedegbe, G., Pbert, L., Rao, G., Ruiz, J. M., Stevermer, J. J., Tsevat, J., Underwood, S. M., & Wong, J. B. (2023). Screening for depression and suicide risk in adults: US Preventive Services Task Force recommendation statement. *JAMA, 329*(23), 2057–2067. https://doi.org/10.1001/jama.2023.9297.

Bell, R. A., Franks, P., Duberstein, P. R., Epstein, R. M., Feldman, M. D., Fernandez y Garcia, E., & Kravitz, R. L. (2011). Suffering in silence: Reasons for not disclosing depression in primary care. *Annals of Family Medicine, 9*(5), 439-446. https://doi.org/10.1370/afm.1277.

Buelt, A., & McQuaid, J. R. (2023). Comparing clinical guidelines for the management of major depressive disorder. *American Family Physician, 107*(2), 123-124. https://pubmed.ncbi.nlm.nih.gov/36791452/.

Buelt, A. (2023). Management of major depression: Guidelines from the VA/DoD. *American Family Physician, 107*(3), 323–325. https://pubmed.ncbi.nlm.nih.gov/36920804/.

Campbell, L. F., Norcross, J. C., Vasquez, M. J., & Kaslow, N. J. (2013). Recognition of psychotherapy effectiveness: The APA resolution. *Psychotherapy (Chic), 50*(1), 98-101. https://doi.org/10.1037/a0031817.

Centers for Disease Control and Prevention. (2023). *Data and statistics on children's mental health*. https://www.cdc.gov/childrensmentalhealth/data.html#print.

Cipriani, A., Furukawa, T. A., Salanti, G., Chaimani, A., Atkinson, L. Z., Ogawa, Y., Leucht, S., Ruhe, H. G., Turner, E. H., Higgins, J. P. T., Egger, M., Takeshima, N., Hayasaka, Y., Imai, H., Shinohara, K., Tajika, A., Ioannidis, J. P. A., & Geddes, J. R. (2018). Comparative efficacy and acceptability of 21 antidepressant drugs for the acute treatment of adults with major depressive disorder: A systematic review and network meta-analysis. *The Lancet, 391*(10128), 1357–1366. https://doi.org/10.1016/S0140-6736(17)32802-7.

Coupland, C., Hill, T., Morriss, R., Moore, M., Arthur, A., & Hippisley-Cox, J. (2018). Antidepressant use and risk of adverse outcomes in people aged 20-64 years: Cohort study using a primary care database. *BMC Medicine, 16*(1), 36. https://doi.org/10.1186/s12916-018-1022-x.

Cox, J. L., Holden, J., & Henshaw, C. (2014). *Perinatal mental health: The Edinburgh postnatal depression scale (EPDS) manual*. RCPsych publications, London.

Cuijpers, P., Quero, S., Dowrick, C., & Arroll, B. (2019). Psychological treatment of depression in primary care: Recent developments. *Current Psychiatry Reports, 21*(12), 129. https://doi.org/10.1007/s11920-019-1117-x.

Falk, D. E., Yi, H. Y., & Hilton, M. E. (2008). Age of onset and temporal sequencing of lifetime DSM-IV alcohol use disorders relative to comorbid mood and anxiety disorders. *Drug and Alcohol Dependence, 94*(1-3), 234-245. https://doi.org/10.1016/j.drugalcdep.2007.11.022.

Ferenchick, E. K., Ramanuj, P., & Pincus, H. A. (2019). Depression in primary care: Part 1-screening and diagnosis. *BMJ, 365*, l794. https://doi.org/10.1136/bmj.l794.

Garcia, M. E., Hinton, L., Neuhaus, J., Feldman, M., Livaudais-Toman, J., & Karliner, L. S. (2022). Equitability of depression screening after implementation of general adult screening in primary care. *JAMA Network Open, 5*(8), e2227658. https://doi.org/10.1001/jamanetworkopen.2022.27658.

Gartlehner, G., Gaynes, B. N., Hansen, R. A., Thieda, P., DeVeaugh-Geiss, A., Krebs, E. E., Moore, C. G., Morgan, L., & Lohr, K. N. (2008). Comparative benefits and harms of second-generation antidepressants: Background paper for the American College of Physicians. *Annals of Internal Medicine, 149*(10), 734–750. https://doi.org/10.7326/0003-4819-149-10-200811180-00008.

Gartlehner, G., Dobrescu, A., Chapman, A., Toromanova, A., Emprechtinger, R., Persad, E., Affengruber, L., Pieh, C., Klerings, I., & Wagner, G. (2023). Nonpharmacologic and pharmacologic treatments of adult patients with major depressive disorder: A systematic review and network meta-analysis for a clinical guideline by the American College of Physicians. *Annals of Internal Medicine, 176*(2), 196–211. https://doi.org/10.7326/M22-1845.

Gilbody, S., Sheldon, T., & House, A. (2008). Screening and case-finding instruments for depression: A meta-analysis. *CMAJ, 178*(8), 997-1003. https://doi.org/10.1503/cmaj.070281.

GBD 2019 Diseases and Injuries Collaborators. (2020). Global burden of 369 diseases and injuries in 204 countries and territories, 1990-2019: A systematic analysis for the Global Burden of Disease Study 2019. *The Lancet, 396*(10258), 1204–1222. https://doi.org/10.1016/S0140-6736(20)30925-9.

GBD 2017 Disease and Injury Incidence and Prevalence Collaborators. (2018). Global, regional, and national incidence, prevalence, and years lived with disability for 354 diseases and injuries for 195 countries and territories, 1990-2017: A systematic analysis for the Global Burden of Disease Study 2017. *The Lancet, 392*(10159), 1789–1858. https://doi.org/10.1016/S0140-6736(18)32279-7.

Greenberg, P. E., Fournier, A. A., Sisitsky, T., Pike, C. T., & Kessler, R. C. (2015). The economic burden of adults with major depressive disorder in the United States (2005 and 2010). *Journal of Clinical Psychiatry, 76*(2), 155-162. https://doi.org/10.4088/JCP.14m09298.

Greenberg, P. E., Fournier, A. A., Sisitsky, T., Simes, M., Berman, R., Koenigsberg, S. H., & Kessler, R. C. (2021). The economic burden of adults with major depressive disorder in the United States (2010 and 2018). *Pharmacoeconomics, 39*(6), 653-665. https://doi.org/10.1007/s40273-021-01019-4.

Hasin, D. S., Sarvet, A. L., Meyers, J. L., Saha, T. D., Ruan, W. J., Stohl, M., & Grant, B. F. (2018). Epidemiology of adult DSM-5 major depressive disorder and its specifiers in the United States. *JAMA Psychiatry, 75*(4), 336-346. https://doi.org/10.1001/jamapsychiatry.2017.4602.

Kendler, K. S., & Gardner, C. O. (2014). Sex differences in the pathways to major depression: A study of opposite-sex twin pairs. *American Journal of Psychiatry, 171*(4), 426-435. https://doi.org/10.1176/appi.ajp.2013.13101375.

Kessler, R. C., Berglund, P., Demler, O., Jin, R., Merikangas, K. R., & Walters, E. E. (2005). Lifetime prevalence and age-of-onset distributions of DSM-IV disorders in the National Comorbidity Survey Replication. *Archives of General Psychiatry, 62*(6), 593-602. https://doi.org/10.1001/archpsyc.62.6.593.

Kessler, R. C., Ormel, J., Petukhova, M., McLaughlin, K. A., Green, J. G., Russo, L. J., Stein, D. J., Zaslavsky, A. M., Aguilar-Gaxiola, S., Alonso, J., Andrade, L., Benjet, C., de Girolamo, G., de Graaf, R., Demyttenaere, K., Fayyad, J., Haro, J. M., Hu, C. Y., Karam, A., Lee, S., Lepine, J. P., Matchsinger, H., Mihaescu-Pintia, C., Posada-Villa, J., Sagar, R., & Ustün, T. B. (2011). Development of lifetime comorbidity in the World Health Organization world mental health surveys. *Archives of General Psychiatry, 68*(1), 90–100. https://doi.org/10.1001/archgenpsychiatry.2010.180.

Kovich, H., Kim, W., & Quaste, A. M. (2023). Pharmacologic treatment of depression. *American Family Physician, 107*(2), 173–181. https://pubmed.ncbi.nlm.nih.gov/36791444/.

Lam, R. W., McIntosh, D., Wang, J., Enns, M. W., Kolivakis, T., Michalak, E. E., Sareen, J., Song, W. Y., Kennedy, S. H., MacQueen, G. M., Milev, R. V., Parikh, S. V., Ravindran, A. V., & CANMAT Depression Work Group. (2016). Canadian Network for Mood and Anxiety Treatments (CANMAT) 2016 clinical guidelines for the management of adults with major depressive disorder: Section 1. Disease burden and principles of care. *Canadian Journal of Psychiatry. Revue Canadienne de Psychiatrie, 61*(9), 510–523. https://doi.org/10.1177/0706743716659416.

Mangione, C. M., Barry, M. J., Nicholson, W. K., Cabana, M., Chelmow, D., Coker, T. R., Davidson, K. W., Davis, E. M., Donahue, K. E., Jaén, C. R., Kubik, M., Li, L., Ogedegbe, G., Pbert, L., Ruiz, J. M., Silverstein, M., Stevermer, J., & Wong, J. B. (2022). Screening for depression and suicide risk in children and adolescents: US Preventive Services Task Force recommendation statement. *JAMA, 328*(15), 1534–1542. https://doi.org/10.1001/jama.2022.16946.

Maund, E., Stuart, B., Moore, M., Dowrick, C., Geraghty, A. W. A., Dawson, S., & Kendrick, T. (2019). Managing antidepressant discontinuation: A systematic review. *Annals of Family Medicine, 17*(1), 52-60. https://doi.org/10.1370/afm.2336.

Maurer, D. M., Raymond, T. J., & Davis, B. N. (2018). Depression: Screening and diagnosis. *American Family Physician, 98*(8), 508-515. https://pubmed.ncbi.nlm.nih.gov/30277728/.

McHugh, R. K., Whitton, S. W., Peckham, A. D., Welge, J. A., & Otto, M. W. (2013). Patient preference for psychological vs pharmacologic treatment of psychiatric disorders: A meta-analytic review. *Journal of Clinical Psychiatry, 74*(6), 595-602. https://doi.org/10.4088/JCP.12r07757.

Mitchell, A. J., Vaze, A., & Rao, S. (2009). Clinical diagnosis of depression in primary care: A meta-analysis. *The Lancet, 374*(9690), 609-619. https://doi.org/10.1016/s0140-6736(09)60879-5.

National Institute of Mental Health. (2023). *Major depression.* https://www.nimh.nih.gov/health/statistics/major-depression.

National Institute for Health and Care Excellence. (2022). *Depression in adults: Treatment and management.* https://www.nice.org.uk/guidance/cg90.

O'Connor, E., Rossom, R. C., Henninger, M., Groom, H. C., & Burda, B. U. (2016). Primary care screening for and treatment of depression in pregnant and postpartum women: Evidence report and systematic review for the US Preventive Services Task Force. *JAMA, 315*(4), 388-406. https://doi.org/10.1001/jama.2015.18948.

O'Connor, E. A., Perdue, L. A., Coppola, E. L., Henninger, M. L., Thomas, R. G., & Gaynes, B. N. (2023). Depression and suicide risk screening: Updated evidence report and systematic review for the US Preventive Services Task Force. *JAMA, 329*(23), 2068-2085. https://doi.org/10.1001/jama.2023.7787.

Olfson, M., & Marcus, S. C. (2010). National trends in outpatient psychotherapy. *American Journal of Psychiatry, 167*(12), 1456-1463. https://doi.org/10.1176/appi.ajp.2010.10040570.

Park, L. T., & Zarate, C. A., Jr. (2019). Depression in the primary care setting. *New England Journal of Medicine, 380*(6), 559-568. https://doi.org/10.1056/NEJMcp1712493.

Pearce, M., Garcia, L., Abbas, A., Strain, T., Schuch, F. B., Golubic, R., Kelly, P., Khan, S., Utukuri, M., Laird, Y., Mok, A., Smith, A., Tainio, M., Brage, S., & Woodcock, J. (2022). Association between physical activity and risk of depression: A systematic review and meta-analysis. *JAMA Psychiatry, 79*(6), 550–559. https://doi.org/10.1001/jamapsychiatry.2022.0609.

Prasitlumkum, N., Cheungpasitporn, W., Tokavanich, N., Ding, K. R., Kewcharoen, J., Thongprayoon, C., Kaewput, W., Bathini, T., Vallabhajosyula, S., & Chokesuwattanaskul, R. (2021). Antidepressants and risk of sudden cardiac death: A network meta-analysis and systematic review. *Medical Sciences (Basel, Switzerland), 9*(2), 26. https://doi.org/10.3390/medsci9020026.

Pyne, J. M., Rost, K. M., Zhang, M., Williams, D. K., Smith, J., & Fortney, J. (2003). Cost-effectiveness of a primary care depression intervention. *Journal of General Internal Medicine, 18*(6), 432-441. https://doi.org/10.1046/j.1525-1497.2003.20611.x.

Qaseem, A., Owens, D. K., Etxeandia-Ikobaltzeta, I., Tufte, J., Cross, J. T., Jr., Wilt, T. J. (2023). Nonpharmacologic and pharmacologic treatments of adults in the acute phase of major depressive disorder: A living clinical guideline from the American College of Physicians. *Annals of Internal Medicine, 176*(2), 239–252. https://doi.org/10.7326/M22-2056.

Ramanuj, P., Ferenchick, E. K., & Pincus, H. A. (2019). Depression in primary care: Part 2-management. *BMJ, 365*, l835. https://doi.org/10.1136/bmj.l835.

Santo, L., & Kang, K. (2023). *National Hospital Ambulatory Medical Care Survey: 2019 National Summary Tables* (76). https://dx.doi.org/10.15620/cdc:123251.

Shorey, S., Ng, E. D., & Wong, C. H. J. (2022). Global prevalence of depression and elevated depressive symptoms among adolescents: A systematic review and meta-analysis. *British Journal of Clinical Psychology, 61*(2), 287-305. https://doi.org/10.1111/bjc.12333.

Simon, G. E., VonKorff, M., Piccinelli, M., Fullerton, C., & Ormel, J. (1999). An international study of the relation between somatic symptoms and depression. *New England Journal of Medicine, 341*(18), 1329-1335. https://doi.org/10.1056/nejm199910283411801.

Sjöberg, L., Karlsson, B., Atti, A. R., Skoog, I., Fratiglioni, L., & Wang, H. X. (2017). Prevalence of depression: Comparisons of different depression definitions in population-based samples of older adults. *Journal of Affective Disorders, 221*, 123-131. https://doi.org/10.1016/j.jad.2017.06.011.

Strakowski, S. M., Keck, P. E., Jr., Arnold, L. M., Collins, J., Wilson, R. M., Fleck, D. E., Corey, K. B., Amicone, J., & Adebimpe, V. R. (2003). Ethnicity and diagnosis in patients with affective disorders. *Journal of Clinical Psychiatry, 64*(7), 747–754. https://doi.org/10.4088/jcp.v64n0702.

Teply, R. M., Packard, K. A., White, N. D., Hilleman, D. E., & DiNicolantonio, J. J. (2016). Treatment of depression in patients with concomitant cardiac disease. *Progress in Cardiovascular Diseases, 58*(5), 514-528. https://doi.org/10.1016/j.pcad.2015.11.003.

Thornicroft, G., Chatterji, S., Evans-Lacko, S., Gruber, M., Sampson, N., Aguilar-Gaxiola, S., Al-Hamzawi, A., Alonso, J., Andrade, L., Borges, G., Bruffaerts, R., Bunting, B., de Almeida, J. M., Florescu, S., de Girolamo, G., Gureje, O., Haro, J. M., He, Y., Hinkov, H., Karam, E., Kawakami, N., Lee, S., Navarro-Mateu, F., Piazza, M., Posada-Villa, J., de Galvis, Y. T., & Kessler, R. C. (2017). Undertreatment of people with major depressive disorder in 21 countries. *The British Journal of Psychiatry: The Journal of Mental Science, 210*(2), 119–124. https://doi.org/10.1192/bjp.bp.116.188078.

Tylee, A., & Gandhi, P. (2005). The importance of somatic symptoms in depression in primary care. *Primary Care Companion Journal of Clinical Psychiatry, 7*(4), 167-176. https://doi.org/10.4088/pcc.v07n0405.

United States Department of Veterans Affairs. (2020). *Managing depression in primary care.* https://www.pbm.va.gov/PBM/AcademicDetailingService/Documents/508/IB10-1406DEP-Provider-DepressioninPrimaryCare_508Ready.pdf.

VA/DoD Clinical Practice Guideline. (2022). *The management of major depressive disorder.* https://www.healthquality.va.gov/guidelines/MH/mdd/VADoDMDDCPGFinal508.pdf.

Valenstein, M., Vijan, S., Zeber, J. E., Boehm, K., & Buttar, A. (2001). The cost-utility of screening for depression in primary care. *Annals of Internal Medicine, 134*(5), 345-360. https://doi.org/10.7326/0003-4819-134-5-200103060-00007.

Villarroel, M. A., & Terlizzi, E. P. (2020). Symptoms of depression among adults: United States, 2019. *NCHS Data Brief*(379), 1-8. https://pubmed.ncbi.nlm.nih.gov/33054920/.

Wang, J., Wu, X., Lai, W., Long, E., Zhang, X., Li, W., Zhu, Y., Chen, C., Zhong, X., Liu, Z., Wang, D., & Lin, H. (2017). Prevalence of depression and depressive symptoms among outpatients: A systematic review and meta-analysis. *BMJ Open, 7*(8), e017173. https://doi.org/10.1136/bmjopen-2017-017173.

Weinberger, A. H., Gbedemah, M., Martinez, A. M., Nash, D., Galea, S., & Goodwin, R. D. (2018). Trends in depression prevalence in the USA from 2005 to 2015: Widening disparities in vulnerable groups. *Psychological Medicine, 48*(8), 1308-1315. https://doi.org/10.1017/s0033291717002781.

Weissman, M. M., Bland, R. C., Canino, G. J., Faravelli, C., Greenwald, S., Hwu, H. G., Joyce, P. R., Karam, E. G., Lee, C. K., Lellouch, J., Lépine, J. P., Newman, S. C., Rubio-Stipec, M., Wells, J. E., Wickramaratne, P. J., Wittchen, H., & Yeh, E. K. (1996). Cross-national epidemiology of major depression and bipolar disorder. *JAMA, 276*(4), 293–299. https://pubmed.ncbi.nlm.nih.gov/8656541/.

World Health Organization. (2023, March 30). *Depression*. https://www.who.int/news-room/fact-sheets/detail/depression.

Chapter 13

Anxiety

Gözde Bacik Yaman*, MD

Department of Psychiatry, Süleyman Demirel University, Isparta, Turkey

Abstract

Anxiety is worry and tension accompanied by increased sympathetic system activity. It is a symptom that can be seen in many psychiatric disorders and is the main symptom of anxiety disorders. General medical conditions can initiate and increase anxiety; sometimes anxiety causes and exacerbates general medical conditions. Anxiety disorders impair patients' quality of life and lead to a deterioration in their occupational, family, and social functioning. According to systemic analyzes, the worldwide prevalence of anxiety disorders is estimated to be 7.3%. The main aim of treatment is to improve the mental and physical symptoms of anxiety disorder and functionality. Various treatment guidelines have been developed to eliminate the differences between research and clinical practice in anxiety disorders. According to current treatment guidelines, selective serotonin reuptake inhibitor antidepressants constitute the first-line treatment option in the pharmacological treatment of anxiety disorders.

Keywords: anxiety disorder, practice guidelines, mental disorders

Introduction

Anxiety is worry and tension accompanied by increased sympathetic system activity. It is an emotion that is phenomenologically similar to fear. It is also called fear with uncertain objects or fear disproportionate to the real danger. Mental and bodily reactions that are activated for the self-protection of the organism against an objective danger and threat situation are defined as normal anxiety. Pathological anxiety, on the other hand, refers to a condition that is disproportionate to the apparent danger and threat, or even experienced as if there is no danger, accompanied by clinically significant, exaggerated mental symptoms such as fear, anxiety, uneasiness, restlessness, and somatic symptoms due to autonomic nervous system hyperactivation, leading to impaired functioning (Sala et al., 2008).

Anxiety is a symptom seen in many psychiatric disorders and is the main symptom of anxiety disorders. When physical symptoms of anxiety are reviewed, its relationship with

* Corresponding Author's Email: yaman.eg@gmail.com.

In: Common Diseases According to Family Medicine Practice Guidelines
Editors: Esra Meltem Koç and Hilal Aksoy
ISBN: 979-8-89530-302-3

general medical conditions is also understood (Table 1) (Sala et al., 2008). General medical conditions can initiate and increase anxiety, and sometimes anxiety causes and exacerbates general medical conditions. Family physicians are in an essential position to diagnose patients with mental illness early and to refer them to health services, where their treatment and rehabilitation will be provided. Anxiety disorders are among the most frequently observed psychiatric disorders in patients applying to primary health care services. For this reason, it is essential to know the risk factors, symptoms, and signs associated with anxiety and treatment management by current guidelines in family medicine practices (Kroenke et al., 2007).

Epidemiology

According to the results of the study in which applications to institutions providing primary health care services were evaluated, it was observed that 19.5% of 965 patients had at least one anxiety disorder diagnosis, and 41% of these patients were not receiving treatment during the evaluation (Kroenke et al., 2007). Anxiety disorders are one of the leading causes of disability and contribute to the global burden on the patient (Baxter et al., 2014). According to the results of systemic reviews, the worldwide prevalence of anxiety disorders is estimated to be 7.3% (4.5% to 10.9%) (Stein et al., 2022). Anxiety disorders impair patients' quality of life and lead to a deterioration in their occupational, family, and social functioning. Data from epidemiological studies emphasize the importance of comorbidity between anxiety disorders and physical diseases. There is evidence of a relationship between anxiety disorders and cerebrovascular disease, coronary heart disease, and diabetes (Roest et al., 2010; Scott, 2014). Additionally, anxiety disorders are known to be comorbid with mental illnesses such as depression and alcohol and substance abuse (Saha et al., 2021). It is also reported that anxiety disorders increase mortality risk (Meier et al., 2016).

Classification of Anxiety Disorders

Many patients with anxiety disorders present to the physician because of physical complaints. Medically unexplained symptoms make it difficult to determine the correct diagnosis. Tachycardia, tachypnoea, chest pain, breathlessness, feeling of suffocation, difficulty in swallowing, headache, sweating, tremors, nausea, dizziness, and diffuse body aches are common physical symptoms. The fact that patients present to the physician with physical complaints instead of reporting their mental complaints leads to misdiagnosis, unnecessary investigations, and inappropriate and inadequate treatment. Recognition of anxiety disorders is essential to reduce the burden of the disease on the health system to increase labor productivity and the quality of life of patients (Vermani et al., 2011).

Different categories of anxiety disorders have been defined by evaluating anxiety symptoms with clinical features such as specific triggers, emergence, course, and disability (Guha, 2014; Janca & Hiller, 1996). In the fifth edition of the Diagnostic and Statistical Manual of Mental Disorders (DSM-5), the main subtypes of anxiety disorders are shown in Table 2 (Guha, 2014).

Table 1. Physical symptoms of anxiety

- Tachycardia
- Tachypnoea
- Chest pain
- Breathlessness
- Feeling of suffocation
- Difficulty in swallowing
- Headache
- Sweating
- Tremors
- Nausea
- Dizziness
- Diffuse body ache.

Table 2. DSM-5 classification of anxiety disorders

- Separation anxiety disorder
- Selective Mutism
- Specific Phobia
- Social Anxiety Disorder (social phobia)
- Panic disorder
- Agarophobia
- Generalized anxiety disorder
- Drug-induced anxiety disorder
- Anxiety disorder due to another health condition
- Another recognized anxiety disorder
- Unspecified anxiety disorder.

Separation Anxiety Disorder

In separation anxiety disorder, incompatible with the developmental process, persistent, excessive anxiety, and fear are observed for separation from essential attachment figures. This anxiety leads to non-participation in activities where the attachment figure is separated. Separation anxiety disorder can cause problems in many areas of life, such as academic performance, work, social interactions, and close relationships. Lifetime prevalence rates vary between 4.1% and 5.1%. It is one of the most common anxiety disorders in childhood. The lifetime age of onset of the disease varies regionally. According to the data of a recent study, it was observed that 43.1% of those with separation anxiety disorder had onset in adulthood (Silove et al., 2015).

It is reported that those with a family history of separation anxiety disorder have a higher rate of the disorder than the general population. Mutual and complex interactions of genetic and environmental factors are thought to play a role in the development of the disorder. Loss of caregiver in childhood, conflict between parents, history of anxiety and alcohol/substance use disorder in parents, and traumatic life events are considered the risk factors for the disease. In the differential diagnosis, agoraphobia, panic disorder, and generalized anxiety disorder should be considered (Baldwin et al., 2016).

Selective Mutism

Selective Mutism is characterized by the inability to speak in unfamiliar environments, usually in childhood. People with this disorder can speak in environments where they feel comfortable. It is reported that the prevalence rate of selective non-speech points varies between 0.03% and 0.79% (Elizur & Perednik, 2003; Karakaya et al., 2008). The average age of onset varies between 2.7 and 4.6 years. It is more common in girls than in boys (Kristensen, 2000; Sharkey & McNicholas, 2012).

Genetic, environmental, and developmental factors play a role in the etiology of the disease. Autism spectrum, other neurodevelopmental disorders, and communication problems should be considered in the differential diagnosis of selective non-speaking (Hua & Major, 2016).

Specific Phobia

Specific phobia is a state of excessive and irrational fear of particular objects and situations at a level disproportionate to the real danger. Specific phobias have animal, natural environment, blood-injection-injury, and situational subtypes. For patients, encountering the phobic stimulus always causes them to experience intense fear. Generally, specific phobias are accompanied by mood disorders, other anxiety disorders, and substance use disorders (Stinson et al., 2007).

The lifetime prevalence of specific phobia varies between 3% and 15% (Eaton et al., 2018). The most common types of phobias are height and animal phobia (Stinson et al., 2007). Although the symptoms of the disease often begin in childhood, it is observed that the disease has a second peak in older age due to changing conditions (Wardenaar et al., 2017; El-Gabalawy et al., 2011). In addition to environmental factors such as trauma, genetic factors are thought to play a role in the etiology of the disease (Muris, 2002). Specific risk factors for phobia include female gender and low education level. Differential diagnoses should be made for post-traumatic stress disorder, agoraphobia, and panic disorder (Eaton et al., 2018).

Social Anxiety Disorder (Social Phobia)

Social Anxiety Disorder is a state of intense fear and anxiety about being criticized, ridiculed, and rejected in social activities requiring interaction with people. Patients avoid situations and environments where they can contact others because they think that their anxiety, shyness, and physical symptoms (sweating, trembling, and blushing) will be noticed by others. The possibility of comorbidity with other anxiety disorders is high (Guha, 2014).

The lifetime prevalence rate of social anxiety disorder is estimated to be 4%. It usually starts in childhood (Stein et al., 2017). It is thought that genetic and biological factors, temperament characteristics, cognitive components, peer and parental relationships, adverse life events, and cultural variables play a role in the disorder's etiology (Spence & Rapee, 2016). Risk factors associated with social anxiety disorder include young age, female gender, low education level, low income, being single, and being widowed. In the differential diagnosis, timid personality disorder, agoraphobia, and post-traumatic stress disorder should be considered (Stein et al., 2017).

Panic Disorder

Panic attacks are seizures that occur suddenly and unexpectedly, terrify people, cause intense fear and distress, and are accompanied by physical symptoms due to sympathetic activation of the nervous system. Panic attacks do not only occur in panic disorder. Sudden situations that arouse intense fear and terror can activate the sympathetic system and panic attacks to react to threats and danger. Panic disorder occurs when recurrent and unexpected symptoms of panic attack are accompanied by anticipatory anxiety (anticipation and fear of having a panic attack). Symptoms and findings in the clinical course of the disease show individual differences. Physical findings during panic attacks cause patients to fear and worry that they will have a heart attack, stroke, epileptic seizure, die, lose their mind, harm themselves and others. Patients may avoid situations and activities that they think trigger panic attacks, and their occupational, social, and family functioning is seriously impaired. Furthermore, patients exhibit safety-enhancing behaviors, such as carrying medication with them constantly, having their blood pressure measured frequently, and checking their pulse to control and calm physical symptoms of panic attacks. Their anxiety about physical illness causes them to apply to health institutions, especially emergency services, frequently and to have unnecessary examinations (Guha, 2014).

The lifetime prevalence rate of panic attacks is estimated to be 13.2%. It was observed that only 12.8% of people who had previously experienced panic attacks met the DSM-5 diagnostic criteria for panic disorder. The prevalence rate of panic disorder in countries is 1.7% (de Jonge et al., 2018). It is reported that panic disorder has a prevalence of approximately 10% in primary health care services (King et al., 2008).

Abnormalities of the central and peripheral nervous systems have been shown to play a role in the etiopathogenesis of panic disorder. It is thought that impairment in fear processing circuits in the brain, increased sympathetic response of the autonomic nervous system, early life negative experiences, and genetic factors contribute to the disease. Female gender, early age, low education level, unemployment, and low-income level are important risk factors for panic disorder (de Jonge et al., 2018). Patients frequently present to the clinics with somatic symptoms. In the differential diagnosis, conditions such as pheochromocytoma, thyroid, parathyroid diseases, cardiac, and pulmonary diseases, intracranial tumors, and epilepsy, which overlap clinically with panic symptoms, should be excluded. Additionally, it should be considered that the drugs and illegal substances that patients use can trigger panic attacks (Giomi et al., 2021).

Agoraphobia

People with agoraphobia experience fear and anxiety about being in places or situations that they think they cannot escape. They may fear and avoid public transport, visiting a shopping center, leaving home, or being in public places. In DSM-5, agoraphobia is classified as a separate clinical diagnosis from the spectrum of panic disorder. Depending on the severity of the disease, individuals' social and professional lives are negatively affected. Agoraphobia can accompany significant depression, dysthymia, and substance use disorders (Guha, 2014).

The lifetime prevalence of agoraphobia is estimated to be 1.3%. There are different data on the association with panic disorder (Paul et al., 2022). According to some studies, cases of agoraphobia that are not accompanied by panic disorder are at a high rate. Symptoms usually start before the age of 35. It is more common in women than in men (Kessler et al., 2006).

It is thought that parental overprotectiveness, night terror, early life negative experiences, age, and genetic predisposition play a role in the etiology of agoraphobia. In the differential diagnosis, specific phobia, separation anxiety, post-traumatic stress disorder, panic disorder, and major depression should be considered (Paul et al., 2022).

Generalized Anxiety Disorder

Generalized anxiety disorder is a chronic, excessive, inappropriate state of worry accompanied by nonspecific physical and mental symptoms (such as muscle tension, fatigue, difficulty concentrating, restlessness, irritability, and sleep disturbances). Anxiety is usually related to simple daily activities, economic situations, health problems, and time management. They are defined as overly anxious people by their close relatives. Although they realize that the anxiety they experience is exaggerated, they have difficulty controlling their worries. Patients with generalized anxiety disorder usually present to primary health care services with vague physical complaints (Roberge et al., 2015). Non-specific symptoms overlapping with physical diseases lead to late diagnosis. Patients with generalized anxiety disorder are also at risk for cardiovascular diseases and suicide (Dang, 2022). It is frequently comorbid with major depression (Katzman, 2014).

The lifetime prevalence of generalized anxiety disorder is more than 6%. It is more common in women than in men (Kroenke et al., 2007). It is reported that environmental, psychological, genetic, and biological factors have been reported to play an essential role in their etiology. Early life negative experiences, parental loss, parental inconsistent behaviors, abuse, personality disorders, and interpersonal problems are associated with symptoms of a generalized anxiety disorder (Newman et al., 2003). Major depressive disorder, panic disorder, generalized anxiety disorder, post-traumatic stress disorder, and obsessive-compulsive disorder are included in the differential diagnosis (Latas, 2018).

Basic Principles in the Treatment of Anxiety Disorders

The main aim of treatment is to improve the psychological and physical symptoms of anxiety disorder and functionality. It is essential to establish a good patient-physician relationship. Treatment options should be explained to the patient, and the patient should be involved in the treatment decision. Patients may be reluctant to start drug treatment with the concern that tolerance to drug treatment may develop or that they will become dependent on drugs. Patients may think that drug treatment is symptomatic and neglect the treatment. Patients with anxiety disorders, especially those with panic disorder, should be informed that they may experience worsening anxiety symptoms at the beginning of antidepressant treatment, and some side effects may occur. Tolerance to these symptoms develops between 7-10 days. Pharmacotherapy should be started at a low dose, and the therapeutic dose should be reached in 1-2 weeks (Table 3) (Katzman et al., 2014; Andrews et al., 2018; Baldwin et al., 2005; Bandelow et al., 2008; Bandelow et al., 2015b).

Table 3. Initial and therapeutic doses of commonly used antidepressants in anxiety disorders

	Initial Dose	Average Dose	Dose Range
Sertraline	25 mg	100 mg	50-200 mg
Paroxetine	10 mg	40 mg	20-50 mg
Fluvoxamine	25-50 mg	100 mg	50-200 mg
Fluoxetine	5-10 mg	20 mg	10-80 mg
Citalopram	20 mg	40 mg	20-60 mg
Venlafaxine	37.5 mg	150 mg	75-225 mg
Clomipramine	10-12.5 mg	75 mg	50-225 mg

Treatment Guidelines for Anxiety Disorders

Various treatment guidelines have been developed to eliminate differences between research and clinical practice in anxiety disorders (Table 4) (Baldwin et al., 2005; Bandelow et al., 2012; Bandelow et al., 2015a; Kendrick & Pilling, 2012; Bisson et al., 2019; Benedek et al., 2009; Katzman et al., 2014; Andrews et al., 2018).

The British Association of Psychopharmacology evidence-based treatment guidelines for anxiety disorders, renewed in 2014, include separation anxiety disorder, specific phobia, social anxiety disorder, panic disorder, and generalized anxiety disorder. Acute and long-term treatment of disorders, psychological interventions, and resistance to treatment are included. Selective serotonin reuptake inhibitor antidepressants (SSRI) are recommended as the first-line treatment option. Benzodiazepines can be used for a short period and in groups of patient that do not respond to other treatment options (Baldwin et al., 2005).

In the treatment guideline for anxiety disorders published by the World Federation of Biological Psychiatry in 2012, recommendations are graded by categories of evidence. Specific phobia, social anxiety disorder, panic disorder, agoraphobia, and generalized anxiety disorder are included. The first-line treatment for panic disorder and agoraphobia is SSRI or venlafaxine; the first-line treatments for generalized anxiety disorder are SSRI, serotonin noradrenalin reuptake inhibitor antidepressants (SNRIs), pregabalin, and SSRI and venlafaxine for social anxiety disorder. This treatment guideline does not recommend discontinuing breastfeeding during SSRI or TSA use, except doxepin. Paroxetine and alprazolam should not be used in pregnant women or those planning a pregnancy (Bandelow et al., 2012).

Table 4. Treatment Guidelines for Anxiety Disorders

British Psychopharmacological Society Guidelines for the Evidence-Based Treatment of Anxiety Disorders
World Federation of Societies of Biological Psychiatry Anxiety Disorders Disorders Treatment Guide
The German guidelines for the treatment of anxiety disorders.
National Institute for Health and Clinical Treatment Guidelines
American Psychiatric Association Treatment Guidelines
Canadian Treatment Guidelines for Anxiety Disorders
Royal Australia and New Zealand Clinical Practice Guideline

The German S3 anxiety disorders treatment guideline was published in 2014. It was stated that treatment should continue for 6-12 months after remission. Cognitive behavioral therapies are recommended among psychotherapy options, and psychodynamic therapies are recommended in cases where it is not possible or ineffective. Among the pharmacotherapy options, SSRIs or SNRIs are recommended in the first place. Benzodiazepine is not recommended in patients at high risk of suicide due to abuse. It has been stated that treatment should be continued for 6-12 months after remission, and treatment can be extended up to 24 months to prevent relapse. In cases where there is no response to the drug between four and six weeks, it is reported that the drug should be discontinued and switched to another drug, and in cases of partial response at the end of 4-6 weeks, the drug dose should be increased. This treatment guideline suggests that exercise can be combined with other standard treatment options (Bandelow et al., 2015a).

The National Institute for Health and Clinical Excellence (NICE) guideline includes treatment algorithms for social anxiety, panic, and generalized anxiety disorders. In all guidelines, cognitive behavioral therapy ranks first as a psychotherapy method. The NICE guideline recommends psychodynamic therapies for social anxiety disorder. While other treatment guidelines emphasize the need to start treatment immediately, NICE recommends psychoeducation and self-help in the first place (Kendrick & Pilling, 2012; Bisson et al., 2019; Benedek et al., 2009).

In the Canadian clinical practice guideline published in 2014, social anxiety disorder, social phobias, panic disorder, agoraphobia, and generalized anxiety disorder were included. SSRIs and SNRIs are recommended for first-line treatment. The use of benzodiazepines is recommended for a short period for the onset of SSRI and SNRI efficacy in the early treatment period, and it is stated that treatment should continue for 12-24 months. It was emphasized that psychotherapies should be planned once a week for the first 12-20 weeks (Katzman et al., 2014).

Conclusion

Anxiety disorders, among the most common psychiatric disorders in primary care, lead to impairments in social, economic, and interpersonal areas. Their chronic course and comorbidity with mental and physical diseases negatively affect patients' quality of life and functionality. The fact that patients mostly present to physicians with somatic complaints, inadequate examination time, and a lack of knowledge and experience about anxiety disorders makes diagnosing the disease difficult. Undiagnosed anxiety disorders lead to unnecessary and costly diagnostic examinations. The diagnosis of the disease in primary health care services and early treatment planning by current treatment guidelines contribute to improving patients' clinical outcomes, increasing their quality of life, and decreasing health care costs.

References

Andrews, G., Bell, C., Boyce, P., Gale, C., Lampe, L., Marwat, O., Rapee, R., & Wilkins, G. (2018). Royal Australian and New Zealand College of Psychiatrists clinical practice guidelines for the treatment of panic disorder, social anxiety disorder and generalised anxiety disorder. *Australian & New Zealand Journal of Psychiatry, 52*(12), 1109-1172. https://doi.org/10.1177/0004867418799453.

Baldwin, D. S., Anderson, I. M., Nutt, D. J., Bandelow, B., Bond, A., Davidson, J. R., Den Boer, J. A., Fineberg, N. A., Knapp, M., Scott, J., & Wittchen, H. U. (2005). Evidence-based guidelines for the pharmacological treatment of anxiety disorders: Recommendations from the British Association for Psychopharmacology. *Journal of Psychopharmacology, 19*(6), 567-596. https://doi.org/10.1177/0269881105059253.

Baldwin, D. S., Gordon, R., Abelli, M., & Pini, S. (2016). The separation of adult separation anxiety disorder. *CNS Spectrums, 21*(4), 289-294. https://doi.org/10.1017/S1092852916000080.

Bandelow, B., Zohar, J., Hollander, E., Kasper, S., Möller, H. J., WFSBP Task Force on Treatment Guidelines for Anxiety Obsessive-Compulsive Post-Traumatic Stress Disorders, Zohar, J., Hollander, E., Kasper, S., Möller, H. J., Bandelow, B., Allgulander, C., Ayuso-Gutierrez, J., Baldwin, D. S., Buenvicius, R., Cassano, G., Fineberg, N., Gabriels, L., Hindmarch, I., Kaiya, H., Klein, D. F., Lader, M., Lecrubier, Y., Lépine, J. P., Liebowitz, M. R., Lopez-Ibor, J. J., Marazziti, D., Miguel, E. C., Oh, K. S., Preter, M., Rupprecht, R., Sato, M., Starcevic, V., Stein, D. J., van Ameringen, M., & Vega, J. (2008). World Federation of Societies of Biological Psychiatry (WFSBP) guidelines for the pharmacological treatment of anxiety, obsessive-compulsive and post-traumatic stress disorders–first revision. *The World Journal of Biological Psychiatry, 9*(4), 248-312. https://doi.org/10.1080/15622970802465807.

Bandelow, B., Sher, L., Bunevicius, R., Hollander, E., Kasper, S., Zohar, J., Möller, H. J., & WFSBP Task Force on Anxiety Disorders, OCD and PTSD. (2012). Guidelines for the pharmacological treatment of anxiety disorders, obsessive–compulsive disorder and posttraumatic stress disorder in primary care. *International Journal of Psychiatry in Clinical Practice, 16*(2), 77-84. https://doi.org/10.3109/13651501.2012.667114.

Bandelow, B., Lichte, T., Rudolf, S., Wiltink, J., & Beutel, M. E. (2015a). The German guidelines for the treatment of anxiety disorders. *European Archives of Psychiatry and Clinical Neuroscience, 265*, 363-373. https://doi.org/10.1007/s00406-014-0563-z.

Bandelow, B., Reitt, M., Röver, C., Michaelis, S., Görlich, Y., & Wedekind, D. (2015b). Efficacy of treatments for anxiety disorders: A meta-analysis. *International Clinical Psychopharmacology, 30*(4), 183-192. https://doi.org/10.1097/YIC.0000000000000078.

Baxter, A. J., Vos, T., Scott, K. M., Ferrari, A. J., & Whiteford, H. A. (2014). The global burden of anxiety disorders in 2010. *Psychological Medicine, 44*(11), 2363-2374. https://doi.org/10.1017/S0033291713003243.

Benedek, D. M., Friedman, M. J., Zatzick, D., & Ursano, R. J. (2009). Guideline watch (March 2009): Practice guideline for the treatment of patients with acute stress disorder and posttraumatic stress disorder. *Focus, 7*(2), 204-213. https://doi.org/10.1176/foc.7.2.foc204.

Bisson, J. I., Berliner, L., Cloitre, M., Forbes, D., Jensen, T. K., Lewis, C., Monson, C. M., Olff, M., Pilling, S., Riggs, D. S., Roberts, N. P., & Shapiro, F. (2019). The international society for traumatic stress studies new guidelines for the prevention and treatment of posttraumatic stress disorder: Methodology and development process. *Journal of Traumatic Stress, 32*(4), 475-483. https://doi.org/10.1002/jts.22421.

Dang, T. T., Patel, K., Farhat, K., Abraldes, J., Ma, M., Bailey, R. J., Burak, K. W., Mitchell, N., & Tandon, P. (2022). Anxiety in cirrhosis: A prospective study on prevalence and development of a practical screening nomogram. *European Journal of Gastroenterology & Hepatology, 34*(5), 553-559. https://doi.org/10.1097/MEG.0000000000002301.

de Jonge, P., Roest, A. M., Lim, C., Levinson, D., & Scott, K. (2018). Panic disorder and panic attacks. In *Mental Disorders Around the World: Facts and Figures from the WHO World Mental Health Surveys* (pp. 93-105). Cambridge University Press. https://doi.org/10.1017/9781316336168.007.

Eaton, W. W., Bienvenu, O. J., & Miloyan, B. (2018). Specific phobias. *The Lancet Psychiatry, 5*(8), 678-686. https://doi.org/10.1016/S2215-0366(18)30169-X.

El-Gabalawy, R., Mackenzie, C. S., Shooshtari, S., & Sareen, J. (2011). Comorbid physical health conditions and anxiety disorders: A population-based exploration of prevalence and health outcomes among older adults. *General Hospital Psychiatry, 33*(6), 556-564. https://doi.org/10.1016/j.genhosppsych.2011.07.005.

Elizur, Y., & Perednik, R. (2003). Prevalence and description of selective mutism in immigrant and native families: A controlled study. *Journal of the American Academy of Child & Adolescent Psychiatry, 42*(12), 1451-1459. https://doi.org/10.1097/00004583-200312000-00012.

Giomi, S., Siri, F., Ferro, A., Moltrasio, C., Ariyo, M., Delvecchio, G., & Brambilla, P. (2021). Executive functions in panic disorder: A mini-review. *Journal of Affective Disorders, 288*, 107-113. https://doi.org/10.1016/j.jad.2021.03.084.

Guha, M. (2014). *Diagnostic and Statistical Manual of Mental Disorders: DSM-5*. Reference Reviews, 28(3), 36-37. https://doi.org/10.1108/RR-10-2013-0256.

Hua, A., & Major, N. (2016). Selective mutism. *Current Opinion in Pediatrics, 28*(1), 114-120. https://doi.org/10.1097/MOP.0000000000000300.

Janca, A., & Hiller, W. (1996). ICD-10 checklists - a tool for clinicians' use of the ICD-10 classification of mental and behavioral disorders. *Comprehensive Psychiatry, 37*(3), 180-187. https://doi.org/10.1016/S0010-440X(96)90034-6.

Karakaya, I., Şişmanlar, Ş. G., Öç, Ö. Y., Memik, N. Ç., Coşkun, A., Ağaoğlu, B., & Yavuz, C. I. (2008). Selective mutism: A school-based cross-sectional study from Turkey. *European Child & Adolescent Psychiatry, 17*, 114-117. https://doi.org/10.1007/s00787-007-0644-x.

Katzman, M. A., Bleau, P., Blier, P., Chokka, P., Kjernisted, K., & Van Ameringen, M. (2014). Canadian clinical practice guidelines for the management of anxiety, posttraumatic stress and obsessive-compulsive disorders. *BMC Psychiatry, 14*(1), 1-83. https://doi.org/10.1186/1471-244X-14-S1-S1.

Kendrick, T., & Pilling, S. (2012). Common mental health disorders - identification and pathways to care: NICE clinical guideline. *British Journal of General Practice, 62*(594), 47-49. https://doi.org/10.3399/bjgp12X616481.

Kessler, R. C., Chiu, W. T., Jin, R., Ruscio, A. M., Shear, K., & Walters, E. E. (2006). The epidemiology of panic attacks, panic disorder, and agoraphobia in the National Comorbidity Survey Replication. *Archives of General Psychiatry, 63*(4), 415-424. https://doi.org/10.1001/archpsyc.63.4.415.

King, M., Nazareth, I., Levy, G., Walker, C., Morris, R., Weich, S., Bellón-Saameño, J. A., Moreno, B., Švab, I., Rotar, D., Rifel, J., Maaroos, H. I., Aluoja, A., Kalda, R., Neeleman, J., Geerlings, M. I., Xavier, M., de Almaida, M. C., Correa, B., & Torres-Gonzalez, F. (2008). Prevalence of common mental disorders in general practice attendees across Europe. *The British Journal of Psychiatry, 192*(5), 362-367. https://doi.org/10.1192/bjp.bp.107.039966.

Kristensen, H. (2000). Selective mutism and comorbidity with developmental disorder/delay, anxiety disorder, and elimination disorder. *Journal of the American Academy of Child & Adolescent Psychiatry, 39*(2), 249-256. https://doi.org/10.1097/00004583-200002000-00026.

Kroenke, K., Spitzer, R. L., Williams, J. B., Monahan, P. O., & Löwe, B. (2007). Anxiety disorders in primary care: prevalence, impairment, comorbidity, and detection. *Annals of Internal Medicine, 146*(5), 317-325. https://doi.org/10.7326/0003-4819-146-5-200703060-00004.

Latas, M., Trajković, G., Bonevski, D., Naumovska, A., Vučinić Latas, D., Bukumirić, Z., & Starčević, V. (2018). Psychiatrists' treatment preferences for generalized anxiety disorder. *Human Psychopharmacology: Clinical and Experimental, 33*(1), e2643. https://doi.org/10.1002/hup.2643.

Meier, S. M., Mattheisen, M., Mors, O., Mortensen, P. B., Laursen, T. M., & Penninx, B. W. (2016). Increased mortality among people with anxiety disorders: Total population study. *The British Journal of Psychiatry, 209*(3), 216-221. https://doi.org/10.1192/bjp.bp.115171975.

Muris, P., Merckelbach, H., de Jong, P. J., & Ollendick, T. H. (2002). The etiology of specific fears and phobias in children: A critique of the non-associative account. *Behaviour Research and Therapy, 40*(2), 185-195. https://doi.org/10.1016/S0005-7967(01)00051-1.

Newman, M. G., Llera, S. J., Erickson, T. M., Przeworski, A., & Castonguay, L. G. (2013). Worry and generalized anxiety disorder: A review and theoretical synthesis of evidence on nature, etiology, mechanisms, and treatment. *Annual Review of Clinical Psychology, 9*, 275-297. https://doi.org/10.1146/annurev-clinpsy-050212-185544.

Paul, T., Varshney, A., & Singh, A. P. (2022). Effectiveness of neurofeedback therapy adjunct to cognitive behavioral therapy in agoraphobia: A case study. *Annals of Neurosciences, 29*(4), 249-254. https://doi.org/10.1177/09727531221145768.

Roberge, P., Normand-Lauzière, F., Raymond, I., Luc, M., Tanguay-Bernard, M. M., Duhoux, A., Christian, B., & Fournier, L. (2015). Generalized anxiety disorder in primary care: Mental health services use and treatment adequacy. *BMC Family Practice, 16*(1), 1-11. https://doi.org/10.1186/s12875-015-0358-y.

Roest, A. M., Martens, E. J., de Jonge, P., & Denollet, J. (2010). Anxiety and risk of incident coronary heart disease: A meta-analysis. *Journal of the American College of Cardiology, 56*(1), 38-46. https://doi.org/10.1016/j.jacc.2010.03.034.

Saha, S., Lim, C. C., Cannon, D. L., Burton, L., Bremner, M., Cosgrove, P., Huo, Y., & McGrath, J. J. (2021). Co-morbidity between mood and anxiety disorders: A systematic review and meta-analysis. *Depression and Anxiety, 38*(3), 286-306. https://doi.org/10.1002/da.23113.

Sala, T., Cox, B. J., & Sareen, J. (2008). Anxiety disorders and physical illness comorbidity: An overview. In *Anxiety in Health Behaviors and Physical Illness. Series in Anxiety and Related Disorders*. Springer. https://doi.org/10.1007/978-0-387-74753-8_6.

Scott, K. M. (2014). Depression, anxiety, and incident cardiometabolic diseases. *Current Opinion in Psychiatry, 27*(4), 289-293. https://doi.org/10.1097/YCO.0000000000000067.

Sharkey, L., & McNicholas, F. (2012). Selective mutism: A prevalence study of primary school children in the Republic of Ireland. *Irish Journal of Psychological Medicine, 29*(1), 36-40. https://doi.org/10.1017/S0790966700017596.

Silove, D., Alonso, J., Bromet, E., Gruber, M., Sampson, N., Scott, K., Andrade, L., Benjet, C., Caldas de Almeida, J. M., De Girolamo, G., de Jonge, P., Demyttenaere, K., Fiestas, F., Florescu, S., Gureje, O., He, Y., Karam, E., Lepine, J. P., Murphy, S., Villa-Posada, J., Zarkov, Z., & Kessler, R. C. (2015). Pediatric-onset and adult-onset separation anxiety disorder across countries in the World Mental Health Survey. *American Journal of Psychiatry, 172*(7), 647-656. https://doi.org/10.1176/appi.ajp.2015.14091185.

Spence, S. H., & Rapee, R. M. (2016). The etiology of social anxiety disorder: An evidence-based model. *Behaviour Research and Therapy, 86*, 50-67. https://doi.org/10.1016/j.brat.2016.06.007.

Stein, D. J., Lim, C. C., Roest, A. M., De Jonge, P., Aguilar-Gaxiola, S., Al-Hamzawi, A., Alonso, J., Benjet, C., Bromet, E. J., Bruffaerts, R., de Girolamo, G., Florescu, S., Gureje, O., Haro, J. M., Harris, M. G., He, Y., Hinkov, H., Horiguchi, I., Hu, C., Karam, A., Karam, E. G., Lee, S., Lepine, J. P., Navarro-Mateu, F., Pennell, B. E., Piazza, M., Posada-Villa, J., ten Have, M., Torres, Y., Viana, M. C., Wojtyniak, B., Xavier, M., Kessler, R. C., Scott, K. M., & WHO World Mental Health Survey Collaborators. (2017). The cross-national epidemiology of social anxiety disorder: Data from the World Mental Health Survey Initiative. *BMC Medicine, 15*(1), 1-21. https://doi.org/10.1186/s12916-017-0889-2.

Stein, D. J., Scott, K. M., De Jonge, P., & Kessler, R. C. (2022). Epidemiology of anxiety disorders: From surveys to nosology and back. *Dialogues in Clinical Neuroscience*, 127-136. https://doi.org/10.31887/DCNS.2017.19.2/dstein.

Stinson, F. S., Dawson, D. A., Chou, S. P., Smith, S., Goldstein, R. B., Ruan, W. J., & Grant, B. F. (2007). The epidemiology of DSM-IV specific phobia in the USA: Results from the National Epidemiologic Survey on Alcohol and Related Conditions. *Psychological Medicine, 37*(7), 1047-1059. https://doi.org/10.1017/S0033291707000086.

Vermani, M., Marcus, M., & Katzman, M. A. (2011). Rates of detection of mood and anxiety disorders in primary care: A descriptive, cross-sectional study. *The Primary Care Companion for CNS Disorders, 13*(2), 27211. https://doi.org/10.4088/PCC.10m01013.

Wardenaar, K. J., Lim, C. C., Al-Hamzawi, A. O., Alonso, J., Andrade, L. H., Benjet, C. D., Bunting, B., de Girolamo, G., Demyttenaere, K., Florescu, S. E., Gureje, O., Hisateru, T., Huang, Y., Karam, E., Kiejna, A., Lepine, J. P., Navarro-Mateu, F., Oakley Browne, M., Piazza, M., Posada-Villa, J., ten Have, M. L., Torres, Y., Xavier, M., Zarkov, Z., Kessler, R. C., Scott, K. M., & De Jonge, P. (2017). The cross-national epidemiology of specific phobia in the World Mental Health Surveys. *Psychological Medicine, 47*(10), 1744-1760. https://doi.org/10.1017/S0033291717000174.

Chapter 14

Psychosis

Mehmet Vatansever*, MD
Department of Family Medicine, Kanuni Training and Research Hospital, Trabzon, Turkey

Abstract

The complex psychiatric condition known as psychosis is defined by a loss of connection to reality and frequently manifests itself as hallucinations, delusions, and cognitive abnormalities. Although it is estimated that between 1.5% and 3.5% of people will satisfy the criteria for a psychotic disorder, a much larger percentage of people will likely have at least one psychotic symptom throughout their lifetime. Numerous psychiatric, neuropsychiatric, neurologic, neurodevelopmental, and medical diseases frequently include psychosis. It is a defining characteristic of schizophrenia spectrum disorders and other psychotic diseases, a factor in many mood and substance use disorders, as well as a difficult symptom in many neurologic and medical conditions. Psychosis can be extremely challenging for both patients and their loved ones, which is why it has become a major focus of medical treatment. Primary care settings, such as family medicine play a crucial role in the early detection, diagnosis, treatment, and ongoing management of individuals with psychosis. This thorough chapter seeks to present an up-to-date summary of the most recent clinical recommendations and research findings for the management of psychosis in primary care settings.

Keywords: schizophrenia, delusions, hallucinations

Introduction

Psychosis is a condition in which an individual experiences a detachment from reality, signifying a combination of psychological symptoms. The prevailing belief suggests that a considerable and fluctuating portion of the population might encounter at least one psychotic symptom during their lifetime, although the percentage of individuals meeting the formal diagnostic criteria for a psychotic disorder is relatively low, ranging from 1.5 to 3.5% (Van Os et al., 2001). Psychosis frequently occurs and significantly impairs functionality as a symptom in various psychiatric, neurodevelopmental, neurological, and medical disorders. It is a critical focus for assessment and therapy in both neurological and psychiatric settings (Ismail et al.,

* Corresponding Author's Email: mysvatan@gmail.com.

In: Common Diseases According to Family Medicine Practice Guidelines
Editors: Esra Meltem Koç and Hilal Aksoy
ISBN: 979-8-89530-302-3

2011; Jellinger, 2012; Sultzer et al., 2014). It is a hallmark of schizophrenia spectrum disorders and other psychotic illnesses, plays a role in numerous mood and substance use disorders, and represents a challenging symptom across a range of neurological and medical conditions (Fiorentini et al., 2021). Psychosis has evolved into a key focus of treatment for medical experts due to the significant amounts of misery it can cause for patients and loved ones. Primary care settings, such as family medicine, also play a significant role in the early detection, diagnosis, treatment, and ongoing management of individuals with psychosis. This section defines psychosis and outlines the classification and recent changes in criteria for primary psychotic disorders as described in the Fifth Edition of the Diagnostic and Statistical Manual of Mental Disorders (Bhati, 2013). It encapsulates the contemporary evidence-based strategies for evaluating and managing both primary and secondary forms of psychosis. The definitions of psychosis in DSM-5 and the Tenth Revision of the International Classification of Diseases, encompassing hallucinations, delusions, and delusional misidentification syndromes, are presented. Additionally, it reviews the existing classification, updated criteria, and approaches for assessing psychoses in neurological conditions. Psychosis is a key characteristic of schizophrenia spectrum disorders and presents with consistent but fluctuating traits in mood and substance use disorders. Additionally, it frequently occurs in a range of developmental, acquired, and degenerative neurological and medical conditions. In these contexts, psychosis leads to impairment and acts as an obstacle to productivity and engagement (C. Morgan et al., 2014). Therefore, assessment and treatment of patients receiving care from neurologists, psychiatrists, and family physicians are important goals. This part not only delineates psychosis but also examines the basic clinical attributes of primary psychotic disorders and secondary psychoses in neurological conditions. It concludes by offering pragmatic, evidence-based guidelines for the evaluation and management of both primary and secondary psychotic disorders.

Main Body

A dramatic change in perception, behavior, and thought processes, known as psychosis, causes a person to lose their sense of reality. Hallucinations (sensory experiences that are not anchored in reality), delusions (persistent false beliefs that are resistant to logical reasoning), disorganized thinking, and obviously abnormal behavior are typical characteristics of psychosis. Frequently, these traits are referred to as positive symptoms.

Psychosis can present in a variety of clinical settings, including its relationship with mood disorders (such as major depressive disorder or bipolar disorder), during the times between episodes of mood disorders (as shown in schizoaffective disorder), or alone, as in the case of schizophrenia. People who are predisposed to them due to their personality qualities, developmental phases, or genetic predispositions are especially likely to experience transient psychotic episodes at times of psychological or physical stress.

In conclusion, psychosis represents a severe and complex mental condition characterized by a detachment from reality, with symptoms most commonly including delusions, hallucinations, and disorganized thinking and behavior.

Etiology

A fundamental mental disorder, substance abuse, or other neurologic or medical problem can all lead to psychosis. Dopaminergic overactivity (particularly in the mesocortical, mesolimbic, and nigrostriatal systems), and brain abnormalities, such as decreased prefrontal, superior, and medial temporal gray matter, have been linked to first-episode psychotic diseases (Pantelis et al., 2003). Psychotic symptoms and the onset of the disease often align with genetic and epigenetic predispositions, as well as environmental influences (such as substance abuse, stress, trauma, migration, infections, the postpartum period, or other medical reasons). However, primary psychotic disorders are viewed as neurodevelopmental anomalies that are believed to originate during prenatal development. There is substantial evidence indicating that genetic predispositions contribute significantly to the onset of psychotic disorders (Cardno et al., 1999).

Epidemiology

When compared to schizophrenia, which affects about 15 people per 100,000 people, the rate of a first episode of psychosis is roughly 50 per 100,000 (McGrath et al., 2004). The onset of psychosis primarily occurs in males during their teens to mid-20s, while in females, it often happens from their teens to late 20s. The early onset of psychosis is linked to poorer prognoses, yet early intervention can lead to more favorable results. It is exceedingly rare for psychosis to manifest in children.

Pathophysiology

The neurotransmitter dopamine has the strongest association with the pathophysiology of psychotic diseases. The positive symptoms in psychotic disorders are thought to result from an overabundance of dopamine in the mesolimbic pathway. Additional factors include glutamate, an excitatory neurotransmitter. The N-methylD-aspartate (NMDA) glutamate receptor was found to be less functional in numerous investigations (Geddes et al., 2011; Kehrer et al., 2008). Gamma-amino-butyric acid (GABA), a crucial neurotransmitter that acts as an inhibitor, has recently come under the spotlight in studies (Kinon et al., 2011). According to certain research, patients with schizophrenia exhibit signs of dysfunction. Asymmetry in acetylcholine is the final implication (Freedman et al., 2008; Olincy et al., 2006). Given that nicotine has been demonstrated to improve cholinergic function, this discovery was made while examining the smoking habits of schizophrenic patients. Studies showed that cognition had also improved, and observers observed some changes in the smokers deficiencies (Potasiewicz et al., 2017).

Schizophrenia Spectrum and Other Psychotic Disorders

Schizophrenia spectrum and other psychotic disorders encompass schizotypal (personality) disorders and various psychotic conditions. These disorders are characterized by one or more of the following five categories: hallucinations, disorganized thinking (speech), delusions, and negative symptoms.

Fundamental Characteristics that Define Psychotic Disorders

Delusions

Delusions are unchangeable fixed beliefs that cannot be altered in the face of contradictory information. They may cover a range of subjects in their content. Persecutory delusions are the most prevalent type, where people think they will be hurt or harassed by someone, a company, or a group. Referential illusions are also common, where people think that certain gestures, remarks, environmental clues, and so on are directed at them specifically. Erotomanic delusions involve the false notion that someone else is in love with them, whereas grandiose delusions involve people feeling they have outstanding talents, fortune, or renown. Somatic delusions are preoccupations with one's physical well-being and organ function, while nihilistic delusions center on the expectation of a big disaster (Bhati, 2013).

Hallucinations

Hallucinations occur in the absence of any external input. They are distinguished by their clarity and vividness, approximating normal perceptions, and being outside of the person's deliberate control. While hallucinations can manifest in any sensory modality, auditory hallucinations are particularly prevalent in schizophrenia and related disorders. Hearing voices, whether familiar or unknown, is a common aspect of auditory hallucinations. These voices are distinguished from the person's own thoughts. Hallucinations are typically experienced during full consciousness, with those occurring during the transition into sleep (hypnagogic) or upon waking up (hypnopompic) considered normal human experiences. Additionally, hallucinations might be seen as a typical aspect of religious experiences in some cultural situations (Bhati, 2013).

Disorganized Thinking (Speech)

Speech patterns are frequently used to detect disordered thinking, also known as formal thought disorder. This may entail changing the subject, responding to queries in a way that is unconnected to them, or even speaking in an incoherent manner. It is important to remember that somewhat slurred speech is frequent and not unique to any one ailment; as a result, for something to be called a symptom, it must materially interfere with efficient communication. When the person making the diagnosis and the patient speak different languages, it can be difficult to determine the severity of the impairment. Certain religious or cultural practices may involve disorganized speech, but they do not necessarily indicate psychosis unless accompanied by other clear psychotic symptoms. Less severe forms of disorganized thinking or speech can also occur during the prodromal and residual stages of schizophrenia (Bhati, 2013).

Disorganized or Abnormal Motor Behavior (Including Catatonia)

Severe disorganization or abnormal movements, ranging from childish playfulness to sudden restlessness, may result in challenges with everyday tasks because of disruptions in purposeful actions. Catatonic behavior involves a significant reduction in responsiveness to the environment, including resistance to instructions, maintaining rigid or bizarre postures, or a complete lack of verbal and motor responses. Catatonia may also involve aimless and heightened physical movements that lack an obvious reason. These symptoms historically associated with schizophrenia are not specific and may occur in other mental disorders and medical conditions (Bhati, 2013).

Catatonia is another expression of psychosis that can manifest as either extreme resistance or increased excitement (Bhati, 2013).

Negative Symptoms

Reduced emotional expression and avolition are negative symptoms that are prevalent in schizophrenia but are comparatively less pronounced in other psychotic disorders. Reduced emotional display in the face, eye contact, speech intonation (prosody), and hand, head, and facial movements that generally transmit emotions during speaking are all examples of diminished emotional expressiveness. The hallmark of avolition is a drop in self-motivated, worthwhile activities, which frequently results in protracted periods of inactivity and a loss of interest in job or social involvement. Alogia (reduced speech output), anhedonia (diminished capacity for pleasure, though people can still engage in pleasurable activities at the moment), and asociality (apparent disinterest in social interactions, occasionally linked to avolition or restricted social opportunities) are additional negative symptoms (Bhati, 2013).

Psychosis Symptoms and Clinical Phenomena Assessment

The variety of psychotic diseases makes it possible to forecast key elements of the condition, such as the severity of cognitive or neurobiological abnormalities. The treatment approach is determined based on the intensity of mood symptoms in psychosis, which also serves as a predictive indicator. Therefore, for all psychotic diseases, dimensional assessments of depression and mania alert doctors to mood pathology and the need for treatment when necessary. Many individuals diagnosed with psychotic disorders exhibit cognitive deficits across various domains, which serve as indicators of their functional abilities. Clinical neuropsychological evaluation can aid in guiding diagnosis and therapy, although quick evaluations without a thorough neuropsychological evaluation can still yield valuable data that may be adequate for a diagnosis. When formal neuropsychological tests are performed, they should be done by people who have been trained to use the testing devices (Bhati, 2013).

Primary Psychotic Disorders

When exposed to specific social and environmental dangers, a portion of the population can become more susceptible to chronic psychotic symptoms due to genetic, epigenetic, and developmental variables (Arnedo et al., 2015; Linscott & Van Os, 2013; V. A. Morgan et al., 2011). This concept, sometimes referred to as the psychosis proneness-persistence model, aids in explaining how hallucinations and delusions can manifest in a variety of neurologic and psychiatric diseases. It adheres to the Research Domain Criteria (RDoC) framework of the National Institute of Mental Health (NIMH), which investigates these phenomena in connection with underlying neurological systems in a variety of contexts rather than in terms of particular diagnostic classifications (Ford et al., 2014; Insel et al., 2010).

Given this, it is not unexpected that the DSM-5 lists psychosis as a symptom of a number of psychiatric diseases. Psychosis predominantly manifests in schizophrenia spectrum disorders, such as schizophrenia, brief psychotic disorder, schizophreniform disorder, schizoaffective disorder, and delusional disorder. However, it can also emerge in people with bipolar disorder during either manic or depressive episodes and in individuals undergoing a major depressive episode within major depressive disorder. In these instances, the psychotic features, especially delusions, might align with or contradict the current emotional state.

Schizophrenia Spectrum Disorders

Following the DSM-5 release, schizophrenia is no longer considered the prototype of psychotic disorders; instead, it is seen as one of many psychotic conditions that fall under a wider spectrum of psychopathology. The kind, quantity, complexity, intensity, and duration of the psychotic symptoms and other characteristics that characterize the many disorders on the schizophrenia spectrum vary from one disorder to the next. Hallucinations, delusions, disordered thinking (formal thought disorder, typically deduced from a person's speech), wildly chaotic or aberrant motor action (including catatonia), and negative symptoms are all signs of schizophrenia spectrum disorders (Bhati, 2013).

Schizotypal (Personality) Disorder

Social and interpersonal deficiencies that limit the ability to see and cause pronounced discomfort with close interactions are characteristics of schizotypal disorder. These impairments often co-occur with unsettling perceptual experiences (such as illusions) and cognitive distortions, including ideas of reference, suspicion or paranoia, odd beliefs, or magical thinking without the full conviction of delusions. These experiences are similar to but less intense than those encountered by individuals with schizophrenia (Chemerinski et al., 2013).

Delusional Disorder

In comparison to the DSM-4, the DSM-5 includes a wider spectrum of psychotic intensity when defining delusional illness. This diagnostic calls for the presence of one or more delusions that endure for at least a month without the presence of overt hallucinations, according to both the DSM-IV-TR and the DSM-5. If hallucinations are experienced, they must be connected to the delusional topic, such as tactile hallucinations of insects crawling on the skin in a patient with parasitosis beliefs. As a result, although the existence of odd content is utilized as a specifier in this diagnostic, the existence of either common or bizarre delusions (or both) is now in line with a diagnosis of delusional disorder.

Brief Psychotic Disorder

This condition is marked by the presence of symptoms such as delusions, hallucinations, disorganized thinking (manifested through disorganized speech), or unusual psychomotor activities (such as severe disorganization or catatonia), not explainable by other mental, substance-related, or medical disorders. The symptoms persist for a minimum of one day and no more than one month, after which there is a full restoration of the person's prior functional level. Negative symptoms are not among the diagnostic criteria for this condition.

Schizophreniform Disorder

Schizophreniform disorder serves as an intermediate condition within the continuum that includes brief psychotic disorder and schizophrenia, characterized by two or more psychotic-related symptoms. Such symptoms encompass delusions, hallucinations, incoherent speech (a sign of disorganized thought processes), and highly disordered or catatonic actions, with at least one being either delusions, hallucinations, or incoherent speech. This disorder's timeframe spans from a minimum of one month up to less than six months. The DSM-5 differentiates from the DSM-IV-TR by permitting an early tentative diagnosis of schizophreniform disorder within this period, eliminating the need to delay for a possible improvement.

Schizophrenia

The DSM-5 has made significant revisions to the diagnostic criteria for schizophrenia. The fundamental criteria now require two or more psychotic and related symptoms (such as delusions, hallucinations, disorganized speech, grossly disorganized or catatonic behavior, and negative symptoms), each persisting for a substantial part of a 1-month period (or shorter if treated effectively). At least one of these symptoms must be delusions, hallucinations, or disorganized speech. Additionally, these symptoms must lead to reduced functioning in one or more major life areas, including self-care, work, interpersonal relationships, or academic performance.

In contrast to earlier DSM versions, the DSM-5 no longer recognizes schizophrenia subgroups. The major symptom at the time of an evaluation previously served to categorize these subtypes (paranoid, disorganized, catatonic, undifferentiated, residual). Given their longitudinal instability, overlap of traits, and inability to consistently predict outcomes, these the validity of these classifications was questioned. The DSM-5 eliminates schizophrenia subtyping in favor of utilizing the Clinician-Rated Dimensions of Psychosis Symptom Severity scale to describe the characteristics of schizophrenia. This change acknowledges the challenges associated with schizophrenia subtypes and reflects the reduced use of subtypes in both clinical and research settings.

Schizoaffective Disorder

The psychiatric field has grappled with defining schizoaffective disorder. Some researchers view it as a variant of schizophrenia with prominently prominent mood symptoms that are not atypical. Others characterize it as a mood disorder where psychotic symptoms linked to mood episodes do not reoccur. Others still believe that schizophrenia and a mood disorder simply co-occur since they are two relatively prevalent but etiologically different forms of psychiatric illnesses. Although the DSM-5's criteria have been altered in a way that is expected to result in a decrease in the number of diagnoses of schizoaffective disorder, the issue nonetheless remains unsolved.

Under the DSM-IV-TR, the diagnostic criteria for schizoaffective disorder require an uninterrupted illness phase during which a significant mood episode aligns with certain diagnostic features. These features, referred to as Criteria A for schizophrenia, include experiences of delusions, hallucinations, chaotic speech (reflecting disturbed thought processes), erratic psychomotor activities, and negative symptoms, necessitating the presence of delusions, hallucinations, or chaotic speech them. Schizoaffective disorder diagnosis mandates the occurrence of delusions or hallucinations for a minimum duration of two weeks, regardless of manic or depressive episodes' presence. This duration of psychosis, independent of mood disturbances, sets schizoaffective disorder apart from bipolar or depressive disorders with psychotic elements, where psychotic features are tied to the beginning or end of the mood episode.

Secondary Psychotic Disorders

The DSM-5 acknowledges the common co-occurrence of psychotic phenomena such as delusions and hallucinations with a range of neurocognitive disorders stemming from various medical conditions, including Alzheimer's disease, Parkinson's disease, Lewy body disease, frontotemporal lobar degeneration, Huntington's disease, prion disease, cerebrovascular disease, traumatic brain injury, and HIV, among others. In instances where these psychotic features coincide with cognitive impairments due to these conditions, the DSM-5 recommends classifying the neurocognitive disorder as having "behavioral disturbance (psychosis)" rather than attributing it to a separate schizophrenia spectrum disorder. When hallucinations or delusions are significant, not explained by other mental disorders, extend beyond delirium symptoms, cause significant distress or functional decline, and are linked to a neurological or medical condition, or arise from substance use or medication, the diagnosis of a "psychotic disorder due to another medical condition" or a "substance/medication-induced psychotic disorder" is considered more appropriate. A thorough exploration of the clinical aspects of psychosis in neurological conditions exceeds this summary's scope, given the significant expansion in the research covering the clinical presentation, epidemiology, and potential neurobiological underpinnings of hallucinations and delusions in these disorders over the last two decades.

Evaluation

The interview is crucial in helping determine the course of treatment, similar to other medical or psychiatric issues. As usual, getting a complete history comes first. This includes documenting the timeline and severity of symptoms, previous psychiatric conditions, medical history, hospitalizations, medications (both psychiatric and non-psychiatric), detailed social background, substance use history, history of trauma (emotional, physical, sexual), suicidal thoughts with any prior attempts, and experiences of auditory/visual hallucinations. While these elements are essential, they are not exhaustive, and medical professionals should recognize that psychiatric patients may have difficulties providing a concise history due to their underlying condition.

The mental state exam (MSE), which is a crucial part of the psychiatric interview and of equal importance to the history, is conducted. It is important to pay close attention to how the patient appears, behaves, speaks, feels, thinks, and processes his or her thoughts. A conventional medical examination, in addition to a urine toxicology test, can assist in ruling out non-psychiatric origins of psychosis as can a few further tests if clinical suspicion allows. One of these is:

- Complete blood count and metabolic panel
- Urinalysis, urine cultures
- Thyroid-stimulating hormone (TSH), T4, T3
- Liver function tests
- Vitamin B12
- HIV
- CT, MRI
- EEG
- Lumbar puncture
- Rheumatologic or immunological workup.

It should be emphasized that certain substances, such as psychedelics, certain synthetic forms of cannabis, and bath salts, may not be identifiable through standard drug screening panels (Freudenreich et al., 2009).

Treatment

Depending on the underlying factors contributing to the disorder, several approaches are taken while treating patients who are experiencing psychosis. Any patient having a psychotic episode has to be evaluated by a psychiatrist. The primary and most effective treatment for psychotic episodes and illnesses connected to them is antipsychotic medication, with the choice, dose, and method of administration primarily depending on the unique clinical circumstances.

Antipsychotic medications are frequently chosen as the therapy of choice for diseases that fall within the spectrum of schizophrenia. Usually, the initial dosage is started at a modest level and is increased as necessary. It is important to note that there has been continuous discussion regarding the relative effectiveness of second-generation antipsychotics against their first-generation counterparts (Hartling et al., 2012; Saha et al., 2016; Temmingh et al., 2018).

Drug-induced psychosis, mania, delirium (Wang et al., 2013), psychotic aspects of depression, and the psychotic features of dementia and other neurological conditions have all shown positive responses to antipsychotic treatment. However, it is important to note that addressing the root cause remains the optimal course of action beyond the acute phase of psychosis.

Antipsychotic medications have demonstrated their efficacy primarily in alleviating the positive symptoms of psychosis, such as hallucinations, delusions, disorganized thinking, and behavior. However, they are generally less effective in addressing the negative symptoms of psychosis (Buchanan et al., 2010). Significant adverse effects such as extrapyramidal symptoms and risky QT prolongation might also be seen in them. In particular, clozapine and olanzapine have been proven to lower the risk of suicide in patients with psychosis (Ringbäck Weitoft et al., 2014).

There is evidence that benzodiazepines are a successful treatment for the catatonic symptoms of psychosis.

In addition to drugs, family members and other caregivers are crucial in the management of a psychotic patient. This includes providing the patient with a secure and therapeutic environment and communicating with them in a collected and sympathetic way (Price et al., 2015).

An acutely psychotic patient who is agitated, perhaps hostile, and at risk of hurting oneself or another person should be admitted to the hospital and placed under the supervision of medical personnel. In this instance, an injectable form of a standard antipsychotic containing a benzodiazepine is most efficient (Clinton et al., 1987). Physical restrictions should never be used since they increase death rates.

Patients with psychotic symptoms may benefit greatly from cognitive behavioral therapy in addition to medication (Taylor et al., 2020).

Finally, it is crucial to remember that early care may enhance clinical outcomes for patients with acute onset psychosis who later develop a schizophrenia-spectrum psychotic disease. Poorer treatment outcomes are statistically associated with treatment delays (Perkins et al., 2005).

Antipsychotic Medications

Antipsychotic medications, also known as neuroleptic drugs, constitute a class of pharmaceuticals primarily that are used to alleviate or manage the symptoms of psychotic disorders, enhance the quality of life, and support individuals in their path to recovery. Psychotic disorders are characterized by the presence of psychotic symptoms, which can encompass hallucinations, delusions, disorganized thinking, and impaired insight. Schizophrenia is the most prevalent and well-known among psychotic disorders. However, other psychotic conditions, such as schizoaffective disorder and bipolar disorder with psychotic symptoms, also exist.

Antipsychotic medications, or neuroleptics, are widely recognized as a fundamental treatment approach for addressing psychotic symptoms, allowing for symptom attenuation and improved functioning in individuals. These drugs are prescribed by psychiatrists or specialist physicians and their usage necessitates vigilant monitoring and individualized adjustments, tailored to meet the specific needs and tolerances of the patient."

Psychotic medications are broadly categorized into two main groups: typical (first-generation) antipsychotics and atypical (second-generation) antipsychotics. Each category has its own mechanism of action and potential side effects:

1. Typical Antipsychotics (First-Generation Antipsychotics):

Typical antipsychotics, such as haloperidol, chlorpromazine, and fluphenazine, primarily function by blocking dopamine receptors in the brain, specifically targeting the D2 receptors. This helps reduce the overactivity of dopamine, which is thought to contribute to psychotic symptoms.

Common side effects include extrapyramidal symptoms (EPS) such as dystonia, akathisia, and parkinsonism, as well as tardive dyskinesia (involuntary movements), sedation, weight gain, and elevated prolactin levels.

2. Atypical Antipsychotics (Second – Generation Antypsychotics):

Examples include Aripiprazole, Risperidone, Olanzapine, Quetiapine, Clozapine. Atypical antipsychotics also affect dopamine receptors but to a lesser extent than typical antipsychotics. They also target serotonin receptors, which can help alleviate negative and mood symptoms associated with psychosis. Atypical antipsychotics tend to have a lower risk of EPS and tardive dyskinesia compared to typical antipsychotics. However, they may be associated with metabolic side effects, such as weight gain, diabetes, and lipid abnormalities.

The choice of antipsychotic medication depends on various factors, including the specific symptoms and diagnosis of the individual, their medical history, and their response to previous treatments. In some cases, a combination of medications may be used to achieve the best results.

It is important to note that antipsychotic medications are typically prescribed by a psychiatrist or mental health professional and should be closely monitored for their effectiveness and side effects. Additionally, these medications are often just one component of a comprehensive treatment plan for psychotic disorders, which can also include psychotherapy, support groups, and lifestyle modifications.

It is crucial for individuals with psychotic disorders to work closely with their healthcare providers to find the most suitable medication and treatment plan to manage their condition and improve their overall well-being. The choice of medication and treatment approach may need to be adjusted over time based on an individual's response and changing needs (Gründer et al., 2016; Lally & MacCabe, 2015; Leucht et al., 2021).

Differential Diagnosis

To separate psychoses that are the result of a fundamental psychiatric illness from those that emerge from medical or neurological issues, the following standards should be examined:

Age of onset: This factor holds paramount significance in the determination of the etiology behind a psychotic episode. Primary psychotic disorders typically manifest during the late teenage years up to the early thirties, with men often presenting symptoms at an earlier age than women. On the contrary, psychotic symptoms linked to medical or neurological conditions typically manifest after the age of 40. The advanced age of the patient correlates with an increased risk of medical or neurological psychosis, a correlation particularly notable within hospital settings.

The pattern of onset: In contrast, primary psychotic disorders can present with subtle symptoms initially, including a prodromal phase that can resemble those of other psychiatric disorders. For instance, schizophrenia's early stages can be mistaken for depression. On the other hand, medical or neurological psychosis typically presents abruptly.

Genetics: There exists a substantial correlation between primary psychotic disorders and a family history of the condition, which is more pronounced than the link between psychosis and medical/neurological conditions.

Presentation: Primary psychotic disorders frequently manifest during periods of significant life stressors such as relocation, changes in employment, or the termination of a relationship. Conversely, psychosis associated with medical/neurological conditions tends to manifest predominantly within healthcare settings.

Hallucinations: Primary psychotic disorders are typically characterized by auditory hallucinations, whereas psychosis associated with medical/neurological conditions often involves various forms of hallucinations, except auditory (e.g., visual, tactile, olfactory) (Freudenreich, 2012; Lauterbach et al., 2008).

Prognosis

While schizophrenia was once thought to invariably result in a poor prognosis, recent studies have demonstrated the potential for favorable outcomes. The introduction of numerous newer medications, as well as the availability of long-acting injectable antipsychotics, has expanded the range of treatment options for patients while addressing issues related to treatment adherence. As mentioned earlier, early intervention and intensive treatment appear to play a crucial role in achieving favorable long-term outcomes. Limited data exists to support either positive or negative prognoses for a single psychotic episode linked to a medical or neurological condition, with the outlook being dependent on the specific underlying condition. In such cases, the optimal course of action typically involves addressing the current episode while concurrently treating the underlying disease (Blackburn, 2019; Freudenreich et al., 2007).

Complications

In any episode of psychosis, regardless of its underlying cause, there exists a potential risk of harm to oneself or others. Consequently, these patients necessitate admission to a secure and therapeutic medical environment. The criteria for involuntary admission may vary depending on the state or country's legal regulations. Symptoms such as paranoia, suspicion, fear, or other manifestations of psychosis can impede initial help-seeking behavior and hinder a patient's ability to comply with medication and treatment regimens. Antipsychotic medications are linked to notable side effects, including extrapyramidal symptoms (EPS), metabolic syndrome, cardiac irregularities, sexual dysfunction, anticholinergic effects, and tardive dyskinesia, among others. Psychotic disorders can significantly impact daily functioning and increase the risk of suicide compared to the general population. For instance, the suicide rate among individuals with schizophrenia is around 5%. (Hor & Taylor, 2010).

Pearls and Other Problems

- Psychosis constitutes a constellation of symptoms that lead to a detachment from reality.
- Approximately 1.5% to 3.5% of individuals will meet the diagnostic criteria for a primary psychiatric disorder during their lifetime, while a larger population will experience varying degrees of psychotic symptoms.
- Anomalies in temporal gray matter have been associated with the onset of first-episode psychosis.
- The occurrence of initial psychotic episodes often correlates with epigenetic or environmental stressors.
- A psychotic episode or disorder manifests through one or more of these five key features: delusions, hallucinations, incoherent thinking, chaotic behavior, and negative symptoms.
- The occurrence rate of a psychotic episode is estimated to be approximately 50 cases per 10,000 individuals. Typically, males experience the onset of psychotic disorders earlier than females.
- Neurotransmitters such as dopamine, glutamate, GABA, and acetylcholine play a crucial role in the development of psychotic conditions.
- Delusions can be classified as 'bizarre,' which are completely irrational, or 'non-bizarre,' which are extremely improbable, yet not impossible.
- A comprehensive patient history and a thorough mental status examination (MSE) are of paramount importance in establishing a diagnosis.
- In addition to a urine toxicology screen, a standard medical workup is essential for excluding non-psychiatric causes of psychosis. It is important to note that not all drugs will be detectable through routine screening.
- When distinguishing primary psychotic disorders from those related to medical or neurological issues, it is important to consider factors such as the age at onset, onset pattern, genetic predispositions, symptomatology, and the type of hallucinations experienced.

- The initial phase of schizophrenia is often confused with major depressive disorder.
- A psychiatric evaluation is essential for anyone experiencing psychotic symptoms.
- Antipsychotic medications are considered the standard of care for treating psychotic episodes and related disorders.
- These medications are particularly effective against the positive symptoms of psychosis.
- However, it is crucial to acknowledge that antipsychotic medications can lead to significant side effects, including QTc prolongation, extrapyramidal symptoms (EPS), metabolic syndrome, sexual side effects, and tardive dyskinesia, among others."
- Clozapine and olanzapine are the sole antipsychotic agents demonstrated to reduce suicidality in individuals with psychosis.
- Creating a secure and therapeutic setting characterized by tranquil and empathetic patient interactions is indispensable in addressing psychotic symptoms.
- There exists the possibility of achieving favorable outcomes in patients diagnosed with psychotic disorders.
- Timely intervention plays a pivotal role in securing favorable long-term results.
- The risk of suicide in individuals with schizophrenia is higher compared to the general population (Bansal & Chatterjee, 2021; Rössler et al., 2005; J. van Os et al., 2009).

"Psychosis Management in Primary Care"

The complex psychiatric condition known as psychosis is defined by a loss of connection to reality and frequently manifests itself as hallucinations, delusions, and cognitive abnormalities. Primary care settings, such as family medicine play a crucial role in the early detection, diagnosis, treatment, and ongoing management of individuals with psychosis. This thorough review seeks to present an up-to-date summary of the most recent clinical recommendations and research findings for the management of psychosis in primary care settings. Due to its complexity, psychosis presents considerable obstacles in primary care. Recent research has led to a better understanding of the underlying causes, treatment modalities, and strategies for long-term care. The goal of this study is to offer primary care physicians with the knowledge and resources needed for efficient psychosis management by compiling the most recent advancements in the field.

The following are important details about managing psychosis in primary care (Abdel-Baki et al., 2012; Maj et al., 2021; Spencer et al., 2001):

Early Detection and Assessment

- It is critical to spot the first indications of psychosis.
- Screening instruments and evaluation techniques.
- Red flags for specialist referral.

Pharmacological Management

- The function of antipsychotic drugs in the treatment of psychosis.
- Recent developments in pharmaceutical treatments.
- Controlling adverse effects and drug adherence.

Psychotherapy

- Integrating psychotherapy into primary care is one of the psychosocial interventions.
- Psychosocial therapies supported by evidence.
- Models of collaborative care.

Participation of the Support Network

- The family's support of those suffering from psychosis.
- Using available community resources.
- Eliminating stigma and increasing awareness.

Ongoing Monitoring and Follow-Up

- The significance of routine follow-up visits.
- Tracking the development of symptoms and the impact of treatment.
- Modifying treatment programs as necessary.

Initiatives in Education and Public Health

- Increasing knowledge of psychosis in contexts of primary care.
- Programs for community education.
- Lowering inequities in healthcare access.

Conclusion

This comprehensive review emphasizes the pivotal role that primary care physicians play in the management of psychosis and illuminates recent strides in the realms of diagnosis, treatment, and continual care. Remaining abreast of the most current research discoveries and guidelines stands as a cornerstone for enhancing outcomes and augmenting the quality of life for individuals who grapple with psychosis. Through the dedicated adherence to evidence-based methodologies and the nurturing of cooperative relationships with mental health experts, primary care practitioners are empowered to exert a profound influence on the overall well-being of their patients navigating the complexities of psychosis.

References

Abdel-Baki, A., Ouellet-Plamondon, C., & Malla, A. (2012). Pharmacotherapy challenges in patients with first-episode psychosis. *Journal of Affective Disorders, 138*, S3–S14. https://doi.org/10.1016/j.jad.2012.02.029.

Arnedo, J., Svrakic, D. M., Del Val, C., Romero-Zaliz, R., Hernández-Cuervo, H., Fanous, A. H., Pato, M. T., Pato, C. N., De Erausquin, G. A., Cloninger, C. R., & Zwir, I. (2015). Uncovering the hidden risk architecture of the schizophrenias: Confirmation in three independent genome-wide association studies. *The American Journal of Psychiatry, 172*(2), 139–153. https://doi.org/10.1176/APPI.AJP.2014.14040435.

Bansal, V., & Chatterjee, I. (2021). Role of neurotransmitters in schizophrenia: A comprehensive study. *Kuwait Journal of Science, 48*(2). https://doi.org/10.48129/kjs.v48i2.9264.

Bhati, M. T. (2013). Defining psychosis: The evolution of DSM-5 schizophrenia spectrum disorders. *Current Psychiatry Reports, 15*(11). https://doi.org/10.1007/S11920-013-0409-9.

Blackburn, T. P. (2019). Depressive disorders: Treatment failures and poor prognosis over the last 50 years. *Pharmacology Research & Perspectives, 7*(3). https://doi.org/10.1002/prp2.472.

Buchanan, R. W., Kreyenbuhl, J., Kelly, D. L., Noel, J. M., Boggs, D. L., Fischer, B. A., Himelhoch, S., Fang, B., Peterson, E., Aquino, P. R., & Keller, W. (2010). The 2009 schizophrenia PORT psychopharmacological treatment recommendations and summary statements. *Schizophrenia Bulletin, 36*(1), 71–93. https://doi.org/10.1093/SCHBUL/SBP116.

Cardno, A. G., Marshall, E. J., Coid, B., Macdonald, A. M., Ribchester, T. R., Davies, N. J., Venturi, P., Jones, L. A., Lewis, S. W., Sham, P. C., Gottesman, I. I., Farmer, A. E., McGuffin, P., Reveley, A. M., & Murray, R. M. (1999). Heritability estimates for psychotic disorders: The Maudsley twin psychosis series. *Archives of General Psychiatry, 56*(2), 162–168. https://doi.org/10.1001/ARCHPSYC.56.2.162.

Chemerinski, E., Triebwasser, J., Roussos, P., & Siever, L. J. (2013). Schizotypal personality disorder. *Journal of Personality Disorders, 27*(5), 652–679. https://doi.org/10.1521/PEDI_2012_26_053.

Clinton, J. E., Sterner, S., Stelmachers, Z., & Ruiz, E. (1987). Haloperidol for sedation of disruptive emergency patients. *Annals of Emergency Medicine, 16*(3), 319–322. https://doi.org/10.1016/S0196-0644(87)80179-8.

Fiorentini, A., Cantù, F., Crisanti, C., Cereda, G., Oldani, L., & Brambilla, P. (2021). Substance-induced psychoses: An updated literature review. *Frontiers in Psychiatry, 12*, 694863. https://doi.org/10.3389/FPSYT.2021.694863.

Ford, J. M., Morris, S. E., Hoffman, R. E., Sommer, I., Waters, F., McCarthy-Jones, S., Thoma, R. J., Turner, J. A., Keedy, S. K., Badcock, J. C., & Cuthbert, B. N. (2014). Studying hallucinations within the NIMH RDoC framework. *Schizophrenia Bulletin, 40*(Suppl 4). https://doi.org/10.1093/SCHBUL/SBU011.

Freedman, R., Olincy, A., Buchanan, R. W., Harris, J. G., Gold, J. M., Johnson, L., Allensworth, D., Guzman-Bonilla, A., Clement, B., Ball, M. P., Kutnick, J., Pender, V., Martin, L. F., Stevens, K. E., Wagner, B. D., Zerbe, G. O., Soti, F., & Kem, W. R. (2008). Initial phase 2 trial of a nicotinic agonist in schizophrenia. *The American Journal of Psychiatry, 165*(8), 1040–1047. https://doi.org/10.1176/APPI.AJP.2008.07071135.

Freudenreich, O. (2012). Differential diagnosis of psychotic symptoms: Medical. *Psychiatric Times*. http://www.psychiatrictimes.com.

Freudenreich, O., Charles Schulz, S., & Goff, D. C. (2009). Initial medical work-up of first-episode psychosis: A conceptual review. *Early Intervention in Psychiatry, 3*(1), 10–18. https://doi.org/10.1111/J.1751-7893.2008.00105.X.

Freudenreich, O., Holt, D. J., Cather, C., & Goff, D. C. (2007). The evaluation and management of patients with first-episode schizophrenia: A selective, clinical review of diagnosis, treatment, and prognosis. *Harvard Review of Psychiatry, 15*(5), 189–211. https://doi.org/10.1080/10673220701679804.

Geddes, A. E., Huang, X. F., & Newell, K. A. (2011). Reciprocal signalling between NR2 subunits of the NMDA receptor and neuregulin1 and their role in schizophrenia. *Progress in Neuro-Psychopharmacology & Biological Psychiatry, 35*(4), 896–904. https://doi.org/10.1016/J.PNPBP.2011.02.017.

Gründer, G., Heinze, M., Cordes, J., Mühlbauer, B., Juckel, G., Schulz, C., Rüther, E., & Timm, J. (2016). Effects of first-generation antipsychotics versus second-generation antipsychotics on quality of life in schizophrenia: A double-blind, randomised study. *The Lancet Psychiatry, 3*(8), 717–729. https://doi.org/10.1016/S2215-0366(16)00085-7.

Hartling, L., Abou-Setta, A. M., Dursun, S., Mousavi, S. S., Pasichnyk, D., & Newton, A. S. (2012). Antipsychotics in adults with schizophrenia: Comparative effectiveness of first-generation versus second-generation medications: A systematic review and meta-analysis. *Annals of Internal Medicine, 157*(7), 498–511. https://doi.org/10.7326/0003-4819-157-7-201210020-00525.

Hor, K., & Taylor, M. (2010). Suicide and schizophrenia: A systematic review of rates and risk factors. *Journal of Psychopharmacology (Oxford, England), 24*(4 Suppl), 81–90. https://doi.org/10.1177/1359786810385490.

Insel, T., Cuthbert, B., Garvey, M., Heinssen, R., Pine, D. S., Quinn, K., Sanislow, C., & Wang, P. (2010). Research domain criteria (RDoC): Toward a new classification framework for research on mental disorders. *The American Journal of Psychiatry, 167*(7), 748–751. https://doi.org/10.1176/APPI.AJP.2010.09091379.

Ismail, Z., Nguyen, M. Q., Fischer, C. E., Schweizer, T. A., Mulsant, B. H., & Mamo, D. (2011). Neurobiology of delusions in Alzheimer's disease. *Current Psychiatry Reports, 13*(3), 211–218. https://doi.org/10.1007/S11920-011-0195-1.

Jellinger, K. A. (2012). Cerebral correlates of psychotic syndromes in neurodegenerative diseases. *Journal of Cellular and Molecular Medicine, 16*(5), 995. https://doi.org/10.1111/J.1582-4934.2011.01311.X.

Kehrer, C., Maziashvili, N., Dugladze, T., & Gloveli, T. (2008). Altered excitatory-inhibitory balance in the NMDA-hypofunction model of schizophrenia. *Frontiers in Molecular Neuroscience, 1*. https://doi.org/10.3389/NEURO.02.006.2008.

Kinon, B. J., Zhang, L., Millen, B. A., Osuntokun, O. O., Williams, J. E., Kollack-Walker, S., Jackson, K., Kryzhanovskaya, L., & Jarkova, N. (2011). A multicenter, inpatient, phase 2, double-blind, placebo-controlled dose-ranging study of LY2140023 monohydrate in patients with DSM-IV schizophrenia. *Journal of Clinical Psychopharmacology, 31*(3), 349–355. https://doi.org/10.1097/JCP.0B013E318218DCD5.

Lally, J., & MacCabe, J. H. (2015). Antipsychotic medication in schizophrenia: A review. *British Medical Bulletin, 114*(1), 169–179. https://doi.org/10.1093/bmb/ldv017.

Lauterbach, M. D., Stanislawski-Zygaj, A. L., & Benjamin, S. (2008). The differential diagnosis of childhood- and young adult-onset disorders that include psychosis. *Journal of Neuropsychiatry and Clinical Neurosciences, 20*(4), 409–418. https://doi.org/10.1176/JNP.2008.20.4.409/ASSET/IMAGES/LARGE/AL0133T5.JPEG.

Leucht, S., Huhn, M., & Davis, J. M. (2021). Should 'typical,' first-generation antipsychotics no longer be generally used in the treatment of schizophrenia? *European Archives of Psychiatry and Clinical Neuroscience, 271*(8), 1411–1413. https://doi.org/10.1007/s00406-021-01335-y.

Linscott, R. J., & Van Os, J. (2013). An updated and conservative systematic review and meta-analysis of epidemiological evidence on psychotic experiences in children and adults: On the pathway from proneness to persistence to dimensional expression across mental disorders. *Psychological Medicine, 43*(6), 1133–1149. https://doi.org/10.1017/S0033291712001626.

Maj, M., van Os, J., De Hert, M., Gaebel, W., Galderisi, S., Green, M. F., Guloksuz, S., Harvey, P. D., Jones, P. B., Malaspina, D., McGorry, P., Miettunen, J., Murray, R. M., Nuechterlein, K. H., Peralta, V., Thornicroft, G., van Winkel, R., & Ventura, J. (2021). The clinical characterization of the patient with primary psychosis aimed at personalization of management. *World Psychiatry, 20*(1), 4–33. https://doi.org/10.1002/wps.20809.

McGrath, J., Saha, S., Welham, J., El Saadi, O., MacCauley, C., & Chant, D. (2004). A systematic review of the incidence of schizophrenia: The distribution of rates and the influence of sex, urbanicity, migrant status and methodology. *BMC Medicine, 2*(1), 1–22. https://doi.org/10.1186/1741-7015-2-13/COMMENTS.

Morgan, C., Lappin, J., Heslin, M., Donoghue, K., Lomas, B., Reininghaus, U., Onyejiaka, A., Croudace, T., Jones, P. B., Murray, R. M., Fearon, P., Doody, G. A., & Dazzan, P. (2014). Reappraising the long-term course and outcome of psychotic disorders: The AESOP-10 study. *Psychological Medicine, 44*(13), 2713–2726. https://doi.org/10.1017/S0033291714000282.

Morgan, V. A., Valuri, G. M., Croft, M. L., Griffith, J. A., Shah, S., Young, D. J., & Jablensky, A. V. (2011). Cohort profile: Pathways of risk from conception to disease: The Western Australian schizophrenia high-risk e-Cohort. *International Journal of Epidemiology, 40*(6), 1477–1485. https://doi.org/10.1093/IJE/DYQ167.

Olincy, A., Harris, J. G., Johnson, L. L., Pender, V., Kongs, S., Allensworth, D., Ellis, J., Zerbe, G. O., Leonard, S., Stevens, K. E., Stevens, J. O., Martin, L., Adler, L. E., Soti, F., Kem, W. R., & Freedman, R. (2006). Proof-of-concept trial of an alpha7 nicotinic agonist in schizophrenia. *Archives of General Psychiatry, 63*(6), 630–638. https://doi.org/10.1001/ARCHPSYC.63.6.630.

Pantelis, C., Velakoulis, D., McGorry, P. D., Wood, S. J., Suckling, J., Phillips, L. J., Yung, A. R., Bullmore, E. T., Brewer, W., Soulsby, B., Desmond, P., & McGuire, P. K. (2003). Neuroanatomical abnormalities before and after onset of psychosis: A cross-sectional and longitudinal MRI comparison. *The Lancet, 361*(9354), 281–288. https://doi.org/10.1016/S0140-6736(03)12323-9.

Perkins, D. O., Gu, H., Boteva, K., & Lieberman, J. A. (2005). Relationship between duration of untreated psychosis and outcome in first-episode schizophrenia: A critical review and meta-analysis. *The American Journal of Psychiatry, 162*(10), 1785–1804. https://doi.org/10.1176/APPI.AJP.162.10.1785.

Potasiewicz, A., Nikiforuk, A., Hołuj, M., & Popik, P. (2017). Stimulation of nicotinic acetylcholine alpha7 receptors rescue schizophrenia-like cognitive impairments in rats. *Journal of Psychopharmacology (Oxford, England), 31*(2), 260–271. https://doi.org/10.1177/0269881116675509.

Price, O., Baker, J., Bee, P., & Lovell, K. (2015). Learning and performance outcomes of mental health staff training in de-escalation techniques for the management of violence and aggression. *The British Journal of Psychiatry: The Journal of Mental Science, 206*(6), 447–455. https://doi.org/10.1192/BJP.BP.114.144576.

Ringbäck Weitoft, G., Berglund, M., Lindström, E. A., Nilsson, M., Salmi, P., & Rosén, M. (2014). Mortality, attempted suicide, re-hospitalisation and prescription refill for clozapine and other antipsychotics in Sweden-a register-based study. *Pharmacoepidemiology and Drug Safety, 23*(3), 290–298. https://doi.org/10.1002/PDS.3567.

Rössler, W., Joachim Salize, H., van Os, J., & Riecher-Rössler, A. (2005). Size of burden of schizophrenia and psychotic disorders. *European Neuropsychopharmacology, 15*(4), 399–409. https://doi.org/10.1016/j.euroneuro.2005.04.009.

Saha, K. B., Bo, L., Zhao, S., Xia, J., Sampson, S., & Zaman, R. U. (2016). Chlorpromazine versus atypical antipsychotic drugs for schizophrenia. *The Cochrane Database of Systematic Reviews, 4*(4). https://doi.org/10.1002/14651858.CD010631.PUB2.

Spencer, E., Birchwood, M., & McGovern, D. (2001). Management of first-episode psychosis. *Advances in Psychiatric Treatment, 7*(2), 133–140. https://doi.org/10.1192/apt.7.2.133.

Sultzer, D. L., Leskin, L. P., Melrose, R. J., Harwood, D. G., Narvaez, T. A., Ando, T. K., & Mandelkern, M. A. (2014). Neurobiology of delusions, memory, and insight in Alzheimer disease. *The American Journal of Geriatric Psychiatry: Official Journal of the American Association for Geriatric Psychiatry, 22*(11), 1346–1355. https://doi.org/10.1016/J.JAGP.2013.06.005.

Taylor, C. D. J., Haddock, G., Speer, S., & Bee, P. E. (2020). Characterizing core beliefs in psychosis: A qualitative study. *Behavioural and Cognitive Psychotherapy, 48*(1), 67–81. https://doi.org/10.1017/S1352465819000274.

Temmingh, H. S., Williams, T., Siegfried, N., & Stein, D. J. (2018). Risperidone versus other antipsychotics for people with severe mental illness and co-occurring substance misuse. *The Cochrane Database of Systematic Reviews, 1*(1). https://doi.org/10.1002/14651858.CD011057.PUB2.

Van Os, J., Hanssen, M., Bijl, R. V., & Vollebergh, W. (2001). Prevalence of psychotic disorder and community level of psychotic symptoms: An urban-rural comparison. *Archives of General Psychiatry, 58*(7), 663–668. https://doi.org/10.1001/ARCHPSYC.58.7.663.

van Os, J., Linscott, R. J., Myin-Germeys, I., Delespaul, P., & Krabbendam, L. (2009). A systematic review and meta-analysis of the psychosis continuum: Evidence for a psychosis proneness–persistence–

impairment model of psychotic disorder. *Psychological Medicine, 39*(2), 179–195. https://doi.org/10.1017/S0033291708003814.

Wang, H. R., Woo, Y. S., & Bahk, W. M. (2013). Atypical antipsychotics in the treatment of delirium. *Psychiatry and Clinical Neurosciences, 67*(5), 323–331. https://doi.org/10.1111/PCN.12066.

Chapter 15

Autism Spectrum Disorder

Ayça Asma Sakalli[1,*], MD
and H. Seda Küçükerdem[2], MD
[1]Department of Family Medicine, Balıkesir City Hospital, Balıkesir, Turkey
[2]Department of Family Medicine, Izmir City Hospital, Izmir, Turkey

Abstract

Autism spectrum disorder (ASD) is a progressively prevalent form of developmental issue that has a global impact. Family physicians provide services to protect the health of individuals during the prenatal period and provide early diagnosis. During the healthy growth monitoring of infants and children, autism spectrum disorder and other developmental disorders should also be monitored. Family physicians are the first point of contact for lifelong follow-up of children, young people, and adults diagnosed with autism. Family physicians apply evidence-based practices in the early symptoms, diagnosis, treatment, and follow-up of autism. Although there are not yet many evidence-based data available, studies on autism have gained momentum in recent years.

Keywords: autism spectrum disorder, evidence-based medicine, family practice, guideline

Introduction

Autism spectrum disorder, which falls under the umbrella of neurodevelopmental disorders, is marked by social and communicative challenges and repetitive behaviors, and interests. Signs often begin early in life, classifying it as a developmental issue. Although autism can be diagnosed at any age, it is defined as a "developmental disorder" as symptoms usually appear in the first two years of life (American Psychiatric Association, 2013). The term "Autism Spectrum Disorder" entered the literature with the DSM-V published in 2013. Before this, DSM-IV-R included five different special needs groups under the umbrella of Pervasive Developmental Disorders (Autistic Disorder, Rett Syndrome, Asperger Syndrome, Pervasive Developmental Disorder, Not Otherwise Specified Childhood Disintegrative Disorder). Rett Disorder was removed from the five subgroups defined in DSM-IV, and the other four categories were named "Autism Spectrum Disorder" under the same umbrella. The term

* Corresponding Author's Email: draycaasma@gmail.com.

In: Common Diseases According to Family Medicine Practice Guidelines
Editors: Esra Meltem Koç and Hilal Aksoy
ISBN: 979-8-89530-302-3

"spectrum" denotes the wide variety of symptoms, abilities, and degrees of functional impairment that can manifest in individuals with ASD. Some individuals with ASD can fully work in all activities of daily living, while others require significant support to perform basic daily activities (Mughal et al., 2020).

Family doctors play a crucial role in early detection, help people recognize the early warning signs of autism spectrum disorders (ASD), support the guiding families through treatment, conduct cause-related evaluations, and provide therapeutic support. To effectively participate in shared decision-making and manage co-occurring medical disorders that can impact outcomes and everyday functions, the family must be informed about the evidence supporting various approaches (The American Academy of Pediatrics [AAP], 2020).

There is no standard worldwide view of the cause, assessment, diagnosis, and management of Autism Spectrum Disorder, which was only defined as recently as 2013. When deciding on the applications for individuals with ASD, scientifically based applications should be preferred. Using non-scientifically based interventions can cause a loss of time, effort, and economic resources and harm the individual with ASD or their family. With the increasing prevalence of ASD, national guidelines have been published in some countries.

This text will include the recommendations of the American Academy of Pediatrics (AAP), European Child & Adolescent Psychiatry (ESCAP), NICE (National Institute for Health and Care Excellence), and the *Australian* Government's Cooperative Research Centre (ACRC).

Epidemiology

When autism was first described, it was considered a rare developmental disorder. However, in recent studies, the prevalence of autism has been shown to be on the rise, with current estimates suggesting that it affects at least 1% of children. This increased prevalence has increased the demand for health services for children and youth of all ages (NICE, 2017).

The Autism and Developmental Disabilities Monitoring Network (ADDM) was founded by the Centers for Disease Control and Prevention, an agency under the United States Department of Health, to collect routine data on autism and other developmental disorders. In 2020, the ADDM Network found that 1 in 36 children aged 8 (2.8%) had ASD, following follow-up in 11 communities in the United States. According to ADMM data, the prevalence of ASD was reported as 1/150 in 2006, 1/69 in 2012, 1/59 in 2014, and 1/44 in 2018. The likelihood of diagnosing ASD at 48 months for children born in 2016 (4 years) was found to be 1.6 times greater in 2020 compared to children born in 2012 (8 years) (ADDM, 2023). More children are being diagnosed at an earlier age. The widening of diagnostic criteria, early intervention for children with ASD, widespread screening recommendations, public knowledge of the disorder and its symptoms, and increasing accessibility to school-based treatments all contribute to this increase. It is critical to make advancements in ASD early diagnosis to provide assistance and support sooner (AAP, 2020).

86.5% of ASD cases reported to date have been reported from High-Income Countries, representing only 20% of the world's population. Insufficient population-based studies conducted in Low-to-Middle-Income Countries may under-represent the impact of ASD. Determining the prevalence of Autism Spectrum Disorder (ASD) is complicated by factors such as the level of public awareness, the diagnostic capabilities of the studies, and the comparability and cross-cultural appropriateness of ASD screening, measurement, and epidemiological findings (Styles et al., 2020).

Risk Factors

No single factor has been identified that causes ASD. It is a heterogeneous disorder resulting from the combination of genetic, epigenetic, and environmental factors. Interactions between several genes, expression variability due to epigenetic factors, and exposure to environmental factors are likely responsible for ASD (Rylaarsdam et al., 2019).

The first evidence for genetic factors in autism spectrum disorder is based on studies with twins and families. Siblings, especially twins, exhibit a higher incidence of ASD compared to the broader population. Research involving twins reveals that identical twins have a notably greater probability of sharing ASD traits than fraternal twins. (AAP, 2020). Today, genetic diseases that cause autism spectrum disorder have been identified due to chromosome abnormalities and genetic linkage analysis studies related to the genetics of autism spectrum disorder. The AAP guideline recommends conducting specialized tests or consulting a pediatric geneticist when there is suspicion of a distinct syndrome or metabolic disorder (Fragile X, Neurofibromatosis 1, Rett syndrome, Smith-Lemli-Opitz syndrome, Timothy, PTEN hamartoma tumor syndrome). For example, all children with ASD should have DNA testing for Fragile X syndrome, especially boys and children with a family history of male intellectual disability (AAP, 2020). The NICE guidelines do not recommend any routine medical investigations. However, it states that if there is evidence of certain dysmorphic features, congenital anomalies, and/or learning (intellectual) disability, genetic testing recommended by the regional genetic center may be conducted (NICE, 2017).

Table 1. Factors associated with an increased prevalence of autism (NICE)

- A sibling with ASD.
- Congenital disabilities associated with central nervous system malformation and/or dysfunction, including cerebral palsy.
- Preterm gestational age, precisely less than 35 weeks.
- Psychosis or emotional illness resembling schizophrenia in parents.
- Maternal use of sodium valproate in pregnancy.
- A learning (intellectual) disability.
- Attention deficit hyperactivity disorder.
- Neonatal encephalopathy/epileptic encephalopathy, including infantile spasms.
- Chromosomal disorders.
- Genetic disorders.
- Muscular dystrophy.
- Neurofibromatosis.
- Tuberous sclerosis.

Among 8-year-old children, boys are approximately four times as likely as girls to be diagnosed with ASD. However, 2020 was the first year in which the rate of girls diagnosed with ASD by the ADDM Network was above 1% (ADDM, 2023). The atypical presentation of symptoms in girls with autism may lead to girls being underdiagnosed. Women often exhibit more nuanced social and communication challenges, and they may be better at concealing or compensating for their differences (ESCAP, 2019).

Improving early autism detection could be aided by professionals being more aware of risk factors beyond just being male. High-risk groups include siblings of diagnosed individuals, children of older fathers and mothers who are either older or very young, and those with a history of poor pre- or perinatal development (e.g., pregnancy medication usage, obesity, hypertension, or infection) (ESCAP, 2019). Research shows no link between vaccinations and a higher risk of ASD, and vaccines should be given to children with ASD as per the standard schedule (AAP, 2020). Factors that increase the prevalence of autism included in the NICE guide are shown in Table 1.

Clinical Symptoms

The behavioral characteristics that constitute ASD are frequently present before the age of three. However, these symptoms may not emerge until the school years or even later in adulthood. The nature and severity of developmental challenges, signs, and symptoms can greatly differ from one person to another. They can also change in the same individual over time (ACRC, 2018). Despite advances in neurobiology and genetics, ASD diagnosis is still focusing on recognizing and documenting behaviorally defined clinical symptoms.

The American Psychiatric Association's Diagnostic and Statistical Manual of Mental Disorders from 2013 and the WHO International Classification of Diseases (ICD-11) of 2018 are used to diagnose ASD. The criteria for diagnosing ASD in the DSM-5 are shown in Table 2. There are many similarities between the DSM-5 and ICD-11 autism classifications. DSM-V and ICD-11 include ASD under the classification of neurodevelopmental disorders. In the DSM-5 and ICD-11, autism symptoms fall into two main categories: ongoing challenges with back-and-forth social interaction and communication and various consistent, repetitive behaviors and interests that show limited adaptability. The deficits should significantly disrupt functioning in personal, family, social, educational, occupational, or other crucial domains (APA, 2013; WHO, 2019). The principal distinctions are outlined in Table 3.

Observation of difficulties in non-verbal behaviors that govern social interaction, inability to establish peer relationships commensurate with the child's developmental stage, and incapacity to spontaneously share enjoyment and interests with others (such as showing, offering, or indicating objects of interest to others) are noted (Rosello et al., 2020). Children with ASD often engage in non-verbal communication such as eye contact, gestures, body language, and facial expressions less often than their typically developing peers. Speech delay is expected in ASDs and is often parents' first concern. While children with other developmental characteristics and sensory disabilities who have speech problems try to compensate for this with non-verbal means, such as gestures, to communicate, children with ASD do not show this compensation effort (Cui et al., 2023).

Table 2. ASD Diagnostic criteria - DSM-5

A. All of the following symptoms describing persistent deficits in social communication/interaction across contexts (not accounted for by general developmental delays) must be met: • Challenges in engaging in social or emotional interaction, such as struggling to have balanced and ongoing talks, difficulty initiating interactions, and issues with focusing on and expressing feelings and interests with others. • Individuals have significant challenges in maintaining relationships, which can manifest as disinterest in others, struggles with imaginative play and participation in social activities appropriate for their age, and issues adapting to varying social norms. • Non-verbal communication problems such as abnormal eye contact, posture, facial expressions, tone of voice, and gestures, as well as an inability to understand these.
B. At least two out of the four signs associated with restricted and repetitive behavior must be present: • Characterized by stereotyped or repetitive verbal patterns, physical motions, or the usage of things. • Excessive adherence to routines, ritualized patterns of verbal or nonverbal behavior, or excessive resistance to change • Intense and focused interests that are highly limited and deviate from the norm. • Excessive or deficient response to sensory stimuli or abnormal fascination with sensory characteristics of the surroundings.

Repetition of someone else's words (echolalia) is common in ASD. Individuals with ASD might speak in a tone that is unusually high, low, rapid, slow, or monotone. They may create unique words or repeat specific phrases inappropriately. A strong preference for certain non-functional routines or rituals is common in ASD. Challenges with small changes in daily activities or slight alterations in their environment can lead to significant disruptions for them and their families, such as intense outbursts (Hodges et al., 2020).

Table 3. Differences between ASD classification systems

DSM-V	ICD-11
acknowledges that autism and intellectual disability can co-occur.	*differentiates autism with and without intellectual disability and assigns a severity rating to intellectual disability*
requires that individuals meet all three criteria for social communication and interaction and at least 2 of 4 criteria for restricted and repetitive behaviors	lists essential (required) features but does not specify a minimum number or combination of features an individual must possess
uses the specifier 'with or without accompanying language impairment' to assess the current level of language	records the degree of impairment of functional language at three levels (with mild or no impairment, with impaired, with complete, or almost complete absence of functional language)
The severity of social communication difficulties and restricted, repetitive behaviors are graded according to the person's need for support.	There is no classification based on a person's support needs.
the implies that it is possible that ASD could be confused with other diagnoses, such as selective mutism or ADHD	recognizes that conditions such as ADHD and selective mutism occur together.

Early Detection and Screening

Early identification of children with autism is vital to providing family support and securing the right educational and therapeutic services. The full long-term advantages of early intervention programs have yet to be determined, but there is strong evidence that early intervention can improve social communication skills, reduce the severity of symptoms, optimize child development, and reduce parental stress and well-being (ESCAP, 2019).

No single procedure can be recommended for early detection of autism; however, there are several widely available screening tools. All guidelines stress that these screening tools are intended to alert doctors to the possibility of autism, not to confirm the diagnosis. The objective of screening tools is to aid caregivers in identifying and reporting symptoms observed in children at high risk for ASD. One fundamental and highly effective way to improve detection might be to have healthcare professionals promptly address parents' concerns, especially those about early delays or abnormalities in social interactions such as looking, smiling, and making sounds to communicate (ESCAP, 2019).

Screenings, which focus on early indicators of fundamental challenges in social communication. Certain early symptoms that could signal to a doctor or parent the potential for ASD are often called "red flags" (Table 4) (AAP, 2018).

The AAP recommends screening all children for ASD symptoms when they reach 18 - 24 months old during their routine primary care visits by combining both developmental surveillance throughout all appointments and standardized screening exams designed explicitly for autism. Primary care providers must identify all children who would benefit from early intervention. The AAP guide mentions M-CHAT, SCQ, STAT, Promising Autism Screening Tests, The Infant/Toddler Checklist, Early Screening for Autism, and Communication Disorders screening tests.

The M-CHAT is the most researched and commonly utilized tool for screening toddlers for autism spectrum disorder. M-CHAT is a screening tool that uses a parent-completed questionnaire, clinic-administered follow-up examinations, and repeated questionnaires to identify children at risk of autism in the overall population. It is valid for children aged 16 to 30 months. Children who do not pass the ASD screening tests or who are flagged as potential diagnoses should be recommended for further diagnostic analysis and support programs. Presently, there are no established screening instruments for use in pediatric settings for children older than 30 months, and there are no AAP guidelines for routine ASD screening for this group. AAP currently advises implementing continuous monitoring within the primary healthcare framework. Improved accuracy and culturally sensitive screening methods are required. According to the AAP guideline, primary care providers should know the diagnostic criteria for ASD, appropriate etiological evaluation, and the co-occurring medical and behavioral conditions that affect the child's function and quality of life.

ESCAP states that it is necessary to complete the availability and robustness of screening and diagnostic tools for individuals from economic or social challenged backgrounds, or for members of ethnic or racial minoriti communities.

The NICE guidelines do not recommend a universal ASD screening. However, it recommends improving early recognition of autism by establishing local autism teams and, increasing recognition of characteristics suggestive of potential autism through collaborative institutional training (NICE, 2017). Appropriate personnel from the health, mental health, education, and social care sectors should comprise the local autism team, a multidisciplinary group tasked with overseeing the identification, management, and follow-up of individuals with autism. While other causes should also be considered, NICE advises clinicians to consider the possibility of autism when development or behavior concerns arise. NICE recommends that the clinician should think about autism as a potential diagnosis when observing issues with a child's growth or actions, while also evaluating other potential causes. behavior or development should be taken seriously. Additionally, the observations and apprehensions of parents or caregivers regarding a child's or adolescent's actions or developmental milestones should be regarded with seriousness. The NICE guidance sets out characteristics by age group to help identify findings suggestive of possible autism. NICE recommends directing children under the age of 3 to the autism specialists should there be a noticeable decline in their linguistic or social abilities. Children over the age of 3 experiencing a setback in language skills and people of any age who exhibit a decline in motor abilities should first be referred to a pediatrician or pediatric neurologist.

In England and Northern Ireland, assessments for children typically occur between the ages of 2 and 2.5 years using the Ages and Stages Questionnaire-3. Similarly, the "Scottish Child Health Programme" evaluates child development between 27 to 30 months, andthe "Healthy Child Wales Programme" conducts assessments around the 27-month milestone. It is important to note that these assessments are not part of the formal UK National Screening Committee (UK NSC) recommended screening program. While these assessments are not explicitly designed to detect Autism Spectrum Disorder (ASD) in children, there is the possibility that certain behaviors, and signs indicative of undiagnosed ASD could be observed during these assessments (UK NSC, 2023).

ACRC guidance recommends referral for assessment when a person demonstrates characteristics of autism. The primary care provider should begin the referral process for an autism evaluation. (Recommendation Level: Strong). Practitioners should gather details to help them understand whether referral for an assessment considering autism is appropriate and desirable for the client (Recommendation Level: Strong). When evaluating a referral, practitioners must consider the client's characteristics, functioning, and context, including strengths and support needs. Standardized developmental screening measures administered to children may also be helpful. The decision to refer a patient for evaluation requires clinical judgment based on all available information (ACRC, 2023).

Table 4. Red flags (AAP)

At the age of 12 months	• Exhibits a lack of response to their given name
At the age of 14 months	• Does not indicate interest by gesturing toward objects
At the age of 18 months	• Does not pretend play
General	• Potentially avoids eye contact and desires solitude • Develops difficulty comprehending and discussing the emotions of others • Exhibits impaired verbal communication and linguistic abilities. • Engages in repetitive use of words or phrases (echolalia) • Provides irrelevant responses to questions • Experiences emotional distress due to minor alterations • Has obsessive interests • Exhibits repetitive motor behaviors such as hand flapping and rocking. • Has unusual reactions to the way things sound, smell, taste, look, or feel.

Diagnosis

Autism diagnosis is a multi-stage process. Evaluation of current symptoms with a multidisciplinary approach requires stages such as obtaining the developmental history of the primary caregiver and excluding other possible diagnoses.

Symptoms can present and be interpreted in different ways depending on environmental settings. The physician making the diagnosis should consider whether the current adjustment disorder is due to a medical or psychiatric disorder. Intellectual abilities should be routinely evaluated for the presence of medical diseases and psychiatric disorders with a high prevalence of ASD. In addition, cognitive, language, and neuropsychological evaluations provide information about the person's strengths and weaknesses and facilitate the management of the disease.

Given the complex nature and severity of ASD symptoms, as well as their similarity to symptoms of other psychiatric conditions, it is essential to employ the right diagnostic tools and scales for precise ASD diagnosis to enhance patient management. The evaluation process includes interviews with parents or caregivers, patient interviews, observations of the patient, and a differential diagnosis of other neurodevelopmental disorders, all conducted through comprehensive clinical assessments and family history reviews.

The standard view in all guidelines is that specific diagnostic tools should be used for diagnosis according to the DSM-V and ICD-11 criteria, and the clinician should make a decision based on the patient's medical history, physical examination, observations, and observations of parents and teachers. Furthermore, all guidelines emphasize that the diagnosis should not be based solely on specific diagnostic tools (AAP, 2020; ESCAP, 2019; ACRC, 2023; NICE, 2017).

The AAP recommends that primary care providers discuss with families the significance of evaluating both the developmental status and the potential for an autism spectrum disorder (ASD) diagnosis. They should also assist the family in connecting with community resources throughout the process. Evaluating the historical symptoms of ASD can be facilitated by instruments such as the SCQ or the Social Responsiveness Scale (SRS). For generating structured data that supports a confirmed diagnosis, recognized observational instruments such as the Autism Diagnostic Observation Schedule, Second Edition (ADOS-2), and the Childhood Autism Rating Scale, Second Edition (CARS-2) are frequently employed (AAP, 2020).

The NICE guideline recommends not excluding autism for the presence of adequate eye contact, the expression of smiles and affection toward family members, engagement in pretend play activities, and typical development of language skills, and challenges that seem to be resolved after a needs-based intervention. A previous assessment concluded that autism does not exist. If the diagnosis remains unclear following the autism diagnostic evaluation, it may be prudent to continue monitoring the child or adolescent, taking into account any emerging information (NICE, 2017).

ESCAP recommends that the clinical diagnosis be personalized and contextualized, focusing on individual limitations and strengths (ESCAP, 2019).

According to the guidance provided by ACRC, individuals who display symptoms of autism as suspected by primary healthcare professionals should be referred for a Comprehensive Needs Assessment. This assessment process is divided into two main components: the assessment of functioning and the medical evaluation. In conducting an assessment of functioning, practitioners should collect data to enhance their understanding of the client's attributes, capabilities, and broader situational factors. This process involves identifying their strengths and determining the support needed for different life activities. (Grade of Recommendation: Strong). On the other hand, the medical evaluation concentrates on assessing the client's health status, and functional capabilities, and overall well-being. It often involves taking a comprehensive case history, conducting physical examinations, and conducting further clinical evaluations when necessary. The goal of the medical evaluation is to contribute to the recognition of traits potentially relevant to diagnosing autism and related disorders (ACRC, 2023).

Management and Treatment

The goals of ASD treatment are to minimize core deficits and co-occurring related disorders, enhance functional independence by promoting the development and mastery of adaptive skills, and address disruptive behaviors that may hinder the application of these skills. Treatment goals should be individualized and developmentally appropriate, considering performance data on scales used at diagnosis. Families should participate in the choice of intervention strategies and choosing intervention strategies and continue to be engaged in subsequent decisions regarding education and treatment (AAP, 2019).

ESCAP suggests that interventions should primarily focus on implementing strategies that create a more accommodating environment for individuals with autism. It is crucial to understand and promote diverse methods to facilitate the inclusion of children and adults with autism and their families. This necessitates collaboration not only from the healthcare, education, and social care sectors but also from all community services that play a significant role in ensuring a good quality of life. Due to the limited number of large-scale randomized control trials for autism interventions, it is insufficient to rely solely on such evidence to provide treatment and support for autistic individuals. Interventions should be grounded in scientific and empirical evidence. However, given the limitations of existing research studies, overall treatment approaches should also incorporate recommendations from international expert panels, be consistent with societal norms, and receive the endorsement of the individual with autism and their legal guardians.

The Comprehensive Treatment Model (CTM) and Focused Interventions are the primary classifications of evidence-based interventions introduced by the AAP guideline (Wong et al., 2015). The National Professional Development Center for ASD (NPDC) is affiliated with the U.S. Department of Education. The center is a collaborative effort between multiple universities aimed at advancing the use of evidence-based methods for children and adolescents diagnosed with ASD. NPDC dedicated to Autism Spectrum Disorder has identified a total of 27 evidence-based practices that have been proven effective in enhancing outcomes for students with ASD (Table 5).

Many evidence-based treatment models are founded on Applied Behaviour Analysis principles. ABA, or Applied Behaviour Analysis, is the methodical use of interventions anchored in the principles of learning theory to enhance socially important behaviors significantly and to confirm that the interventions implemented are effective in improving behavior. The application of ABA techniques in addressing ASD symptoms indicates that observable behaviors can be altered through systematically reinforcing communication skills and other skill developments. Therefore, ABA interventions may focus on fostering new abilities (e.g., social participation) and minimizing negative behaviors such as aggression. Speech-language therapy is commonly recognized as a primary intervention for children diagnosed with ASD (AAP, 2019).

In the United States of America, the Food and Drug Administration (FDA) has approved two drugs, Risperidone and Aripiprazole, for agitation and irritability in autism. In Europe, the European Medicines Agency (EMEA) has sanctioned the use of Haloperidol for managing persistent and severe aggression in children and adolescents with autism where alternative therapies have failed or have led to intolerable side effects. Additionally, a prolonged-release melatonin formulation has received recent approval for the treatment of insomnia associated with autism (ESCAP, 2019).

NICE recommends that to reduce the fundamental characteristics of autism, a social communication intervention should be considered by involving play-based techniques with parents, caregivers, and educators to enhance shared focus, involvement, and reciprocal communication in the child or young individual. Do not use antipsychotics, antidepressants, or anticonvulsants to manage the core features of autism. However, consider antipsychotic medication to work with challenging behavior when psychosocial or other interventions are inadequate. It is advisable for a pediatrician or psychiatrist to initially prescribe and oversee the use of antipsychotic medication (NICE, 2021).

Table 5. Evidence-based practices

- Antecedent-based intervention
- Cognitive behavioral intervention
- Differential reinforcement of alternative, incompatible, or other behavior
- Discrete trial teaching
- Exercise
- Extinction
- Functional behavior assessment (FBA)
- Functional communication training
- Modeling
- Naturalistic intervention
- Parent-implemented intervention
- Peer-mediated instruction and intervention
- Picture Exchange Communication System (PECS)
- Pivotal response training
- Prompting
- Reinforcement
- Response interruption/ redirection
- Scripting
- Self-management
- Social narratives
- Social skills training
- Structured playgroup
- Task analysis
- Technology-aided instruction and intervention
- Time delay
- Video modeling
- Visual support.

While the ACRC does not include a section on intervention and treatment, the remaining three guidelines all suggest that there are currently no medications available to address the core symptoms of autism. Additionally, interventions often referred to as "alternative" treatments, such as neurofeedback, facilitated communication, auditory integration training, omega-3 fatty acids, secretin, chelation, hyperbaric oxygen therapy, exclusion diets, and others, are not considered appropriate approaches to treatment basic features of autism.

Co-Occurring Conditions and Follow-Up

ASD often coexists with physical, mental, neurodevelopmental, and functional conditions that, while not included in the diagnostic criteria, can significantly and adversely affect the well-being of both the child and their family. Medical and other conditions frequently associated with autism include seizures, sleep disturbances, gastrointestinal issues, feeding difficulties, obesity, and catatonia, among others (AAP, 2019).

The AAP recommends that primary care clinicians should inform families of children diagnosed with ASD about the increased risk and the signs and symptoms of seizures and consult a pediatric neurologist when concerned about the possibility of atypical regressions or seizures. Screening EEGs are generally not advised for patients without symptoms. However, an overnight EEG is recommended if the clinical history indicates the possibility of seizures or atypical regression. Children diagnosed with ASD face an increased risk of developing obesity. To address this concern, AAP recommends that primary care providers regularly assess a child's body mass index percentile, taking into account their age. This assessment should be integrated into routine health supervision care.

ASD is frequently associated with intellectual disability and structural language disorders. Roughly 70% of individuals fulfill the diagnostic criteria for at least one psychiatric disorder who have autism. Additionally, approximately 50% of young and child with autism have co-occurring conditions such as intellectual disability, defined as having an IQ below 70.

Attention deficits and hyperactivity are common in people with autism spectrum disorder. When attentional difficulties or hyperactivity exceed that seen in people of comparable mental age, a diagnosis of attention-deficit/hyperactivity disorder (ADHD) should be considered (APA, 2013). ACRC recommends that practitioners should employ methods that enhance the emotional and mental health of their clients (Grade of Recommendation: Strong). The clinician should be aware that disorders such as anxiety, eating, and mood disorders will present differently in autism. According to the NICE guideline, cognitive behavioral therapy may be considered to treat anxiety (NICE, 2019).

AAP recommends screening for depression in patients over the age of 12. Until interventions specifically tailored for ASD are developed, strategies commonly used for all other adolescents at high risk of depression should be considered (AAP, 2019).

NICE recommends psychosocial and pharmacological interventions in line with the guidelines prepared for ADHD, constipation, etc., for managing accompanying mental health or medical problems in autistic children and young people. In case of sleep problems, it recommends taking a detailed history of sleep habits, snoring, and making a regular sleep plan. If these are inadequate, melatonin treatment can be started with the recommendation of a pediatrician or psychiatrist. The US Food and Drug Administration currently approves no medication for treating insomnia in children with or without ASD. Nutritional evaluation for feeding problems, questioning the existence of a strict diet, and blood tests can be performed if necessary (NICE, 2019).

ASD in Adults

ASD is a lifelong disorder; some individuals can be recognized in adulthood. ASD affects an estimated 2.21% of individuals in the United States (Dietz et al., 2020). Although most studies have been done on children, adult autism is also on the agenda. NICE has specific guidance on adult autism.

Autism symptoms can be less apparent in adulthood compared to childhood, particularly among cognitively capable individuals who have mastered strategies to mask or bypass specific challenges. The NICE guideline recommends assessing possible autism in the presence of the symptoms listed in Table 6.

Particularly complicated is the diagnosis of autism in adult women who did not receive a diagnosis during infancy. Numerous individuals are erroneously ascribed to diverse mental health disorders, including borderline personality disorders. Professionals must refrain from promptly rejecting the diagnosis of autism in females, disregarding the fact that symptoms can fall below the diagnostic criteria (ESCAP).

NICE recommends the use of the Autism Spectrum Quotient-10 items (AQ-10) as a diagnostic tool for adults who may have autism, provided that they do not have moderate or severe learning difficulties (Table 7) (NICE, 2021). Each item 1, 7, 8, and 10 in this tool is given 1 point for "Strongly Agree" or "Slightly Agree." For each item 2, 3, 4, 5, 6, and 9, 1 point are given for "Strongly Disagree" or "Slightly Disagree." Consider referring the individual for a specialized diagnostic assessment if they score six or higher (Allison et al., 2012).

A 'health passport' comprising details to inform all staff regarding the individual's care and support requirements is advised by NICE to be provided for adults with autism; the individual should carry this passport at all times (NICE, 2017).

The AAP recommends that the planning of the medical transition to adulthood for every component of health care begins between the ages of 12 and 14 years. Similarly, NICE recommends reassessment at around age 14 to determine the need for treatment to continue into adulthood.

Table 6. Signs of ASD in adults

At least one of the following: -Persistent difficulties in social interaction -Persistent difficulties in social communication - Characterized by stereotypic behaviors, inflexibility, repeated actions, an aversion to change, or a limited range of interests.
At least one of the following: -Difficulties in acquiring or maintaining employment or an education -Challenges in forming or maintaining social connections - Prior or ongoing engagement with mental health or learning disability services -An account of a neurodevelopmental ailment encompassing learning difficulties and attention deficit hyperactivity disorder or a mental disorder.

Table 7. Autism Spectrum Quotient (AQ-10)

1	I often notice small sounds when others do
2	I usually concentrate more on the whole picture rather than on the small details.
3	I find it easy to do more than one thing at once
4	If there is an interruption, I can quickly switch back to what I was doing.
5	I find it easy to 'read between the lines' when someone is talking to me.
6	I know how to tell if someone listening to me is getting bored.
7	When I am reading a story, I find it challenging to work out the characters' intentions.
8	I like to collect information about categories of things (e.g., types of cars, types of birds, types of trains, types of plants, etc.).
9	I find it easy to work out what someone is thinking or feeling just by looking at their face.
10	I find it challenging to work out people's intentions.

Turkey and Autism Spectrum Disorder

According to the report published in 2020, it is estimated that "there are around 550 thousand individuals with autism in Turkey and the number of children with autism in the 0-14 age group in our country is 140 thousand" (Grand National Assembly of Turkey, 2020).

There is not yet a national guideline for ASD in Turkey. The "ASD Screening and Follow-up Program" was established in 2017 by the General Directorate of Public Health of the Ministry of Health within the scope of the Autism Action Plan. In Turkey, autism screening is performed by family physicians between 18 and 36 months. An evaluation is made that includes the five early signs of autism (Table 8). If even one question on the evaluation form favors the presence of autism, the person is referred to a child psychiatrist.

Within the scope of the Turkey National Autism Action Plan 2016-2019, autism training was given to primary healthcare workers by the provincial autism team, a trained child psychiatrist, and two coordinators, using an interactive video-based training method. On December 31, 2019, 98.8% (n = 53,768) of family physicians nationwide were trained (Dursun et al., 2022). Screening data were collected by adding five early findings (delayed speech, repetitive behaviors, absence of joint attention, reduced eye contact, and non-responsiveness to verbal cues by name) to the family medicine registry system. The data obtained from this program are included in Table 9.

Table 8. ASD Assessment Questions

Does he/she look when his name is called?	☐ Yes	☐ No
Does he/she make eye contact?	☐ Yes	☐ No
Does he/she look at an object you point with your finger at?	☐ Yes	☐ No
Does he/she have repetitive behaviors?	☐ Yes	☐ No
Is there any speech delay? (From the 12th month onward, it is expected to make a meaningful expression consisting of one word, and from the 24th month onward, it is expected to make a sentence consisting of 2 words).	☐ Yes	☐ No

Table 9. Screening and Follow-up Programme

Years	Number of children screened	Number of children diagnosed with ASD as a result of referral
2018	667.323	805
2019	733.898	1.484
2020	461.875	937
Total	1.863.096	3226

As recommended in the AAP guidelines, screening is also performed in primary care in Turkey. The training of health workers, providing all kinds of social support to the child and family, preparation of the "Diagnosis Informing and Individual Counselling Protocol," preparation of the "transition to adulthood clinics" report on the problems experienced in medical follow-up during the transition to adulthood, preparation of a guide for families, sharing the information of the individual with ASD with other official institutions are similar to the guidelines in other countries.

The 2023-2030 action plan aims to develop or adapt new screening and diagnostic scales. For early symptoms of ASD, it aims to screen for typically developing children aged 18-36 and 36-72 months, with priority given to siblings diagnosed with ASD. Furthermore, Applied Behaviour Analysis in Autism (ABA) training will be given to personnel to work as supervisors in the Provincial Directorates of Family and Social Services. However, there is no mention of a local and regional autism team as recommended in the NICE and ACRC guidelines. Unlike other guidelines, "mobile child monitoring for home examination-screening and health services" is planned.

Conclusion

There are not enough evidence-based medical practices on autism spectrum disorder that are accepted worldwide. National guidelines should be developed for the screening, diagnosis, treatment, and follow-up processes. Family physicians should provide services in line with these guidelines.

References

Allison, C., Auyeung, B., & Baron-Cohen, S. (2012). Toward brief "Red Flags" for autism screening: The Short Autism Spectrum Quotient and the Short Quantitative Checklist for Autism in toddlers in 1,000 cases and 3,000 controls [corrected]. *Journal of the American Academy of Child and Adolescent Psychiatry, 51*(2), 202–212.e7. https://doi.org/10.1016/j.jaac.2011.11.003.

Autism and Developmental Disabilities Monitoring (ADDM) Network. (2023). *Community Report on Autism* (Updated March 2023). https://www.cdc.gov/ncbddd/autism/pdf/ADDM-Community-Report-SY2020-h.pdf.

Autism spectrum disorder in under 19s: recognition, referral, and diagnosis. (2017). In PubMed. National Institute for Health and Care Excellence (NICE). https://pubmed.ncbi.nlm.nih.gov/31999412/.

American Psychiatric Association. (2013). *Diagnostic and statistical manual of mental disorders* (5th ed.). https://doi.org/10.1176/appi.books.9780890425596.

Cui, M., Ni, Q., & Wang, Q. (2023). Review of intervention methods for language and communication disorders in children with autism. *PeerJ, 11,* e15735. https://doi.org/10.7717/peerj.15735.

Dietz, P. M., Rose, C. E., McArthur, D., & Maenner, M. (2020). National and State Estimates of Adults with Autism Spectrum Disorder. *Journal of Autism and Developmental Disorders, 50*(12), 4258–4266. https://doi.org/10.1007/s10803-020-04494-4.

Dursun, O. B., Turan, B., Ögütlü, H., Binici, N. C., Örengül, A. C., Alatas, E., Özdemir, R. M., Taşlıbeyaz, E., Karaman, S., Mukaddes, N. M., & on behalf of Turkish Autism Workgroup (2022). A new model for recognition, referral, and follow-up of autism spectrum disorder: A nationwide program. *Autism Research,* 1–10. https://doi.org/10.1002/aur.2813.

Fuentes, J., Hervás, A., Howlin, P., & (ESCAP ASD Working Party) (2021). ESCAP Practice Guidance for Autism: A Summary of Evidence-Based Recommendations for Diagnosis and Treatment. *European Child & Adolescent Psychiatry, 30*(6), 961–984. https://doi.org/10.1007/s00787-020-01587-4.

Goodall, E., Dargue, N., Hinze, E., Sulek, R., Varcin, K., Waddington, H., Whitehouse, A. J. O., Wicks, R., Allen, G., Best, J., Eapen, V. Evans, K., Hiremath, M, Hinze, W., Lawson, W., Toby, S., & Trembath, D. (2023). A National Guideline for the Assessment and Diagnosis of Autism in Australia: 2023 Update. *Autism CRC*. Brisbane.

Grand National Assembly of Turkey. (2020). *Down Syndrome, Autism and Other Developmental Disorders Report of the Parliamentary Investigation Established to Determine the Prevalence and the Measures to be Taken to Solve the Problems of Individuals and Their Families.*

Hodges, H., Fealko, C., & Soares, N. (2020). Autism spectrum disorder: definition, epidemiology, causes, and clinical evaluation. *Translational Pediatrics, 9*(Suppl 1), S55–S65. https://doi.org/10.21037/tp.2019.09.09.

Maenner, M. J., Warren, Z., Williams, A. R., Amoakohene, E., Bakian, A. V., Bilder, D. A., Durkin, M. S., Fitzgerald, R. T., Furnier, S. M., Hughes, M. M., Ladd-Acosta, C. M., McArthur, D., Pas, E. T., Salinas, A., Vehorn, A., Williams, S., Esler, A., Grzybowski, A., Hall-Lande, J., Nguyen, R. H. N., & Shaw, K. A. (2023). Prevalence and Characteristics of Autism Spectrum Disorder Among Children Aged 8 Years - Autism and Developmental Disabilities Monitoring Network, 11 Sites, United States, 2020. *Morbidity and Mortality Weekly Report. Surveillance Summaries (Washington, D.C.: 2002), 72*(2), 1–14. https://doi.org/10.15585/mmwr.ss7202a1.

Mughal, S., Faizy, R. M., & Saadabadi, A. (2022, July 19). Autism Spectrum Disorder. In StatPearls. StatPearls Publishing. https://www.ncbi.nlm.nih.gov/books/NBK525976/.

National Institute for Health and Care Excellence (NICE). (2017). *Autism spectrum disorder in under 19s: Recognition, referral and diagnosis.*

National Institute for Health and Care Excellence (NICE). (2021). *Autism Spectrum Disorder in Under 19s: Support and Management.*

Republic Of Turkey Ministry Of Family And Social Services. (2023). *For Indıvıduals Wıth Autısm Spectrum Dısorder 2. National Action Plan 2023-2030.* https://aile.gov.tr/media/134582/otizm_eylem_plani.pdf.

Republic of Turkey Ministry of Health General Directorate of Public Health. (June 23, 2020). Letter dated 23.6.2020 and numbered 80166981 sent to the General Directorate of Disabled and Elderly Services.

Rosello, B., Berenguer, C., Baixauli, I., García, R., & Miranda, A. (2020). Theory of Mind Profiles in Children With Autism Spectrum Disorder: Adaptive/Social Skills and Pragmatic Competence. *Frontiers in Psychology, 11,* 567401. https://doi.org/10.3389/fpsyg.2020.567401.

Rylaarsdam, L., & Guemez-Gamboa, A. (2019). Genetic Causes and Modifiers of Autism Spectrum Disorder. *Frontiers in Cellular Neuroscience, 13,* 385. https://doi.org/10.3389/fncel.2019.00385.

Styles, M., Alsharshani, D., Samara, M., Alsharshani, M., Khattab, A., Qoronfleh, M. W., & Al-Dewik, N. I. (2020). Risk factors, diagnosis, prognosis and treatment of autism. *Frontiers in Bioscience (Landmark edition), 25*(9), 1682–1717. https://doi.org/10.2741/4873.

The American Academy of Pediatrics [AAP]. Hyman, S. L., Levy, S. E., & Myers, S. M. (2020). Identification, Evaluation, and Management of Children With Autism Spectrum Disorder. *Pediatrics, 145*(1). https://doi.org/10.1542/peds.2019-3447.

UK National Screening Committee. (2023). *A review of screening for autism spectrum disorders in pre-school children under the age of 5 years.* https://view-health-screeningrecommendations.service.gov.uk/document/606/download.

Whitehouse, A. J. O., Evans, K., Eapen, V., & Wray, J. (2018). *A national guideline for the assessment and diagnosis of autism spectrum disorders in Australia.* Cooperative Research Centre for Living with Autism.

World Health Organization. (2019). 6A02 Autism spectrum disorder. In *International statistical classification of diseases and related health problems* (11th ed.). http://id.who.int/icd/entity/437815624.

Wong, C., Odom, S. L., Hume, K. A., Cox, A. W., Fettig, A., Kucharczyk, S., Brock, M. E., Plavnick, J. B., Fleury, V. P., & Schultz, T. R. (2015). Evidence-Based Practices for Children, Youth, and Young Adults with Autism Spectrum Disorder: A Comprehensive Review. *Journal of Autism and Developmental Disorders, 45*(7), 1951–1966. https://doi.org/10.1007/s10803-014-2351-z.

Part 5

Hematological Diseases

Chapter 16

Iron Deficiency Anemia

Gülseren Pamuk[*], PhD
Department of Family Medicine, Izmır Katip Celebi University, Izmır, Turkey

Abstract

Iron deficiency anemia (IDA) is a common health problem worldwide, particularly prevalent in developing countries. This article provides a comprehensive review of the prevalence, causes, diagnostic methods, clinical findings, treatment options, and prevention strategies of iron deficiency anemia. In addition to explaining fundamental topics such as iron metabolism, absorption, and storage, the article provides information on laboratory tests and treatment options used in the diagnosis of iron deficiency anemia. It is important to consider clinical findings in addition to laboratory test results during the diagnosis and treatment process. Treatment options include oral iron preparations and parenteral iron therapy. However, before starting treatment, it is necessary to determine the underlying cause of iron deficiency anemia. Long-term follow-up and recurrence assessment are crucial for monitoring patients' health status. Early diagnosis, effective treatment, and the implementation of prevention strategies are of great importance in combating iron deficiency anemia.

Keywords: anemia, iron deficiency, iron deficiency anemia, hemoglobin

Introduction

Anemia is a common public health issue, with iron deficiency anemia being the most prevalent type. The Global Burden of Disease Study evaluating the years 1990-2021 has revealed that anemia is the leading cause of years of lived with disability worldwide (Global Burden of Disease Study 2021).

Epidemiology of Iron Deficiency Anemia

As the level of development of the countries decreases, the frequency of iron deficiency anemia increases. Particularly at risk are children under the age of 5, women of reproductive age

[*] Corresponding Author's Email: drgulpmk@gmail.com.

In: Common Diseases According to Family Medicine Practice Guidelines
Editors: Esra Meltem Koç and Hilal Aksoy
ISBN: 979-8-89530-302-3

between 15-49 years, pregnant and postpartum women, and adolescents who have started their menstrual cycle. According to the World Health Organization (WHO), it is estimated that 40% of children aged 6-59 months, 37% of pregnant women, and 30% of women aged 15-49 years are affected by anemia worldwide (World Health Organization, 2023). Additionally, 2-5% of men and postmenopausal women experience iron deficiency anemia (Goddard et al., 2021). Data from the National Health and Nutrition Examination Survey (NHANES) and the Centers for Disease Control and Prevention (CDC) in the United States indicate that iron deficiency and iron deficiency anemia are prevalent (Centers for Disease Control and Prevention (CDC), 2002). Subsequent studies in the selected population have shown that iron deficiency has not decreased (Gupta, P. M. et al., 2017).

Definition of Iron Deficiency Anemia

Iron deficiency anemia is a condition where the number of erythrocytes and the hemoglobin concentration are lower than normal. According to the WHO, anemia is defined as a hemoglobin (Hb) level of less than 13 g/dl in men and less than 12 g/dl in women (Herbert, V., 1968). However, certain exceptions must be considered regarding this definition. In dehydrated patients, hemoglobin levels may appear normal even if they have anemia. Additionally, pregnant women may experience a dilutional decrease in erythrocyte mass due to an increase in plasma volume. Patients with chronic obstructive pulmonary disease (COPD) and individuals living at high altitudes can have normal hemoglobin levels despite blood loss (Higgins, P. D. R., & Rockey, D. C., 2003).

Etiological Factors of Iron Deficiency Anemia

The causes of iron deficiency anemia can vary depending on age, race, and the development level of the country of residence. The main causes of iron deficiency anemia are insufficient dietary iron intake, malabsorption, and blood loss.

Insufficient Dietary Iron Intake: In developing countries, nutritional deficiencies leading to insufficient dietary intake are a common cause of iron deficiency. Vegetarian diets can also cause deficiencies in dietary intake. Conditions that reduce iron absorption include celiac disease, atrophic (autoimmune) gastritis, Helicobacter pylori infection, bariatric surgery, proton pump inhibitors, histamine 2 receptor blockers, and antacids. Additionally, tannins in tea and phytates in whole grains can cause absorption deficiencies. In patients who do not respond to iron treatment, malabsorption should be considered. However, bleeding should also be considered based on the patient's age and gender.

In developed countries, the significant causes of iron deficiency anemia are gastrointestinal and gynecological bleeding (Camaschella, C., 2015). Additionally, pregnancy, intestinal parasites, and frequent blood donation can cause iron deficiency anemia due to blood loss (Auerbach, M. et al., 2024).

In men and postmenopausal women, iron deficiency anemia is a significant symptom of gastrointestinal malignancies. In 16% of individuals with iron deficiency anemia who underwent endoscopy, gastrointestinal cancers and high-risk adenomas were detected.

Similarly, malignant gastrointestinal cancer was found in 12% of another group who underwent endoscopy.

Iron Metabolism

Iron, an essential inorganic nutrient in the human body, plays a crucial role in numerous biological processes, including DNA and RNA synthesis, oxygen transport, cellular respiration, the activity of many enzymes, heme synthesis, detoxification processes, and immune function and metabolism (Shen, Z. et al., 2018). Iron homeostasis is tightly regulated by balancing absorption, systemic transport, cellular uptake, and storage in healthy cells (Zhang, L. et al., 2017). Iron is not synthesized during physiological processes, so iron levels must be maintained through diet. Dietary iron is primarily absorbed by duodenal enterocytes (90%). Since iron absorption is ≤2% of total intake, the stomach does not significantly contribute to iron assimilation (Laskar, A. et al., 2013). There are two types of dietary iron that can be absorbed: heme iron from the breakdown of hemoglobin and myoglobin in red meat, and non-heme inorganic iron released primarily from vegetables and grains (Recuenco M. C. et al., 2013; Sokolov, A. V. et al., 2017).

Iron absorption occurs in the duodenum through two different mechanisms. One mechanism involves the absorption of heme iron found in hemoglobin and myoglobin. The other pathway is for the absorption of ferrous iron. The digestion of heme-containing foods begins in the stomach. The acidic environment and protease enzymes release iron from heme, converting it to ferric (Fe^{3+}) form. Ferric iron then becomes heme and enters the cell. The other pathway involves the absorption of non-heme iron, which usually reaches the duodenum in ferric form and must be converted to ferrous form for absorption (Hallberg, L., & Hulthen, L., 2002). Iron absorption is influenced by various factors. Heme iron absorption is less affected by the diet's composition, while non-heme iron absorption is more related to the individual's iron levels, the amount of iron in the food, and other nutrients present. For example, ascorbic acid, meat, fish, and alcohol increase iron absorption, while phytates, polyphenols, calcium, zinc, and some plant components decrease it (Reddy, M. B. et al., 2000).

Iron is notable for its unique properties. Its ability to exchange electrons allows it to easily switch between ferric (Fe^{2+}) and ferrous (Fe^{3+}) forms. This flexibility enables it to integrate into heme structures such as hemoglobin and myoglobin, thereby fulfilling oxygen-binding functions. It also plays a critical role in many enzymes, and in the maintenance of cell membranes, proteins, and DNA. Besides hemoglobin and myoglobin, iron is necessary for the production of enzymes such as cytochromes and several others. Additionally, iron can cause cellular damage by facilitating reactions that produce free radical ions from hydrogen peroxide. Therefore, iron balance in the body is delicate, and both iron deficiency and excess are common conditions in humans (Carley, A., 2003). Iron-protoporphyrin (heme) and iron-sulfur compounds act as cofactors in the catalytic activities of many enzymes. Consequently, the cellular functions and metabolic effects of iron become more evident. Iron is essential for the body's healthy functioning, but imbalances can lead to severe health problems (Andrews, N. C., 1999).

The normal iron content of an adult body is approximately 3 to 4 grams. Most of the iron is found in circulating erythrocytes; additional iron is present in myoglobin and certain enzymes, as well as in storage and transport forms (Auerbach, M. et al., 2024). Iron requirements and storage vary by age and gender. For example, in the late stages of pregnancy, a fetus may contain about 75 mg/kg of iron. However, after birth, infants' iron stores rapidly decrease, leading to a negative iron balance in most children. Therefore, iron intake should be encouraged in growing children. After adolescence, iron requirements decrease, and lifetime iron stores may increase in men. A normal adult male may have 35-45 mg/kg of iron, whereas iron stores in women typically decrease from postpubertal to menopausal periods. Postmenopausal women's iron stores usually reach levels observed in adult men (Andrews, N. C., & Bridges, K. R., 1998). Most of the body's iron is found in the form of hemoglobin and myoglobin, while a small amount is present in enzymes such as peroxidase, catalase, and ribonucleotide reductase. The amount of non-heme-bound iron in adult males is about 1 gram, stored in macrophages and hepatocytes as ferritin or hemosiderin. Only 0.1% of the body's iron is found in the plasma bound to transferrin (Andrews, N. C., 2004). In the development of iron deficiency anemia, iron stores are initially depleted. This condition appears in laboratory data as low ferritin, indicating iron deficiency. If this negative iron balance continues, hemoglobin production decreases, erythrocytes decrease, and anemia develops. This condition appears in the laboratory as microcytic anemia (Auerbach, M. et al., 2024).

Clinical Findings

The symptoms of iron deficiency anemia can vary depending on the rate of anemia's progression. If anemia develops slowly, the body's adaptation mechanisms can enable patients to tolerate very low hemoglobin levels (<7.0 g/dl) with almost no symptoms (Hugman, A., 2006). In iron deficiency, there is inadequate oxygen supply to tissues, often leading to symptoms such as weakness, fatigue, and difficulty concentrating (Camaschella, C., 2015; Lopez, A. et al., 2016). The most common symptom is loss of appetite. Angular stomatitis and atrophic glossitis, where the tongue is painfully swollen, can occur in iron deficiency anemia. Plummer-Vinson syndrome can develop as a complication of iron deficiency anemia, characterized by the formation of esophageal webs and difficulty swallowing. Other symptoms of iron deficiency anemia include irritability, difficulty concentrating, attention deficits, and breath-holding spells. Patients may also present with palpitations, exertional dyspnea, or reduced exercise tolerance, and restless legs syndrome characterized by leg pain and the need to move the legs. The clinical findings of iron deficiency anemia may also include pica, characterized by the craving to eat substances such as soil, clay, ice, or chalk (Fleming, M. D., 2015).

Diagnosis of Iron Deficiency Anemia

The patient's medical history and physical examination are crucial to both diagnosing and identifying the underlying cause. Dietary habits, potential sources of bleeding, malabsorption conditions, infections, and symptoms such as pica should be carefully evaluated. In the physical examination, common findings of anemia such as tachycardia, murmur, and pale skin should be noted, along with non-specific findings for iron deficiency. Symptoms such as jaundice, hepatosplenomegaly, and lymphadenopathy can indicate iron deficiency anemia and should be observed.

Iron deficiency is examined in three stages:

Prelatent Phase: In the first stage, tissue iron stores may be depleted. Hematocrit and serum iron levels remain unchanged, but ferritin levels are low.

Latent Phase: In this stage, the iron stores of macrophages are reduced. Serum iron levels are low, total iron-binding capacity (TIBC) increases, but hematocrit is not yet reduced. This stage is diagnosed by a low transferrin saturation measured in the morning. Erythropoiesis begins to be limited by iron deficiency, leading to increased levels of free transferrin receptors. Reticulocyte hemoglobin concentration decreases, and newly produced erythrocytes are iron-deficient.

Iron Deficiency Anemia: In the third stage, iron deficiency becomes more pronounced. Hemoglobin levels decrease, and erythrocytes become microcytic and hypochromic. Even if iron deficiency anemia has not yet developed, it should be treated. Iron therapy can lead to a reversible improvement in the stages of iron deficiency.

In the laboratory diagnosis of iron deficiency, a complete blood count (CBC), which shows hematological parameters, is frequently used. However, diagnosing iron deficiency solely based on CBC may not be possible.

In CBC, low hemoglobin values are detected. The mean corpuscular volume (MCV) and the mean corpuscular hemoglobin (MCH) are reduced. The red cell distribution width (RDW), measured by automated blood counters, increases. Although the white blood cell count is usually normal, an increase in platelet count is often observed. In peripheral blood smear, anisocytosis is prominent; erythrocytes may initially be normal in size but become microcytic and hypochromic as the condition progresses.

In iron deficiency, serum iron levels are typically reduced, while serum total iron-binding capacity (TIBC) is generally increased. However, sometimes TIBC may be normal or decreased. Serum ferritin levels, which indicate the body's iron stores, are a sensitive and straightforward test. Low levels of ferritin usually indicate iron deficiency. However, because ferritin is also an acute phase reactant, it may be normal in the presence of infection, cancer, or chronic inflammatory diseases, even in iron deficiency. Unlike low ferritin values, low serum iron cannot be used to diagnose or exclude iron deficiency. Chronic disease anemia may also show low serum iron. According to the Centers for Disease Control and Prevention (CDC) in the United States, serum ferritin is the gold standard test in anemic adults (Guyatt, G. H. et al., 1992). According to the American Gastroenterological Association (AGA) guidelines, ferritin is used to diagnose iron deficiency in anemia patients, with a recommended cutoff value of 45 ng/mL instead of 15 ng/mL (Ko, C. W. et al., 2020). Endoscopy is recommended for gastrointestinal bleeding in postmenopausal women and men with iron deficiency anemia (Snook, J. et al., 2021). If endoscopy is not possible, computed tomographic colonography is recommended (Snook, J. et al., 2021). According to the AGA guidelines, bidirectional endoscopy is recommended for postmenopausal women and men with asymptomatic iron deficiency anemia. The guidelines also recommend testing for Helicobacter pylori during endoscopy. Routine gastric biopsy for atrophic gastritis diagnosis is not recommended in patients with iron deficiency anemia (Ko, C. W. et al., 2020). If there is a waiting period for endoscopy, iron therapy should be started in the meantime (Snook, J. et al., 2021).

In patients with suspected celiac disease and iron deficiency anemia, serology should be checked before small bowel biopsy, and biopsy should be considered if the serology is positive (Ko, C. W. et al., 2020).

In asymptomatic patients with uncomplicated iron deficiency anemia and negative endoscopy results, iron supplementation should be tried before the routine use of video capsule endoscopy (Ko, C. W. et al., 2020).

The importance of serum ferritin levels in the diagnosis of iron deficiency anemia has been reported. Other iron parameters can be evaluated when serum ferritin levels are inconclusive. Additionally, even if laboratory results are uncertain, a rise in hemoglobin levels by the second week of iron therapy confirms the diagnosis (Snook, J. et al., 2021).

Age, gender, and hemoglobin concentration are independent variables in assessing the risk of gastrointestinal cancer in iron deficiency anemia, and fecal immunochemical testing is not recommended for risk assessment (Snook, J. et al., 2021).

Prevention of Iron Deficiency Anemia

In healthcare delivery, preventing disease is more important than treating it. To prevent iron deficiency anemia (IDA), breastfeeding should be encouraged. From the sixth month onward, complementary feeding with balanced iron content should be recommended for infant nutrition. This dietary approach should continue in child and adult nutrition. To prevent IDA, low-dose preventive iron supplementation of 1-2 mg/kg/day should be started at the end of the fourth month for full-term infants and at the end of the first month for preterm infants (Turkish Ministry of Health, General Directorate of Public Health, 2018). Additionally, pregnant women should undergo complete blood count screenings during their follow-ups. Those diagnosed with anemia should receive therapeutic doses of iron, while those without anemia should receive prophylactic doses from the end of the fourth month until three months postpartum (Turkish Ministry of Health, General Directorate of Public Health, 2018).

Treatment

The aim of iron deficiency treatment is to replenish depleted iron stores. However, to prevent the recurrence of anemia, the underlying cause must be treated.

Oral Iron Therapy

Iron therapy is usually administered orally or parenterally. The most commonly recommended and used oral iron preparations are ferrous salts. However, the absorption of ferrous salts is low and variable due to food products and free radical-mediated mucosal damage. Ferric compounds were developed to overcome these problems but are generally less soluble, reducing bioavailability. To address these issues, new molecules, such as the iron polymaltose complex (IPC), which can dissolve at neutral pH and are not chelated by other substances, have been developed (Kavakli, K. et al., 2004). In adults, the best response is usually achieved with a daily intake of 200 mg of elemental iron. Iron therapy should be taken on an empty stomach, as taking it with food can reduce iron absorption. Iron absorption increases with the consumption of iron-rich foods such as orange juice, meat, and fish, and decreases with the consumption of certain foods such as grains, tea, and milk. Milk intake can particularly reduce iron absorption in infants during the breastfeeding period. In children, iron therapy is typically administered as 1.5-2 mg/kg of elemental iron three times a day. Studies have shown no difference in efficacy between taking the appropriate dose of iron once a day or dividing it into multiple doses throughout the day (Stoltzfus, R. J. et al., 2004). Although daily iron therapy is recommended, if the patient cannot tolerate it, an alternative option of every other day treatment can be considered (Snook, J. et al., 2021). The duration of treatment is 3-6 months. Hemoglobin levels should be evaluated at the end of the first 4 weeks. Iron therapy should continue for an additional 3 months after hemoglobin levels normalize (Snook, J. et al., 2021). If hemoglobin levels do not reach normal within a month, there may be a problem. It should be reviewed whether the treatment is being taken correctly, if there are any additional losses, and if the diagnosis is correct. Approximately 12% of patients on oral iron therapy experience side effects such as upper abdominal burning, nausea, abdominal cramps, and diarrhea. There is no difference in side effects between ferrous sulfate, fumarate, or gluconate salts.

Iron absorption decreases when taken with antacids, proton pump inhibitors, histamine 2 receptor antagonists, or medications containing aluminum, magnesium, calcium, or zinc. Similarly, iron can reduce the absorption of medications such as bisphosphonates, tetracycline, quinolones, levodopa, methyldopa, levothyroxine, and penicillamine. Therefore, it is recommended to allow at least a 2-hour interval between these medications and iron supplements. Iron and zinc should not be taken simultaneously.

The patient's anemia usually improves within 1-2 months with appropriate iron medication and treatment of the underlying condition. After the anemia improves, it is advised to continue treatment for another 2-3 months to replenish the body's iron stores. For patients who do not respond to iron therapy and have negative endoscopy results, small bowel biopsy and kidney examination should be considered (Snook, J. et al., 2021). In cases where this is not possible, magnetic resonance imaging can be an alternative (Snook, J. et al., 2021). For patients in whom the underlying cause cannot be identified despite all investigations, long-term iron therapy should be provided (Snook, J. et al., 2021). Anemia usually resolves after iron therapy, but it can recur in some patients over the long term (Snook, J. et al., 2021). Periodic testing should be conducted to evaluate recurrence after treatment (Snook, J. et al., 2021).

Parenteral Iron Therapy

Parenteral iron therapy is used for patients who cannot tolerate oral iron therapy, have severe iron deficiency, and in cases where iron is rapidly lost from the gastrointestinal system and cannot be replaced orally (e.g., hereditary hemorrhagic telangiectasia), have exacerbations of conditions (e.g., ulcerative colitis), or where iron cannot be absorbed from the gastrointestinal system (e.g., duodenal resection) or in hemodialysis patients where sufficient iron cannot be provided (Andrews, N. C., 2004; Snook, J. et al., 2021). However, if it is determined that oral iron therapy will not be effective or if it is urgent to correct iron deficiency anemia, parenteral therapy should be considered at an earlier stage (Snook, J. et al., 2021).

Screening

Routine screening for iron deficiency anemia is not recommended. Screening is recommended for premenopausal women, women with hypermenorrhea, individuals with conditions that can cause iron malabsorption, and pregnant women (Auerbach, M. et al., 2024). Routine screening is not recommended for individuals taking antithrombotic medications such as aspirin. Screening should be planned based on individual risk factors. The Centers for Disease Control and Prevention (CDC) of the United States recommends screening women of childbearing age every five years. However, a more frequent (annual) screening is recommended in the presence of hypermenorrhea, low iron intake, or a history of iron deficiency (Centers for Disease Control and Prevention, 1998).

Conclusion

Iron deficiency anemia (IDA) is a widespread health issue globally, particularly prevalent in developing countries. The primary causes of IDA include nutritional deficiencies, malabsorption disorders, and blood loss. Particularly at risk are children under the age of 5, women of reproductive age, pregnant and postpartum women, and adolescents who have started their menstrual cycles. Therefore, early diagnosis and appropriate interventions are crucial for preventing and treating IDA.

In diagnosis, the patient's medical history and physical examination are as important as laboratory tests. Common tests used in the diagnosis of IDA include complete blood count (CBC), serum ferritin level, serum iron level, and total iron-binding capacity (TIBC). Oral iron therapy is an effective treatment option for most cases of IDA. However, there are factors that can reduce the absorption of oral iron preparations, and it is important to consider these factors.

Success in the treatment of IDA is related to the administration of the treatment in the appropriate dose and duration. Parenteral iron therapy may be considered for patients who do not respond to treatment or cannot tolerate oral iron preparations. Regular follow-up after treatment is important to monitor the patient's recovery process and prevent recurrences.

To prevent IDA, it is necessary to provide nutritional education and supplements, especially for high-risk groups. Effective preventive measures include breastfeeding infants, choosing iron-rich foods during the transition to solid foods, and providing regular follow-up and iron supplements to pregnant women.

In conclusion, IDA is a significant public health issue worldwide that can be controlled with accurate diagnosis, treatment, and preventive measures. Therefore, greater emphasis should be placed on prevention and treatment strategies for IDA in health policies and practices.

References

Andrews, N. C. (1999). Disorders of iron metabolism. *The New England Journal of Medicine, 341*(26), 1986-199. https://doi.org/10.1056/NEJM199912233412607.

Andrews, N. C. (2004). Iron deficiency and related disorders. In J. P. Greer, J. Foerster, J. N. Lukens, G. M. Rodgers, F. Paraskevas, & B. Glader (Eds.), *Wintrobe's Clinical Hematology* (11th ed., Vol. 1, pp. 979-1009). Philadelphia: Lippincott Williams & Wilkins.

Andrews, N. C., & Bridges, K. R. (1998). Disorders of iron metabolism and sideroblastic anemia. In D. G. Nathan & S. H. Orkin (Eds.), *Nathan and Oski's Haematology of Infancy and Childhood* (5th ed., Vol. 1, pp. 423-461). Philadelphia: W.B. Saunders.

Auerbach, M., DeLoughery, T. G., Means, R. T., Jr., Elmore, J. G., & others. (2024). Causes and diagnosis of iron deficiency and iron deficiency anemia in adults.

Camaschella, C. (2015). Iron-deficiency anemia. *The New England Journal of Medicine, 372*(19), 1832-1843. https://doi.org/10.1056/NEJMra1401038.

Carley, A. (2003). Anemia: When is it iron deficiency? *Pediatric Nursing, 29*(2), 127-133.

Centers for Disease Control and Prevention (CDC). (2002). Iron deficiency—United States, 1999-2000. *MMWR Morbidity and Mortality Weekly Report, 51*(29), 897.

Centers for Disease Control and Prevention. (1998). Recommendations to prevent and control iron deficiency in the United States. *MMWR Recommendations and Reports, 47*(RR-3), 1.

Fleming, M. D. (2015). Disorders of iron and copper metabolism, the sideroblastic anemias and lead toxicity. In S. H. Orkin, D. Nathan, D. Ginsburg, T. Look, D. E. Fisher, & D. Lux (Eds.), *Nathan and Oski's Hematology and Oncology of Infancy and Childhood* (8th ed., pp. 344-380). Philadelphia: Elsevier Inc.

GBD 2021 Anaemia Collaborators. (2023). Prevalence, years lived with disability, and trends in anaemia burden by severity and cause, 1990-2021: Findings from the Global Burden of Disease Study 2021. *The Lancet Haematology, 10*(10), e713.

Goddard, A. F., James, M. W., McIntyre, A. S., Scott, B. B., & British Society of Gastroenterology. (2011). Guidelines for the management of iron deficiency anaemia. *Gut, 60*(10), 1309-1316. https://doi.org/10.1136/gut.2010.228874.

Gupta, P. M., Hamner, H. C., Suchdev, P. S., et al., (2017). Iron status of toddlers, nonpregnant females, and pregnant females in the United States. *The American Journal of Clinical Nutrition, 106*(6), 1640S.

Guyatt, G. H., Oxman, A. D., Ali, M., & others. (1992). Demir eksikliği anemisinin laboratuvar tanısı: Genel bakış. *Journal of General Internal Medicine, 7*(2), 145.

Hallberg, L., & Hulthen, L. (2002). Perspectives on iron absorption. *Blood Cells, Molecules, and Diseases, 29*(3), 562–573.

Herbert, V. (1968). Megaloblastic anemia as a problem in world health. *The American Journal of Clinical Nutrition, 21*(11), 1115-1120.

Higgins, P. D. R., & Rockey, D. C. (2003). Iron-deficiency anemia. *Techniques in Gastrointestinal Endoscopy, 5*(3), 134-141.

Hugman, A. (2006). Hepcidin: An important new regulator of iron homeostasis. *Clinical Laboratory Haematology, 28*(2), 75-83. https://doi.org/10.1111/j.1365-2257.2006.00768.x.

Kavakli, K., Yilmaz, D., & Cetinkaya, B. (2004). Safety profiles of Fe2+ and Fe3+ oral preparations in the treatment of iron deficiency anemia in children. *Pediatric Hematology Oncology, 21*(5), 403-410.

Ko, C. W., Siddique, S. M., Patel, A., Harris, A., Sultan, S., Altayar, O., ... & Sultan, S. (2020). AGA clinical practice guidelines on the gastrointestinal evaluation of iron deficiency anemia. *Gastroenterology, 159*(3), 1085-1094.

Laskar, A., Eilertsen, J., Li, W., & Yuan, X. M. (2013). SPION primes THP1 derived M2 macrophages towards M1-like macrophages. *Biochemical and Biophysical Research Communications, 441*(4), 737–742. https://doi.org/10.1016/j.bbrc.2013.10.115.

Lopez, A., Cacoub, P., Macdougall, I. C., & Peyrin-Biroulet, L. (2016). Iron deficiency anaemia. *The Lancet, 387*(10021), 907.

Recuenco, M. C., Rahman, M. M., Takeuchi, F., Kobayashi, K., & Tsubaki, M. (2013). Electron transfer reactions of candidate tumor suppressor 101F6 protein, a cytochrome b561 homologue, with ascorbate and monodehydroascorbate radical. *Biochemistry, 52*(21), 3660–3668. https://doi.org/10.1021/bi301607s.

Reddy, M. B., Hurrell, R. F., & Cook, J. D. (2000). Estimation of nonheme-iron bioavailability from meal composition. *The American Journal of Clinical Nutrition, 71*(4), 937-943.

Shen, Z., Liu, T., Li, Y., Lau, J., Yang, Z., Fan, W., ... & Chen, X. (2018). Fenton-reaction-acceleratable magnetic nanoparticles for ferroptosis therapy of orthotopic brain tumors. *ACS Nano, 12*(11), 11355–11365. https://doi.org/10.1021/acsnano.8b06201.

Snook, J., Bhala, N., Beales, I. L. P., Cannings, D., Kightley, C., Logan, R. P., ... & Logan, R. P. (2021). British Society of Gastroenterology guidelines for the management of iron deficiency anaemia in adults. *Gut, 60*(10), 1309-1316.

Sokolov, A. V., Voynova, I. V., Kostevich, V. A., Vlasenko, A. Y., Zakharova, E. T., & Vasilyev, V. B. (2017). Comparison of interaction between ceruloplasmin and lactoferrin/transferrin: To bind or not to bind. *Biochemistry. Biokhimiia, 82*(9), 1073–1078. https://doi.org/10.1134/S0006297917090115.

Stoltzfus, R. J., Chway, H. M., Montresor, A., & others. (2004). Low dose daily iron supplementation improves iron status and appetite but not anemia, whereas quarterly anthelminthic treatment improves growth, appetite and anemia in Zanzibari preschool children. *Journal of Nutrition, 134*(2), 348-356.

Turkish Ministry of Health, General Directorate of Public Health. (2018). *Follow-up Protocols for Infants, Children, and Adolescents*. Ankara.

Turkish Ministry of Health, General Directorate of Public Health. (2018). *Prenatal Care Guide*. Ankara.

World Health Organization. (2023). *Health-topics Anaemia.* Retrieved from https://www.who.int/health-topics/anaemia#tab=tab_1.

Zhang, L., Reyes, A., & Wang, X. (2017). The role of DNA repair in maintaining mitochondrial DNA stability. *Advances in Experimental Medicine and Biology, 1038*, 85–105. https://doi.org/10.1007/978-981-10-6674-0_7.

Chapter 17

Vitamin B12 Deficiency

Serap Öksüz*, MD
Department of Family Medicine, İzmir Katip Çelebi University, İzmir, Turkey

Abstract

Vitamin B12 (cobalamin) is one of the common causes of macrocytic anemia, which manifests with hematological and neuropsychiatric disorders. The diagnosis of vitamin B12 deficiency, which increases in frequency with age, is based on the measurement of serum B12 levels. Vitamin B12 acts as a cofactor in the enzymatic reactions necessary for folate metabolism and DNA synthesis. While B12 deficiency is more common in elderly populations, studies conducted in different age groups and geographical regions show variability in the prevalence of the deficiency. B12 deficiency can present with anemia, neurological symptoms, and gastrointestinal signs. It can cause nerve damage, cognitive disorders, and behavioral disturbances. B12 deficiency is associated with malabsorption, autoimmune diseases, poor nutrition, stomach surgeries, infections, and the prolonged use of certain medications. Particularly, drugs such as metformin and proton pump inhibitors can adversely affect B12 absorption. Treating B12 deficiency is especially important for the elderly and at-risk groups. With early diagnosis and appropriate treatment, hematological and neurological responses can be achieved, improving overall health and quality of life.

Keywords: anemia, Vitamin B12, cobalamin

Introduction

Vitamin B12 (cobalamin) is a nutrient that plays a critical role in hematological and nervous system diseases, such as macrocytic anemia and neuropsychiatric disorders. B12 deficiency is a common problem that increases with age and is usually diagnosed by measuring serum B12 levels (Robert & Brown, 2003). Since B12 is primarily found in animal products, women who are vegetarians or vegans are at risk for B12 deficiency (Pepper & Black, 2011). Vitamin B12 functions as a cofactor in the enzymatic reactions necessary for folate metabolism and DNA synthesis (Dror & Allen, 2018). The deficiency is associated with malabsorption, autoimmune diseases, poor nutrition, stomach surgeries, infections, and the prolonged use of certain

* Corresponding Author's Email: dr-serap10@hotmail.com.

In: Common Diseases According to Family Medicine Practice Guidelines
Editors: Esra Meltem Koç and Hilal Aksoy
ISBN: 979-8-89530-302-3

medications (Means & Fairfield, 2024). Neurological and cognitive disorders caused by the deficiency can lead to serious health problems, making early recognition and treatment of the deficiency crucial.

Synthesis and Absorption of Vitamin B12

Vitamin B12 (cobalamin) deficiency, which presents with hematological and neuropsychiatric disorders, is one of the most common causes of macrocytic anemia. The diagnosis of vitamin B12 deficiency, which increases with age, is based on the measurement of serum B12 levels (Robert & Brown, 2003).

Vitamin B12 cannot be synthesized by plants or animals. It is synthesized by specific bacteria and archaea and then transferred to animal tissues through microbial interactions. Ruminants obtain essential vitamin B12 through a symbiotic relationship with bacteria in their bodies. Therefore, we depend on B12-producing bacteria in the stomachs of ruminants. Meat (beef, veal, lamb) and milk from herbivorous ruminants are good sources of vitamin B12 for humans. Numerous studies on the relationship between dietary B12 sources and plasma B12 levels indicate that higher consumption of meat, milk, and fish is associated with higher plasma B12 levels, especially in Western countries (Watanabe & Bito, 2018).

Vitamin B12, a nutrient synthesized only by prokaryotes, acts as a cofactor in the essential enzymatic reactions necessary for folate metabolism and DNA synthesis (Dror & Allen, 2018).

Vitamin B12 binds to two proteins: haptocorrin, a glycoprotein that carries the majority of circulating B12 and its inactive form, and transcobalamin, which is responsible for transporting B12 to all cells in the body (Nexo & Hoffmann-Lücke, 2011). B12 obtained through food binds to haptocorrin (HC) in the saliva. In the small intestine, pancreatic proteases separate B12 from haptocorrin, allowing it to bind to the intrinsic factor (IF) secreted by the stomach's parietal cells. The IF-B12 complex then binds to receptors in the terminal ileum, where it dissociates from IF and binds to transcobalamin (TC) to be released from ileal mucosal cells into the plasma. TC delivers B12 to the cells' TC receptors, and B12 is released from transcobalamin to act as a cofactor in enzymatic reactions (Green, 2017). After stopping B12 intake, the liver stores it for one to three years before it is completely depleted (Ghazal, Zur & Silver, 2023).

The impact of vitamin B12 on the gut microbiota is not yet fully understood. Approximately 50% of a 1 μg oral dose of B12 is absorbed into the ileum, but absorption decreases as the dose increases. B12 not absorbed in the ileum passes into the colon, where it is metabolized by gut bacteria into B12 analogs (Guetterman et al., 2022).

In addition to the cyano form used in supplements, vitamin B12, or cobalamin, exists in various forms such as methyl-, deoxyadenosyl-, and hydroxy-cobalamin. Forms other than the cyano form are converted into methyl- or 5-deoxyadenosyl forms, which are necessary cofactors for methionine synthase and L-methylmalonyl-CoA mutase, essential for purine and pyrimidine synthesis. The reaction depends on methylcobalamin as a cofactor and also relies on folate, where the methyl group from methyltetrahydrofolate is transferred to homocysteine to form methionine and tetrahydrofolate. Disruptions in these metabolic steps due to B12 deficiency lead to megaloblastic anemia. The accumulation of methylmalonyl CoA in B12 deficiency is believed to be responsible for neurological effects (O'Leary & Samman, 2010).

Pregnancy and Vitamin B12

During pregnancy, vitamin B12 is transferred to the fetus through the placenta. Therefore, in pregnant women with B12 deficiency, the levels of B12 transferred to the fetus are reduced. Since B12 is found primarily in animal products, women who are vegetarians or vegans are at risk for B12 deficiency (Pepper & Black, 2011).

Myelination and synaptogenesis, which are critical stages of the central nervous system and brain development, begin in the third trimester of pregnancy and continue to influence neuronal development during infancy and early childhood. Vitamin B12 plays an essential role in these critical stages, including neural myelination, synaptogenesis, and neurotransmitter synthesis, which are crucial for cell division and growth of the fetus. Therefore, vitamin B12 has significant effects on cognitive development and functionality. B12 deficiency can lead to nerve damage and brain atrophy (Venkatramanan et al., 2016).

In cases of maternal B12 deficiency, unrecognized neonatal B12 deficiency can worsen if the baby is breastfed without B12 supplementation. The clinical presentation of B12 deficiency in infants is often nonspecific, such as developmental delay, which can lead to delayed diagnosis and treatment. The neurological damage caused by prolonged B12 deficiency depends on the severity and duration of the deficiency, making early diagnosis and treatment of B12 deficiency critical (Hinton et al., 2010).

The recommended daily doses of vitamin B12 are 0.4 mcg for infants up to 6 months, 0.5 mcg from 6 months to 1 year, and the daily requirement increases with age until reaching 2.4 mcg at 14 years old, which is the adult dose. During pregnancy and lactation, the daily requirement for vitamin B12 increases further, with recommended doses of 2.6 mcg during pregnancy and 2.8 mcg during lactation (Institute of Medicine (US) Standing Committee on the Scientific Evaluation of Dietary Reference Intakes, 1998).

Epidemiology

In a study involving 100 pediatric patients, which aimed to determine the B12 levels and associated risk factors in children from the age of 6 months (when complementary feeding starts) to the preschool period (72 months), B12 deficiency was found to be 25% in the 6-11 month age group, 5.8% in the 12-23 month age group, and 2.8% in the 24-47 month age group (Elgormus et al., 2023). In a study group consisting of 3,478 children aged 0.5 to 12.9 years from four geographical regions of Thailand and Bangkok, 25.1% of the population was found to have insufficient B12 intake (Pongcharoen et al., 2024).

According to a study conducted by NHANES (The National Health and Nutrition Examination Survey), the prevalence of B12 deficiency in individuals over 60 years old was approximately 3% to 5%. Another NHANES study reported that the prevalence of B12 deficiency in the general population was between 1.6% and 2.6% (Pfeiffer et al., 2007). Epidemiological studies targeting the elderly population in industrialized countries indicate that the prevalence of B12 deficiency is around 20%, and this rate can reach up to 50% depending on the reference cobalamin levels. A study focused on the elderly population living in institutions reported that B12 deficiency ranged between 30% and 40% (Andrès et al., 2007).

Clinical Findings

The typical presentation of vitamin B12 deficiency can include non-specific complaints such as fatigue and weakness due to anemia, or it can present as mild anemia incidentally detected without symptoms due to improved diagnostic capabilities. Vitamin B12 deficiency can also present with glossitis-related symptoms such as tongue pain, swelling, tenderness, papilla loss, and hyperpigmentation (Means & Fairfield, 2024).

In adults, clinical neurological manifestations can include demyelination of the dorsal column, loss of vibration sense, proprioception (ataxia), and stereognosis, as well as demyelination of the lateral corticospinal system leading to hyperreflexia. In neonates, it can present with neural tube defects, developmental delay, and hypotonia (Al-Awami et al., 2023).

The classic neurological clinical appearance of B12 deficiency is subacute combined degeneration of the spinal cord, which causes both motor and sensory deficits. It can also cause neurological symptoms such as optic neuropathy, paresthesia, and myelopathy. Behavioral disorders are the most common psychiatric complaint, but cognitive disorders such as dementia or delirium can also be observed in these patients (Ghazal et al., 2023).

Severe symptomatic B12 deficiency is known to cause various neuropsychiatric symptoms, including cognitive impairment, depression, and psychosis. However, no causal relationship has been established between low or borderline low B12 levels and widespread psychiatric disorders. Psychiatrists are advised to refer patients with neurological symptoms suggestive of B12 deficiency, such as paresthesia, weakness, numbness, unsteady gait, pallor, and fatigue, and accompanying hematological findings, to a primary care doctor for further investigation (Kennedy et al., 2024).

Hyperhomocysteinemia refers to high levels of homocysteine in the blood, a metabolite produced during methionine metabolism. Folate or B12 deficiency is one of the causes of hyperhomocysteinemia. Studies indicate that elevated homocysteine levels are associated with atherosclerosis, endothelial damage, and stroke. It is believed that the accumulation of homocysteine and its metabolites, homocysteinylated proteins, mediates toxicity by inducing cytotoxicity, inflammation, protein aggregation, and apoptosis (Reddy et al., 2007).

Over 90% of circulating homocysteine is found in an oxidized form bound to proteins, while only 2% of total homocysteine is in a free reduced form. Normal plasma homocysteine levels are below 10 mmol/L. Mild hyperhomocysteinemia is defined as levels below 16 mmol/L, while severe hyperhomocysteinemia is defined as levels above 100 mmol/L. Only protein-unbound homocysteine is subject to glomerular filtration, and most are reabsorbed in the tubules. The renal elimination of homocysteine is minimal. Additionally, homocysteine undergoes transsulfuration in the kidney, and thus an increase in plasma homocysteine is expected in the case of renal transsulfuration deficiency (Capelli et al., 2019).

Both retrospective and prospective cohort studies on B12 metabolism have shown a positive relationship between decreased B12 or folate levels, or elevated methylmalonic acid levels due to deficiency, and the risk of stroke. Secondary increases in homocysteine have been identified in patients with coronary artery disease, thromboembolism, stroke, and transient ischemic attacks. The Diabetic Intervention with Vitamins to Improve Nephropathy (DIVINe) study revealed that the administration of vitamins B6, folate, and B12 increased the incidence of cardiovascular events in patients with diabetic nephropathy. Similarly, another study showed that high-dose B12 supplementation did not reduce stroke risk and was detrimental. Meta-analysis of the data from these two studies indicated that the harmful effects of cyanocobalamin dosage and resultant high toxic thiocyanate levels in patients with impaired renal function masked the benefits of B vitamin supplementation in other groups. The subgroup analysis showed that B vitamin treatment reduced the risk of stroke and cardiovascular events in patients with normal renal function. Clinical data from these studies do not provide much insight into the mechanism by which B12 and other B vitamins reduce stroke risk (Rotha & Mohamadzadeh, 2021).

Causes of Vitamin B12 Deficiency

Vitamin B12 deficiency can be caused by malabsorption, autoimmune diseases, poor nutrition, stomach surgeries, infections, and various drug-related reasons.

Food-cobalamin malabsorption is defined as B12 deficiency despite normal dietary intake of B12 from food. Conditions that prevent the dissociation of B12 from food proteins, such as atrophic gastritis, stomach surgery, chronic H. pylori infection, pancreatic insufficiency, long-term use of medications such as antacids, H2 receptor blockers, and proton pump inhibitors, as well as alcoholism, can lead to this form of deficiency. B12 bound to proteins in food cannot be easily absorbed (Means & Fairfield, 2024).

Autoimmune gastritis, characterized by atrophy of the oxyntic mucosa due to antibodies against parietal cells, is estimated to occur in 0.3% to 2.7% of the general population. This condition is often asymptomatic but can sometimes present with dyspeptic or reflux symptoms. The diagnosis of autoimmune atrophic gastritis, a chronic disease, relies on serological tests and histopathological examination of stomach biopsies. Atrophy of the oxyntic mucosa leads to malabsorption of B12, resulting in its deficiency (Castellana et al., 2024).

Pernicious anemia is an autoimmune gastritis that presents with B12 deficiency and consequent megaloblastic anemia due to the lack of intrinsic factor (IF), a glycoprotein that binds cobalamin and enables its absorption in the terminal ileum (Vaqar et al., 2023). The Clinical Practice Update Expert Review recommends evaluating anemia due to B12 deficiency in patients with histology consistent with autoimmune gastritis. Pernicious anemia should be considered a late-stage indicator of B12 deficiency in autoimmune gastritis. Newly diagnosed patients with pernicious anemia should undergo endoscopic imaging and biopsy to confirm corpus-predominant atrophic gastritis, rule out gastric malignancies, and perform risk stratification. Healthcare providers should evaluate iron and B12 deficiencies in individuals with atrophic gastritis, and consider atrophic gastritis in patients with unexplained iron or B12 deficiencies (Shah et al., 2021).

One of the most common side effects of metformin, used in the treatment of type 2 diabetes mellitus, is vitamin B12 deficiency. Although mechanisms such as reduced secretion of intrinsic factor, inhibition of intrinsic factor-B12 complex absorption, or effects on the binding of the intrinsic factor-B12 complex to its receptor have been proposed, the exact mechanism by which metformin causes B12 deficiency is still not fully understood. Prolonged B12 deficiency can lead to anemia, and the resulting neuropathy is often confused with diabetic peripheral neuropathy (Huynh et al., 2024).

In a cross-sectional study involving 1,111 patients with type 2 diabetes who had been taking metformin for at least six months, the prevalence of B12 deficiency was found to be 22.2%. The study also showed a significant association between increasing daily doses of metformin and B12 deficiency (Kim et al., 2019). Proton pump inhibitors (PPIs) have been the subject of numerous studies regarding electrolyte and vitamin imbalances, including those of calcium, magnesium, and B12 (Alblooshi et al., 2024). A case-control study comparing 25,956 patients with B12 deficiency to 184,199 patients without deficiency found that the risk of B12 deficiency increased by 65% in patients who had been on PPI therapy for more than two years compared to those who had not (Bhatnagar et al., 2024).

Laboratory Findings

In vitamin B12 deficiency, laboratory results can show macrocytosis (increased MCV), pancytopenia, or bicytopenia (leukopenia with anemia or thrombocytopenia with anemia). There is often an increase in the red cell distribution width (RDW), and peripheral blood smears can reveal macro-ovalocytes, hypersegmented neutrophils, and decreased reticulocyte count. In cases where both iron deficiency and B12 deficiency coexist, MCV may remain within the normal range. Ineffective erythropoiesis due to B12 deficiency can lead to intramedullary hemolysis, resulting in elevated bilirubin and LDH levels without reticulocytosis. In any case, the assessment should include serum iron, transferrin or transferrin saturation, ferritin, B12 vitamin, and folate levels. Additionally, when B12 deficiency is suspected, it is recommended to evaluate both B12 vitamin levels and methylmalonic acid (MMA) levels (Means & Brodsky, 2024; Pelling et al., 2022).

In B12 deficiency, ineffective erythropoiesis due to intramedullary apoptosis of megaloblastic erythroid precursors can cause hemolysis. This may be accompanied by increased plasma bilirubin and serum lactate dehydrogenase (LDH) levels, as well as elevated iron, ferritin, and soluble transferrin receptor levels (Costanzo et al., 2023).

Diagnosis

A threshold value of 150 pmol/L is typically used to define vitamin B12 deficiency, although some argue that this value is too low to reflect adequate B12 levels. This viewpoint arises from the observation that clinical symptoms of B12 deficiency can occur even when serum B12 levels are above 150 pmol/L. The sensitivity to diagnosing B12 deficiency based on elevated serum homocysteine and MMA levels is 95.9% and 98.4%, respectively. Therefore, it has been suggested to consider a B12 deficiency threshold of 220 to 258 pmol/L (298-350 pg/mL), since high serum homocysteine and MMA levels are indicative of B12 deficiency. Using the 150 pmol/L threshold, the prevalence of B12 deficiency is estimated to be between 5% and 15%. However, when the threshold is set at 258 pmol/L along with elevated serum homocysteine or MMA levels, the prevalence can increase to 40.5%. It is noteworthy that serum MMA and homocysteine levels increase with age and these tests are expensive (Wong, 2015). There are also differing opinions on the cutoff points for diagnosing B12 deficiency and its auxiliary markers such as methylmalonic acid and homocysteine. A review of many studies suggests that the reference values currently used to detect mild, moderate, and severe forms of B12 deficiency need to be re-evaluated (Aparicio-Ugarriza et al., 2015).

Treatment

For most individuals with vitamin B12 deficiency, the initial treatment typically involves intramuscular (IM) injections, despite the significant workload of healthcare professionals. Although case-control and case series studies report that oral administration of B12 is as effective as IM administration, healthcare providers often choose IM injections due to concerns about efficacy. A systematic review evaluating the response of patients with hematological and neurological symptoms due to B12 deficiency showed that high daily doses of oral B12 supplementation (up to 2000 mcg) are as effective as IM administration. Another observation indicated that starting with daily high-dose oral B12 (1000 mcg), followed by weekly and then monthly doses, is also as effective as IM administration. Oral B12 therapy has benefits, such as reducing frequent visits to healthcare providers and minimizing injection-related side effects, yet the data has not been sufficient to change daily practice in most countries (Vidal-Alabal et al., 2005).

In another randomized controlled trial evaluating the questions of oral versus IM administration, uncertainties in treatment protocols were expected to persist due to low levels of evidence, methodological deficiencies, insufficient outcome data, and participant variability. There is a need for studies focusing on B12 metabolism, including participants with poor oral B12 absorption due to factors such as pernicious anemia or gastrointestinal diseases, regardless of ethnicity, age, or region (Wang et al., 2018).

For adults, the recommended dose is 1000 mcg intramuscularly in the cyanocobalamin form weekly, then monthly, or 1000 mcg of hydroxocobalamin every two months. If there are symptoms of anemia and/or neurological symptoms, 1000 mcg can be administered weekly one to three times, or daily, followed by weekly administration. For children, evidence on the optimal dose and regimen for B12 deficiency treatment is limited. A regimen of 100 mcg daily for one week, then 1000 mcg every other day for one week, followed by twice weekly and then weekly doses, has been shown to be safe and effective for symptomatic children. Some experts believe that a parenteral dose of 50 or 100 mcg is sufficient for infants and young children. There is no intravenous administration of B12 (Means & Fairfield, 2024).

The United Kingdom recommends treating B12 deficiency with IM hydroxocobalamin. The standard initial treatment, if there is no neurological involvement, is 1000 µg IM three times a week for two weeks. The British National Formulary (BNF) recommends that patients with neurological symptoms receive 1000 µg IM every other day until recovery. The guidelines developed by the British Committee for Standards in Haematology's (BCSH) General Haematology Task Force, composed of members of the executive committee and UK hematologists, suggest continuing every-other-day treatment for patients with neurological symptoms after three weeks of therapy. For maintenance therapy without neurological deficits, 1000 µg of hydroxocobalamin IM is given every three months. If neurological deficits are present at the time of presentation, 1000 µg IM hydroxocobalamin should be administered every two months. At this stage, no further tests for B12 levels are necessary. For patients with absorption issues such as pernicious anemia who cannot tolerate IM injections but are adherent to treatment, high-dose oral cobalamin may be a reasonable option. However, IM administration remains the recommended route. Hydroxocobalamin is generally well-tolerated, with rare hypersensitivity reactions such as anaphylaxis in individuals sensitive to cobalt or the active ingredients in the medication. A reticulocyte response should be observed within 7-10 days in the treatment of anemia due to B12 deficiency alone when folate and iron levels are normal. If there is no response, the diagnosis should be re-evaluated for other causes of anemia (Devalia et al., 2014).

Conclusion

Vitamin B12 deficiency is one of the most common causes of megaloblastic anemia, and its prevalence increases with age. Besides anemia, B12 deficiency causes neurological, gastrointestinal, and cardiovascular symptoms. Evaluating the significance of the deficiency and its clinical outcomes begins with assessing cobalamin levels, but there is no 'gold standard' test for defining the deficiency. Measuring plasma methylmalonic acid and homocysteine levels can assist in diagnosis, although the availability of these tests is currently limited. It is recommended to do not delay treatment to prevent neurological disorders.

References

Al-Awami, H. M., Raja, A., & Soos, M. P. (2023). Physiology, gastric intrinsic factor. In *StatPearls* [Internet]. Treasure Island (FL): StatPearls Publishing. Retrieved from https://b151d261525caba499e7105a46a9e75760825l3d.vetisonline.com/books/NBK546655/.

Alblooshi, A. J., Baig, M. R., & Anbar, H. S. (2024). Patients' knowledge and pharmacists' practice regarding the long-term side effects of proton pump inhibitors: A cross-sectional study. *Archives of Academic Emergency Medicine, 12*(1), e35. https://doi.org/10.22037/aaem.v12i1.2305.

Andrès, E., Vidal-Alaball, J., Federici, L., Henoun Loukili, N., Zimmer, J., & Kaltenbach, G. (2007). Vitamin B12 deficiency: An important and often neglected problem in the elderly. *European Journal of Internal Medicine, 18*(6), 456-462. https://doi.org/10.1016/j.ejim.2007.02.013.

Aparicio-Ugarriza, R., Gonzalo Palacios, Monika Alder, Marcela González-Gross (2015). A review of the cut-off points for the diagnosis of vitamin B12 deficiency in the general population. *Clinica Chimica Acta, 53*(8), 1149–1159. https://doi.org/10.1515/cclm-2014-0784.

Barcellini, W. (2024). Macrocytosis/Macrocytic anemia. In *UpToDate*. Retrieved from https://www.uptodate.com.

Bhatnagar, M. S., Choudhari, S., Pawar, D., & Sharma, A. (2024). Long-term use of proton-pump inhibitors: Unravelling the safety puzzle. *Cureus, 16*(1), e52773. https://doi.org/10.7759/cureus.52773.

Capelli, I., Cianciolo, G., Gasperoni, L., Zappulo, F., Tondolo, F., Cappuccilli, M., & La Manna, G. (2019). Folic acid and vitamin B12 administration in CKD, why not? *Nutrients, 11*(2), 383. https://doi.org/10.3390/nu11020383.

Castellana, C., Eusebi, L. H., Dajti, E., Iascone, V., Vestito, A., Fusaroli, P., Fuccio, L., D'Errico, A., & Zagari, R. M. (2024). Autoimmune atrophic gastritis: A clinical review. *Cancers, 16*(7), 1310. https://doi.org/10.3390/cancers16071310.

Costanzo, G., Sambugaro, G., Mandis, G., Vassallo, S., & Scuteri, A. (2023). Pancytopenia secondary to vitamin B12 deficiency in older subjects. *Journal of Clinical Medicine, 12*(5), 2059. https://doi.org/10.3390/jcm12052059.

Devalia, V., Hamilton, M. S., & Molloy, A. M. (2014). Guidelines for the diagnosis and treatment of cobalamin and folate disorders. *British Journal of Haematology, 166*(4), 496-513. https://doi.org/10.1111/bjh.12959.

Dror, D. K., & Allen, L. H. (2018). Vitamin B-12 in human milk: A systematic review. *Advances in Nutrition, 9*(Suppl 1), 358S-366S. https://doi.org/10.1093/advances/nmx019.

Elgormus, Y., Okuyan, O., Dumur, S., Sayili, U., & Uzun, H. (2023). The epidemiology of deficiency of vitamin B12 in preschool children in Turkey. *Medicina (Kaunas), 59*(10), 1809. https://doi.org/10.3390/medicina59101809.

Ghazal, F., Zur, M., & Silver, A. (2023). Combined presentation of acute confusion and severe pancytopenia in vitamin B12 deficiency. *Cureus, 15*(6), e40236. https://doi.org/10.7759/cureus.40236.

Green, R. (2017). Vitamin B12 deficiency from the perspective of a practicing hematologist. *Blood, 129*(19), 2603-2611. https://doi.org/10.1182/blood-2016-10-569186.

Guetterman, H. M., Huey, S. L., Knight, R., Fox, A. M., Mehta, S., & Finkelstein, J. L. (2022). Vitamin B-12 and the gastrointestinal microbiome: A systematic review. *Advances in Nutrition, 13*(2), 530-558. https://doi.org/10.1093/advances/nmab123.

Hinton, C. F., Ojodu, J. A., Fernhoff, P. M., Rasmussen, S. A., Scanlon, K. S., & Hannon, W. H. (2010). Maternal and neonatal vitamin B12 deficiency detected through expanded newborn screening--United States, 2003-2007. *Journal of Pediatrics, 157*(1), 162-163. https://doi.org/10.1016/j.jpeds.2010.03.006.

Huynh, D. T., Nguyen, N. T., & Do, M. D. (2024). Vitamin B12 deficiency in diabetic patients treated with metformin: A cross-sectional study. *PLoS One, 19*(4), e0302500. https://doi.org/10.1371/journal.pone.0302500.

Institute of Medicine (US) Standing Committee on the Scientific Evaluation of Dietary Reference Intakes and its Panel on Folate, Other B Vitamins, and Choline. (1998). *Dietary reference intakes for thiamin, riboflavin, niacin, vitamin B6, folate, vitamin B12, pantothenic acid, biotin, and choline*. Washington, DC: National Academies Press. https://doi.org/10.17226/6015.

Kennedy, K. P., Alexander, J. L., & Garakani, A., et al. (2024). Vitamin B12 supplementation in psychiatric practice. *Current Psychiatry Reports*. https://doi.org/10.1007/s11920-024-01505-4.

Kim, J., Ahn, C. W., Fang, S., Lee, H. S., & Park, J. S. (2019). Association between metformin dose and vitamin B12 deficiency in patients with type 2 diabetes. *Medicine (Baltimore), 98*(46), e17918. https://doi.org/10.1097/MD.0000000000017918.

Langan, R. C., & Goodbred, A. J. (2007). Vitamin B12 deficiency: Recognition and management. *American Family Physician, 96*(6), 384-389.

Means, R. T., Jr., & Brodsky, R. A. (2024). Diagnostic approach to anemia in adults. In *UpToDate*. Retrieved from https://www.uptodate.com.

Means, R. T., Jr., & Fairfield, K. M. (2024). Causes and pathophysiology of vitamin B12 and folate deficiencies. In *UpToDate*. Retrieved from https://www.uptodate.com.

Means, R. T., Jr., & Fairfield, K. M. (2024). Clinical manifestations and diagnosis of vitamin B12 and folate deficiency. In *UpToDate*. Retrieved from https://www.uptodate.com.

Means, R. T., Jr., & Fairfield, K. M. (2024). Treatment of vitamin B12 and folate deficiencies. In *UpToDate*. Retrieved from https://www.uptodate.com.

Nexo, E., & Hoffmann-Lücke, E. (2011). Holotranscobalamin, a marker of vitamin B-12 status: Analytical aspects and clinical utility. *American Journal of Clinical Nutrition, 94*(1), 359S-365S. https://doi.org/10.3945/ajcn.111.013458.

O'Leary, F., & Samman, S. (2010). Vitamin B12 in health and disease. *Nutrients, 2*(3), 299–316. https://doi.org/10.3390/nu2030299.

Pelling, M. M., Kimura, S. T., Han, E. J., & Shin, Y. M. (2022). Severe vitamin B12 deficiency presenting as pancytopenia, hemolytic anemia, and paresthesia: Could your B12 be any lower? *Cureus, 14*(9), e29225. https://doi.org/10.7759/cureus.29225.

Pepper, M. R., & Black, M. M. (2011). B12 in fetal development. *Seminars in Cell & Developmental Biology, 22*(6), 619-623. https://doi.org/10.1016/j.semcdb.2011.05.005.

Pereira Fontes, C., & Fonseca, S. (2021). Pseudothrombotic microangiopathy as a rare presentation of cobalamin deficiency. *Cureus, 13*(8), e17184. https://doi.org/10.7759/cureus.17184.

Pfeiffer, C. M., Johnson, C. L., Jain, R. B., Yetley, E. A., Picciano, M. F., Rader, J. I., ... & Osterloh, J. D. (2007). Trends in blood folate and vitamin B-12 concentrations in the United States, 1988–2004. *The American Journal of Clinical Nutrition, 86*(3), 718-727. https://doi.org/10.1093/ajcn/86.3.718.

Pongcharoen, T., Rojroongwasinkul, N., Tuntipopipat, S., et al. (2024). South East Asian Nutrition Surveys II (SEANUTS II) Thailand: Triple burden of malnutrition among Thai children aged 6 months to 12 years. *Public Health Nutrition*, 1-39. https://doi.org/10.1017/S1368980024000053

Reddy, V. S., Jamma Trinath, G. Bhanuprakash Reddy (2019). Implication of homocysteine in protein quality control processes. *Biochimie, 165*, 19-31. https://doi.org/10.1016/j.biochi.2019.06.017.

Robert, C., & Brown, D. L. (2003). Vitamin B12 deficiency. *American Family Physician, 67*(5).

Rotha, W., & Mohamadzadeh, M. (2021). Vitamin B12 and gut-brain homeostasis in the pathophysiology of ischemic stroke. *EBioMedicine, 73*, 103676. https://doi.org/10.1016/j.ebiom.2021.103676.

Shah, S. C., Piazuelo, M. B., Kuipers, E. J., & Li, D. (2021). AGA clinical practice update on the diagnosis and management of atrophic gastritis: Expert review. *Gastroenterology, 161*(4), 1325-1332.e7. https://doi.org/10.1053/j.gastro.2021.06.078.

Vaqar, S., Shackelford, K. B., & Rudolph, S. (2023). Pernicious anemia (Nursing). In *StatPearls* [Internet]. Treasure Island (FL): StatPearls Publishing. Retrieved from https://b151d261525caba499e7105a46a9e757608251 3d.vetisonline.com/books/NBK568700/.

Venkatramanan, S., Armata, I. E., Strupp, B. J., & Finkelstein, J. L. (2016). Vitamin B-12 and cognition in children. *Advances in Nutrition, 7*(5), 879-888. https://doi.org/10.3945/an.115.012021.

Vidal-Alaball, J., Butler, C. C., Cannings-John, R., Goringe, A., Hood, K., McCaddon, A., ... & Papaioannou, A. (2005). Oral vitamin B12 versus intramuscular vitamin B12 for vitamin B12 deficiency. *Cochrane Database of Systematic Reviews, 3*, CD004655. https://doi.org/10.1002/14651858.CD004655.pub2.

Wang, H., Li, L., Qin, L. L., Song, Y., Vidal-Alaball, J., & Liu, T. H. (2018). Oral vitamin B12 versus intramuscular vitamin B12 for vitamin B12 deficiency. *Cochrane Database of Systematic Reviews, 3*(3), CD004655. https://doi.org/10.1002/14651858.CD004655.pub3.

Watanabe, F., & Bito, T. (2018). Vitamin B12 sources and microbial interaction. *Experimental Biology and Medicine, 243*(2), 148–158. https://doi.org/10.1177/1535370217746612.

Wong, C. W. (2015). Vitamin B12 deficiency in the elderly: Is it worth screening? *Hong Kong Medical Journal, 21*(2), 155–164. https://doi.org/10.12809/hkmj144383.

Chapter 18

Lymphoma

Ramazan Oğuz Yüceer*, MD
Department of Medical Pathology, Batman Training and Research Hospital, Batman, Turkey

Abstract

Lymphomas represent malignancies arising from the diverse differentiation stages of B, T, and Natural Killer cells, which collectively constitute the essential components of the immune system. Generally classified as Hodgkin and non-Hodgkin lymphoma. Although its etiology is not fully understood, genetic, infectious, inflammatory, and modifiable factors such as obesity and tobacco use have been implicated. Patients are usually presented with painless lymphadenopathy and B symptoms (unexplained weight loss, high fever, and night sweats). The gold standard in the diagnosis of lymphoma is based on the histopathological examination of the affected lymph nodes. Treatment modalities such as chemotherapy, radiotherapy, immunotherapy, and stem cell transplantation depend on histological features, the clinical staging of the disease, and prognostic features. Short-term effects of chemotherapy and radiotherapy include nausea, vomiting, neuropathy, and alopecia, whereas long-term effects include cardiotoxicity, infertility, and secondary cancers such as lung and breast. After remission or complete cure is achieved, patients should undergo NCCN-recommended age-appropriate screenings and routine surveillance to monitor for complications and relapse. Due to lymphoma being an immunosuppressive condition, patients should be vaccinated for pneumococcal, Haemophilus influenzae type b, influenza, and COVID-19, following the NCCN Prevention and Treatment of Cancer-Related Infections guidelines. Additionally, individuals in contact with the patient should ensure that they have up-to-date vaccinations.

Keywords: lymphoma, family practice, guideline

Introduction

Lymphoma represent a diverse group of neoplasms, constituting approximately 5% of all malignancies. They are the result of the clonal proliferation of B cells, T cells, and natural killer (NK) cell subsets at various maturation stages. The World Health Organization (WHO) classification of lymphoid tumors encompasses more than 90 distinct subtypes. Lymphoma are generally categorized into 10% Hodgkin lymphoma (HL) and 90% non-Hodgkin lymphoma

* Corresponding Author's Email: r.yuceer66@hotmail.com.

In: Common Diseases According to Family Medicine Practice Guidelines
Editors: Esra Meltem Koç and Hilal Aksoy
ISBN: 979-8-89530-302-3

(NHL). HL is further divided into classical and nodular lymphocyte-predominant types, while NHL is classified based on the cell origin as B-cell, T-cell, or NK-cell lymphoma (Mugnaini & Ghosh, 2016; Armitage & Weisenburger, 1998; Alaggio et al., 2022). In this chapter section of our book, we provide information on the diagnosis, follow-up, and treatment modalities for HL and NHL according to current guidelines.

Epidemiology

Lymphoma accounted for 4.6% of all new cancer cases in 2023. HL is a rare neoplasm with an estimated incidence rate in the USA of 2.6 cases per 100,000 people. It exhibits a bimodal distribution, with peaks between the ages of 20-40 and older than 55 (National Institutes of Health, National Cancer Institute, 2023a). Men are more commonly affected than women. NHL is more prevalent in individuals aged 65 to 74 years, with a median age of 67 years. The incidence is higher in men and among Caucasians. Geographical variations may lead to differences in the incidence of individual subtypes. For example, follicular lymphoma is more common in Western countries, while T-cell lymphoma is more prevalent in Asia (National Institutes of Health, National Cancer Institute, 2023b; Chu et al., 2023). Globally, in 2020, HL accounted for 0.4% of newly reported cancer cases and 0.2% of cancer-related deaths. NHL, on the other hand, represented 2.8% of new cancer cases and 2.6% of cancer-related deaths (Sung et al., 2021).

Etiology and Risk Factors

The definitive etiology of lymphoma remains unknown. Lymphoma can be associated with various factors, including genetics, infections, environmental factors, immunodeficiency conditions, and chronic inflammation. A family history of lymphoma has also been associated with an increased risk of its development. Infectious agents, such as Epstein-Barr virus (EBV), human immunodeficiency virus (HIV), Helicobacter pylori, Borrelia burgdorferi, Chlamydia psittaci, Campylobacter jejuni, Human T-cell lymphotropic virus (HTLV), Hepatitis C, and Human herpesvirus 8 (HHV8), as well as immunosuppressive diseases such as rheumatoid arthritis, systemic lupus erythematosus, Sjögren's syndrome, dermatomyositis, and celiac disease, are known to elevate the risk of lymphomagenesis (Chu et al., 2023). Additionally, chronic use of immunosuppressive drugs increases the susceptibility to lymphoma. Tobacco use, obesity, breast implants, and long-term exposure to pesticides have also been associated with an increased risk of developing lymphoma (Sergentanis et al., 2013; U.S. Food & Drug Administration, 2023; Schinasi & Leon, 2014).

Clinical Presentation

Patients typically present with painless superficial lymphadenopathy and B symptoms, including unexplained weight loss, high fever, night sweats, and chronic pruritus. On physical examination, supradiaphragmatic lymph nodes are typically observed in HL (Vaillant & Stang,

2022). Patients with NHL may present with symptoms specific to the affected localization, such as the gastroenteric system (epigastric pain or discomfort, anorexia, weight loss, nausea, and/or vomiting, as well as occult GI bleeding), skin, or central nervous system (headache, lethargy, focal neurologic deficits, seizures, paralysis, spinal cord compression, or lymphomatous meningitis). High-grade lymphoma can lead to oncological emergencies, including superior vena cava syndrome, malignant epidural spinal cord compression, or malignant pericardial effusion. Additionally, patients may experience paraneoplastic syndromes such as dermatomyositis, polymyositis, and cerebellar degeneration (Vaillant & Stang, 2022; Higdon et al., 2018).

Diagnosis

To diagnose lymphoma, a biopsy of the affected area is necessary. A definitive diagnosis is achieved through the examination of morphology, immunohistochemistry, and flow cytometry. While fine needle aspiration and core needle biopsy are components of the evaluation process, they are not sufficient to diagnose lymphoma (Lewis et al., 2020).

Staging

The Modified Ann Arbor staging system is the most widely used system for staging Hodgkin and non-Hodgkin lymphoma. This staging system is based on the localization of lymphadenopathy, the number and size of lymph nodes, and whether there is systemic involvement of extranodal lymph nodes. The Lugano classification system, which was introduced in 2007, modified the staging approach by incorporating the results of positron emission tomography and computed tomography (PET-CT) to determine the stage of lymphoma. The Lugano staging system is classified based on the presence or absence of two symptoms: A (absence of symptoms) and B (unexplained weight loss, high fever, and night sweats) for Hodgkin lymphoma. The previously recommended bone marrow biopsy is now only recommended for diffuse large B-cell lymphoma when a negative PET-CT result is obtained (Cheson et al., 2014).

Prognosis

The International Prognostic Index (IPI) is used to predict the prognosis of non-Hodgkin lymphoma. It is scored considering the following factors: Age> 60, Elevated serum lactate dehydrogenase, Eastern Cooperative Oncology Group (ECOG) performance status≥ 2, Ann Arbor stage III or IV disease, and Extranodal sites>1. The 5-year overall survival is approximately 90% in the low stages of NHL lymphoma and 60% in the advanced stages (Koyuncu et al., 2022).

In Hodgkin lymphoma, the International Prognostic Score (IPS) is used for prognosis. The IPS takes into account the following factors: Age> 45, Male sex, Serum albumin concentration <4.0 g per dL, Hemoglobin concentration <10.5 g per dL, Ann Arbor stage IV disease,

Leukocytosis ≥ 15,000 µL, Lymphopenia < 600 lymphocytes µL, < 8% of total white blood cell count (Townsend & Linch, 2012).

In low-grade non-Hodgkin lymphoma, overall survival is generally high, but for those with high-grade lymphoma, it is considerably lower.

Treatment

The treatment of lymphoma depends on histological features, the clinical staging of the disease, and prognostic factors. Treatment options include chemotherapy, radiotherapy, immunotherapy, stem cell transplantation, and surgical intervention. The goal of lymphoma treatment is to cure the disease while managing short- and long-term complications. The National Comprehensive Cancer Network (NCCN) recommends that patients over the age of 60 should avoid certain chemotherapeutic agents due to their side effects.

The initial treatment for Hodgkin lymphoma varies based on three subgroups of patients. Early-stage patients (stage I to IIA) are treated with ABVD (doxorubicin, bleomycin, vinblastine, and dacarbazine) followed by limited-involved field radiation therapy (IFRT). For patients in advanced stages (stage IIB-IV), treatment options can include Stanford V (doxorubicin, vinblastine, mechlorethamine, etoposide, vincristine, bleomycin, and prednisone) and escalated-BEACOPP (bleomycin, etoposide, doxorubicin, cyclophosphamide, vincristine, procarbazine, and prednisone). Additionally, autologous stem cell transplantation and allogeneic stem cell transplantation can be considered in suitable cases. In patients for whom autologous stem cell transplantation is not successful, treatments such as brentuximab vedotin, PD-1 blockade, and non-myeloablative allogeneic transplantation can be applied (National Comprehensive Cancer Network, 2023a).

In the treatment of non-Hodgkin lymphoma, a combination of chemoimmunotherapy and rituximab is commonly used, often in conjunction with CHOP (cyclophosphamide, doxorubicin, vincristine, and prednisone) and rituximab (R-CHOP). For advanced-stage patients, bone marrow transplantation or Chimeric Antigen Receptor T (CAR-T) cell therapy can be suitable (National Comprehensive Cancer Network, 2023b; National Comprehensive Cancer Network, 2023c).

Short-term complications of chemotherapy and radiotherapy may include nausea, vomiting, headache, alopecia, anemia, leukopenia, fatigue, and dermatitis. Long-term complications can include heart and lung toxicity, hypothyroidism, infertility, sterility, and the risk of secondary cancers such as breast or lung cancer (National Comprehensive Cancer Network, 2023a; National Comprehensive Cancer Network, 2023b; National Comprehensive Cancer Network, 2023c).

Surveillance

Patients who achieve remission after treatment should undergo age-appropriate screenings in addition to routine follow-up to monitor complications and relapse. Complications of lymphoma treatment include secondary malignancies, cardiac disease, infertility, and endocrine, neurological, and psychiatric dysfunction.

The extent and frequency of lymphoma follow-up vary depending on the histological subtype. Patients should be followed by a hematologist every three to six months for the first two years, every six to twelve months through year three, and annually thereafter. If there is no recurrence after five years, the patient can see a primary care physician. In the presence of symptoms, imaging is recommended for patients. NCCN recommends chest radiography or chest CT every six to twelve months for the first two years after treatment and then annually for three to five years after treatment. Tumor-specific DNA sequences, which are not used routinely but are becoming increasingly common, can serve as markers.

Pneumococcal vaccination should be administered at baseline and 5 years after a lymphoma diagnosis is made. Patients receiving anti-B cell antibodies should not receive an annual influenza vaccination. The administration of live vaccines (such as Zoster, etc.) during chemotherapy is contraindicated. The recommended inactivated or live vaccines can be administered three months after chemotherapy or six months after anti-B cell antibody therapy. Three doses of the Haemophilus influenzae type b vaccine should be administered starting six to twelve months after hematopoietic stem cell transplantation. Contacts from the household should receive the recommended vaccinations. Everyone should receive influenza vaccinations, including COVID-19 (National Comprehensive Cancer Network, 2023d; National Comprehensive Cancer Network, 2023e; National Comprehensive Cancer Network, 2023f). The surveillance for lymphoma for up to five years is summarized in Table 1.

Table 1. Lymphoma Surveillance for up to five years

Physical exam: Patients should undergo physical examinations every three to six months during the first one to two years, followed by examinations every six to 12 months until the fifth year. *Imaging screening:* During the first two years after treatment, you may have a computed tomography (CT) scan of your neck, chest, abdomen, and pelvis every six months or the presence of symptoms or when the doctor suspects. *Laboratory screening:* Complete blood count, chemistry profile, fasting blood glucose, TSH level, and lipid panel (total cholesterol level, triglyceride level, the levels of HDL and LDL cholesterol) annually. Cytomegalovirus (CMV) antibody testing. *Counseling:* Survivorship counseling, including long-term treatment effects, prevention of new cancers, and healthy living. Annual depression screening. Neurocognitive impairment screening *Cardiac screening:* Annual blood pressure screening is especially recommended, particularly for patients undergoing doxorubicin treatment. *Cancer screening:* Annual breast magnetic resonance imaging (MRI) or mammography should be conducted eight to ten years after breast or armpit radiotherapy treatment, or at age 40 for individuals who received radiation during their treatment, especially between the ages of ten and 30. Screening for cervical, colorectal, endometrıal, lung, skin, and prostate cancer *Immunizations:* Live vaccines should not be administered during chemotherapy. They should be given at least three months after chemotherapy has been completed. Pneumococcal vaccination is particularly important for patients with splenectomy and should be administered at least eight weeks after the procedure, with a follow-up dose at least five years later. For Haemophilus influenzae type b, patients who have undergone hematopoietic stem cell transplantation should receive three doses. Annual influenza and COVID-19 vaccines should be administered, and live vaccines can be resumed at least three months after the completion of chemotherapy.

(National Comphrensive Network, 2023).

Conclusion

Lymphoma account for approximately 5% of all malignancies and encompass many subtypes. The diagnosis and follow-up of lymphoma require multidisciplinary management, involving physical examination, laboratory tests, and imaging methods. Post-treatment screening and vaccination programs for patients are particularly important, especially in family medicine.

References

Alaggio, R., Amador, C., Anagnostopoulos, I., Attygalle, A. D., Araujo, I. B. D. O., Berti, E., ... & Xiao, W. (2022). The 5th edition of the World Health Organization classification of haematolymphoid tumours: Lymphoid neoplasms. *Leukemia, 36*(7), 1720-1748. https://doi.org/10.1038/s41375-022-01620-2.

Armitage, J. O., & Weisenburger, D. D. (1998). New approach to classifying non-Hodgkin's lymphomas: Clinical features of the major histologic subtypes. *Journal of Clinical Oncology, 16*(8), 2780-2795. https://doi.org/10.1200/JCO.1998.16.8.2780.

Cheson, B. D., Fisher, R. I., Barrington, S. F., Cavalli, F., Schwartz, L. H., Zucca, E., & Lister, T. A. (2014). Recommendations for initial evaluation, staging, and response assessment of Hodgkin and non-Hodgkin lymphoma: The Lugano classification. *Journal of Clinical Oncology, 32*(27), 3059-3068. https://doi.org/10.1200/JCO.2013.54.8800.

Chu, Y., Liu, Y., Fang, X., Jiang, Y., Ding, M., Ge, X., ... & Wang, X. (2023). The epidemiological patterns of non-Hodgkin lymphoma: Global estimates of disease burden, risk factors, and temporal trends. *Frontiers in Oncology, 13*, 1059914. https://doi.org/10.3389/fonc.2023.1059914.

Higdon, M. L., Atkinson, C. J., & Lawrence, K. V. (2018). Oncologic emergencies: Recognition and initial management. *American Family Physician, 97*(11), 741-748.

Koyuncu, M. B., Guler, E., Koseci, T., Ucar, M. A., Tombak, A., Akdeniz, A., ... & Cavusoglu, C. (2022). Integration of low muscle mass into the IPS system and its prognostic significance in patients with Hodgkin's lymphoma. *Biomarkers in Medicine, 16*(2), 57-67. https://doi.org/10.2217/bmm-2021-0696.

Lewis, W. D., Lilly, S., & Jones, K. L. (2020). Lymphoma: Diagnosis and treatment. *American Family Physician, 101*(1), 34-41.

Mugnaini, E. N., & Ghosh, N. (2016). Lymphoma. *Primary Care: Clinics in Office Practice, 43*(4), 661-675. https://doi.org/10.1016/j.pop.2016.07.012.

National Comprehensive Cancer Network. (2023a). *NCCN guidelines & clinical resources: Hodgkin lymphomas guideline.* Retrieved October 14, 2023, from https://www.nccn.org/professionals/physician_gls/pdf/hodgkins.pdf.

National Comprehensive Cancer Network. (2023b). *NCCN guidelines & clinical resources: B-Cell lymphomas guideline.* Retrieved October 14, 2023, from https://www.nccn.org/professionals/physician_gls/pdf/b-cell.pdf.

National Comprehensive Cancer Network. (2023c). *NCCN guidelines & clinical resources: T-Cell lymphomas guideline.* Retrieved October 14, 2023, from https://www.nccn.org/professionals/physician_gls/pdf/t-cell.pdf.

National Comprehensive Cancer Network. (2023d). *NCCN guidelines & clinical resources: Prevention and treatment of cancer-related infections.* Retrieved October 14, 2023, from https://www.nccn.org/professionals/physician_gls/pdf/infections.pdf.

National Comprehensive Cancer Network. (2023e). *NCCN guidelines & clinical resources: Hodgkin lymphomas patient guide.* Retrieved October 15, 2023, from https://www.nccn.org/patients/guidelines/content/PDF/hodgkin-patient.pdf.

National Comprehensive Cancer Network. (2023f). *NCCN guidelines & clinical resources: Non-Hodgkin lymphomas patient guide.* Retrieved October 16, 2023, from https://www.nccn.org/patients/guidelines/content/PDF/nhl-diffuse-patient.pdf.

National Institutes of Health, National Cancer Institute. (2023a). *Surveillance, epidemiology, and end results program cancer stat facts: Hodgkin lymphoma.* Retrieved October 12, 2023, from https://seer.cancer.gov/statfacts/html/hodg.html.

National Institutes of Health, National Cancer Institute. (2023b). *Surveillance, epidemiology, and end results program cancer stat facts: Non-Hodgkin lymphoma.* Retrieved October 12, 2023, from https://seer.cancer.gov/statfacts/html/nhl.html.

Schinasi, L., & Leon, M. E. (2014). Non-Hodgkin lymphoma and occupational exposure to agricultural pesticide chemical groups and active ingredients: A systematic review and meta-analysis. *International Journal of Environmental Research and Public Health, 11*(4), 4449-4527. https://doi.org/10.3390/ijerph110404449.

Sergentanis, T. N., Kanavidis, P., Michelakos, T., & Petridou, E. T. (2013). Cigarette smoking and risk of lymphoma in adults. *European Journal of Cancer Prevention, 22*(2), 131-150. https://doi.org/10.1097/CEJ.0b013e328355ed08.

Sung, H., Ferlay, J., Siegel, R. L., Laversanne, M., Soerjomataram, I., Jemal, A., & Bray, F. (2021). Global cancer statistics 2020: GLOBOCAN estimates of incidence and mortality worldwide for 36 cancers in 185 countries. *CA: A Cancer Journal for Clinicians, 71*(3), 209-249. https://doi.org/10.3322/caac.21660.

Townsend, W., & Linch, D. (2012). Hodgkin's lymphoma in adults. *The Lancet, 380*(9844), 836-847.

U.S. Food & Drug Administration. (2023). *Questions and answers about breast implant-associated anaplastic large cell lymphoma.* Retrieved October 17, 2023, from https://www.fda.gov/medical-devices/breast-implants/medical-device-reports-breast-implant-associated-anaplastic-large-cell-lymphoma.

Vaillant, A. A. J., & Stang, C. M. (2022). Lymphoproliferative disorders. In *StatPearls* [Internet]. StatPearls Publishing.

Part 6

Ophthalmological Diseases

Chapter 19

Conjunctivitis

Pinar Fakirullahoğlu*, PhD
Department of Family Medicine, Kayakyolu Family Health Center, Erzurum, Turkey

Abstract

Most of the patients who go to primary care with eye-related complaints have conjunctivitis. Defined as inflammation of the conjunctiva layer of eye conjunctivitis, it is classified as infectious (viral, bacterial) and non-infectious (allergic, chemical, or nonspecific) conjunctivitis. Among these, viral and bacterial conjunctivitis usually have a good course and resolve spontaneously, and the rate of complications is low. The clinical presentation of conjunctivitis is often eye redness, pain, discharge, itching, vision changes, and sensitivity to light. Treatment should be planned according to the factor. Another important point in primary care treatment is to distinguish conditions that require referral of the patient to an ophthalmologist.

Keywords: primary care, conjunctivitis, inflammation

Introduction

Conjunctivitis is inflammation of the conjunctiva. Although conjunctivitis can be caused by many causes, it can be grouped into four basic groups: bacteria, viruses, allergens, and irritants (Visscher et al., 2009). According to Western sources, the most common reason for eye-related applications in primary care is acute eye infection, with a rate of 1-2% (Rietveld et al., 2007; Visscher et al., 2009).

When evaluating a patient with conjunctivitis, the environment in which the patient lives must be considered due to factors such as the age of the patient and the presence of any associated systemic disease presence of a previous eye disease, duration of symptoms, whether the disease affects both eyes, if there is discharge, its amount and type, history of contact lens use, whether there is itching, pain, and sensitivity to light, whether there is lymphadenopathy around the ear, history of trauma, and environment (Cronau et al., 2010; Galor & Jeng, 2008; Sethuraman & Kamat, 2009).

* Corresponding Author's Email: fakirullahoglupinar@gmail.com.

In: Common Diseases According to Family Medicine Practice Guidelines
Editors: Esra Meltem Koç and Hilal Aksoy
ISBN: 979-8-89530-302-3

When the etiological agents in conjunctivitis are examined, differences are observed between childhood and adulthood (Weiss et al., 1993). While 78% of childhood conjunctivitis is bacterial, 20% is adenoviral. Among bacterial agents, Hemophilus influenza ranks first with a rate of 58%; Streptococcus pneumonia, Staphylococcus aureus, and Moraxella catarrhalis are among the most common agents (Patel et al., 2007).

Viral conjunctivitis is more common in adults. The most common etiological agents in adult bacterial conjunctivitis are Staphylococcus aureus and Hemophilus influenza (Cronau et al., 2010; Patel et al., 2007). Bacterial conjunctivitis can be associated with upper respiratory tract infections, such as otitis media, and can sometimes affect one eye or sometimes both eyes. Although bacterial conjunctivitis can heal spontaneously, treatment directed at the agent shortens the disease process, provides less labor loss, and results in greater patient satisfaction.

Viral Conjunctivitis

The most common cause of viral conjunctivitis is Adenoviruses. Adenoviruses are involved in the etiology of conjunctivitis with many serological subtypes (Roba et al., 1995). Conjunctivitis usually starts unilaterally and continues in both eyes. Early symptoms of upper respiratory tract infection, such as fever and preauricular lymphadenopathy, can be observed. Viral conjunctivitis is highly contagious and can spread rapidly through the patient, the patient's secretions, or objects contaminated by the patient (Azar et al., 1996).

In viral conjunctivitis, the discharge is typically watery and mucous, and patients may experience a lump when they wake up in the morning. However, burning eyes, conjunctival hyperemia, and sandy eyes are common symptoms.

Viral conjunctivitis does not require specific treatment, as it can heal on its own. Similar to the course of a cold, there may be an exacerbation on the third or fifth day, and the symptoms usually regress in the following second week.

Adenoviral Conjunctivitis

Pharyngoconjunctival Fever

Adenovirus type 3 is responsible, and it progresses with upper respiratory tract findings such as unilateral or bilateral conjunctivitis, high fever, pharyngitis, preauricular lymphadenopathy. It is highly contagious.

Epidemic Keratoconjunctivitis

Adenovirus types 8,19,37 are responsible (Jernigan et al., 1993). It has a fulminant course. Because both the cornea and the conjunctival epithelium can be affected, keratitis resulting in vision loss may occur. It should be evaluated by an eye specialist.

Herpes Simplex Conjunctivitis

Usually, the involvement is unilateral. There are dendritic keratitis and conjunctiva involvement with typical herpetic vesicular skin lesions (Green & Pavan-Langston, 2006). Steroids are contraindicated because active keratitis worsens with steroid treatment.

Herpes Zoster Conjunctivitis

This occurs as a result of the involvement of the ophthalmic branch of the trigeminal nerve (V1). It is seen in adults and the involvement is unilateral.

Varicella Zoster Conjunctivitis

This occurs as a result of chickenpox infection affecting one or both eyes. It appears as a papular lesion in the conjunctiva and limbus. It regresses along with the symptoms of chickenpox.

Acute Hemorrhagic Conjunctivitis

Clinically, there is a significant subconjunctival hemorrhage, and it develops due to Enterovirus and Coxsackie viruses.

Bacterial Conjunctivis

The most commonly accused factors of bacterial conjunctivitis are Staphylococcus aureus, Streptococcus pneumoniae, Haemophilus influenzae, and Moraxella catarrhalis. While S. aureus infection is more common in adults, other factors are more common in children (Friedlaender, 1995). Bacterial conjunctivitis is highly contagious. As with viral conjunctivitis, the disease can easily be transmitted through the secretions of the patient or objects contaminated by the patient. Outbreaks due to S.pneumoniae have been reported (Martin et al., 2003).

In bacterial conjunctivitis, one or both eyes can be affected. Clinically, there is bursing and conjunctival hyperemia in the mornings, similar to viral conjunctivitis. However, unlike viral conjunctivitis, the discharge is purulent and continuous. The discharge is yellow, green, or white in color and has a darker consistency.

Hyperacute Bacterial Conjunctivitis

This is an infection caused by Neisseria Gonorrea that has a rapid and severe course and requires immediate referral to an ophthalmologist (Ullman et al., 1987). It occurs as a result of contact between contaminated hands and eyes in sexually active adults and is often accompanied by urethritis. It can also be transmitted from mother to baby during birth. Abundant purulent discharge that develops in the patient within 12 hours after infection is typical (Wan et al., 1986). Pain, hyperemia, preauricular lymphadenopathy, conjunctival edema, and vision loss can develop. Gram staining and Polymerase chain reaction (PCR) are used to see gram-negative diplococci in diagnosis (McAnena et al., 2015).

Acute Bacterial Conjunctivitis

This is the most common type of bacterial conjunctivitis. The most common agents are S. Aureus, S.epidermidis and pneumococci among Gr(+) species, while H.influenza and Moraxella lacunata are among Gr(-) species (Chung & Cohen, 2000; Mannis et al., 1990). It usually starts with burning, redness, and stinging in one eye and affects the other eye after a few days.

The most common cause of neonatal conjunctivitis is bacterial conjunctivitis. In studies, the most common agent was found to be S.aureus (Mani & Vidya, 1997; Mannis et al., 1990; Verma et al., 1994).

Chronic Bacterial Conjunctivitis

The most common causes of chronic bacterial conjunctivitis are S.aureus and Moraxella lacunata bacteria. Complications may develop in staphylococcal conjunctivitis and keratoconjunctivitis and keratitis can also be seen (Mannis et al., 1990). In addition to the use of appropriate topical antibiotics in the treatment, maintenance of the eyelids is also important. Cases that do not respond to treatment should be referred to an eye specialist.

Chlamidia Conjunctivitis

There are two forms: Trachoma and adult inclusion conjunctivitis.

Trachoma

This infection, which is endemic in underdeveloped countries, is a chronic table of keratoconjunctivitis caused by recurrent infection of Chlamydia trachomatis. While it can appear asymptomatic active trachoma that is often seen in children, it can present with redness, sensitivity to light, and mucopurulent discharge. This issue will be discussed in a separate section.

Adult Inclusion Conjunctivitis

This form, seen in developed countries, is sexually transmitted and causes chronic follicular conjunctivitis. It can be found asymptomatically in the genital system and can be transmitted through the birth canal in newborns. It usually presents with unilateral mucopurulent discharge, tenderness, and redness. On days 5 to 12 in newborns, bilateral discharge is seen (Lietman et al., 1998). Diagnosis is made by culture of conjunctival samples with Giemza or direct fluorescent antibody staining.

Allergic Conjunctivitis

This is a condition of conjunctivitis characterized by complaints of itching in both eyes, usually in patients with a history of atopy (asthma, allergic rhinitis, etc.). It is more common in developed countries. It is the most common cause of chronic conjunctivitis, and rates are reported to be 15-25% in the American population and up to 50% in Europe (Burbach et al., 2009; Rosario & Bielory, 2011; Utz & Kaufman, 2014). Itching is the most typical symptom and in studies conducted, it has been seen in 88% of patients (Dykewicz & Fineman, 1998; Granet, 2008). However, itching can cause other symptoms to worsen. Symptoms are often accompanied by rhinitis (Cronau et al., 2010; Granet, 2008). Clinically, similar to viral conjunctivitis, bilateral redness, watery or stringy discharge, foreign body sensation, and itching are present. A history of atopy and recent contact help differentiate viral and allergic conjunctivitis.

Mast cells are mainly responsible for the clinical appearance of allergic conjunctivitis. Mast substances such as histamine, chymase, and heparin are released from the cells. Therefore, topical mast cell stabilizers, and antihistamines can be used in the treatment of allergic conjunctivitis.

Seasonal and Perennial Allergic Conjunctivitis

This is the most common type of allergic conjunctivitis, with a rate of 90-95%. While it affects 50% of the population in Europe, it has a rate of 15-25% in America (Burbach et al., 2009; Rosario & Bielory, 2011; Utz & Kaufman, 2014). It is an example of a type 1 hypersensitivity reaction. In seasonal allergic conjunctivitis, symptoms vary depending on exposure to the allergen. For example, those due to tree pollen are seen in spring, whereas those due to environmental molds can show symptoms from August to October (Leonardi, 2013). In perennial allergic conjunctivitis, there are allergens that cause symptoms throughout the year, such as house dust and the animal epithelium. Chronic inflammation can sometimes develop as a result of year-round allergen exposure (Moloney & McCluskey, 2007).

Giant Papillary Conjunctivitis

This is a condition that usually develops as a result of contact lens use. It is a hypersensitivity reaction. It presents with symptoms such as redness, itching, foreign body sensation in the eye, and increased complaints with lens use. It is characterized by giant papillae in the tarsal conjunctiva of the upper eyelid. Sometimes ptosis can be observed as a result of inflammation of the eyelid (Ackerman et al., 2016; Leonardi, 2013). Although topical steroids are used in the treatment, long-term use should be avoided (Srinivasan et al., 1979; Sugar & Meyer, 1981). Additionally, the patient should take a break from contact lens use and be informed about lens cleaning.

Vernal Conjunctivitis

This is often seen in regions where the equatorial climate prevails. It is proportionally more common in men and, when looked at by age, it is more common in children and adolescents. 50% of patients have a history of atopy (De Smedt et al., 2013; Gomes, 2014). A cobblestone appearance on the upper eyelid is typical, and ptosis, keratoconus, and vision loss can be observed.

Atopic Keratoconjunctivitis

Atopic conjunctivitis, like other types of allergic conjunctivitis, is a hypersensitivity reaction. It is often seen between the ages of 30-50. A history of atopy is also present in this type of patient. Inflammation can be seen in the conjunctiva and cornea. It can lead to complications such as keratoconus, vision loss, and cataracts (Moloney & McCluskey, 2007; Utz & Kaufman, 2014).

Diagnosis

The diagnosis of conjunctivitis is a diagnosis of exclusion based on a history and physical examination. Cultures often do not need to be taken at the first examination. Culture, direct antibody, or PCR tests are generally used in conjunctivitis outbreaks to detect N. Gonorrhoeae, the causative agent of hyperacute bacterial conjunctivitis, and in atypical or chronic cases that do not respond to treatment (Rapuano, 2008).

On clinical examination, bacterial conjunctivitis is usually not accompanied by systemic symptoms, whereas viral conjunctivitis is usually accompanied by signs of upper respiratory tract infection, such as fever and preauricular lymphadenopathy. Adenoviral conjunctivitis can be accompanied by pharyngitis in children (Yen et al., 2009). Allergic conjunctivitis is accompanied by localized symptoms such as sneezing and nasal congestion (Hara, 1996).

While itching is the primary complaint in allergic conjunctivitis, it can also be seen in viral and bacterial conjunctivitis. Furthermore, stinging and burning in the eyes may often accompany viral and allergic conjunctivitis (Ackerman et al., 2016; O'Brien, 2013).

Discharge and burring are especially important in bacterial conjunctivitis. In bacterial conjunctivitis, there is a yellow, green, white, and purulent discharge. After the discharge is wiped off, it recurs on the edges of the lid and corners of the eyes. While the discharge is watery and mucoid in viral conjunctivitis, it is watery in allergic conjunctivitis (Hara, 1996; Morrow & Abbott, 1998).

Conjunctival hyperemia and edema can be seen in all three types of conjunctivitis. In conjunctivitis, hyperemia does not extend to the limbus. If conjunctival hyperemia extends to the limbus, keratitis, or uveitis comes to mind. Evaluation of the bulbar and tarsal conjunctiva is important in distinguishing allergic conjunctivitis. Especially in allergic conjunctivitis, there is a bumpy appearance in the tarsal conjunctiva (Moloney & McCluskey, 2007). Additionally, allergic conjunctivitis is frequently seen together with diseases such as allergic rhinitis and asthma (Granet, 2008).

In the case of contact lens use, the diagnosis of conjunctivitis should be made with care. For those who wear soft contact lenses, especially long-term lenses, the risk of pseudomonal keratitis is high (Cheng et al., 1999; Tabbara et al., 2000). Although keratitis is present here, it is characterized by redness and discharge similar to clinical conjunctivitis. Since ulcerative keratitis can lead to corneal perforation within 24 hours, keratitis should be excluded before conjunctivitis is suspected and treated. In keratitis, the patient cannot open their eyes or keep them open on their own, and there is dullness in the cornea. Another issue as important as the diagnosis of conjunctivitis is which patients should be referred to. The light reflex is not affected in conjunctivitis. If it is affected, diseases such as uveitis and optic neuropathy should be considered. Significant redness in the limbus, severe foreign body sensation that prevents the patient from keeping his eyes open, photophobia, decreased visual acuity, corneal opacity, fixed pupils, severe headache with nausea, hyperacute bacterial conjunctivitis, or suspicion of epidemic keratoconjunctivitis (EKC) are among the conditions that require referral (Khaw et al., 2004; Kunimoto et al., 2004; Limberg, 1991; Saw et al., 2003).

Treatment

Since conjunctivitis is highly contagious, the first thing we do in primary care for patients with conjunctivitis is general recommendations to prevent transmission. Personal belongings of infected people, such as towels, bed linens, and handkerchiefs, should never be used. The second most important issue is the inappropriate use of corticosteroids in cases of conjunctivitis. The use of ophthalmic corticosteroids in the treatment of acute conjunctivitis is not recommended (Wilkins et al., 2011). While inappropriate corticosteroid use can cause threatening conditions for seeing, chronic corticosteroid use may cause cataracts and glaucoma (Renfro & Snow, 1992). Bacterial conjunctivitis usually heals on its own. However, there are publications stating that topical antibiotic therapy applied in the first week after the onset of symptoms has some benefits, such as rapid healing and shortening the duration of the disease (Azari & Barney, 2013; Chen et al., 2023). Acute conjunctivitis in contact lens wearers, inclusion conjunctivitis, or hyperacute bacterial conjunctivitis in adults are cases where antibiotic treatment is required. Among the most frequently preferred agents in antibiotic therapy are erythromycin ophthalmic ointment or trimethoprim-polymyxin B drops because they are widely available, non-toxic, and inexpensive. Furthermore, the combination of bacitracin or bacitracin-polymyxin B is also used. While the drop form is more preferred in adults; Ointment forms are preferred in children and patients with poor compliance due to their ease of use. Azithromycin is used from the age of one in the United States, but it should not be forgotten that it is expensive and opens the door to the formation of resistant infections (Opitz & Harthan, 2012). Aminoglycosides should be used with caution because they are toxic to the corneal epithelium and may cause reactive keratoconjunctivitis. Although chloramphenicol drops are a widely used and low-cost treatment option in the treatment of bacterial conjunctivitis; Due to their topical use, and serious side effects such as bone marrow hypoplasia and aplastic anemia, it is not used in the United States for the treatment of ocular infections (Fraunfelder & Fraunfelder, 2013). Fluoroquinolones are antibiotics that should be used with caution. It is not as effective as aminoglycosides and should not be used during the neonatal period. However, fluoroquinolones are used in conjunctivitis seen in contact lens wearers due to the high incidence of Pseudomonas infection. Systemic antibiotic therapy (doxycycline, tetracycline, erythromycin, or azithromycin) should be administered in inclusion of conjunctivitis in adults. In hyperacute bacterial conjunctivitis due to Neisseria, systemic and topical treatment must be applied together. In hyperacute bacterial conjunctivitis, a single dose of ceftriaxone should be administered intramuscularly, and topical fluoroquinolones should be used. Additionally, the patient's partner must also receive treatment (Guidelines for Treatment of Sexually Transmitted Diseases, 1998).

Topical or systemic antiviral treatments have no place in the treatment of viral conjunctivitis. Cold compresses and topical decongestants can be used to relieve the patient. In the presence of secondary bacterial infection, topical antibiotic drops can be added to the treatment. Topical antiviral treatment can be used in herpes simplex keratoconjunctivitis (Shiuey et al., 2000). There are many treatment options available for the treatment of allergic conjunctivitis, such as topical mast cell stabilizers, topical antihistamines (naphazoline-pheniramine, ketotifen, olopatadine), topical corticosteroids, immunosuppressants (cyclosporine A) (Bielory & Friedlaender, 2008; Ciprandi et al., 1996). Caution should be exercised in terms of corneal side effects in the use of topical NSAID (non-steroidal anti-inflammatory) Ketorolac drops (the only FDA-approved) which are used to relieve itching in viral or allergic conjunctivitis (Ballas et al., 1993; Flach, 1992). Patients with acute bacterial conjunctivitis usually respond to treatment by showing a decrease in symptoms within one or two days, and patients with viral or allergic conjunctivitis usually show a decrease in symptoms within two weeks. Patients who do not respond should be referred to an ophthalmologist.

Conclusion

Conjunctivitis is a frequently encountered clinical condition in primary health care. Although conjunctivitis usually has a benign course and can resolve spontaneously, serious diseases can be differentiated with appropriate diagnosis, treatment, and recommendations, so the patient can be protected from serious complications such as permanent vision loss. Another important point here is that the patient's misinformation that his condition will not improve if he does not use antibiotics should be corrected by providing appropriate education to the patient. Another important point is that topical steroids should be used under the supervision of an ophthalmologist because it will be more effective and reliable. Although there are different recommendations for the use of contact lenses, warnings about hand hygiene storage conditions, and the duration of lenses should be taken into account.

References

Ackerman, S., Smith, L. M., & Gomes, P. J. (2016). Ocular itch associated with allergic conjunctivitis: latest evidence and clinical management. *Therapeutic advances in chronic disease*, *7*(1), 52-67.

Azar, M. J., Dhaliwal, D., Bower, K. S., Kowalski, R. P., & Gordon, Y. (1996). Possible consequences of shaking hands with your patients with epidemic keratoconjunctivitis. *American journal of ophthalmology*, *121*(6), 711-712.

Azari, A. A., & Barney, N. P. (2013). Conjunctivitis: a systematic review of diagnosis and treatment. *Jama*, *310*(16), 1721-1730.

Ballas, Z., Blumenthal, M., Tinkelman, D. G., Kriz, R., & Rupp, G. (1993). Clinical evaluation of ketorolac tromethamine 0.5% ophthalmic solution for the treatment of seasonal allergic conjunctivitis. *Survey of ophthalmology*, *38*, 141-148.

Bielory, L., & Friedlaender, M. H. (2008). Allergic conjunctivitis. *Immunology and allergy clinics of North America*, *28*(1), 43-58.

Burbach, G. J., Heinzerling, L., Röhnelt, C., Bergmann, K., Behrendt, H., & Zuberbier, T. (2009). Ragweed sensitization in Europe-GA (2) LEN study suggests increasing prevalence. *Allergy*, *64*(4), 664-665.

Chen, Y.-Y., Liu, S.-H., Nurmatov, U., van Schayck, O. C., & Kuo, I. C. (2023). Antibiotics versus placebo for acute bacterial conjunctivitis. *Cochrane Database of Systematic Reviews*(3).

Cheng, K. H., Leung, S. L., Hoekman, H. W., Beekhuis, W. H., Mulder, P. G., Geerards, A. J., & Kijlstra, A. (1999). Incidence of contact-lens-associated microbial keratitis and its related morbidity. *The Lancet*, *354*(9174), 181-185.

Chung, C. W., & Cohen, E. J. (2000). Clinical Evidence: Eye disorders: bacterial conjunctivitis. *Western Journal of Medicine*, *173*(3), 202.

Ciprandi, G., Buscaglia, S., & Canonica, G. W. (1996). Management of allergic conjunctivitis. *Clinical Immunotherapeutics*, *5*, 374-391.

Cronau, H., Kankanala, R. R., & Mauger, T. (2010). Diagnosis and management of red eye in primary care. *American family physician*, *81*(2), 137-144.

De Smedt, S., Wildner, G., & Kestelyn, P. (2013). Vernal keratoconjunctivitis: an update. *British Journal of Ophthalmology*, *97*(1), 9-14.

Dykewicz, M. S., & Fineman, S. (1998). Executive summary of joint task force practice parameters on diagnosis and management of rhinitis. *Annals of Allergy, Asthma & Immunology*, *81*(5), 463-468.

Flach, A. J. (1992). Cyclo-oxygenase inhibitors in ophthalmology. *Survey of ophthalmology*, *36*(4), 259-284.

Fraunfelder, F. W., & Fraunfelder, F. T. (2013). Restricting topical ocular chloramphenicol eye drop use in the United States. Did we overreact? *American journal of ophthalmology*, *156*(3), 420-422.

Friedlaender, M. H. (1995). A review of the causes and treatment of bacterial and allergic conjunctivitis. *Clinical therapeutics*, *17*(5), 800-810.

Galor, A., & Jeng, B. H. (2008). Red eye for the internist: when to treat, when to refer. *Cleveland Clinic journal of medicine*, *75*(2), 137-144.

Gomes, P. J. (2014). Trends in prevalence and treatment of ocular allergy. *Current opinion in allergy and clinical immunology*, *14*(5), 451-456.

Granet, D. (2008). Allergic rhinoconjunctivitis and differential diagnosis of the red eye. Allergy and Asthma Proceedings,

Green, L. K., & Pavan-Langston, D. (2006). Herpes simplex ocular inflammatory disease. *International ophthalmology clinics*, *46*(2), 27-37.

Guidelines for Treatment of Sexually Transmitted Diseases. (1998). (Morbidity and Mortality Weekly Report, Issue.

Hara, J. H. (1996). The red eye: diagnosis and treatment. *American family physician*, *54*(8), 2423-2430.

Jernigan, J. A., Lowry, B. S., Hayden, F. G., Kyger, S. A., Conway, B. P., Groschel, D. H., & Farr, B. M. (1993). Adenovirus type 8 epidemic keratoconjunctivitis in an eye clinic: risk factors and control. *Journal of Infectious Diseases*, *167*(6), 1307-1313.

Khaw, P., Shah, P., & Elkington, A. (2004). Injury to the eye. *Bmj*, *328*(7430), 36-38.

Kunimoto, D. Y., Kanitkar, K. D., & Makar, M. S. (2004). The Wills eye manual: office and emergency room diagnosis and treatment of eye disease. *(No Title)*.

Leonardi, A. (2013). Allergy and allergic mediators in tears. *Experimental Eye Research*, *117*, 106-117.

Lietman, T., Dawson, C., & Osaki, S. (1998). Ocular chlamydial infections. *International ophthalmology clinics*, *38*(4), 125-135.

Limberg, M. (1991). A review of bacterial keratitis and bacterial conjunctivitis. *American journal of ophthalmology*, *112*(4 Suppl), 2S-9S.

Mani, V., & Vidya, K. (1997). A microbiological study of ophthalmia neonatorum in hospital-born babies. *Journal of the Indian Medical Association*, *95*(7), 416-417, 421.

Mannis, M., Tasman, W., & Jaeger, E. (1990). *Duane's Clinical Ophtalmology*. In.

Martin, M., Turco, J. H., Zegans, M. E., Facklam, R. R., Sodha, S., Elliott, J. A., Pryor, J. H., Beall, B., Erdman, D. D., & Baumgartner, Y. Y. (2003). An outbreak of conjunctivitis due to atypical Streptococcus pneumoniae. *New England Journal of Medicine*, *348*(12), 1112-1121.

McAnena, L., Knowles, S., Curry, A., & Cassidy, L. (2015). Prevalence of gonococcal conjunctivitis in adults and neonates. *Eye*, *29*(7), 875-880.

Moloney, G., & McCluskey, P. J. (2007). Classifying and managing allergic conjunctivitis. *Medicine today*, *8*(11), 16-21.

Morrow, G. L., & Abbott, R. L. (1998). Conjunctivitis. *American family physician*, *57*(4), 735-746.

O'Brien, T. P. (2013). Allergic conjunctivitis: an update on diagnosis and management. *Current opinion in allergy and clinical immunology*, *13*(5), 543-549.

Opitz, D. L., & Harthan, J. S. (2012). Review of azithromycin ophthalmic 1% solution (AzaSite®) for the treatment of ocular infections. *Ophthalmology and eye Diseases*, *4*, OED. S7791.

Patel, P. B., Diaz, M. C. G., Bennett, J. E., & Attia, M. W. (2007). Clinical features of bacterial conjunctivitis in children. *Academic Emergency Medicine*, *14*(1), 1-5.

Rapuano, C. (2008). American Academy of Ophthalmology Cornea/External Disease Panel. *Preferred Practice Pattern Guidelines. Conjunctivitis*.

Renfro, L., & Snow, J. S. (1992). Ocular effects of topical and systemic steroids. *Dermatologic clinics*, *10*(3), 505-512.

Rietveld, R. P., Ter Riet, G., Bindels, P. J., Schellevis, F. G., & Van Weert, H. C. (2007). Do general practitioners adhere to the guideline on infectious conjunctivitis? Results of the Second Dutch National Survey of General Practice. *BMC family practice*, *8*, 1-7.

Roba, L. A., Kowalski, R. P., Gordon, A. T., Romanowski, E. G., & Gordon, Y. J. (1995). Adenoviral ocular isolates demonstrate serotype-dependent differences in in vitro infectivity titers and clinical course. *Cornea*, *14*(4), 388-393.

Rosario, N., & Bielory, L. (2011). Epidemiology of allergic conjunctivitis. *Current opinion in allergy and clinical immunology*, *11*(5), 471-476.

Saw, S.-M., Gazzard, G., & Friedman, D. S. (2003). Interventions for angle-closure glaucoma: an evidence-based update. *Ophthalmology*, *110*(10), 1869-1879.

Sethuraman, U., & Kamat, D. (2009). The red eye: evaluation and management. *Clinical pediatrics*, *48*(6), 588-600.

Shiuey, Y., Ambati, B. K., Adamis, A. P., & Group, V. C. S. (2000). A randomized, double-masked trial of topical ketorolac versus artificial tears for treatment of viral conjunctivitis. *Ophthalmology*, *107*(8), 1512-1517.

Srinivasan, B. D., Jakobiec, F. A., Iwamoto, T., & DeVoe, A. G. (1979). Giant papillary conjunctivitis with ocular prostheses. *Archives of Ophthalmology*, *97*(5), 892-895.

Sugar, A., & Meyer, R. F. (1981). Giant papillary conjunctivitis after keratoplasty. *American journal of ophthalmology*, *91*(2), 239-242.

Tabbara, K. F., El-Sheikh, H. F., & Aabed, B. (2000). Extended wear contact lens related bacterial keratitis. *British Journal of Ophthalmology*, *84*(3), 327-328.

Ullman, S., Roussel, T. J., & Forster, R. K. (1987). Gonococcal keratoconjunctivitis. *Survey of ophthalmology*, *32*(3), 199-208.

Utz, V. M., & Kaufman, A. R. (2014). Allergic eye disease. *Pediatric Clinics*, *61*(3), 607-620.

Verma, M., Chhatwal, J., & Varughese, P. (1994). Neonatal conjunctivitis: a profile. *Indian pediatrics*, *31*(11), 1357-1361.

Visscher, K. L., Hutnik, C. M., & Thomas, M. (2009). Evidence-based treatment of acute infective conjunctivitis: Breaking the cycle of antibiotic prescribing. *Canadian family physician, 55*(11), 1071-1075.

Wan, W. L., Farkas, G. C., May, W. N., & Robin, J. B. (1986). The clinical characteristics and course of adult gonococcal conjunctivitis. *American journal of ophthalmology, 102*(5), 575-583.

Weiss, A., Brinser, J. H., & Nazar-Stewart, V. (1993). Acute conjunctivitis in childhood. *The Journal of pediatrics, 122*(1), 10-14.

Wilkins, M. R., Khan, S., Bunce, C., Khawaja, A., Siriwardena, D., & Larkin, D. F. (2011). A randomised placebo-controlled trial of topical steroid in presumed viral conjunctivitis. *British Journal of Ophthalmology, 95*(9), 1299-1303.

Yen, K., Steinkuller, P., & Chilakopati, M. (2009). Ocular infections. *Textbook of pediatric infectious diseases. 6th edition. Philadelphia: WB Saunders*, 817-821.

Chapter 20

Trachoma

Feriște Yetkin*, MD
Department of Ophtalmology, University of Health Sciences, Bursa, Turkey

Abstract

Trachoma is an overlooked tropical infectious ailment resulting from Chlamydia trachomatis strains A, B, and C. From a pathophysiological standpoint, trachoma constitutes a disease complex featuring two intertwined chronic processes: a recurring, generally mild infectious-inflammatory condition primarily affecting children, and a non-contagious, scarring affliction emerging later in life, ultimately leading to blindness. Typically prevalent in impoverished, rural communities in developing regions, particularly sub-Saharan Africa, trachoma has prompted the World Health Organization (WHO) to advocate for its control through a comprehensive approach that includes surgery, widespread antibiotic distribution, encouragement of facial cleanliness, and environmental enhancements. These combined interventions constitute the effective SAFE strategy, correlating with noteworthy reductions in the prevalence of active disease over the past two decades. Nevertheless, there remains a considerable population with trachoma still susceptible to the risk of blindness.

Keywords: trachoma, chlamydia trachomatis, blindness

Introduction

Trachoma is the most common infectious disease-causing blindness, triggered by the ancient organism Chlamydia trachomatis bacterium. It poses a global public health problem, particularly in regions with limited access to healthcare resources. Trachoma is currently an endemic disease in developing countries. The disease is most prevalent in Africa, the Middle East, Asia, and Central and South America. Currently, trachoma is endemic in developing regions worldwide. It affects the vision of approximately 2.1 million people globally, with 1.1 million of them considered totally blind (Mohammadpour et al., 2016). Most infections are transmitted from eye to eye. Transmission can also occur through contact with flies or any object in households that has contact with the infection and has the ability to transmit it (Taylor et al., 2014).

* Corresponding Author's Email: feristeyetkin@gmail.com.

In: Common Diseases According to Family Medicine Practice Guidelines
Editors: Esra Meltem Koç and Hilal Aksoy
ISBN: 979-8-89530-302-3

The disease manifests itself with intense conjunctival inflammation characterized by prominent follicles. This inflammation persists due to recurrent infections and an immune response against chlamydial antigens. Over time, this inflammation leads to scarring and, due to the inward turning of the eyelids (entropion), the eyelashes come into contact with the cornea (trichiasis), causing blindness. The fundamental event in trachoma is the progression from recurrent reinfection and inflammation to the complication of blindness. Trachoma is more prevalent in crowded and unsanitary living conditions, where access to clean water and proper hygiene practices is limited. The World Health Organization (WHO) has launched a global initiative called the "SAFE" strategy to control and eliminate trachoma, which includes surgery for advanced cases, treating active infections with antibiotics, promotion of facial hygiene to mitigate transmission, and environmental improvements such as improving sanitation to reduce the breeding grounds for the flies that spread the infection (Kuper et al., 2003). This section offers a detailed examination of trachoma, including its origins, prevalence, clinical presentations, diagnostic approaches, available treatments, and preventive measures.

Etiology and Pathogenesis

Trachoma is induced by Chlamydia trachomatis, a gram-negative bacterium characterized by a singular chromosome and functioning as a virulence factor, with multiple copies of a plasmid residing within obligatory intracellular spaces. It belongs to the Chlamydiaceae family. This disease primarily affects conjunctival epithelial cells and is characterized by a versatile interaction between the pathogen and the host. The cause of endemic trachoma is C trachomatis serotypes A, B, and C. Infections of Chlamydia trachomatis transmitted through the genital tract typically arise from serotypes ranging from D to K, and in addition, these serotypes can trigger ophthalmic neonatorum in infants or inclusion conjunctivitis in adults (Clarke, 2011).

The developmental cycle of Chlamydia trachomatis consists of two main stages: the elementary body and the reticulate body stages. The elementary body stage begins with a small, round structure known as the elementary body, which is infectious and resistant to the external environment, with a diameter of approximately 0.3 micrometers. The elementary body serves the function of transmitting from an infected person to a healthy person, often occurring through contact or contaminated objects. After entering the cell, the elementary body transforms into the reticulate body stage, located within a specialized vesicle inside the cell. The reticulate body becomes more metabolically active, undergoes replication, and participates in various intracellular functions within the infected cell. This stage is critical for the spread and maintenance of the infection. The transformation of reticulate bodies into elementary bodies occurs through cell lysis, allowing the newly formed elementary bodies to spread to surrounding cells. This process is crucial for infecting new cells and ensuring the continuation of the infection (Elwell et al., 2016).

The cell wall of Chlamydia trachomatis, particularly in the infectious form called the elementary body, exhibits distinctive features. This cell wall encompasses crucial structural characteristics that support the pathogen's resilience to environmental conditions and its life cycle within the host cell. The elementary body possesses a rigid cell wall, a trait that aids in its prolonged survival in the external environment and improves resistance against external factors. OmpA is the primary outer membrane protein of the cell wall, constituting approximately 60% of the mass of the cell wall. OmpA plays a critical role in binding to the surface of the host cell, facilitating the attachment of the infected cell to the host cell and initiating the infection. The proteins in the cell wall lead to genetic variations that characterize different Chlamydia trachomatis serovars. Specific serovars, particularly those associated with the eyes, have tissue-specific characteristics. For instance, serovars linked to the eyes have lost the capacity for tryptophan synthesis and exhibit polymorphism in specific genes (Carlson et al., 2005).

Long-term studies indicate that scar tissue is associated with chronic conjunctival inflammation. This inflammation may persist for an extended period even after the infection has cleared. This suggests that the impact of the disease extends not only during the active infection period, but also in the subsequent phase after the infection has been resolved (Hu et al., 2013). Therefore, it can be stated that blinding trachoma is not merely a result of an infection but is also significantly influenced by the long-term effects of the immune system response and the subsequent development of scar tissue in the disease process.

Epidemiology

Trachoma, a communicable eye infection triggered by the bacterium Chlamydia trachomatis, stands as a primary contributor to blindness, especially in underprivileged, rural areas where the availability of clean water and fundamental healthcare services may be restricted. The disease is often transmitted through direct contact with the eyes of an infected person, sharing of communal items, and exposure to insect bites. It is more prevalent in regions with inadequate access to clean water, crowded living conditions, and poor hygiene, commonly found in low-income countries. Trachoma is endemic in developing regions such as Africa, the Middle East, Asia, and Central and South America. It is especially prevalent in hyperendemic regions. Among preschool children, trachoma has the highest transmission rate, showing a significant decline in both boys and girls after the age of ten. The occurrence of chronic trachoma, marked by scarring and trichiasis, tends to increase with advancing age. In general, the persistent formation of scar tissue due to recurring infections can lead to enduring damage to the eyes. This manifestation becomes evident as the trachoma advances. As a general trend, females appear to have a higher risk of experiencing any form of trachoma symptoms, including stages leading to blindness such as trichiasis and corneal opacities, compared to males. The increased risk observed among these women is commonly related to their ongoing close interactions with small children, who are identified as the primary reservoir of infection (Congdon et al., 1993). The World Health Organization (WHO) has categorized trachoma as one of the disregarded tropical diseases within the United Nations and estimates that nearly 100 million individuals are at risk of infection. Approximately 1.2 million individuals experience blindness due to trachoma, and there is a likelihood of vision impairment for around 2 million people. Trachoma is particularly prevalent in regions such as Africa, the Middle East, and Asia (Resnikof et al., 2002). According to the weekly epidemiological records of the World Health Organization, in 2018, there were 158 million individuals living in regions where active trachoma posed a public health threat, and 88% of them were located in Africa. More than half of these individuals reside in Ethiopia (WHO, 2020). In a study conducted in Ethiopia, positive Chlamydia trachomatis (Ct) DNA test results were obtained from some flies captured while leaving households with Ct infection. This implies that flies could potentially facilitate the transmission of conjunctival Ct both between households and within them (Last et al., 2020). In a study based on PCR tests, it has been suggested that Chlamydia trachomatis may persist on skin, cotton fabric, and plastic for more than a day. (Versteeg et al., 2020). This further underscores the significance of fingers and tainted objects during the transmission process.

The World Health Organization (WHO) outlines specific objectives to eradicate trachoma as a public health concern: sustaining a prevalence of active trachoma in children aged 1-10 below 5% for at least two years without treatment; lowering the prevalence of trachomatous trichiasis in adults to under 0.2%; and implementing an effective monitoring program for trachomatous trichiasis (WHO 2015). These goals aim to reduce the impact of trachoma and maintain long-term control, preventing the spread of the disease among communities and improving individuals' quality of life.

Clinical Manifestations

Disease Progression

An active trachoma is a chronic form of follicular conjunctivitis that develops due to recurrent infections during childhood. In children with active trachoma, follicles and papillae are observed; papillae serve as an indicator of the severity of inflammation. Follicles appear as yellow and white dots under the eyelids. Follicles are composed of lymphoid tissue containing B lymphocytes. The large tarsal follicles seen in trachoma eventually undergo necrosis, heal with scarring, and are observed in a linear or star-shaped pattern, known as the Arlt's line. Limbal follicles can emerge, and new vessels develop, leading to the formation of the corneal pannus. As trachoma progresses, incorrect growth of eyelashes toward the wrong direction (trichiasis) and repeated irritation can lead to damage to the cornea. This damage may appear as small pits or depressions on the cornea, and these pits are referred to as 'Herbert's pits (Thylefors et al., 1987).

The community reservoir of active trachoma is found in children who are exposed to recurrent infections. In children consistently exposed to C. trachomatis, symptoms often do not resolve. In a cynomolgus monkey model of trachoma, it has been observed that severe inflammatory response decreases after two months in animals receiving weekly C. trachomatis injections, but follicular response continues as long as re-administration takes place (Taylor et al., 1982). Prolonged, recurrent, severe infections often leave scars on the conjunctiva, which is a sign of advanced trachoma. Scarring can be pronounced in the late childhood, masking the symptoms of an active disease. By middle age, scarring in some cases can be significant enough to lead to entropion or trichiasis, where the eyelashes turn inward. Recognizing these stages is crucial for early intervention and management. To prevent the development of corneal opacification resulting from trichiasis and inward turning of the eyelid, eyelid surgery is required (Thylefors et al., 1987).

Complications

Vision loss due to trachoma results from irreversible corneal damage. It is believed that this damage occurs as a result of multiple processes. Scarring can affect the meibomian openings, leading to gland atrophy and the development of dry eye features; similarly, scarring in the conjunctiva and lacrimal ducts due to chronic trachoma can lead to aqueous tear deficiency and tear drainage dysfunction. The inward-turned eyelashes irritate the cornea, which can become drier than normal and can allow for secondary infections. As a result, corneal opacities develop, and the damage is irreversible.

The World Health Organization has implemented a grading system to evaluate the intensity of trachoma, taking into account the presence or absence of five fundamental indicators (Muñoz and West, 1997) (Table 1).

The WHO grading system is used by non-ophthalmic trained personnel to assess the prevalence of trachoma and determine treatment needs in endemic areas.

Diagnosis and Assessment

A comprehensive clinical examination, including slit lamp biomicroscopy, is important in the diagnosis of trachoma.

To make a clinical diagnosis of trachoma, at least two of the specified clinical characteristics following should be present:

1. Follicles (small nodules) and papillary hypertrophy (swollen papillae) in the superior tarsal conjunctiva
2. Limbic follicles and sequel (Herbert's pits)
3. Tarsal conjunctiva with typical scarring (Arlt line)
4. The vascular pannus is located most prominently in the superior limbus, visible macroscopically.

Chronic trachoma can lead to insufficient tear production due to blockage of the tear ducts, causing trichiasis and entropion.

Chlamydia trachomatis can be detected through Immunofluorescence Antibody Tests, Polymerase Chain Reaction (PCR), Giemsa staining, and cell culture isolation (Solomon et al., 2004).

The diagnosis of trachoma is generally made by combining clinical symptoms. However, laboratory tests can be used, especially in ambiguous cases or situations where treatment resistance is suspected, to establish a definitive diagnosis and formulate an effective treatment plan.

Table 1. Trachoma grading system

Grade	Implication
1.	Follicular conjunctival inflammation
2.	Severe intensity of inflammation
3.	Scarring in the tarsal conjunctiva
4.	Trichiasis
5.	Corneal opacity

Treatment Modalities

The treatment for trachoma involves the use of antibiotics to eliminate the infection caused by Chlamydia trachomatis. The World Health Organization (WHO) recommends two main antibiotic regimens:

Tetracycline Eye Ointment: A 1% tetracycline eye ointment is applied to both eyes twice daily to the lower conjunctival fornix for a duration of six weeks.
Azithromycin: A single oral dose of azithromycin is administered, limited to 1 gram based on body weight, with a dosage of 20 mg/kg (Munoz et al., 2003).

Treatment for complications of trachoma may include artificial tears for dry eyes and eyelid surgery for ectropion or trichiasis (Burton et al., 2015).

Prevention and Control

Blindness resulting from trachoma is frequently witnessed in areas marked by insufficient personal and community hygiene. Several factors contributing to the increased risk of trachoma among individuals include limited access to clean water, the absence of fundamental sanitation amenities, residence within the same household as a confirmed trachoma case, densely populated living environments, and pervasive poverty. A shared factor appears to be the close proximity of children with unclean faces. This situation, combined with the presence of infections from eye and nasal secretions, creates an environment conducive to transmission.

The SAFE strategy is a comprehensive approach developed for the control and prevention of trachoma. It is implemented by the World Health Organization (WHO), particularly in regions where trachoma is prevalent. The SAFE strategy includes the following components:

Surgery (S): Involves surgical intervention to correct trichiasis, a condition where eyelashes turn inward, causing irritation and damage to the eyes.
Antibiotics (A): Includes the distribution of antibiotics to treat infections caused by the bacterium Chlamydia trachomatis and prevent its spread.
Facial Cleanliness (F): Encourages regular facial cleanliness to prevent the transmission of bacteria and the spread of trachoma.
Environmental Improvements (E): This involves addressing environmental factors such as improving access to clean water, enhancing sanitation facilities, and preventing the breeding of flies, which can contribute to the spread of trachoma (Gaynor et al., 2002).

A study conducted with children in Ethiopia revealed that developing a habit of face washing, combined with three rounds of azithromycin treatment, led to a reduction in the prevalence of active disease (Ngondi et al., 2008). While antibiotic treatment is acknowledged as the most effective element for overall outcomes, the incorporation of health education has been observed to offer additional benefits in further reducing the risk of active Chlamydia trachomatis infection (Cumberland et al., 2008).

Conclusion

Trachoma can be prevented by addressing environmental factors such as improving access to clean water, enhancing sanitation facilities, and preventing the breeding of flies. Simultaneously, raising awareness among the community about the causes, symptoms, and prevention methods of trachoma is crucial.

Infections often start at a young age and become less frequent as age increases. Infections are usually acquired through family contact and contact with others who have an active disease. Repeated infections lead to the most severe symptoms of the disease. The discovery of an effective Water, Sanitation, and Hygiene (WASH) strategy can expedite control, but even when known to be effective against a disease, WASH may not act quickly. A Chlamydia vaccine could be beneficial, but it is still in the development stage. The real hope may lie in a more frequent Mass Drug Administration (MDA). MDA administered twice a year or more frequently can eliminate infection in the most severely affected areas. In this scenario, by 2030, trachoma may not only be eliminated as a public health concern, but it may also be completely eradicated.

References

Burton, M., Habtamu, E., Ho, D., & Gower, E. W. (2015). Interventions for trachoma trichiasis. *Cochrane Database of Systematic Reviews, 2015*(11), CD004008. https://doi.org/10.1002/14651858.CD004008.pub3.

Caldwell, H. D., Kromhout, J., & Schachter, J. (1981). Purification and partial characterization of the major outer membrane protein of *Chlamydia trachomatis*. *Infection and Immunity, 31*, 1161–1176. https://doi.org/10.1128/IAI.31.3.1161-1176.1981.

Carlson, J. H., Porcella, S. F., McClarty, G., & Caldwell, H. D. (2005). Comparative genomic analysis of *Chlamydia trachomatis* oculotropic and genitotropic strains. *Infection and Immunity, 73*, 6407–6418. https://doi.org/10.1128/IAI.73.10.6407-6418.2005.

Clarke, I. N. (2011). Evolution of *Chlamydia trachomatis*. *Annals of the New York Academy of Sciences, 1230*, E11–E18. https://doi.org/10.1111/j.1749-6632.2011.06194.x.

Congdon, N., West, S., Vitale, S., Katala, S., & Mmbaga, B. B. (1993). Exposure to children and risk of active trachoma in Tanzanian women. *American Journal of Epidemiology, 137*, 366–372. https://doi.org/10.1093/oxfordjournals.aje.a116683.

Cumberland, P., Edwards, T., Hailu, G., Harding-Esch, E., Andreasen, A., Mabey, D., & Todd, J. (2008). The impact of community-level treatment and preventative interventions on trachoma prevalence in rural Ethiopia. *International Journal of Epidemiology, 37*, 549–558. https://doi.org/10.1093/ije/dyn045.

Elwell, C., Mirrashidi, K., & Engel, J. (2016). Chlamydia cell biology and pathogenesis. *Nature Reviews Microbiology, 14*, 385–400. https://doi.org/10.1038/nrmicro.2016.30.

Gaynor, B. D., Yi, E., & Lietman, T. (2002). Rationale for mass antibiotic distribution for trachoma elimination. *International Ophthalmology Clinics, 42*(1), 85–92. https://doi.org/10.1097/00004397-200201000-00012.

Hu, V. H., Holland, M. J., & Burton, M. J. (2013). Trachoma: Protective and pathogenic ocular immune responses to *Chlamydia trachomatis*. *PLoS Neglected Tropical Diseases, 7*, e2020. https://doi.org/10.1371/journal.pntd.0002020.

Kuper, H., Solomon, A. W., Buchan, J., Zondervan, M., Foster, A., & Mabey, D. (2003). A critical review of the SAFE strategy for the prevention of blinding trachoma. *The Lancet Infectious Diseases, 3*, 372–381. https://doi.org/10.1016/S1473-3099(03)00659-5.

Last, A., Versteeg, B., Shafi Abdurahman, O., Robinson, A., Dumessa, G., Abraham Aga, M., Shumi Bejiga, G., Negussu, N., Greenland, K., Czerniewska, A., Thomson, N., Cairncross, S., Sarah, V., Macleod, D., Solomon, A. W., Logan, J., & Burton, M. J. (2020). Detecting extra-ocular *Chlamydia trachomatis* in a trachoma-endemic community in Ethiopia: Identifying potential routes of transmission. *PLoS Neglected Tropical Diseases, 14*, e0008120. https://doi.org/10.1371/journal.pntd.0008120.

Mohammadpour, M., Abrishami, M., Masoumi, A., & Hashemi, H. (2016). Trachoma: Past, present, and future. *Journal of Current Ophthalmology, 28*, 165–169. https://doi.org/10.1016/j.joco.2016.08.011.

Muñoz, B., & West, S. (1997). Trachoma: The forgotten cause of blindness. *Epidemiologic Reviews, 19*(2), 205–217. https://doi.org/10.1093/oxfordjournals.epirev.a017953.

Muñoz, B., Solomon, A. W., Zingeser, J., Barwick, R., Burton, M., Bailey, R., Mabey, D., Foster, A., & West, S. K. (2003). Antibiotic dosage in trachoma control programs: Height as a surrogate for weight in children. *Investigative Ophthalmology & Visual Science, 44*, 1464–1469. https://doi.org/10.1167/iovs.02-0234.

Ngondi, J., Matthews, F., Reacher, M., Baba, S., Brayne, C., & Emerson, P. (2008). Associations between active trachoma and community intervention with antibiotics, facial cleanliness, and environmental improvement (A,F,E). *PLoS Neglected Tropical Diseases, 2*, e229. https://doi.org/10.1371/journal.pntd.0000229.

Resnikoff, S., Pascolini, D., Etya'ale, D., Kocur, I., Pararajasegaram, R., Pokharel, G. P., & Mariotti, S. P. (2004). Global data on visual impairment in the year 2002. *Bulletin of the World Health Organization, 82*, 844–851.

Solomon, A. W., Holland, M. J., Alexander, N. D., Massae, P. A., Aguirre, A., Natividad-Sancho, A., Molina, S., Safari, S., Shao, J. F., Courtright, P., Peeling, R. W., West, S. K., Bailey, R. L., Foster, A., & Mabey, D. C. (2004). Mass treatment with single-dose azithromycin for trachoma. *The New England Journal of Medicine, 351*(19), 1962–1971. https://doi.org/10.1056/NEJMoa040979.

Taylor, H. R., Burton, M. J., Haddad, D., West, S., & Wright, H. (2014). Trachoma. *The Lancet, 384*(9960), 2142–2152. https://doi.org/10.1016/S0140-6736(13)62182-0.

Taylor, H. R., Johnson, S. L., Prendergast, R. A., Schachter, J., Dawson, C. R., & Silverstein, A. M. (1982). An animal model of trachoma. II. The importance of repeated reinfection. *Investigative Ophthalmology & Visual Science, 23*, 507–515.

Thylefors, B., Dawson, C. R., Jones, B. R., West, S. K., & Taylor, H. R. (1987). A simple system for the assessment of trachoma and its complications. *Bulletin of the World Health Organization, 65*(4), 477–483.

Versteeg, B., Vasileva, H., Houghton, J., Last, A., Shafi Abdurahman, O., Sarah, V., Macleod, D., Solomon, A. W., Holland, M. J., Thomson, N., & Burton, M. J. (2020). Viability PCR shows that nonocular surfaces could contribute to transmission of *Chlamydia trachomatis* infection in trachoma. *PLoS Neglected Tropical Diseases, 14*, e0008449. https://doi.org/10.1371/journal.pntd.0008449.

World Health Organization. (2015). *Strategic and Technical Advisory Group on Neglected Tropical Diseases. Technical consultation on trachoma surveillance, 11−12 September 2014, Task Force for Global Health, Decatur, USA*. Geneva, Switzerland: World Health Organization.

World Health Organization. (2017). *Alliance for the Global Elimination of Trachoma by 2020: Progress report on elimination of trachoma, 2014–2016. Weekly Epidemiological Record, 92*(26), 359–368.

Chapter 21

Periorbital and Orbital Cellulitis

Osman Tecir[*], MD

Department of Emergency Medicine, Trabzon Kanuni Training and Research Hospital, Trabzon, Turkey

Abstract

Orbital infections are classified anatomically and based on the spread of the infection. The orbital septum is a barrier, and infections located anterior to the orbital septum are termed periorbital or preseptal cellulitis. In contrast, infections posterior to the orbital septum are called orbital cellulitis. Bacterial infections are the most common causes of both periorbital and orbital cellulitis, and if left untreated or inadequately treated, they can lead to severe ophthalmic, cranial, and systemic complications. Periorbital cellulitis common findings include widespread eyelid edema, pain, erythema, and increased warmth. In orbital cellulitis, limitations in eye movements, reduced vision, and proptosis can be observed. The diagnosis of periorbital cellulitis is made by clinical evaluation, and radiological imaging is not always necessary. However, in cases where differentiation from orbital cellulitis is challenging, radiological imaging becomes necessary. In treatment, appropriate antibiotic regimens are selected, and patients are closely monitored. Preseptal cellulitis can be managed in outpatient settings, whereas orbital cellulitis requires inpatient treatment. Surgical interventions in orbital cellulitis are indicated in the presence of subperiosteal, orbital abscesses, and cavernous sinus thrombosis. In cases of severe sinusitis, drainage of the infected sinuses should be considered. Orbital cellulitis can lead to severe complications and requires a multidisciplinary approach.

Keywords: cellulitis, antibacterial agents, tomography

Introduction

Orbital infections are named based on the anatomical areas affected and the mode of infection spread. The membranous layer known as the orbital septum acts as a barrier, and infections in front of the orbital septum are referred to as periorbital or preseptal cellulitis. In contrast, infections behind the orbital septum are termed orbital cellulitis. Bacterial infections are the most common cause of periorbital and orbital cellulitis, and if left untreated or inadequately managed, they can lead to severe ophthalmological, cranial, and systemic complications.

---

[*] Corresponding Author's Email: osmantecir@hotmail.com.

In: Common Diseases According to Family Medicine Practice Guidelines
Editors: Esra Meltem Koç and Hilal Aksoy
ISBN: 979-8-89530-302-3

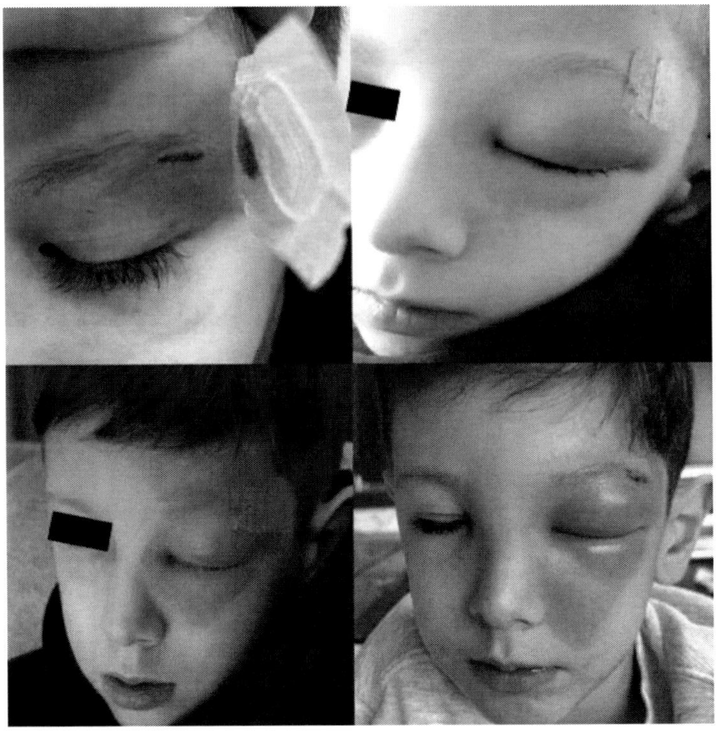

Figure 1. Periorbital cellulitis secondary to skin trauma day by day (Case courtesy of Murat Aykut).

Main Body

Periorbital (Preseptal) Cellulitis

Periorbital cellulitis can occur at any age, but it is most commonly observed in children (Mejia et al., 2023). Its prevalence is higher compared to orbital cellulitis. The most frequent symptoms are widespread edema, pain, erythema, and increased warmth in the eyelids. Unlike orbital cellulitis, periorbital cellulitis does not exhibit limitations in eye movements, visual impairment, or proptosis. Periorbital cellulitis typically occurs from skin infections resulting from the spread of sinusitis infection or regional trauma (Clarke, 2004) (Figure 1). In the etiology of periorbital cellulitis, infections of surrounding tissues such as hordeolum, dacryocystitis, conjunctivitis, or sinusitis, the hematogenous or lymphatic spread of distant infections in the upper respiratory tract or middle ear, and surgical factors can be listed as contributing factors.

Understanding the anatomy of the orbit can help to comprehend the causes of periorbital cellulitis. Above the orbit lies the frontal sinus, medially the ethmoid sinus, and below it the maxillary sinus. Among sinusitis infections, ethmoid sinus infection is the most common cause of periorbital cellulitis (Atfeh & Khalil, 2015). The thin and porous structure of the lamina papyracea between the ethmoid sinus and the orbit can explain this. Additionally, the foramina through which the ethmoid arteries pass also promotes the spread of infection. The probability of periorbital cellulitis leading to severe complications is low. More commonly encountered issues include the confusion between orbital cellulitis and periorbital cellulitis, as well as inadequate or incorrect treatment. The lack of valves in the orbital venous system can lead to the progression of periorbital infections and their spread to orbital infections through the venous system. More severe complications occur by connecting the superior and ophthalmic veins to the cavernous sinus. In valveless veins, infection can spread retrogradely into the intracranial space.

Among the most common bacterial causes of periorbital cellulitis are Staphylococcus aureus, Streptococcus pneumoniae, and Streptococcus pyogenes. With the widespread use of the Haemophilus influenzae type B (Hib) vaccine, cases caused by Haemophilus influenzae have decreased (Atfeh & Khalil, 2015). The increasing prevalence of methicillin-resistant Staphylococcus aureus (MRSA) should also be considered a potential pathogen in cases of periorbital cellulitis. Other causative agents include Acinetobacter, Nocardia, Bacillus, Pseudomonas, Neisseria, Proteus, Pasteurella, and Mycobacterium. Rarely, fungi of the Mucorales and Aspergillus genera can also be responsible.

Diagnosis

History and physical examination, as in many diseases, are crucial. In most cases, there is a history that can lead the physician to a diagnosis. The points to inquire about in the history include recent upper respiratory tract infection or sinusitis, as well as a history of insect bites or trauma-related infections in areas near the orbit. Periorbital cellulitis typically presents with redness, swelling, and eyelid puffiness (Figure 2). It does not demonstrate symptoms such as reduced eye movements and vision loss. The infection is anterior to the ocular tissues and does not reach the extraocular muscles. Findings are generally unilateral. Fever is more commonly associated with orbital cellulitis. However, these distinctions may only sometimes be very clear-cut.

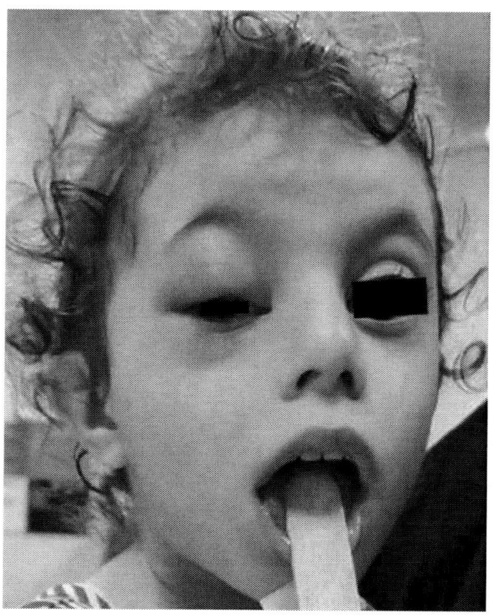

Figure 2. Redness in the right eye, swelling of the eyelid. (Case courtesy of Gizem Topaloglu Cicek).

In some cases of orbital cellulitis, there may be no fever. In contrast, some cases of periorbital cellulitis, fever, chemosis, eye tearing, conjunctivitis, discharge, and mild vision loss may be present. This complicates the differentiation between periorbital and orbital cellulitis (Gonçalves et al., 2016).

The diagnosis of periorbital cellulitis is made through a clinical assessment. Radiological imaging is not necessary in all cases. Radiological imaging should be performed in cases where there is suspicion of orbital cellulitis, subperiosteal abscess, orbital abscess, or cavernous sinus thrombosis, or when an adequate response is not achieved within 24-48 hours with appropriate antibiotics (Jabarin et al., 2018). Contrast-enhanced Orbital CT helps distinguish between periorbital and orbital cellulitis and provides information on the extent of infection spread (Okonkwo et al., 2018) (Figure 3-4). In cases where differentiation cannot be made with all tests, patients should be treated as if they have been diagnosed with orbital cellulitis.

Inadequate or insufficient treatment of periorbital cellulitis can lead to the progression of orbital complications. Orbital complications are categorized into five groups under the Chandler Classification (Table 1) (Chandler et al., 1970). This classification should not be considered a potential course if the infection progresses. Reviewing these groups during the diagnostic stage can be beneficial in determining the severity of the disease and aiding in differential diagnosis.

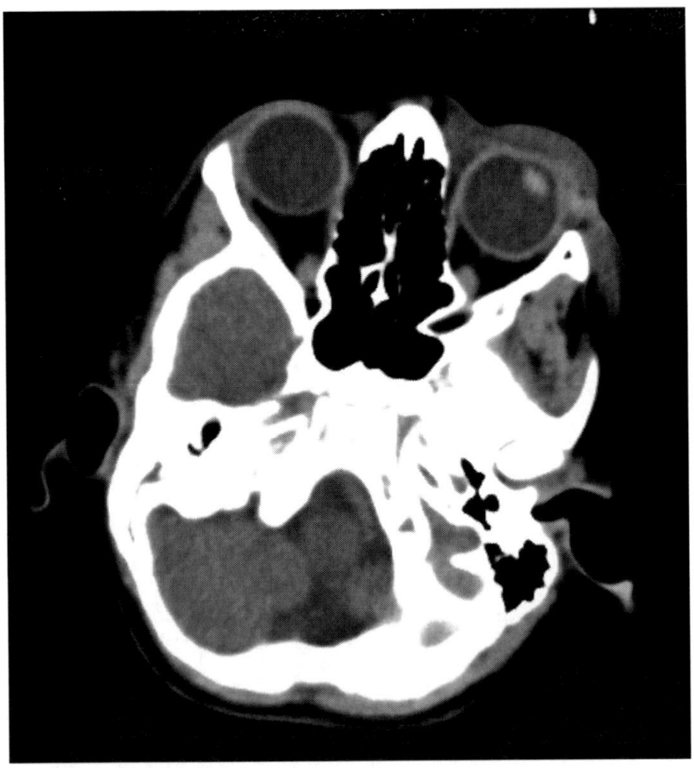

Figure 3. Thickening and increased density in the soft tissues of the left preorbital area. Inflammation-related thickening of the mucosal wall in the left maxillary sinus. (Case courtesy of Melih Imamoglu).

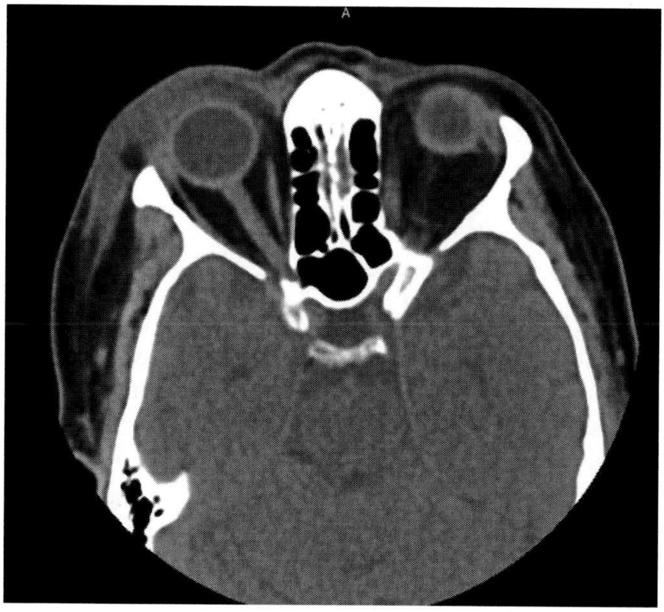

Figure 4. Increased reticular density in the right preorbital area and subcutaneous fat planes. Thickening of the subcutaneous tissue. (Case courtesy of Melih Imamoglu).

Treatment

The selection of antibiotics for the treatment of periorbital cellulitis is made to cover common pathogens, including S. aureus, Streptococcus species, and anaerobes. The planning of the treatment should consider the patient's age and the severity of the disease. In this condition, which is often seen in the pediatric population, infants or those with severe disease should be treated in the hospital using intravenous therapy. Patients with mild disease and those over one year of age can be treated on an outpatient basis with oral antibiotic therapy. For oral use, antibiotics effective against gram-positive and gram-negative bacteria, such as Ampicillin, Amoxicillin/clavulanate, Levofloxacin, Azithromycin, and Clindamycin, can be used. In the cases of evident eyelid trauma or suspected Staphylococcus infection, oral antibiotics such as Dicloxacillin, Flucloxacillin, Cephalexin, or Cefazolin can be used. For intravenous antibiotic selection, broad-spectrum agents effective against gram-positive and gram-negative bacteria are chosen, such as Ceftriaxone, Cefotaxim, Ceftazidime, or Ampicillin/sulbactam. However, with the increasing incidence of MRSA infections in recent years, treatment recommendations have expanded to include Trimethoprim-sulfamethoxazole (TMP-SMX), Clindamycin, or Doxycycline (Bae & Bourget, 2023). It is essential to note that TMP-SMX and Doxycycline do not cover Group A Streptococci, and Doxycycline is not recommended for children under eight years of age. In the cases of hospital-acquired MRSA infections, Vancomycin or Linezolid should be preferred (Sweeney & Yen, 2020). If there is an eyelid injury resulting from contact with organic material, agents that cover anaerobic organisms should be added, such as Metronidazole, Clindamycin, or Piperacillin-Tazobactam. Response to periorbital cellulitis treatment is typically observed within 24-48 hours, and the treatment is usually planned for 5-7 days.

Table 1. Chandler classification

1.	Periorbital Cellulitis
2.	Orbital Cellulitis
3.	Subperiosteal Abscess
4.	Orbital Abscess
5.	Cavernous Sinus Thrombosis

In some cases, this duration may be extended. If there is no response to appropriate antibiotic therapy, a CT scan should be performed to evaluate possible orbital complications and assess the severity of the infection (Howe & Jones, 2004). Even if a CT scan is performed and the differentiation between periorbital and orbital cellulitis cannot be made, patients should be treated in the hospital setting as if they have orbital cellulitis. The routine use of steroids is not part of periorbital cellulitis treatment. In the cases of infection resulting from trauma, the patient's tetanus prophylaxis should be evaluated. In Chandler's classification Groups 3, 4, and 5, drainage is necessary, and surgical consultation should be requested. Complicated cases should be managed with a multidisciplinary approach involving a team of eye specialists, pediatricians, and ENT specialists (*Preseptal Cellulitis - EyeWiki*, n.d.).

Orbital Cellulitis

Orbital cellulitis is an infection of the muscle and fat tissues behind the orbital septum, and it can result in severe consequences ranging from vision loss to life-threatening conditions. It is also known as postseptal cellulitis and can occur at any age, but is commonly seen in children (Tsirouki et al., 2018). Among the most common causes are bacteria such as Staphylococcus aureus, Streptococcus pneumoniae, and Streptococcus pyogenes. It can also be polymicrobial, involving multiple types of bacteria. Rare cases of orbital cellulitis caused by non-spore-forming anaerobic bacteria such as Aeromonas hydrophila, Pseudomonas aeruginosa, and Eikenella corrodens have been reported (Hamed-Azzam et al., 2018). Another rare set of causes includes fungal pathogens, particularly Mucorales and Aspergillus, which are more commonly seen in immunosuppressive patients (Sagiv et al., 2018).

In cases of orbital cellulitis, the most common source of infection is acute rhinosinusitis. However, it should be noted that orbital cellulitis is a rare complication of rhinosinusitis. Due to its anatomical structure, the development of orbital cellulitis is most likely in infections originating from the ethmoid sinus (El Mograbi et al., 2019). Other conditions that can lead to orbital cellulitis include infections in areas close to the orbit (such as dental, middle ear, and facial infections), dacryocystitis, trauma, various ophthalmic surgical procedures, and immunodeficiency. In some cases, orbital cellulitis can also result from the hematogenous spread of infection originating from any part of the body.

Diagnosis

The diagnosis of orbital cellulitis is based primarily on patient history and physical examination findings. Patients often present with complaints of fatigue, visual disturbances, diplopia, eye pain aggravated by eye movements, eyelid swelling, redness, and discomfort. Elevated body temperature may be noticeable during the physical examination. These findings typically occur unilaterally, but edema can also extend to involve the other eyelids. The most distinguishing features of orbital cellulitis are pain with eye movements, proptosis (bulging of the eye), and ophthalmoplegia (paralysis of eye movement) (Hamed-Azzam et al., 2018). Eyelid swelling can also occur in preseptal cellulitis. However, it is essential to note that ophthalmic symptoms are absent in preseptal cellulitis. Chemosis (conjunctival swelling) is more frequently observed in orbital cellulitis than in preseptal cellulitis. Redness of the eyelid can also occur in cases of orbital cellulitis, complications such as optic nerve involvement, rapid-onset atrophy leading to papilledema, or optic neuritis can occur, potentially resulting in blindness. The reasons for the development of optic atrophy in orbital cellulitis include mechanical compression as a factor. The second factor is the constriction of the central retinal and other nourishing arteries, although orbital inflammation can spread directly to the inner structure of the nerve. This can lead to the formation of abscesses and necrotic areas.

Laboratory tests and imaging methods can be helpful in the diagnosis. A complete blood count (CBC), blood cultures, and nasal and throat swabs should be requested. In cases of orbital cellulitis, particularly in pediatric patients, magnetic resonance imaging (MRI) may be superior to computed tomography (CT) due to the absence of radiation exposure and its ability to visualize the soft tissue involvement (Basraoui et al., 2018). However, the use of MRI can be challenging due to limited accessibility, longer scan times, and a greater need for sedation during the procedure compared to CT. In patients with suspected orbital cellulitis, contrast-enhanced CT imaging of the orbit, paranasal sinuses, and brain is the preferred method for distinguishing between preseptal and orbital cellulitis and identifying potential complications (Figure 5). The differential diagnoses for orbital cellulitis are presented in Table 2.

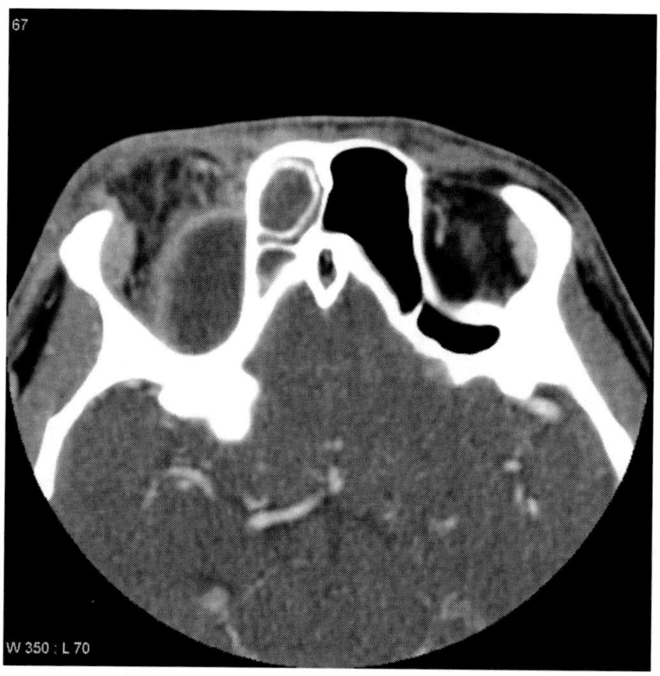

Figure 5. Sub-periosteal abscess in the right orbital area. (Case courtesy of Frank Gaillard, Radiopaedia.org, rID: 4052).

Table 2. Differential diagnosis

• Complications of Acute Sarcoidosis
• Adenoviral Conjunctivitis
• Carotid-Cavernous Fistula
• Langerhans Cell Histiocytosis
• Orbital İnflamatory Syndrome
• Pediatric Mucormycosis
• Retinoblastoma
• Retrobulbar Hemorrhage
• Thyroid Ophthalmopathy

Treatment

Orbital cellulitis, when not immediately diagnosed and treated, can progress and lead to severe complications. Patients diagnosed with orbital cellulitis should be admitted to the hospital and initiated on appropriate broad-spectrum antibiotics. A comprehensive evaluation of the orbit and sinuses should involve consultations with the ophthalmology and otolaryngology (ENT) departments. In managing pediatric patients, pediatric specialists should provide guidance, and consultations with the infectious disease department are recommended. Patients should be closely monitored, including systemic parameters (pulse, blood pressure, fever, neurological evaluation), and ocular evaluations (proptosis, pupil reactions, eye movement, and visual acuity) should be performed every 4 hours. Uncomplicated orbital cellulitis can be managed with antibiotics alone (Danishyar & Sergent, 2023). Pain relief can be achieved with the use of NSAIDs and acetaminophen, either alone or in combination, for palliative purposes. In treating pediatric orbital cellulitis, some studies suggest that corticosteroids may be beneficial (Chen et al., 2018). Antibiotics should be administered intravenously until ocular symptoms return to normal, after which they can be switched to oral administration. Commonly used intravenous antibiotic regimens include ceftriaxone, cefotaxim, ampicillin-sulbactam, or piperacillin-tazobactam. In cases where anaerobic pathogens are suspected, metronidazole should be added to the treatment. For patients with a penicillin allergy, ciprofloxacin or levofloxacin can be preferred. In the cases where MRSA (Methicillin-resistant Staphylococcus aureus) is suspected, vancomycin should be added to the treatment. Antibiotic selection should be adjusted based on the culture and sensitivity results. If patients show improvement with intravenous antibiotics within 48 hours, the transition to oral antibiotics can be considered. Oral antibiotics that can be used include clindamycin, amoxicillin-clavulanate, cefpodoxime, and cefdinir.

Surgical methods for treating orbital cellulitis are indicated in cases of a subperiosteal abscess (most commonly along the medial orbital wall), orbital abscess, and cavernous sinus thrombosis. In cases of severe sinusitis, drainage of the infected sinuses can also be considered. Surgical methods can also be used to obtain culture material for diagnosis. External approaches (through the orbit) and endoscopic transcaruncular surgery can be used.

Orbital cellulitis typically responds completely and rapidly to appropriate antibiotic therapy. However, complications can lead to permanent consequences, and in rare cases, death can result from the complications of orbital cellulitis (Ruíz Carrillo et al., 2017).

Conclusion

Periorbital cellulitis and orbital cellulitis are two important ophthalmological conditions. Periorbital cellulitis is more commonly encountered, responds more rapidly to antibiotic treatment, and can generally be managed in an outpatient setting. In contrast, orbital cellulitis can progress to severe complications, such as visual loss, and therefore requires hospitalization and close monitoring. Imaging techniques can be helpful in the diagnosis and follow-up stages. A multidisciplinary approach should be applied in cases of orbital cellulitis. In conclusion, both periorbital and orbital cellulitis are severe conditions that pose a risk to eye health. Early diagnosis, appropriate antibiotic therapy, and informed care can help mitigate these risks.

References

Atfeh, M. S., & Khalil, H. S. (2015). Orbital infections: five-year case series, literature review and guideline development. *The Journal of Laryngology and Otology*, *129*(7), 670–676. https://doi.org/10.1017/S0022215115001371.

Bae, C., & Bourget, D. (2023). *Periorbital Cellulitis*. StatPearls Publishing.

Basraoui, D., Elhajjami, A., & Jalal, H. (2018). [Imaging of orbital cellulitis in children: about 56 cases]. *The Pan African Medical Journal*, *30*. https://doi.org/10.11604/PAMJ.2018.30.94.14672.

Chandler, J. R., Langenerunner, D. J., & Stevens, E. R. (1970). The pathogenesis of orbital complications in acute sinusitis. *The Laryngoscope*, *80*(9), 1414–1428. https://doi.org/10.1288/00005537-197009000-00007.

Chen, L., Silverman, N., Wu, A., & Shinder, R. (2018). Intravenous Steroids With Antibiotics on Admission for Children With Orbital Cellulitis. *Ophthalmic Plastic and Reconstructive Surgery*, *34*(3). https://doi.org/10.1097/IOP.0000000000000910.

Clarke, W. N. (2004). Periorbital and orbital cellulitis in children. *Paediatrics & Child Health*, *9*(7), 471–472. https://doi.org/10.1093/PCH/9.7.471.

Danishyar, A., & Sergent, S. R. (2023). *Orbital Cellulitis*. StatPearls Publishing.

El Mograbi, A., Ritter, A., Najjar, E., & Soudry, E. (2019). Orbital Complications of Rhinosinusitis in the Adult Population: Analysis of Cases Presenting to a Tertiary Medical Center Over a 13-Year Period. *The Annals of Otology, Rhinology, and Laryngology*, *128*(6), 563–568. https://doi.org/10.1177/0003489419832624.

Gonçalves, R., Menezes, C., Machado, R., Ribeiro, I., & Lemos, J. A. (2016). Periorbital cellulitis in children: Analysis of outcome of intravenous antibiotic therapy. *Orbit (Amsterdam, Netherlands)*, *35*(4), 175–180. https://doi.org/10.1080/01676830.2016.1176205.

Hamed-Azzam, S., AlHashash, I., Briscoe, D., Rose, G. E., & Verity, D. H. (2018). Common Orbital Infections ~ State of the Art ~ Part I. *Journal of Ophthalmic & Vision Research*, *13*(2), 175–182. https://doi.org/10.4103/JOVR.JOVR_199_17.

Howe, L., & Jones, N. S. (2004). Guidelines for the management of periorbital cellulitis/abscess. *Clinical Otolaryngology and Allied Sciences*, *29*(6), 725–728. https://doi.org/10.1111/J.1365-2273.2004.00889.X.

Jabarin, B., Eviatar, E., Israel, O., Marom, T., & Gavriel, H. (2018). Indicators for imaging in periorbital cellulitis secondary to rhinosinusitis. *European Archives of Oto-Rhino-Laryngology : Official Journal of the European Federation of Oto-Rhino-Laryngological Societies (EUFOS) : Affiliated with the German Society for Oto-Rhino-Laryngology - Head and Neck Surgery*, *275*(4), 943–948. https://doi.org/10.1007/S00405-018-4897-4.

Mejia, E., Vohra, V., & Braiman, M. (2023). *Ocular Cellulitis*. StatPearls Publishing.

Okonkwo, A. C. O., Powell, S., Carrie, S., & Ball, S. L. (2018). A review of periorbital cellulitis guidelines in Fifty-One Acute Admitting Units in the United Kingdom. *Clinical Otolaryngology : Official Journal of ENT-UK ; Official Journal of Netherlands Society for Oto-Rhino-Laryngology & Cervico-Facial Surgery*, *43*(2), 718–721. https://doi.org/10.1111/COA.13020.

Preseptal Cellulitis - EyeWiki. (n.d.). Retrieved November 8, 2023, from https://eyewiki.aao.org/Preseptal_Cellulitis.

Ruíz Carrillo, J. D., Vázquez Guerrero, E., & Mercado Uribe, M. C. (2017). [Orbital cellulitis complicated by subperiosteal abscess due to Streptococcus pyogenes infection]. *Boletin Medico Del Hospital Infantil de Mexico*, *74*(2), 134–140. https://doi.org/10.1016/J.BMHIMX.2017.01.006.

Sagiv, O., Thakar, S. D., Kandl, T. J., Kontoyiannis, D. P., Debnam, J. M., & Esmaeli, B. (2018). Clinical Course of Preseptal and Orbital Cellulitis in 50 Immunocompromised Patients with Cancer. *Ophthalmology*, *125*(2), 318–320. https://doi.org/10.1016/J.OPHTHA.2017.10.006.

Sweeney, A. R., & Yen, M. T. (2020). Eyelid Infections. In *Albert and Jakobiec's Principles and Practice of Ophthalmology* (pp. 1–12). Springer International Publishing. https://doi.org/10.1007/978-3-319-90495-5_75-1.

Tsirouki, T., Dastiridou, A. I., Ibánez flores, N., Cerpa, J. C., Moschos, M. M., Brazitikos, P., & Androudi, S. (2018). Orbital cellulitis. *Survey of Ophthalmology*, *63*(4), 534–553. https://doi.org/10.1016/J.SURVOPHTHAL.2017.12.001.

Part 7

Others

Chapter 22

Otitis Media

Dursun Tüzün
Provincial Health Director, Ordu Provincial Health Directorate, Ordu, Turkey

Abstract

Otitis media (OM) is one of the most common diseases in young children. It is a set of diseases that includes acute otitis media (AOM), otitis media with effusion (OME), and chronic suppurative otitis media (CSOM). It is among the causes of hearing loss in developing countries. OM, which can be of bacterial or viral origin, can occur as a result of the transfer of pathogens to the nasopharynx through the eustachian tube. Acute earache, edema of the tympanic membrane, and typical symptoms of hearing loss are among the symptoms. The risk of OM is affected by many environmental and individual factors. In addition to individual factors such as young age, race and ethnicity, male gender, family history, immunodeficiency, craniofacial abnormalities, adenoid hypertrophy, and recurrent upper respiratory tract infections; environmental factors such as low socio-cultural status, crowded population, limited access to healthcare, and lack of hygiene are situations that increase the risk of OM and affect the incidence of chronicity (Schilder et al., 2016; Harmes et al., 2013). In the diagnosis of CSOM for diagnostic purposes, tools such as symptom severity scales, otoscopy, pneumatic otoscopy, automicroscopy, tympanometry, and acoustic reflectometry can be used. AOM is characterized by the rapid onset of symptoms, signs of inflammation such as pain in the erythematous and edematous tympanic membrane auricle, a feeling of fullness, and an increased temperature. Recurrent attacks of AOM; may cause rare but serious complications such as mastoiditis, meningitis, and brain abscess. Every year, an average of 21 thousand people die from OM. The prevalence of OM-related hearing loss is 3 in 1000 (Schilder et al., 2016; Mittal et al., 2015).

Keywords: suppurative otitis media, mastoidectomy, tympanoplasty

Introduction

Although CSOM usually occurs in the first years of life, it can also be seen in adult populations. With a worldwide prevalence of 65-330 million people, 22.6% of CSOM cases are under the age of 5. Clinically significant hearing impairment is observed in sixty out of every CSOM case. The most common prevalence is among Canada, Alaska, Greenland, American Indians, and Australian Aborigines (Mittal et al., 2015; Morris, 2012).

In: Common Diseases According to Family Medicine Practice Guidelines
Editors: Esra Meltem Koç and Hilal Aksoy
ISBN: 979-8-89530-302-3

Diagnosis and Treatment

CSOM, which is the most common cause of permanent hearing loss in developing countries, is a chronic inflammatory process of the mastoid cavity and middle ear (Schilder et al., 2016; Xia et al., 2022). It is characterized by otorrhea that occurs for 2-6 weeks. Thickened mucosa and polyps may also be present in the middle ear. Chronic mastoiditis and tympano-mastoiditis can also accompany it (Morris, 2012). CSOM may cause resistant cases through eustachian tube dysfunction and nasal septum deviation, turbinate bullosa, obstructive nasal functions, and chronic ventilation changes in association with chronic rhinosinusitis (Brescia et al., 2023). Complications of CSOM include common conditions ranging from meningitis, temporal lobe abscess, postal abscess, mastoiditis, extradural abscesses, perisinus abscess, inflammation, and thrombus in the transverse sinus (Kirti et al., 2018). Cholesteatoma is an abnormal accumulation of squamous epithelium in the middle ear cavity and mastoid bone and should be considered among CSOM complications in patients with persistent discharge and unresponsive to treatment. Loss of integrity of the tympanic membrane and recurrent effusions are characteristic features. CSOM may cause destruction of the middle ear bones and cause conductive hearing loss by preventing the effusion from passing sound transmission over the middle ear ossicles and over the tympanic membrane. As more serious complications, it can cause intracranial pathologies and sensorineural type hearing loss (SNHL) as a result of inflammatory mediators affecting the inner ear through the loss of hair cells in the cochlea (Schilder et al., 2016; Mittal et al., 2015; Morris, 2012). The incidence of SNHL can increase with long-term exposure to toxins (Elzinga et al., 2021). CSOM and associated pathologies are more common in low- and middle-income countries (Schilder et al., 2016). Pseudomonas aeruginosa (PA) and Staphylococcus aureus (SA) are the most common pathogens of CSOM. Antibiotic resistance and ototoxicity, as well as the role of host immunity, create a potential need for surgery (Mittal et al., 2015). PA, one of the leading pathogens among the causes of CSOM, colonizes the middle ear through perforation of the tympanic membrane and makes it difficult to eliminate the infection through biofilm layers (Xia et al., 2022). OME is characterized by effusion behind the intact tympanic membrane. OME, which causes conductive hearing loss, may cause negative consequences in terms of language, behavior, and school success in patients with frequent recurrences. OME is a very common disease, and 80% of individuals up to the age of 10 experience an OME attack at least once in their lives (Schilder et al., 2016).

The primary approach in the current treatment modalities for CSOM begins with auditory clearance, a combination of topical antimicrobials. The maintenance of the ear as clean and dry as possible for patients with chronic discharge plays an important role in first-line treatment in terms of the effectiveness of topical agents and the prevention of colonization. Antibiotic drops have been shown to be effective in various randomized controlled studies. Quinolones are among the most common topical agents. In cases of failure after 3 weeks of primary treatment, oral antibiotics are the first choice. The most important disadvantage of oral antibiotics is that they cannot reach the required effective concentration in the middle ear. Many factors, such as scarring of the middle ear and decreased vascularization of its mucosa, are effective in this regard. Although intravenous antibiotic therapy is an effective treatment, it is not an option as a first-line treatment method. Caution should be exercised in its use due to the risk of side effects and the development of antibiotic resistance. It is recommended to use it with the opinion of expert in culture and infectious diseases (Mittal et al., 2015).

Antibiotherapy forms the basis for AOM treatment. Untreated OM may develop complications such as chronic effusions, developmental delays, hearing loss, and learning disabilities. In the medical treatment of CSOM, analgesics for symptoms such as earache and fever, and high-dose amoxicillin for antibiotic therapy are offered as the first choice in patients without allergies. Second- and third-generation cephalosporins are widely used in resistant cases (Harmes et al., 2014).

Surgical treatment should be considered as a treatment method in cases of CSOM that is resistant to medical treatment and recurrent. Surgery such as tympanomastoidectomy is an option that should be considered in patients with severe hearing loss and complications such as dural vein sinus thrombosis, facial nerve paralysis, subperiosteal abscess, and meningitis. Surgical treatment is also an option to remove the underlying cholesteatoma that is resistant to treatment. Timaponplasty can be performed within 6-12 months following healing of the infection. However, spontaneous recovery after resolution of the infection should also be considered as a possibility (Mittal et al., 2015). The role of mastoidectomy in cases of complicated CSOm is well defined. Although controversial, it is advocated by many authors in the process of identifying and controlling the underlying pathology. More radical treatments are preferred, especially in cases with cholesteatoma (Heah et al., 2016). Long-standing cases of CSOM benefit significantly from surgery and hearing rehabilitation (Bruchhage et al., 2023). Success in surgical treatment is not only about surgery; it is affected by many factors such as gender, age, previous surgery, the condition of the middle ear mucosa and ossicles, the presence of otorrhea, cholesteatoma, tympanic sclerosis, and perforation (Cebeci et al., 2020). Ventilation tubes and adenoidectomies are commonly used surgical methods for recurrent OM (Schilder et al., 2016). In CSOM cases requiring surgery, typical ear discharge, pain, and hearing impairment that continue even after surgery are observed. Different surgical tympanoplasty techniques have been presented, and there are also many studies supporting mastoid obliteration to overcome symptoms (Lucidi et al., 2022).

Open and closed techniques remain popular today in the treatment of CSOM and cholesteatoma. Closed techniques are becoming more popular day by day, as they eliminate the need for postoperative care and protection from water contact and provide better auditory results. Despite this, recurrence and residue rates in closed techniques still attract attention. While open techniques are recommended for cholesteatomas that reach the ceiling and reach behind the aditus of the facial canal, closed techniques are recommended for limited sinus tympani and pars tensa cholesteatomas if there is no pathology in the mastoid. However, there is no standard technique, but the characteristics of the patient and the surgeon's preference should be taken into consideration (Cebeci et al., 2020). Cochlear implantation for temporal bone with normal anatomy is a technique that can be performed using a transmastoid or transcanal approach. The presence of inactive and active CSOM, cholesteatoma, or previous infections can be encountered as difficulties during surgery. In the presence of infection, this infection can spread to the intracranial spaces and the labyrinth with implantation. In the presence of cholesteatoma, a recurrence of the disease may occur. Some studies recommend that for the treatment of CSOM, tympanoplasty, and tympanomastoidectomy should be performed first, followed by cochlear implantation 3-6 months later (Vincenti et al., 2014).

Hearing difficulties are one of the most common sequelae to CSOM. Two types of hearing loss can be seen: conductive and sensorineural. The type of conduction may occur by blocking the transmission of sound waves from the middle ear. The amount of fluid accumulated in the mid-cunt and the perforation of the tympanic membrane can cause this condition. In some cases of CSOM, this hearing loss may occur irreversibly. In inner ear damage, sensorineural type hearing loss can occur due to damage to the cochlea and conduction pathways to the brain. Any damage to the outer and inner hair cells can cause permanent and irreversible hearing impairment (Mittal et al., 2015). Chronic cholecystoma and inflammatory granulation are an obstacle to surgical success in terms of hearing recovery due to the damage to bone tissue. Perioperative bleeding, hypertrophic lesions in the mucosa, adhesion tendency, and inadequate ventilation with a postoperative ventilation tube are among the negative factors for surgery (Wiatr et al., 2019). The goal of tympanoplasty is a healthy reconstruction of the tympanic cavity, closure of the perforation, and restoration of hearing. Post-aurical and endoaural approaches are techniques commonly used for this purpose (Yang et al., 2022).

Ossiculoplasty is a method used in cases of CSOM with or without cholesteatoma. It can be applied in one stage or in two stages. In single-stage ossiculoplasty, the aim is to prevent additional surgery and loss of time by performing the procedure in the same session after removing the middle ear infection. Various materials can be used to ensure ideal sound propagation and long-term stability for ideal recovery. Titanium, polycell, hydroxyapatite, and autologous cartilages are among these materials (Park et al., 2022).

It is very important to evaluate patient-related factors holistically in the perioperative period. Cochlear implants can cause various complications as a result of CSOM and previous middle ear surgeries (Lailach et al., 2021).

Conclusion

CSOM is still a serious health problem, especially in developing countries. Even in severe cases, early surgical treatment is an important option in preventing complications and providing a cure (Kirti et al., 2019). The ultimate goal of CSOM surgical treatment is to obtain a result that is well-ventilated, has a tympanic membrane with repaired perforation, is permanently dehydrated in terms of infectious and fluid, and hearing loss is corrected, and to achieve these in a way that is complication-free and does not allow a recurrence. To this end, treatment involves eliminating the pathogen and repairing or reconstructing existing damage. Age, gender, location, and size of the defect, and the condition of the ossicles and middle ear mucosa are very important factors affecting the success of this process. In this process, it is critical to make appropriate planning based on the techniques to be chosen for the operation and the experience of the surgeon (Cebeci et al., 2020).

References

Brescia, G., Frosolini, A., Franz, L., Daloiso, A., Fantin, F., Lovato, A., Filippis, C., & Marioni, G. (2023). Chronic Otitis Media in Patients with Chronic Rhinosinusitis: A Systematic Review. *Medicina (Kaunas)*, 59(1), 123. https://doi.org/10.3390/medicina59010123.

Bruchhage, K. L., Lupatsii, M., Möllenkolk, F., Leffers, D., Kurabi, A., Jürgens, T., Graspeuntner, S., Hollfelder, D., & Leichtle, A. (2023). Hearing rehabilitation and microbial shift after middle ear surgery with Vibrant Soundbridge in patients with chronic otitis media. *Eur Arch Otorhinolaryngol*, 280(7), 3107-3118. https://doi.org/10.1007/s00405-022-07795-9.

Cebeci, S., Özbilen, M. S., Bayramoğlu, I., Kemaloğlu, Y. K., Uygur, K. K., & Bayazit, Y. A. (2020). Impact of the demographic and aetiological factors and intraoperative findings on postoperative outcomes in chronic otitis media surgery. *Turk J Med Sci*, 50(1), 155-162. https://doi.org/10.3906/sag-1907-125.

Elzinga, H. B. E., van Oorschot, H. D., Stegeman, I., & Smit, A. L. (2021). Relation between otitis media and sensorineural hearing loss: a systematic review. *BMJ Open*, 11(8), e050108. https://doi.org/10.1136/bmjopen-2021-050108.

Harmes, K. M., Blackwood, R. A., Burrows, H. L., Cooke, J. M., Harrison, R. V., & Passamani, P. P. (2013). Otitis media: diagnosis and treatment. *Am Fam Physician*, 88(7), 435-440.

Heah, H., Soon, S. R., & Yuen, H. W. (2016). A case series of complicated infective otitis media requiring surgery in adults. *Singapore Med J*, 57(12), 681-685. https://doi.org/10.11622/smedj.2016025.

Kirti, Y. K., & Yashveer, J. K. (2019). Dilemmas in Current Management of Complicated Chronic Otitis Media. *Indian J Otolaryngol Head Neck Surg*, 71(2), 155-160. https://doi.org/10.1007/s12070-018-1334-3.

Lailach, S., Langanke, T., Zahnert, T., Garthus-Niegel, S., & Neudert, M. (2021). Impact of depressive disorders on quality of life after middle ear surgery in patients with chronic otitis media. *Eur Arch Otorhinolaryngol*, 278(9), 3217-3225. https://doi.org/10.1007/s00405-020-06397-7.

Lucidi, D., Cantaffa, C., Nocini, R., Martone, A., Alicandri-Ciufelli, M., & Marchioni, D. (2022). Quality of Life after Surgical Treatment for Chronic Otitis Media: A Systematic Review of the Literature. *J Pers Med*, 12(12), 1959. https://doi.org/10.3390/jpm12121959.

Mittal, R., Lisi, C. V., Gerring, R., Mittal, J., Mathee, K., Narasimhan, G., Azad, R. K., Yao, Q., Grati, M., Yan, D., Eshraghi, A. A., Angeli, S. I., Telischi, F. F., & Liu, X. Z. (2015). Current concepts in the pathogenesis and treatment of chronic suppurative otitis media. *J Med Microbiol*, 64(10), 1103-1116. https://doi.org/10.1099/jmm.0.000155.

Morris, P. (2012). Chronic suppurative otitis media. *BMJ Clinical Evidence*, 2012, 0507. PMID: 23870746; PMCID: PMC3412293.

Park, S., Lim, K. H., Lim, S. J., Park, D. H., Rah, Y. C., & Choi, J. (2022). Functional outcomes of single-stage ossiculoplasty in chronic otitis media with or without cholesteatoma. *Journal of International Advanced Otology*, 18(5), 415-419. https://doi.org/10.5152/iao.2022.21360. PMID: 35971270; PMCID: PMC9524377.

Schilder, A. G., Chonmaitree, T., Cripps, A. W., Rosenfeld, R. M., Casselbrant, M. L., Haggard, M. P., & Venekamp, R. P. (2016). Otitis media. *Nature Reviews Disease Primers*, 2(1), 16063. https://doi.org/10.1038/nrdp.2016.63.

Vincenti, V., Pasanisi, E., Bacciu, A., Bacciu, S., & Zini, C. (2014). Cochlear implantation in chronic otitis media and previous middle ear surgery: 20 years of experience. *Acta Otorhinolaryngologica Italica*, 34(4), 272-277. PMID: 25210222; PMCID: PMC4157528.

Wiatr, M., Skladzien, J., Strek, P., Przeklasa-Muszynska, A., & Wiatr, A. (2019). Chronic otitis media with granulation is a poor prognostic factor for hearing improvement and development of intracranial complications. *Journal of International Advanced Otology*, 15(1), 12-17. https://doi.org/10.5152/iao.2019.4786. PMID: 30924775; PMCID: PMC6483446.

Xia, A., Thai, A., Cao, Z., Chen, X., Chen, J., Bacacao, B., Bekale, L. A., Schiel, V., Bollyky, P. L., & Maria, P. L. S. (2022). Chronic suppurative otitis media causes macrophage-associated sensorineural hearing loss. *Journal of Neuroinflammation*, 19(1), 224. https://doi.org/10.1186/s12974-022-02585-w. PMID: 36096817; PMCID: PMC9465898.

Yang, Q., Wang, B., Zhang, J., Liu, H., Xu, M., & Zhang, W. (2022). Comparison of endoscopic and microscopic tympanoplasty in patients with chronic otitis media. *European Archives of Oto-Rhino-Laryngology*, 279(10), 4801-4807. https://doi.org/10.1007/s00405-022-07273-2. PMID: 35122510; PMCID: PMC9474537.

Chapter 23

Smoking Cessation

Hüseyin Can[1,*],
and Hilal Aksoy[2]
[1]Department of Family Medicine, İzmir Tınaztepe Univesity, Faculty of Medicine, Izmir, Turkey
[2]Department of Family Medicine, Hacettepe University, Faculty of Medicine, Ankara, Turkey

Abstract

Quitting smoking is a challenging process, but smoking cessation treatments can help make this process easier. A multimodal approach to smoking cessation is recommended. This includes cognitive and behavioral therapy with close follow-up and pharmacological treatment. The most effective approach to smoking cessation combines pharmacological treatment with behavioral therapy. There is sufficient evidence and Food and Drug Administration (FDA) approval for nicotine replacement therapy, bupropion, and varenicline in pharmacotherapy. Depending on the patient's condition, these medications are prioritized; if necessary, cytisine and second-line medications may also be preferred.

Keywords: smoking cessation, smoking cessation agents, nicotine replacement therapy, cognitive behavioral therapy, motivational interviewing

Introduction

Tobacco/nicotine addiction is a chronic condition that can frequently involve periods of quitting and relapsing, potentially leading to disability and death. It is distinguished from other addictions by a strong craving for smoke, inability to control the urge to smoke, and the appearance of mood disturbances (such as low mood, dysphoria, anxiety) and various physical/somatic symptoms (such as bradycardia, increased appetite) during periods of nicotine deprivation.

Nicotine addiction is examined in three dimensions: biological factors, environmental and social factors, and behavioral and psychological factors. In addition to genetic predisposition, smoking by family members and friends also increases the risk of nicotine addiction. When examining the neurobiology of addiction, nicotine is the substance primarily responsible. Nicotine, a psychoactive, lipophilic, and easily absorbed substance, exerts its effects through

* Corresponding Author's Email: drhuseyincan@hotmail.com.

In: Common Diseases According to Family Medicine Practice Guidelines
Editors: Esra Meltem Koç and Hilal Aksoy
ISBN: 979-8-89530-302-3

nicotinic acetylcholine receptors (nAChR). A single cigarette contains approximately 9-20 mg of nicotine, with a smoker absorbing about 10% of this amount (1-2 mg) (D'Souza & Markau, 2011). When a person experiencing withdrawal smokes, a single puff saturates 33% of nAChRs, three puffs saturate 75%, a full cigarette saturates 88%, and smoking 2.5-3 cigarettes saturates 95% of the nAChRs. As the saturation rate increases, the desire to smoke and the behavior of seeking cigarettes decrease, and the severity of withdrawal symptoms begins to decrease. A dependent person feels comfortable only after smoking 2.5-3 cigarettes (Brody et al., 2006). In chronic smokers, the number of nAChRs increases by 2-4 times (Perry et al., 2009). This increased receptor number does not change in the first 10 days after quitting smoking, but then gradually starts to decrease. This process takes approximately 2 weeks to 2 months. The response to treatment in the addiction treatment plan can only be observed after this period.

Tobacco use is a risk factor for cardiovascular and respiratory diseases, as well as more than twenty types of cancer. It is reported that more than 8 million people die each year due to tobacco use. It is also known that exposure to secondhand smoke leads to negative health outcomes and causes 1.2 million deaths annually (WHO Tobacco, 2024).

Nicotine addiction is classified under "Substance-Related Disorders" as "Tobacco Use Disorder" in the DSM-5. Nicotine in tobacco is highly addictive. Various policies are developed by health organizations, particularly the World Health Organization (WHO), to combat tobacco addiction (WHO, 2023).

Every physician should, during their professional activities, at least inquire whether their patient uses tobacco, strongly advise those who do to quit, and if the patient is willing, direct them to smoking cessation activities.

A multimodal approach is recommended for smoking cessation treatment. This includes evidence-based motivational strategies and counseling, evidence-based pharmacotherapy, and close follow-up with re-treatment if necessary. Combining pharmacological treatment with behavioral therapy is the most effective approach to quit smoking (Shields et al., 2023).

5A and 5R Concepts in Smoking Cessation Treatment

The 5A strategy is recommended for patients willing to attempt quitting, while the 5R strategy is suggested for those unwilling to quit.

The 5A approach to smoking cessation consists of five brief interventions:

A1. Ask: At every clinic visit, the patient's tobacco use status should always be inquired about and recorded. When they started smoking and the number of pack-years should be documented. The use of other tobacco products (pipe, cigar, hookah, etc.) should also be inquired about (Turkish Thoracic Society, 2014).

A2. Advise: Every smoker should be advised to quit. This advice should be clear, specific, strong, and personalized (Turkish Thoracic Society, 2014).

A3. Assess: For patients willing to quit, the reasons for their desire to quit should be reviewed, and their determination assessed. Nicotine dependence should be measured (preferably using the Fagerström test if possible), and carbon monoxide (CO) levels in the breath should be measured if feasible. If there is a history of previous quit attempts, experiences, difficulties faced, the longest period of abstinence, and the methods used in treatment should be reviewed (Turkish Thoracic Society, 2014).

A4. Assist: A quit plan should be prepared together with the patient. A mutual termination date should be established. The patient should be asked to share their decision to quit with their surroundings and to rearrange their environment to remove reminders of smoking. New daily activities that will enhance their resolve during the quitting period should be developed (U.S. Public Health Service Report, 2008).

Patients should be informed about how the medications will work, ensuring that they do not lose confidence in the medications and that while these will help reduce withdrawal symptoms, quitting ultimately depends on their own decision (Turkish Thoracic Society, 2014).

A5. Arrange: Patients should be followed up in person or by phone calls. The first follow-up should occur during the first week after the quit date. The second follow-up should be within the first month. Subsequent follow-ups can be scheduled biweekly, monthly, or quarterly, depending on the patient's condition. The difficulties encountered should be reviewed, and solutions suggested. If a relapse occurs, the reasons should be investigated, and a complete cessation should be aimed for again. Pharmacotherapy should be reviewed, and dose adjustments made if necessary (Turkish Thoracic Society, 2014).

The 5R strategies applied to patients who are unwilling to quit smoking are as follows:

R1. Relevance: The harms of smoking should be related to the patient's current illness and situation to encourage them to quit (Turkish Thoracic Society, 2014).

R2. Risks: Short-term (shortness of breath, respiratory infections, asthma exacerbation, impotence, infertility, fetal harm, etc.) and long-term (myocardial infarction, cerebrovascular events, cancers, chronic obstructive pulmonary disease, osteoporosis, etc.) risks of smoking should be clearly stated. Additionally, the harm that smoking causes not only to the individual but also to the environment should be mentioned. These include increased risks of lung cancer and heart disease in spouses, low birth weight in newborns, sudden infant death syndrome, and increased risks of asthma, otitis media, and respiratory infections in children (Turkish Thoracic Society, 2014).

R3. Rewards: The potential benefits of quitting smoking should be explained to the patient, including how their health will improve (Turkish Thoracic Society, 2014).

R4. Roadblocks: Potential obstacles to smoking cessation should be identified with the patient, and solutions should be sought. The patient should be provided with strategies to overcome these barriers (Turkish Thoracic Society, 2014).

R5. Repetition: Motivational support should be repeatedly provided to unwilling patients at each clinic visit. Patients who have tried and failed multiple times should be reassured that previous failures do not predict future outcomes and that quitting often takes several attempts (Turkish Thoracic Society, 2014).

Behavioral and Cognitive Methods in Smoking Cessation Treatment

Behavior change can be either a conscious and effortful choice of the individual or an unconscious change without effort. Public health interventions focus on environmental changes that lead individuals to alter their behaviors without being consciously aware of them. Not smoking in places where it is legally prohibited is a prime example of effortless change (Araz, 2016). Cognitive therapy primarily aims to identify the connections between emotions, thoughts, and behaviors, helping individuals interpret their experiences more realistically. Our thoughts about events, objects, and individuals determine our emotions, which in turn influence our behaviors (Ozdel, 2012).

Change in thoughts is crucial in smoking addiction. People who cannot alter their positive thoughts about smoking feel a sense of loss and deficiency when they quit, perceive themselves as punished and weak, envy smokers, and long for smoking. Consequently, these feelings typically lead to the resumption of smoking after a period. Conversely, a smoker with negative thoughts about smoking will experience fewer difficulties during the quitting process and have a lower risk of relapse. A person who thinks, "I am poisoning my body by smoking," "I am harming myself," "I will be healthier if I quit," will feel guilty when smoking, desire to quit, and feel happiness and self-confidence when they do quit. Behaviorally, they will avoid smoking and actively seek ways to quit (Kılınc, 2012).

Successful cognitive-behavioral therapy requires strong collaboration with the patient. Smoking habits should be thoroughly investigated. For instance, it is important to learn where, when, with whom, and under what circumstances the patient wants to smoke. Based on this information, behavior modification begins, and assignments are given to the patient. For example, a person who wants to smoke while driving is advised to pull over and smoke outside the car. Once this behavior is reinforced, the desire to smoke in the car diminishes. Smoking is often a habit linked to social events for individuals, and these associations must be addressed in treatment. If the patient smokes after every meal, we can suggest activities such as brushing teeth or exercising after meals (European Smoking Cessation Guidelines, 2013).

Smoking cessation requires a multifaceted treatment approach in which pharmacological therapy plays a critical role. Pharmacological treatments range from nicotine replacement therapies to nicotine receptor antagonists and antidepressants, encompassing a wide range of medications. Medications used for smoking cessation can be divided into two categories: first-line and second-line. First-line medications have been shown to be effective in the treatment of tobacco dependence, are very safe, and are approved by the Food and Drug Administration (FDA). Second-line medications have also been shown to be effective, but either do not have FDA approval or are suspected of having more side effects. Second-line medications are preferred when first-line medications cannot be used (European Smoking Cessation Guidelines, 2013).

Currently, there are three main groups of first-line medications used for smoking cessation: nicotine replacement therapies, bupropion, and varenicline.

Nicotine Replacement Therapy (NRT): Nicotine replacement therapy aims to eliminate nicotine withdrawal symptoms that occur during the period following smoking cessation. This treatment should be applied to individuals who have high or moderate nicotine dependence, those who smoke more than 15 cigarettes a day, or those who, despite having mild dependence, have not benefited from other smoking cessation methods. It is essential to completely stop smoking during the treatment. Currently used forms of nicotine include gum, lozenges, nasal sprays, oral inhalers, sublingual tablets, and transdermal patches. NRT medications are typically reduced and discontinued over a period of 2-8 weeks, with a concurrent reduction in nicotine withdrawal symptoms. The duration of NRT varies depending on the form used, ranging from 3 to 12 months. In cases of treatment failure or when nicotine withdrawal symptoms are not adequately controlled, combination therapy may be used. The most common combination is the patch and gum. NRT should not be used during pregnancy, while breast-feeding, by individuals under 18 years old, those who have had an acute myocardial infarction in the last six weeks, those with unstable angina pectoris, or those with arrhythmias. The patch form is also not recommended for individuals with persistent skin conditions such as psoriasis and eczema (Turkish Thoracic Society, 2014).

Bupropion: Bupropion is a non-tricyclic, aminoketone antidepressant agent with noradrenergic and dopaminergic activity. It is a weak inhibitor of norepinephrine and dopamine reuptake, which helps reduce nicotine withdrawal symptoms. Bupropion is available in 150 mg tablets, and the treatment involves taking 300 mg per day for eight weeks, although it can be extended up to six months. Treatment with bupropion should begin before quitting smoking: 150 mg for the first three days, then 300 mg (150 mg twice a day) from the fourth day onward, with a target quit date set within 7-14 days. The most common side effects are headache, insomnia, and dry mouth. Caution is needed with drugs metabolized in the liver due to potential interactions. Contraindications for bupropion use include individuals with a history of seizures or taking medications that lower the seizure threshold, those with central nervous system (CNS) trauma, a history of monoamine oxidase (MAO) inhibitor use, uncontrolled hypertension, severe hepatic necrosis, eating disorders such as anorexia or bulimia, those under 18, pregnant women, those with hypersensitivity to bupropion, CNS tumors, bipolar patients, and those with severe cirrhosis. In the cases of severe withdrawal symptoms or failure of monotherapy, NRT and bupropion can be combined (Turkish Thoracic Society, 2014).

Varenicline: Varenicline works by binding to the $\alpha 4\beta 2$ nicotinic receptors in the central nervous system, reducing symptoms associated with nicotine withdrawal. The treatment starts with a dose of 0.5 mg per day for the first three days, followed by 0.5 mg twice a day on days 4 to 7, and then 1 mg twice a day on days 8 to 14. Patients initially continue smoking while on the medication, aiming to quit between days 8 and 14, preferably by the end of the first week. The treatment is completed over 12 weeks with a dose of 1 mg twice daily. Varenicline can cause drowsiness, with side effects including mild to moderate nausea, insomnia, and abnormal dreams (Turkish Thoracic Society, 2014). Contraindications to varenicline include allergy to the drug, pregnancy, breastfeeding, and end-stage renal disease (European Smoking Cessation Guidelines, 2013).

Cytisine: Cytisine is a natural alkaloid extracted from the seeds of plants such as Cytisus laburnum and Sophora tetraptera. It acts as a partial agonist on the $\alpha 4\beta 2$ nicotinic acetylcholine receptors in the central nervous system and prevents nicotine from binding to these receptors. Cytisine is historically the first officially approved medication for smoking cessation. However, due to limited clinical studies, its use is restricted in some countries. The treatment starts with one tablet (1.5 mg) every two hours from days 1 to 3 (up to six tablets per day). During this period, smoking should be reduced to avoid nicotine overdose symptoms. If the desired effect is not achieved, the treatment should be discontinued and retried after two to three months. If a positive response is observed, the patient should continue the treatment with up to five tablets per day (one tablet every 2.5 hours) from days 4 to 12, with smoking cessation on the fifth day. From days 13 to 16, four tablets per day (one tablet every three hours), then three tablets per day (one tablet every five hours) from days 17 to 20, and finally one or two tablets per day (one tablet every six to eight hours) from days 21 to 25, after which the medication is discontinued (European Smoking Cessation Guidelines, 2013).

Clonidine: Clonidine reduces central sympathetic activity by stimulating α2-adrenergic receptors. However, it is not FDA-approved for smoking cessation and is only used as a second-line treatment. Clonidine effectively suppresses nicotine withdrawal symptoms such as tension, irritability, anxiety, cravings, and restlessness. It is available in oral or transdermal (TD) forms. Clonidine treatment should start just before (up to three days) or on the quit day. The typical starting dose is 0.10 mg twice daily orally or 0.10 mg per day of TD, with weekly dose increases of 0.10 mg if necessary. The duration of treatment ranges from 3 to 10 weeks. Common side effects include orthostatic hypotension, dry mouth, drowsiness, dizziness, sedation, and constipation. Contraindications to clonidine include pregnancy and breastfeeding (European Smoking Cessation Guidelines, 2013).

Nortriptyline: Nortriptyline is a tricyclic antidepressant that has been shown to be as effective as bupropion and NRT for smoking cessation. It is not FDA-approved for smoking cessation and is recommended only as a second-line treatment. Side effects include dry mouth, blurred vision, constipation, urinary retention, sedation, drowsiness, weight gain, and orthostatic hypotension. It is contraindicated in patients with cardiovascular disease, pregnant women, and those under 18 years old. Patients should start nortriptyline while still smoking, with a quit date set 10 to 28 days later. The starting dose is 25 mg per day, gradually increasing to 75-100 mg per day over 10 days to 5 weeks. The maximum dose is maintained for 8-12 weeks, after which the medication is reduced (European Smoking Cessation Guidelines, 2013).

Follow-Up During Smoking Cessation

Relapse is common among individuals who have quit smoking or are in the process of quitting, particularly within the first few months and frequently within the first year. Therefore, follow-up during the first year after quitting smoking is crucial. These follow-ups are conducted not only to prevent relapse but also to monitor nicotine withdrawal symptoms, assess the side effects and effectiveness of pharmacotherapy, address any other problems the patient may be experiencing, and check for any lapses in smoking.

Groups at high risk of relapse include young people, those with many smokers in their family and social circles, individuals with high alcohol consumption, and those with lower education levels (Turkish Thoracic Society, 2014).

Research indicates that the first two weeks post-cessation are the most intense period for nicotine withdrawal symptoms. Therefore, it is recommended that two patient consultations be held in the first month after quitting. If the patient cannot attend in person, a phone consultation is suggested. During consultations, physicians should not be judgmental or impatient and should help the patient learn from their mistakes (Fiore, 2008). The frequency of consultations should be monthly up to three months after quitting, and then every three months, with follow-up lasting at least one year. However, follow-up visits should be tailored to the individual needs of each patient (Turkish Thoracic Society, 2014).

Common Problems During Smoking Cessation

Anxiety, tension, insomnia, difficulty concentrating, fatigue, irritability, headaches, constipation, tremors, inappropriate emotional responses, decreased appetite, and dry mouth are common issues during the smoking cessation period. It should be emphasized that these issues are temporary and can occur in many individuals. To relieve tension and depressive moods, activities such as taking a shower, walking, exercising, listening to music, and engaging in hobbies can be relaxing. For insomnia and headaches, reducing caffeine intake in the evenings, taking warm showers, and drinking warm milk or herbal teas can be beneficial. Drinking water and chewing gum can help relieve dry mouth.

In managing the urge to smoke, it is important to remind individuals that the desire to smoke will decrease as the smoke-free periods lengthen. Keeping oneself busy, avoiding situations that encourage smoking, and exercising are recommended strategies (Turkish Thoracic Society, 2014).

Conclusion

When assessing addiction, it is essential to take a detailed history of the patient/client, determine the level of nicotine dependence using a dependence scale such as the Fagerström test, and conduct appropriate physical examinations and laboratory evaluations (e.g., ECG, SFT, PAAC graph, breath carbon monoxide measurement, etc.). It should always be kept in mind that nicotine addiction is a multifaceted condition and that the patient/client needs to be assessed holistically.

In addition to motivational interviewing and behavioral therapy, pharmacological treatment is also used in smoking cessation. However, the cessation process is challenging for both the patient and the clinician and requires close cooperation. All smokers should receive appropriate and adequate counseling during this process. Furthermore, effective pharmacological adjunctive treatments should be provided that are proven to be effective and appropriate for the individual, taking into account contraindications and side effects.

References

Araz, A. (2016). Sağlığın geliştirilmesi: Sağlık davranışlarını değiştirmek [Health promotion: Changing health behaviors]. In G. Dirik (Ed.), *Sağlık psikolojisi* (1st ed., pp. 181-211). Nobel Akademik Yayıncılık.

Avrupa Sigara Bırakma Klavuzu. (2013). A. Karalezli & Ş. Börekçi (Eds.), (1st ed., pp. 55-77). Türkiye Solunum Araştırmaları Derneği.

Brody, A. L., Mandelkern, M. A., London, E. D., Olmstead, R. E., Farahi, J., Scheibal, D., Jou, J., Allen, V., Tiongson, E., Chefer, S. I., Koren, A. O., & Mukhin, A. G. (2006). Cigarette smoking saturates brain alpha 4 beta 2 nicotinic acetylcholine receptors. *Archives of General Psychiatry, 63*(8), 907–915. https://doi.org/10.1001/archpsyc.63.8

D'Souza, M., & Markau, A. (2011). Neuronal mechanisms underlying development of nicotine dependence: Implications for novel smoking-cessation treatments. *Addiction Science & Clinical Medicine, July*, 4-15.

Fiore, M. (2008). United States. Tobacco use and dependence guideline panel. *Treating tobacco use and dependence: 2008 update*. Rockville (MD): US Department of Health and Human Services, Public Health Service.

Kılınç, O. (2012). Sigara bırakma tedavisinde davranışçı ve bilişsel yöntemler [Behavioral and cognitive methods in smoking cessation treatment]. *Turkiye Klinikleri J Pulm Med-Special Topics, 5*(2).

Özdel, K. (2015). Dünden bugüne bilişsel davranışçı terapiler: Teori ve uygulama [Cognitive-behavioral therapies from past to present: Theory and practice]. *Turkiye Klinikleri J Psychiatry-Special Topics, 8*(2).

Perry, D. C., Dávila-García, M. I., Stockmeier, C. A., & Kellar, K. J. (1999). Increased nicotinic receptors in brains from smokers: Membrane binding and autoradiography studies. *The Journal of Pharmacology and Experimental Therapeutics, 289*(3), 1545–1552.

Shields, P. G., Bierut, L., Arenberg, D., Balis, D., Cinciripini, P. M., Davis, J., ... & Darlow, S. (2023). Smoking cessation, version 3.2022, NCCN clinical practice guidelines in oncology. *Journal of the National Comprehensive Cancer Network, 21*(3), 297-322.

Turkish Thoracic Society. (2014). Tütün Kontrolü Çalışma Grubu: Sigara bırakma tanı ve tedavi uzlaşı raporu [Tobacco Control Working Group: Smoking cessation diagnosis and treatment consensus report].

U.S. Public Health Service Report. (2008). The clinical practice guideline treating tobacco use and dependence 2008 update panel, liaisons, and staff. *American Journal of Preventive Medicine, 35*(2), 158–176.

WHO Report on the Global Tobacco Epidemic. (2023). Retrieved from https://www.who.int/teams/health-promotion/tobacco-control (accessed on 30.05.2024).

WHO. *Tobacco*. (2024). Retrieved from https://www.who.int/publications/ (accessed on 30.05.2024).

Chapter 24

Immunizations

Ecenur Patoglu Sarcak*, MD
Agrı 6th Family Health Center, Agrı, Turkey

Abstract

Vaccination is an essential component of public health, serving as a crucial defense against a wide variety of contagious diseases. In this chapter, we undertake a comprehensive review of vaccines, including their recommended administration schedules and the critical functions that healthcare professionals perform during the immunization process.

Keywords: vaccination, immunization, public health, infectious disease, healthcare providers, immunization schedule

Introduction

Immunization, which originates from the Greek word 'immune,' which means "protected," denotes the development of immunity subsequent to the introduction of exogenous antibodies or antigens. Moreover, vaccination is a highly efficient and economically viable approach to improve child survival rates and mitigate the incidence of illness, thus gaining financial advantages, preventing lasting impairments, and fostering productivity (Shukla & Shah, 2018; WHO, 2023). There are several types of vaccinations, including live attenuated vaccines such as oral polio vaccines, varicella vaccines, and measles vaccines. Inactivated whole cell vaccines include the inactivated polio vaccine, the pertussis vaccine, the rabies vaccine, and the whole cell typhoid vaccine. Modified exotoxin vaccines, known as toxoids, consist of diphtheria toxoid and tetanus toxoid. Antigen subunit vaccinations encompass Haemophilus influenza type b, Salmonella typhi polysaccharide antigen, and hepatitis B surface antigen (Shukla & Shah, 2018; WHO, 2023).

---

* Corresponding Author's Email: ecenurpatoglu@gmail.com.

In: Common Diseases According to Family Medicine Practice Guidelines
Editors: Esra Meltem Koç and Hilal Aksoy
ISBN: 979-8-89530-302-3

Table 1. WHO Recommendations for Immunization Programs

Antigen		Children	Adolescents	Adults	Considerations
Recommendations for all immunization programs					
BCG		1 dose			Although it is not included by the regular immunization schedules in the USA and the UK, universal BCG vaccination at birth is advised in areas with high rates of leprosy and tuberculosis.
Hepatitis B		3-4-doses	3 doses (for high-risk groups if not previously immunized)		Birth dose Premature and low birth weight Co-administration and combination vaccine Definition high-risk
Polio		3-5 doses (at least 2 doses of IPV) with DTPCV			bOPV birth dose; Type of vaccine; Fractional dose IPV; Transmission and importation risk; Local epidemiology, programmatic implications, and feasibility for "early" option
DTP-containing vaccine (DTPCV)		3 doses; 2 boosters 12-23 months (DTPCV) and 4-7 years	1 booster 9-15 yrs (Td)		Delayed/interrupted schedule Combination vaccine Maternal immunization
Haemophilus influenzae type b	Option 1	3 doses, with DTPCV			Single dose if > 12 months of age, Not recommended for children > 5 yrs old, Delayed/interrupted schedule Co-administration and combination vaccine
	Option 2	2 or 3 doses, with a booster at least 6 months after the last dose			
Pneumococcal (Conjugate)	Option 1	3 primary doses (3p+0) with DTPCV			Schedule options (3p+0 vs 2p+1) Vaccine options, HIV+ and preterm neonate booster, Vaccination in older adults
	Option 2	2 primary doses plus booster dose at 9-18 months of age (2p+1) with DTPCV			
Rotavirus		2-3 doses depending on the product with DTPCV			Not recommended if > 24 months old
Measles		2 doses			Co-administration live vaccines; Combination vaccine; HIV early vaccination; Pregnancy
Rubella		1 dose	1 dose (adolescent girls and women of reproductive age if not previously vaccinated)		Target 9-14 year old girls; Off-label 1 dose schedule; MACs with intro; Pregnancy; HIV and immunocompromised
HPV			1-2 doses (females)		Target 9-14 year old girls; Off-label 1 dose schedule; MACs with intro; Pregnancy; HIV and immunocompromised

Table 2. WHO Recommendations for Immunization Programs Part 2

Antigen	Children	Adolescents	Adults	Considerations
Recommendations for certain regions				
Japanese Encephalitis	*Inactivated Vero cell-derived vaccine:* generally 2 doses *Live attenuated vaccine:* 1 dose *Live recombinant vaccine:* 1 dose			Co-administration live vaccines; Vaccine options and manufacturer's recommendations; Pregnancy; Immunocompromised
Yellow Fever	1 dose, with measles containing vaccine			Co-administration live vaccines
Tick-Borne Encephalitis[13]	3 doses (> 1 yr FSME-Immun and Encepur; > 3 yrs TBE-Moscow and EnceVir) with at least 1 booster dose (every 3 years for TBE-Moscow and EnceVir)			Definition of high-risk Vaccine options Timing of booster
Recommendations for some high-risk populations				
Typhoid	*Typhoid conjugate vaccine (Typbar-TCV®):* 1 dose*; Vi polysaccharide(ViPS):* 1 dose*; Ty21a live oral vaccine:* 3-4 doses ; *Revaccination for ViPS & Ty21a; every 3-7 years*			Definition of high-risk Vaccine options
Cholera	*Dukoral (WC-rBS)*: 3 doses ≥ 2-5 yrs, booster every 6 months; 2 doses adults/children ≥ 6 yrs, booster every 2nd year; *Shanchol, Euvchol & mORCVAX*: 2 doses ≥1 yrs, booster dose after 2 yrs			Minimum age Definition of high-risk
Meningococcal – MenA conjugate	1 dose 9-18 months (5 μg)			2 doses if < 9 months with 8 week interval
Meningococcal – MenC conjugate	2 doses (2-11 months) with booster 1 year after 1 dose (≥12 months)			Definition of high-risk; Vaccine options
Meningococcal – Quadrivalent conjugate	2 doses (9-23 months) 1 dose (≥2 years)			
Hepatitis A	Inactivated: 1 or 2 doses ≥ 12 months Live attenuated: 1 dose >18 months of age		Inactivated: 2 doses if > 40 years of age	Level of endemicity; Vaccine options; Definition of high risk groups
Rabies	2 doses			PrEP vs PEP; definition of high risk; booster
Dengue (CYD-TDV)	3 doses 9-45 years of age			Minimize risk of vaccine among seronegative individuals by pre-vaccination screening; Pregnancy & lactation
Malaria (RTS,S)	4 doses			Moderate to high malaria transmission; Strategy for highly seasonal transmission, see notes at WHO

Antigen	Children	Adolescents	Adults	Considerations
Recommendations for immunization programs with certain characteristics				
Mumps	2 doses, with measles containing vaccine			Coverage criteria > 80% Combination vaccine
Seasonal influenza (inactivated tri-and quadri-valent)	First vaccine use: 2 doses Revaccinate annually: 1 dose only	1 dose $\geq$ 9 years of age	Revaccinate annually	Priority risk groups
Varicella	1-2 doses	2 doses		Achieve & sustain $\geq$ 80% coverage of Pregnancy Co-administration with other live vaccines

The data for these tables were compiled using information from both the CDC and the WHO, as indicated by the sources: https://www.cdc.gov/vaccines/vpd/index.html and https://www.who.int/teams/immunization-vaccines-and-biologicals/policies/who-recommendations-for-routine-immunization-summary-tables (Organization, 2023b; Prevention, 2023i).

Vaccination has emerged as an indispensable healthcare intervention ever since the original smallpox vaccine was developed by Edward Jenner in 1796; it has since been responsible for the preservation of millions of lives. Despite progress, the prevalence of avoidable infectious diseases persists. Vaccines reduce the likelihood of contracting a disease by collaborating with the body's natural defenses to construct immunity. Upon the administration of a vaccine, the immune system will react. More than twenty life-threatening diseases can now be prevented with vaccines, allowing individuals of all ages to live longer and healthier lives. Currently, between 3.5 and 5 million annual fatalities are averted by immunization against diseases such as influenza, tetanus, diphtheria, and measles (Shukla & Shah, 2018; WHO, 2023).

General Rules for Vaccination

To ensure optimal protection, clinicians should vaccinate their patients with proper timing according to guidelines. Universal vaccination schedules and recommendations can be found on the Centers for Disease Control and Prevention (CDC) website and the World Health Organization (WHO) website. These resources provide crucial information guiding healthcare professionals and patients on when and which vaccines should be administered, ultimately enhancing protection against diseases (South-Paul & Matheny, 2020).

Physicians should educate parents regarding the vaccine's composition, dosage, disease prevention, potential adverse reactions, and follow-up schedules during each vaccination visit. It is recommended that they provide a comprehensive explanation of disease risk and vaccine efficacy, with particular emphasis on the fact that complications are more prevalent among younger age groups. Although significant adverse effects are uncommon, vaccinations are generally safe, and the benefit outweighs the risk. While cost may be a factor for parents to consider when selecting vaccines, doctors should emphasize that all vaccines are effective. Before administering immunizations, physicians should also seek parental consent and provide detailed explanations of potential adverse effects and their frequency (Shukla & Shah, 2018).

The extension of the interval between vaccination doses does not need for the restart of the vaccine series, however, it is advised that a dose should not be administered more than four days prior to the required age (South-Paul & Matheny, 2020). It is imperative for physicians to diligently document the vaccination details and any adverse reactions in the medical records of their patients. It is important to document and report any adverse reactions to health authorities and vaccination producers. It is important to have readily accessible resuscitative equipment and to consult with knowledgeable professionals in the event of serious responses. The concurrent administration of numerous vaccinations is possible; however, it is recommended to observe a suggested gap of four to eight weeks between doses. The use of combination vaccinations is generally favored over the administration of individual vaccine components, and it is recommended to provide age-appropriate re-immunization as needed (Shukla & Shah, 2018) (Table 1).

Hepatitis B Vaccine

Hepatitis B (HepB) is transmitted to the liver by the hepatitis B virus (HBV), which can result in hepatocellular carcinoma and chronic liver disease. HBV constitutes a significant global public health concern, as it induces substantial morbidity and mortality. Hepatitis B vaccines are the most effective, secure, and cost-effective instruments currently available to maintain control and prevent the disease. Global coverage for three doses of the hepatitis B vaccine increased to 85% in 2019 from approximately 30% in 2000. Hepatitis B-related morbidity and mortality have decreased significantly as a consequence of the successful implementation of hepatitis B vaccination programs (Pattyn et al., 2021).

A three-dose regimen of the hepatitis B vaccine (HepB) is recommended beginning at the time of birth. In infants whose mothers are hepatitis B surface antigen (HBsAg)-positive or whose hepatitis B immune status is unknown, the birth dose and hepatitis B immunoglobulin are crucial. The hepatitis B vaccine schedule suggests that the initial dose is administered to all neonates within 24 hours of birth, the second dose is administered every 1 to 2 months with a minimum 4-week interval between doses, and the third dose is administered between 6 and 18 months of age, with an 8-week interval between doses. A 4-dose schedule is permissible when the DTaP-HepB-IPV combination vaccine is administered; this schedule consists of the stand-alone hepatitis B vaccine administered at birth and the combination vaccine for the subsequent 3 doses (Kliegman, 2020).

HepB vaccination is quite effective, with more than 95% of children becoming seropositive after the third dosage. Unless the mother is HBsAg-positive or has uncertain HBsAg status, preterm babies weighing 2 kg should be postponed until 1 month of age or hospital release. The Hepatitis B vaccine produces 3-9% discomfort at the injection site, 8-18% minor systemic side effects, and a 1-6% elevation in temperature over 37.7°C. It has no effect on the immune system or causes diabetes (Kliegman, 2020). The USA HBV vaccination policy calls for routine monovalent HepB vaccination for newborns within 24 hours of birth, catch-up immunization for adolescents who have not received all recommended vaccinations, and immunization for unvaccinated adults with diabetes mellitus between the ages of 19 and 59 as soon as a diagnosis is made. In addition to hepatitis B surface antibody (anti-HBs) and HBsAg testing at ages 9 to 18 months for infants born to HBsAg-positive mothers and anti-HBs for healthcare professionals, post-vaccination testing is not recommended. A titer of 10 mIU/mL is considered an acceptable response to HBs. Serum antibody levels that are low or nonexistent do not reliably indicate HBV vulnerability. Most vaccinated individuals can induce a protective anamnestic immune response due to immunologic memory and the extended incubation time. Higher antigen-content vaccinations, however, are required in cases of renal failure requiring dialysis to maintain an annual measurement of 10 mIU/mL for antibodies (Kliegman, 2020).

Hepatitis A Vaccine

Hepatitis A is not a mild disease. The cumulative number of reported cases during the years 2016 to February 7, 2020, amounted to 31,093, of which 18,989 individuals were hospitalized (61% of the total cases), and there were 314 recorded fatalities in the United States (South-Paul

& Matheny, 2020). The escalation can be attributed to significant factors such as homelessness and substance abuse.

Hepatitis A vaccine, which is approved for use in children 12 months old, is recommended for use in all children aged 12 to 23 months, as well as some high-risk populations. The two dosages in the series should be at least 6 months apart. Children who have received one dose of hepatitis A vaccination before the age of 24 months should receive a second dose 6-18 months later. If protection against hepatitis A infection is desired, 2 doses of vaccination separated by 6-18 months can be delivered to anyone 2 years or older who has not yet received the series of 2-dose hepatitis A vaccine. This is especially critical for persons with chronic liver illness, clotting factor problems, males who have sex with men, injection or non-injection drug use, homelessness, people who have been exposed to the hepatitis A virus at work, travel, and those who have had intimate contact with foreign adoptees. Infants aged 6 to 11 months should receive one dose of hepatitis A vaccination prior to any overseas travel. Beginning at 12 months of age, these children should be revaccinated with the generally recommended two doses of hepatitis A vaccination. Before foreign travel to countries with high or moderate endemic hepatitis A, unvaccinated children 12 months and older should receive two doses; the second dosage should be delivered at least six months following the first dose (Kliegman, 2020).

Pertussis Vaccine

Caused by Bordetella pertussis and B. parapertussis, pertussis, often referred to as "whooping cough," is an extremely contagious brief respiratory illness. In the initial half of the 20th century, it constituted a significant contributor to morbidity and mortality among children. Although the incidence of the disease decreased substantially following vaccination, it never reached complete eradication, with epidemic peaks transpiring every two to three years. Recently, even nations with high rates of early childhood immunization have witnessed an increase in pertussis cases (Cherry, 1984; Mattoo & Cherry, 2005; Nieves & Heininger, 2016; Prevention, 2023d). In the year 2018, the global incidence of pertussis exceeded 151,000 reported cases (Organization, 2023a). Pertussis is transmitted through respiratory particles or contact with newly contaminated objects; After exposure, 70–100% of susceptible household contacts and 50–80% of susceptible school personnel become infected. From one week following exposure to three weeks following the onset of symptoms, contamination persists. The main sources of pertussis infection in young infants are adults, including healthcare workers and adolescents (South-Paul & Matheny, 2020). Severe cough and malaise can interfere with daily activities. Complications include seizures and pneumonia, which are the primary cause of mortality. In 1% of cases, cerebral hemorrhages or hypoxia can result in encephalopathy, with one-third being fatal and one-third causing permanent brain injury (Nieves & Heininger, 2016; South-Paul & Matheny, 2020).

Pertussis vaccination should be administered to all children at 2, 4, and 6 months of age, with supplemental doses at 15-18 months and 4-6 years (a total of five doses; maximum age of 6 years). A supplemental dose of the DTaP vaccine is not required if the fourth dose was administered to a child aged four years or older. All currently accessible pertussis-containing vaccines also provide protection against diphtheria and tetanus. The effectiveness of DTaP vaccines varies between 80% and 89%; however, its effectiveness decreases with time. Each adult and adolescent should be administered one-lifetime dose of Tdap. Regardless of prior

Tdap administration, the Advisory Committee on Immunization Practices (ACIP) advises a Tdap dose during each pregnancy, preferably between weeks 27 and 36 of gestation. The CDC has authorized the substitution of the Tdap vaccine for tetanus, and diphtheria (Td) can be administered as the 10-year booster for tetanus protection in 2019 (Kliegman, 2020; Prevention, 2023h; South-Paul & Matheny, 2020).

Diphtheria and Tetanus

These two uncommon yet perilous illnesses require vaccination for all individuals. Tetanus induces severe muscle stiffness. Severe health complications can result from tetanus, including difficulty inhaling, trouble swallowing, or even mortality. Diphtheria can result in cardiac failure, death, paralysis, or difficulty breathing. The regular diphtheria, tetanus, and pertussis (DTaP) immunization schedule involves five doses of the DTaP vaccine provided to children between the ages of 2, 4, 6, and 15-18 months. The fourth dosage can be given as soon as 12 months after the third dose, as long as at least 6 months have passed after the third dose. If the fourth dosage was given at the age of four or older, the booster dose is not required. Even if a dosage was delivered unintentionally or as part of a catch-up series at 7-10 years, adolescents aged 11-12 years should receive one adult Tdap dose (Kliegman, 2020; South-Paul & Matheny, 2020).

It is recommended that individuals who are pregnant receive a single dose of the Tdap vaccine throughout each pregnancy, ideally administered in the early stages of the third trimester. This measure is intended to provide protection to the infant against pertussis. Pertussis poses the greatest risk of serious and perhaps life-threatening consequences in infants. It is recommended that those who have not previously received the Tdap vaccine should receive a single dose of Tdap. Additionally, it is recommended that people have a booster vaccination every 10 years, either with Tdap or Td, the latter being a vaccine that provides protection against tetanus and diphtheria, but not pertussis. In the event of a serious or contaminated lesion or burn, the interval for receiving a booster dose should be reduced to 5 years (Prevention, 2023h).

Pneumococcal Conjugate Vaccine

Before the implementation of the pneumococcal conjugate vaccine, Streptococcus pneumoniae, a gram-positive diplococcus with more than 90 distinct polysaccharide capsules, was responsible for approximately 17,000 instances of invasive disease per year in the United States. These cases included bacteremia, meningitis, or infection at sites that are typically sterile. Among children under the age of five, this resulted in an annual mortality rate of 200. Infection can be transmitted by respiratory tract droplets. Streptococcus pneumoniae continues to be a prevalent etiological agent of community-acquired pneumonia, sinusitis, otitis media, and bacterial meningitis (South-Paul & Matheny, 2020).

The 13-valent pneumococcal conjugate vaccine (PCV13), marketed under the brand name Prevnar13, and the 23-valent pneumococcal polysaccharide vaccine (PPSV23), commonly known as Pneumovax23, are the two primary forms of pneumococcal vaccines. PPSV23 provides coverage for 23 pneumococcal serotypes, whereas PCV13 provides protection against

13 distinct serotypes. Additionally, vaccines with a wider serotype coverage, such as PCV20 and PCV15, have been developed more recently.

Vaccination regimens and practices for pneumococcal vaccinations may differ from country to country. The United Kingdom, for example, advises a single dosage of PPV13 (Prevenar) at 12 weeks and 1 year of age. The Centers for Disease Control and Prevention (CDC) in the United States, on the other hand, recommends PCV15 or PCV20 vaccinations for newborns, given in a course of four doses at 2 months, 4 months, 6 months, and 12-15 months of age. Individuals aged 65 and older may have a different immunization regimen based on their past vaccination history. Each country's health authorities develop their own immunization guidelines and schedules. As a result, it is essential to follow the immunization schedule and protocols established by local health authorities, while considering the patient's age, medical history, and area standards (Excellence, 2023a; Prevention, 2023e).

Haemophilus Influenza Type B Vaccination

Haemophilus influenzae type b (Hib) is a prevalent cause of serious diseases in children worldwide, causing pneumonia, meningitis, and other infections. Despite its prevalence, highly effective protein-polysaccharide conjugated Hib vaccines have almost completely eliminated the disease in both developed and developing countries. These vaccines also reduce asymptomatic nasopharyngeal carriage and significantly protect unvaccinated individuals, even with moderate vaccine coverage (40-50%) (Watt et al., 2009).

Three different types of single-antigen Hib vaccines are approved for use. The PRP-T vaccine, which is linked to tetanus toxoid, should be given four times, at 2, 4, 6, and 12 through 15 months of age. The PRP-OMP vaccine, which is linked to meningococcal outer membrane protein, should be given three times, at 2, 4, and 12 through 15 months of age. The third Hib vaccine can be used as a booster shot for children ages 15 months through 4 years. Along with single-antigen Hib combination vaccines, Hib is a part of a number of other vaccines (Kliegman, 2020).

Poliovirus Vaccine

Despite the fact that the worldwide incidence of cases has decreased by over 99% since eradication efforts began in 1988, when an estimated 350,000 people were rendered paralyzed by wild polio viruses (WPVs), a few hundred cases of paralysis caused by WPVs continue to occur annually (416 cases in 2013 and 359 cases in 2014) (17,18). Wild poliovirus comes in three different types: type 1, type 2, and type 3. Each has a slightly different capsid protein. The last case of type 2 wild poliovirus was found in India in 1999, and it was declared extinct in September 2015. In October 2019, it was announced that type 3 wild poliovirus was no longer present. The last time it was seen was in November 2012. There is still only type 1 wild poliovirus left (Initiative, 2023).

The instruments used to eradicate the wild polio virus include the live attenuated oral polio vaccine (OPV) and the inactivated polio vaccine (IPV). IPV should be given at 2, 4, and 6 through 18 months of age, with a booster dose at 4 to 6 years of age. The final dose in the series should be given at or after the age of 4 years and at least 6 months after the previous dose. The last dosage in the IPV series should be given to children aged 4 years or older, regardless of the number of prior doses, and the minimum interval between doses 3 and 4 is 6 months. The total number of doses required to complete a series containing oral polio vaccine (OPV) is the same as that advised for the US IPV schedule (Bandyopadhyay et al., 2015; Kliegman, 2020).

Influenza Vaccine

During the flu season, hospitalizations and deaths from pneumonia and flu complications increase. Primary viral pneumonia, subsequent bacterial pneumonia, increasing chronic respiratory and heart diseases, sinusitis, otitis media, and Reye syndrome put preschoolers at risk. Children are at increased risk of developing encephalopathy and dying. The influenza is very infectious and spreads through the air. Because of the virus's capacity to evade immunity, it is a persistent threat. As a result, influenza vaccinations should be given once a year (Kim et al., 2018; Kliegman, 2020; South-Paul & Matheny, 2020).

The influenza vaccination is advised for everyone starting at the age of six months, with a minimum age of six months for inactivated influenza vaccine (IIVs) and 24 months for the live attenuated influenza vaccine (LAIV). The FDA has approved several influenza vaccine formulations for various age groups. Children aged 6 months to 8 years who are getting vaccinated for the first time should have two doses at least four weeks apart. If such youngsters only had one dosage of IIV the previous season, they would need two doses the next season. The influenza vaccine is typically administered in October or November, but there are benefits even when administered as late as February or March, because influenza seasons typically peak in February. For comprehensive information on influenza vaccination dosages, age-specific recommendations, contraindications, and the range of available vaccines, please refer to the following website: https://www.cdc.gov/flu/professionals/acip/summary/summary-recommendations.htm#recommend (Prevention, 2023f).

Measles, Mumps, & Rubella Vaccine

The highly contagious diseases measles, mumps, and rubella (MMR) are caused by viral pathogens and can cause fatalities, as well as major complications, sequelae, and congenital abnormalities (CAs) (Lievano et al., 2012). Measles may cause severe morbidity and, in rare instances, fatal encephalopathy. Measles outbreaks usually start in unvaccinated populations. Infected people might be spreading measles from four days before to four days after the rash appears. Mumps may induce severe bilateral parotitis, which causes excruciating agony, as well as high-fatality disorders including pancreatitis and cerebellar ataxia. Rubella, on the other hand, if infected during pregnancy, can result in severe congenital rubella syndrome. As a result, MMR (Measles, Mumps, and Rubella) immunizations are critical to avoid the spread of these illnesses and minimize their severe consequences (South-Paul & Matheny, 2020).

MMR should be administered between the ages of 12 and 15 months, with a subsequent dose between 4 and 6 years. Before all international travel, one dose of the MMR vaccine should be administered to infants aged 6 to 11 months. Commencing at 12 months of age, these children should be revaccinated with the two doses of the MMR vaccine that are routinely recommended. Before international travel, administer two doses to children older than 12 months; The second dose should be administered at least 4 weeks after the initial dose. Females of child-bearing age who have not received 2 doses of a rubella-containing vaccine or who do not have a positive antibody test for rubella should be offered rubella immunization (using the MMR vaccine): exclude pregnancy before immunization, and avoid pregnancy for one month after vaccination (Excellence, 2023a; Kliegman, 2020).

Upon injection, the MMR vaccine may induce moderate discomfort, irritation, and erythema. Fever between days 7 and 12, transient erythema between days 5 and 20, and transient thrombocytopenia are additional possible adverse effects. Rubella may cause arthralgia in young women, lymphadenopathy in infants, and transient orchitis in young men, among other adverse effects. Autism is not caused by MMR (South-Paul & Matheny, 2020).

Varicella Vaccine

Vaccination against the varicella virus is cost-effective since it can lower hospitalization costs. The hospitalization rate is five per thousand people. The virus is very infectious and starts to become contagious two days before the rashes appear. The Varicella-Zoster Virus may be latent in the dorsal root ganglia and eventually may cause shingles. This emphasizes the importance of immunization in not only avoiding chickenpox, but also its possible long-term consequences, such as shingles (South-Paul & Matheny, 2020).

Varicella vaccination is intended to protect those at high risk for serious disease from the varicella-zoster virus. It involves immunizing those who have certain risk characteristics. People with a verified history of chickenpox or shingles are immune, but those born abroad should be tested for immunity on a regular basis. Vaccination is advised for healthcare professionals who have patient contact, laboratory personnel who have been exposed to the virus, and vulnerable people who have close contact with immunocompromised patients. Children between 9-11 months should take two doses separated by three months, while those over one year and adults should have two doses separated by four to eight weeks (Excellence, 2023c).

Individuals without immunity, contraindications to vaccination, and at risk of severe varicella and sequelae should receive postexposure prophylaxis with varicella-zoster immune globulin, namely VariZIG. This medicine should be given to immunocompromised people, pregnant women who do not have immunity, and certain neonates and babies, however, it may be effective if given up to 10 days after exposure (Prevention, 2023j).

Meningococcal Conjugate Vaccine (MENACYW and MENB)

During the period before conjugate vaccines were developed, Neisseria meningitidis, the most common bacterial pathogen causing meningitis in children and young adults in the United States, was accountable for an estimated 2200-3000 cases of invasive disease each year. 11–19% of instances result in sequelae, including limb amputation, neurologic impairment, and hearing loss, while mortality is reduced to less than 10% (3). There are presently three licensed and accessible quadrivalent meningococcal conjugate (MenACWY) vaccines in the United States: 1) Polysaccharide diphtheria toxoid conjugate vaccine for meningococcal groups A, C, W, and Y (MenACWY-D) is designated for Menveo; 2) Oligosaccharide diphtheria CRM197 conjugate vaccine for meningococcal groups A, C, W, and Y is referred to as MenACWY-CRM; and 3) MenACWY-TT is designated for MenQuadfi. Furthermore, two vaccines against serogroup B meningococcal (MenB) are available and licensed in the United States: 1) MenB-4C (Bexsero) and 2) MenB-FHbp (Trumenba) (Prevention, 2023c). Young infants may not produce an optimal antibody response to serogroup C in unconjugated meningococcal polysaccharide vaccines [not available in the UK at this time] (Excellence, 2023b).

The commercial names and availability of meningococcal vaccines may vary by country, and the recommendations can change accordingly. For the recommendations of the World Health Organization, you can refer to Table 2. For more information, you can consult the sources provided at https://www.cdc.gov/vaccines/vpd/mening/index.html and Immunization against infectious disease - GOV.UK (www.gov.uk) (GOV.UK, 2023; Prevention, 2023b).

Rotavirus Vaccine

Rotavirus is a highly contagious virus that causes severe symptoms such as diarrhea, vomiting, fever, and abdominal pain in newborns and young children. While good hygiene is crucial, the rotavirus vaccination is the most effective approach to protect children (Prevention, 2023g). Annually, rotavirus was responsible for 20-60% of fatalities, 60,000 hospitalizations, and 2-3 million cases of gastroenteritis in the United States prior to the introduction of the rotavirus vaccine. The United States has licensed two live oral vaccines, pentavalent (RVS) and monovalent (RVl), which reduce hospitalization by 85-100% and severity by 74-87%, respectively (South-Paul & Matheny, 2020).

In the United States, two rotavirus vaccinations are now available for infants:

1. RotaTeq® (RV5) is given in three doses at the ages of two months, four months, and six months.
2. Rotarix® (RV1) is administered in two doses at the ages of two and four months.

The first dose of either vaccination should be administered before the child reaches the age of 15 weeks. Children should receive all rotavirus vaccination doses before the age of eight months. Both immunizations are administered to children by placing drops in their mouths (Prevention, 2023g).

Human Papilloma Virus Vaccine

5% of all human malignancies are caused by HPV infection; annually, more than 600,000 new cases are identified. The International Agency for Research on Cancer classifies it as the foremost oncogenic virus that impacts human beings, as well as the principal etiological agent of uterine cervical cancer. This correlation exhibits variability in strength (Mariani et al., 2017; OBSERVATORY, 2023). Among the genotypes that provide a high risk of neoplastic transformation, HPV16 and HPV18 display the most significant biologically aggressive characteristics and serve as the main causes of HPV-associated carcinogenesis. Routine immunization is advised for children aged 11 to 12 years; however, it may begin as early as 9 years old. Individuals between the ages of 13 and 26 who have not been sufficiently immunized should receive a catch-up immunization. Certain people aged 27-45 years are eligible for shared clinical decision-making if they have not been adequately immunized (Prevention, 2023a).

The CDC recommends two doses of the vaccine for individuals aged 11-12, with the first dose being given at age 14 or younger. For those with specific immunocompromising conditions or those receiving their first dose after their 15th birthday, a three-dose schedule is recommended. The second dose should be given one to two months after the first dose, and the third dose should be given six months later (Prevention, 2023a; South-Paul & Matheny, 2020).

Adult Vaccination

The recommendations for vaccinations differ according to risk factors and age. A single dose of the meningococcal groups A with C and W135 and Y vaccination (Nimenrix® or Menveo®) is recommended for those under 25 who are about to join college and are at risk of meningococcal illness. This advice is especially relevant for students under 25 years of age who are starting college and who have not had the vaccination by the time they are 10 years old. Adults who have not had their childhood immunizations or who have not completed their 5-dose course should receive the poliomyelitis, tetanus, and diphtheria vaccine. It is advised that those over 65 get the inactivated influenza vaccination starting in September of each year. People should also get the pneumococcal polysaccharide vaccination at this age. It is advised that those aged 70 to 79 get the herpes-zoster vaccination, ideally the live attenuated version (Zostavax®). In the event that this is not possible, the Varicella-zoster vaccinations criteria can be followed to deliver the herpes-zoster vaccine (recombinant, adjuvanted) under the brand name Shingrix ® (Excellence, 2023a). Vaccinations against chickenpox, measles, mumps, and rubella should also be administered to non-immune people. Hepatitis B, hepatitis A, Hib, or meningococcal vaccinations are recommended for certain travel-related illnesses or underlying medical disorders. It is recommended that all women, regardless of their pregnancy status, receive the annual flu vaccine. It can be given during any trimester. Regardless of prior Tdap administration, ACIP advises administering a Tdap dose during each pregnancy, preferable between weeks 27 and 36, to optimize transplacental antipertussis antibody and protect neonates for the first two months of life, or until they can be vaccinated (South-Paul & Matheny, 2020).

Conclusion

The significance of vaccination and its pivotal role in protecting public health and human welfare cannot be overemphasized. Vaccines play a crucial role in the prevention of diseases, and the partnership and knowledge exchange between healthcare practitioners and those seeking healthcare are essential components of this endeavor. The objective of this guide is to provide crucial details about the prompt and precise administration of vaccines. For a more in-depth analysis of various vaccine categories and those designed for specific age cohorts, individuals can consider consulting reliable healthcare platforms such as the Centers for Disease Control and Prevention (CDC), the World Health Organization (WHO), and the National Health Service (NHS) of the United Kingdom. These authoritative sources offer comprehensive information and expert recommendations.

References

Bandyopadhyay, A. S., Garon, J., Seib, K., & Orenstein, W. A. (2015). Polio vaccination: Past, present and future. *Future Microbiology, 10*(5), 791-808. https://doi.org/10.2217/fmb.15.19.

Cherry, J. D. (1984). The epidemiology of pertussis and pertussis immunization in the United Kingdom and the United States: A comparative study. *Current Problems in Pediatrics, 14*(2), 1-78. https://doi.org/10.1016/0045-9380(84)90016-1.

Excellence, N. I. f. H. a. C. (2023a). *Immunisation schedule*. Retrieved 20.10.2023 from https://bnf.nice.org.uk/treatment-summaries/immunisation-schedule/.

Excellence, N. I. f. H. a. C. (2023b). *Meningococcal vaccine*. NICE. https://bnf.nice.org.uk/treatment-summaries/meningococcal-vaccine/#:~:text=Immunisation%20consists%20of%201%20dose%20given%20at%202%20months%20of,(see%20Immunisation%20Schedule%20above).

Excellence, N. I. f. H. a. C. (2023c). *Varicella-zoster vaccines*. NICE. Retrieved 10.20.2023 from https://bnf.nice.org.uk/treatment-summaries/varicella-zoster-vaccines/#:~:text=Children%20aged%201%20year%20and,unless%20protection%20is%20urgently%20required.

GOV.UK. (2023). *Immunisation against infectious disease*. GOV.UK. Retrieved 20.10.2023 from https://www.gov.uk/government/collections/immunisation-against-infectious-disease-the-green-book.

Initiative, G. P. E. (2023). *The virus*. GPEI. Retrieved 20.10.2023 from https://polioeradication.org/polio-today/polio-prevention/the-virus/.

Kim, H., Webster, R. G., & Webby, R. J. (2018). Influenza virus: Dealing with a drifting and shifting pathogen. *Viral Immunology, 31*(2), 174-183. https://doi.org/10.1089/vim.2017.0141.

Kliegman, R., Stanton, Bonita, St. Geme, Joseph W., & Nelson, Waldo E. (2020). *Nelson textbook of pediatrics* (Vol. 2). Elsevier Inc.

Lievano, F., Galea, S. A., Thornton, M., Wiedmann, R. T., Manoff, S. B., Tran, T. N., Amin, M. A., Seminack, M. M., Vagie, K. A., Dana, A., & Plotkin, S. A. (2012). Measles, mumps, and rubella virus vaccine (M-M-R™II): A review of 32 years of clinical and postmarketing experience. *Vaccine, 30*(48), 6918-6926. https://doi.org/10.1016/j.vaccine.2012.08.057.

Mariani, L., Preti, M., Cristoforoni, P., Stigliano, C. M., & Perino, A. (2017). Overview of the benefits and potential issues of the nonavalent HPV vaccine. *International Journal of Gynaecology and Obstetrics, 136*(3), 258-265. https://doi.org/10.1002/ijgo.12075.

Mattoo, S., & Cherry, J. D. (2005). Molecular pathogenesis, epidemiology, and clinical manifestations of respiratory infections due to *Bordetella pertussis* and other *Bordetella* subspecies. *Clinical Microbiology Reviews, 18*(2), 326-382. https://doi.org/10.1128/cmr.18.2.326-382.2005.

Nieves, D. J., & Heininger, U. (2016). *Bordetella pertussis. Microbiology Spectrum, 4*(3). https://doi.org/10.1128/microbiolspec.EI10-0008-2015.

Observatory, G. C. (2023). *Cancer today*. GCO. Retrieved 10.20.2023 from https://gco.iarc.fr/.

Organization, W. H. (2023a). *Pertussis*. WHO. Retrieved 21.10.2023 from https://www.who.int/health-topics/pertussis#tab=tab_1.

Organization, W. H. (2023b). *WHO recommendations for routine immunization - summary tables*. WHO. Retrieved 23.10.2023 from https://www.who.int/teams/immunization-vaccines-and-biologicals/policies/who-recommendations-for-routine-immunization-summary-tables.

Pattyn, J., Hendrickx, G., Vorsters, A., & Van Damme, P. (2021). Hepatitis B vaccines. *The Journal of Infectious Diseases, 224*(12 Suppl 2), S343-S351. https://doi.org/10.1093/infdis/jiaa668.

Prevention, C. f. D. C. a. (2023a). *HPV vaccine schedule and dosing*. CDC. Retrieved 10.20.2023 from https://www.cdc.gov/hpv/hcp/schedules-recommendations.html#:~:text=CDC%20recommends%20two%20doses%20of,%E2%80%9312%2Dmonth%20schedule).

Prevention, C. f. D. C. a. (2023b). *Meningococcal vaccination*. CDC. https://www.cdc.gov/vaccines/vpd/mening/index.html#:~:text=All%2011%20to%2012%20year,increased%20risk%20for%20meningococcal%20disease.

Prevention, C. f. D. C. a. (2023c). *Meningococcal vaccination: Recommendations of the Advisory Committee on Immunization Practices, United States, 2020*. CDC. https://www.cdc.gov/mmwr/volumes/69/rr/rr6909a1.htm.

Prevention, C. f. D. C. a. (2023d). *Pertussis surveillance trend reporting and case definition*. CDC. Retrieved 21.10.2023 from https://www.cdc.gov/pertussis/surv-reporting.html.

Prevention, C. f. D. C. a. (2023e). *Pneumococcal vaccine recommendations*. CDC. Retrieved 20.10.2023 from https://www.cdc.gov/vaccines/vpd/pneumo/hcp/recommendations.html.

Prevention, C. f. D. C. a. (2023f). *Prevention and control of seasonal influenza with vaccines: Recommendations of the Advisory Committee on Immunization Practices (ACIP)—United States, 2022-23*. CDC. Retrieved 20.10.2023 from https://www.cdc.gov/flu/pdf/professionals/acip/acip-2022-23-summary-of-recommendations.pdf.

Prevention, C. f. D. C. a. (2023g). *Rotavirus vaccination*. CDC. Retrieved 10.20.2023 from https://www.cdc.gov/vaccines/vpd/rotavirus/index.html.

Prevention, C. f. D. C. a. (2023h). *Tdap (Pertussis) vaccine and pregnancy*. CDC. Retrieved 21.10.2023 from https://www.cdc.gov/vaccines/pregnancy/hcp-toolkit/tdap-vaccine-pregnancy.html.

Prevention, C. f. D. C. a. (2023i). *Vaccines and preventable diseases*. CDC. Retrieved 22.10.2023 from https://www.cdc.gov/vaccines/vpd/vaccines-diseases.html.

Prevention, C. f. D. C. a. (2023j). *Varicella/Chickenpox. CDC Yellow Book 2024*. CDC. Retrieved 10.20.2023 from https://wwwnc.cdc.gov/travel/yellowbook/2024/infections-diseases/varicella-chickenpox#:~:text=CDC%20recommends%20varicella%20vaccine%20for,administered%20%E2%89%A53%20months%20apart.

Shukla, V. V., & Shah, R. C. (2018). Vaccinations in primary care. *The Indian Journal of Pediatrics, 85*(12), 1118-1127.

South-Paul, J., & Matheny, S. (2020). *Current diagnosis and treatment: Family medicine* (5th ed.). LANGE.

Watt, J. P., Wolfson, L. J., O'Brien, K. L., Henkle, E., Deloria-Knoll, M., McCall, N., Lee, E., Levine, O. S., Hajjeh, R., Mulholland, K., & Cherian, T. (2009). Burden of disease caused by *Haemophilus influenzae* type b in children younger than 5 years: Global estimates. *Lancet, 374*(9693), 903-911. https://doi.org/10.1016/s0140-6736(09)61203-4.

WHO. (2023). *Vaccines and immunization*. WHO. Retrieved 20.10.2023 from https://www.who.int/health-topics/vaccines-and-immunization#tab=tab_1.

Chapter 25

Insomnia

Latife Merve Yildiz, PhD
Department of Family Medicine, Güneysu Tenzile Erdoğan State Hospital, Rize, Turkey

Abstract

Insomnia is the inability to fall asleep for 30 minutes or more or experiencing sleeplessness for more than three nights a week, affecting one-third of adults. Its prevalence increases with age. The prevalence of insomnia in Turkiye is 21.8%, while in Ankara it is 17.6%. Individuals with insomnia are generally female, elderly, and have a lower socioeconomic status. Risk factors include stress, alcohol, and caffeine consumption. While ICSD-3 categorizes insomnia into various categories, DSM-5 classifies it as 'Sleep-Wake Disorders.' Insomnia can be a symptom of physical and mental illnesses. Insomnia reduces quality of life, leads to economic costs, and increases health risks. Family physicians play a crucial role in the diagnosis and treatment of insomnia. The scales are the Pittsburgh Insomnia Rating Scale (PIRS), Pittsburgh Sleep Quality Index (PSQI), Sleep Hygiene Index (SHI), and Insomnia Severity Index (ISI). Some of these scales are used in Turkiye. Non-pharmacological approaches have advantages in terms of cost in the treatment of insomnia. In pharmacological treatment, benzodiazepines, non-benzodiazepine receptor agonists, and antidepressants are used. Family physicians play a critical role in the effective treatment of insomnia by asking patients about their sleep habits and referring them to specialists when necessary.

Keywords: family medicine, insomnia, primary care

Introduction

Sleep is a fundamental physiological need that determines individuals' quality of life and health, being as essential as breathing or eating. This biological necessity is regulated by brain regions, biochemical factors, circadian rhythms, and homeostatic mechanisms (Basner & McGuire, 2018). During sleep, physical and psychological restoration, energy storage, memory consolidation, and strengthening of the immune system occur. Sleep is categorized into two stages: deepening four-stage non-REM sleep and the fifth stage known as REM (Rapid Eye Movement) sleep (Wagner et al., 1998).

Sleep disorders are studied by both neurology and psychiatry specialists as well as encountered frequently in other medical fields such as family physicians (Gamsızkan, 2017).

In: Common Diseases According to Family Medicine Practice Guidelines
Editors: Esra Meltem Koç and Hilal Aksoy
ISBN: 979-8-89530-302-3

Quality, quantity, and timing deviations in sleep, difficulty falling asleep, and disruptions in the night-day cycle characterize sleep disorders. These conditions negatively impact individuals' social and professional lives and pose significant public health problems.

The epidemiology of sleep disorders varies according to populations and age groups. In a general assessment, the prevalence of sleep disorders varies between 5% and 71% (Aysan et al., 2014). In the United States, 10% of the population experience clinical sleep disorders (Ram et al., 2010).

Throughout the population, 40% of adults in the general population experience difficulties in falling asleep and maintaining it, the rate reaches 69% in primary care patients (Aikens & Rouse, 2005). In terms of gender distribution, this rate is 10.5% for men and 20.2% for women (Demir et al., 2015).

In the study by Gamsızkan et al., in 2014, it was observed that sleep disorders are more common in older age and in women (Gamsızkan & Aslan, 2014). Especially in women, the likelihood of a menopausal transition leading to sleep disorders is higher.

Insomnia is quite common, affecting approximately one-third of adults, and approximately 10% of them experience serious daytime dysfunctions due to difficulty in maintaining sleep (Gagnon et al., 2013). According to the criteria of the Diagnostic and Statistical Manual of Mental Disorders (DSM-IV), the prevalence of insomnia in the general population is around 6%, while it varies between 10% and 40% in primary care settings (Gagnon et al., 2013).

Preventive medicine plays a critical role for primary care providers, such as family physicians. Considering the prevalence of sleep disorders and their associated health risks, healthy sleep should also be addressed in preventive medicine. However, only a small fraction of individuals with symptoms of sleep disorders in the community receive diagnosis and treatment. Considering the critical importance of diagnosing and treating insomnia at the primary care level, there is an emphasis on expanding the inquiries of family physicians in this regard and adopting effective diagnostic methods.

Insomnia

Insomnia, one of the most common sleep disorders, is characterized by difficulties in falling asleep and/or staying asleep, with patients typically taking 30 minutes or more to fall asleep or experiencing such problems on more than three nights per week (Yılmaz et al., 2014). This condition negatively affects patients' quality of life and daily functioning, experiencing symptoms such as excessive daytime fatigue, emotional changes, and decreased performance. Insomnia can occur both as a symptom itself and as a precursor or indication of certain diseases (Tümer et al., 2017).

Epidemiology of Insomnia

Insomnia presents itself as a common sleep disorder on a global scale. One-third of adults experience difficulty falling asleep or maintaining sleep on an annual basis (Gagnon et al., 2013). 17% of them consider the problem to be serious (Rakel, 1993). The prevalence of insomnia in the adult population varies between approximately 15-20%, depending on the definition used, and it is observed to increase with age (Rakel, 1993).

According to estimates from the United States, approximately 40 to 70 million individuals experience intermittent insomnia (Bluestein et al., 2010). This rate is twice the prevalence of major depression. According to a Gallup survey in 1995, nearly half of adults reported being dissatisfied with their sleep at least five nights per month (Ringdahl et al., 2004a).

According to a health survey conducted in Canada in 2002, the prevalence of insomnia in the population aged 15 and older was determined to be 13.4% (Tjepkema, 2005).

Similar prevalence rates are also observed on the European continent. For instance, a study conducted in Germany found that the prevalence of severe insomnia is 4%, which is lower compared to other European countries (Hajak & Group, 2001).

According to the Adult Population-based Epidemiology of Sleep in Turkiye (TAPES) study, the prevalence of insomnia was determined to be 21.8% (Demir et al., 2015). In two separate studies conducted specifically in Ankara, it was found that 23.7% and 29.4% of the participants, respectively, reported one or more insomnia symptoms; while 17.6% of the individuals were identified as clinically having insomnia (Aslan et al., 2006).

The literature states that individuals with insomnia are generally women, divorced, unemployed, elderly, with low education levels, and from low socioeconomic backgrounds (Kahraman, 2006). Additionally, risk factors for insomnia include physical inactivity, irregular sleep schedules, a stressful lifestyle, alcohol, and caffeine consumption, as well as the presence of psychiatric or organic diseases (Gamsızkan, 2017).

The Classification of Insomnia

Table 1. The Classification of Insomnia ICSD-3

Chronic Insomnia • Psychophysiological Insomnia • Idiopathic Insomnia • Paradoxical Insomnia • Inadequate Sleep Hygiene • Behavioral Insomnia in Childhood • Insomnia Caused by Mental Conditions • Insomnia Caused by Medical Conditions • Insomnia Caused by Medication or Substance Use	Chronic insomnia leads to difficulties in initiating and maintaining sleep for individuals. These sleep problems occur at least three times a week, persist for at least three months, and result in symptoms such as daytime fatigue, and lack of concentration; however, it cannot be explained by inadequate sleep or other sleep disorders.
Short-term Insomnia	Short-term insomnia is characterized by sleep difficulties lasting less than three months and cannot be fully explained by inadequate sleep conditions leading to daytime symptoms such as fatigue.
Other Insomnia Disorders (Isolated symptoms and Variants) • Overstayed in bed • Short sleep	This diagnosis is defined as individuals complaining of difficulties in initiating sleep and maintaining sleep, but do not meet the diagnostic criteria for chronic insomnia or short-term insomnia.

The classification of insomnia according to the International Classification of Sleep Disorders-3 (ICSD-3) is as follows (Genç & Dikmen, 2017).

According to DSM-5, the diagnostic criteria for insomnia listed under the title 'Sleep-Wake Disorders' include symptoms experienced for at least three days per week and for a minimum duration of three months, causing impairment in the individual's functioning, and not being associated with another sleep disorder, mental condition, medical condition, or substance use (Diagnostic and Statistical Manual of Mental Disorders, (DSM 5), 2013). Symptoms related to sleep are classified as persistent, episodic, or acute based on their duration.

Insomnia and Etiological Factors

Insomnia occurs both as an independent disorder and as a symptom of various physical and mental illnesses. This condition of insomnia is particularly associated with the presence of primary sleep disorders such as sleep apnea and nocturnal myoclonus (Keskin & Tamam, 2018). Circadian rhythm disorders indicate abnormalities in individuals' biological clocks; sleep-wake phase disorder is commonly observed in the elderly and delayed sleep-wake phase disorder is frequently seen in adolescents (Sateia, 2014). With advancing age, there is a decrease in the restorative periods of sleep, while fragmented sleep patterns, commonly seen in old age, contribute to complaints (Morin et al., 1999). However, these complaints can also be attributed to age-related health issues or medication use in elderly individuals.

Among the etiological factors of sleeplessness (insomnia), there are medical disorders, pharmacotherapeutic medications, and psychiatric conditions. Medical conditions such as respiratory disorders, neurological disorders, and hormonal changes disrupt sleep and alter its cycle. Furthermore, certain medications interfere with sleep either through their stimulating effects (such as decongestants and β-agonists) or by altering hormone balance (such as corticosteroids and antidepressants), while psychiatric disorders such as major depression and obsessive-compulsive disorder also negatively impact sleep quality (Ancoli-Israel, 2000).

In a survey conducted in clinics, approximately 30% of patients with complaints of insomnia receive a diagnosis of depression (Buysse et al., 1994; Radecki & Brunton, 1993). Approximately 40% of those who consult sleep specialists are found to be experiencing a psychiatric issue (Buysse et al., 1994). Additionally, 10% to 15% of those experiencing insomnia struggle with substance abuse (Meyer, 1998). These data indicate that insomnia is not just a solitary disorder but is also associated with psychiatric issues. Among the main causes of insomnia are lifestyle changes, emotional issues, and systemic factors. These factors include significant life changes, disruptions in circadian rhythm, and factors such as alcohol or heavy meals before bedtime (Sateia, 2014).

Insomnia and Family Physicians

Insomnia affects approximately 95% of adults, and despite this high prevalence and morbidity, it is often underrecognized and underdiagnosed (Rakel, 1993). In studies conducted in the United States and Singapore, only 9% and 10% of those with complaints of insomnia sought medical help (Ancoli-Israel, 2000; Shochat et al., 1999). In family consultations, although insomnia is a common condition, only 31% of patients share this condition with their physician (Aikens & Rouse, 2005). Family physicians need to actively question to identify patients struggling with this problem. In primary care, the diagnostic process for insomnia can be achieved through evaluating patients' sleep histories and conducting physical examinations. The active approach of family physicians has the potential to reduce the serious health risks associated with insomnia (Aikens & Rouse, 2005).

Family physicians are the most commonly consulted healthcare professionals for sleep problems, and a detailed investigation of sleep difficulties in primary care is important (Bluestein et al., 2010). For effective screening, adopting a sensitive approach with 1 or 2 questions and then conducting a detailed clinical evaluation is necessary (Gagnon et al., 2013). In effectively considering complaints of insomnia, it is essential to take a detailed sleep history, and during this process, it has been found that more than 30% of first-degree female relatives experience insomnia (Bastien & Morin, 2000). The use of alcohol and tranquilizer accounts for 10% to 15% of insomnia cases (Ringdahl et al., 2004b). It is crucial for family physicians to guide cases that do not respond to treatment without an obvious cause to sleep medicine specialists and to take an active role in counseling and follow-up processes (Saygın et al., 2021).

There are various measurements reported by patients to evaluate sleep problems and their impact on daily functioning. The ideal screening tool for primary care should be both reliable and valid, while also requiring minimal burden on patients (Sarısaltık & Topuzoğlu, 2019; Saygın et al., 2021). Especially, it is preferred that application and scoring should be rapid and cost effective. In this context, the Insomnia Severity Index (ISI) is an important tool for evaluating insomnia according to the criteria of DSM-5 and the International Classification of Sleep Disorders (ICSD) (Edinger & Morin, 2012). The reliability and validity of the ISI have been documented not only in the general population, but also specifically in cancer patients with primary insomnia and other patient groups with insomnia (Gagnon et al., 2013; Savard et al., 2005). Furthermore, the sensitivity of the ISI to treatment response is also considered in clinical and research activities (Morin et al., 2011).

Distinguishing Insomnia

Distinguishing insomnia from other sleep disorders can be achieved by obtaining a brief sleep history. This approach is effective in identifying which sleep problem the individual is experiencing and in determining possible causes of this problem. For instance, factors such as returning from a trip to different time zones recently can help diagnose temporary insomnia due to jet lag (Rakel, 1993). Habits such as waking up early in the morning or going to bed early signal an individual's sleep hygiene. Additionally, the evaluation of a patient's bed partner plays a critical role in identifying potential issues such as snoring, airway obstruction, apnea, or nocturnal myoclonus (Aikens & Rouse, 2005).

Daytime drowsiness, morning headaches, irritability, along with high complaints of snoring, raise concerns about sleep apnea or other respiratory disorders. Individuals with sleep apnea often complain of restless sleep due to frequent short awakening periods called 'micro-arousals' that occur hundreds of times throughout the night (Buysse et al., 2015). Although these micro-arousals are often unnoticed by patients, they disrupt sleep. Both sleep apnea and insomnia lead to daytime sleepiness; however, the treatment of these two conditions differs

(Spicuzza et al., 2015). Therefore, an accurate diagnosis and an appropriate treatment approach are of critical importance.

Insomnia Effects

Insomnia significantly impairs individuals' quality of life and interferes with their physical and social interactions. Insomnia patients tend to make more hospital visits and require increased medical tests and medication compared to individuals without insomnia complaints (Hajak & Group, 2001). Research conducted by the American Automobile Association indicates that driver fatigue contributes to half of commercial truck accidents, with 15% to 20% of these accidents occurring due to insomnia, resulting in half of fatal accidents (Garbarino et al., 2017).

From an economic perspective, insomnia costs over $42 billion annually, with total costs related to productivity loss and associated accidents reaching $100 billion. Approximately 20% of motor vehicle accidents are observed to occur due to driver sleepiness (Daley et al., 2009; Ringdahl et al., 2004b).

When evaluated more closely for its health effects, it has been found that short sleep duration increases the prevalence of stroke and ischemic heart disease, impairs glucose tolerance, and raises the risk of diabetes (Holliday et al., 2013; Sabanayagam & Shankar, 2010). In a study conducted in South Korea with 23,878 participants aged 18 and above, it was found that short sleep duration caused to an increase in the prevalence of stroke and ischemic heart disease (Im & Kim, 2017). The relationship between obesity and insomnia is particularly noteworthy. In a community-based study by Bjorvatn et al., involving 8,860 participants, short sleep duration was found to be associated with an increased prevalence of high body mass index and obesity (Bjorvatn et al., 2007). A meta-analysis published in 2008, including a total of 45 studies, demonstrated a higher risk of developing obesity in both children and adults with short durations of sleep (Cappuccio et al., 2008). In a 20-year cohort study involving approximately 48,000 individuals in Sweden, it was found that individuals with sleep problems had a mortality rate from work accidents approximately twice as high as those without (Akerstedt et al., 2002). In the process of medical residency with intense shifts and long working hours, it has been shown that individuals sleeping less than 6 hours per day have reported more serious accidents or injuries and medical errors (Baldwin Jr & Daugherty, 2004).

Insomnia particularly leads to accidents and medical errors in individuals with intense working hours, therefore, increasing the frequency of visits to healthcare facilities and posing a significant challenge in primary healthcare services, especially for family physicians (Kapur et al., 2002).

Insomnia Diagnosis and Screening Scales

There are many methods used for the diagnosis and screening of insomnia. Among these are expensive and complex tests, such as polysomnography, multiple sleep latency tests, and actigraphy, while there are also simpler and more economical screening tools available (Sarısaltık & Topuzoğlu, 2019). Especially in primary healthcare, the use of tools with Turkish validity is recommended to detect sleep disorders (Sarısaltık & Topuzoğlu, 2019). The use of the Pittsburgh Insomnia Rating Scale (PIRS), adapted into Turkish by Aydın et al., for screening purposes is also important in this context (Aydın et al., 2014).

The Pittsburgh Insomnia Rating Scale (PIRS), adapted into Turkish by Aydın et al., in 2014, addresses personal distress related to sleep, parameters, and quality of life (Aydın et al., 2014). Scores of 30 and above obtained with this scale are considered indicative of insomnia symptoms (Aydın et al., 2014). The Pittsburgh Sleep Quality Index (PSQI), developed by Buysse et al., in 1988, was adapted into Turkish by Ağargün et al., in 1996, and scores of 5 and above indicate poor sleep quality (Agargun, 1996; Buysse et al., 1989). In a study by Fujieda et al., it was concluded that poor sleep quality could be a potential indicator of depression for primary care physicians in primary healthcare services (Fujieda et al., 2017). Additionally, the Turkish version of PSQI is used in research on sleep quality among different patient groups, including pregnant women and university students (Aysan et al., 2014; Safer, 2017).

The Sleep Hygiene Index (SHI), created by Mastin et al., in 2006, focuses on the frequency of behaviors that affect sleep hygiene (Mastin et al., 2006). This index is designed based on the criteria for inadequate sleep hygiene in the ICSD, and it evaluates individuals' sleep schedule, pre-sleep behaviors, physical conditions of the sleeping environment, and stress experienced in bed (Chehri et al., 2016). Özdemir et al., completed the validity and reliability study of SHI in Turkish in 2015, indicating that this scale can be used in both clinical practice and in the general population (Ozdemir et al., 2015).

On the other hand, Morin et al., studied on the Insomnia Severity Index (ISI) in 2001, developing an evaluation scale that includes both day and night components of insomnia (Bastien et al., 2001). Boysan et al., conducted the validity and reliability study of ISI in Turkiye in 2010 (Boysan et al., 2010). This scale addresses not only individuals' difficulties in falling asleep and staying asleep but also the impact of insomnia on their daily functioning. Both indices are among the significant tools used by family physicians and primary healthcare services to evaluate individuals' sleep quality and the severity of insomnia (Sarısaltık & Topuzoğlu, 2019).

The Insomnia Severity Index (ISI) is a tool that evaluates individuals' levels of insomnia and determines their severity based on the scores obtained. In this index, a total score ranging from 0 to 28 indicates the severity of insomnia, with higher values reflecting more severe insomnia (Boysan et al., 2010). In a study by Morin et al., the optimal threshold value for screening insomnia in the community was found to be 10 (Morin et al., 2011). However, a study by Gagnon et al., suggests that this threshold value can be more optimal at 14 (Gagnon et al., 2013). The Insomnia Severity Index is considered a reliable and valid method for detecting clinical insomnia in primary healthcare services (Sarısaltık & Topuzoğlu, 2019). In Turkiye, the Turkish version of ISI has been shown to be practicable and to support its relationship with different populations, as demonstrated by Gamsızkan's study (Gamsızkan & Aslan, 2014). These findings are of great importance to family physicians and primary healthcare professionals in terms of early detection and intervention for insomnia.

Insomnia Management

Insomnia leads to significant health issues in individuals, both in its temporary and long-term forms. Especially in primary healthcare services, one of the initial approaches used in treating insomnia is to raise patients consciousness about sleep habits and improve sleep hygiene

(Gamsızkan, 2017). In this context, simple measures against environmental factors to improve sleep quality, such as using earplugs, are recommended (Rakel, 1993). Creating a 'sleep diary' for the patient helps to effectively manage the treatment process (Edinger & Sampson, 2003). It is noted that regular exercise during daytime periods improves sleep quality, but intense exercise in the evening hours can have negative effects (Irish et al., 2015). Although methods such as progressive muscle relaxation, hypnosis, and meditation are recommended for chronic sleep disorders, there is no definitive information on the effectiveness of these techniques (Oğuz et al., 2019). The negative effects of caffeine and alcoholic beverages on insomnia should not be overlooked, and these substances should be avoided within 6 hours before bedtime (Yılmaz et al., 2014). Over-the-counter sleep aids are often preferred among treatment options; however, it is known that these medications have low efficacy and can create paradoxical effects (Yılmaz et al., 2014). It has been found that over-the-counter sleep aids, especially those containing antihistamines, can adversely affect cognitive abilities and create depressive effects on the central nervous system (Pagel & Parnes, 2001). Therefore, family physicians and primary healthcare services should refrain from recommending over-the-counter sleep aids in the treatment of insomnia, considering their potential side effects (J. D. Lie et al., 2015).

Treatment Methods

Insomnia presents itself as a disorder that significantly impacts individuals' quality of life. The strategic steps to be followed in the treatment of this condition should be determined and implemented according to the patient's condition (Gamsızkan, 2017).

- In the first step, before initiating treatment, the patient's medical history is detailed and reviewed along with the factors contributing to insomnia. At this stage, the factors that trigger, initiate, and perpetuate insomnia are determined, and general medical history information is gathered.
- In the second step, potential medical disorders that disrupt the patient's sleep are focused on. Particularly, conditions such as depression that negatively affect nighttime sleep were included primarily in the treatment plan.
- In the third stage, the patient is informed and educated about their sleep habits and the process of falling asleep. With this education, it is aimed at helping the patient maintain a healthier sleep routine.
- Finally, excessive anxiety situations related to the observed insomnia in the patient are interfered with. Treatment methods aimed at reducing concerns about the negative effects of insomnia are evaluated at this stage.

Non-Pharmacological Treatment Methods Applicable in Primary Care

The treatment of insomnia should adopt a personalized approach, considering the severity and characteristics of the symptoms. Non-pharmacological methods are more cost-effective and have a lower risk of side effects, with long-term results achieved through behavioral changes

(Siebern et al., 2012). However, pharmacological treatment is provided for patients seeking a rapid effect.

Non-pharmacological treatments for insomnia are considered successful when they reduce sleep initiation or increase total sleep time by 30 minutes (Siebern et al., 2012). To evaluate treatment effectiveness, sleep diaries of patients are commonly used as a reference. The evaluation considers criteria such as total sleep time, sleep initiation, and number of awakenings during the night (Krystal et al., 2019).

Summary of non-pharmacological management options that can be applied in primary care as follows:

- *Sleep Hygiene Education:* In insomnia, clinical practices and observations emphasize the importance of sleep hygiene. In individuals with mild insomnia complaints, poor sleep hygiene contributes to the development of this problem. Especially family physicians and primary healthcare services provide guidance to individuals on optimizing sleep hygiene (Chung et al., 2018). Sleep hygiene education supports individuals in having a healthy sleep routine. Individuals are informed about the effects of diet, caffeine, alcohol, and smoking on sleep. The conditions of the bedroom, such as temperature, light, and noise, also affect sleep quality (Yılmaz et al., 2014). Scientific research indicates that exercise has a positive effect on sleep quality. However, engaging in physical activity 3-4 hours before bedtime can enable one to fall asleep (Yılmaz et al., 2014). Consumption of caffeinated and alcoholic beverages taken 6 hours before bedtime can lead to insomnia (Drake et al., 2013). For individuals experiencing difficulty falling asleep, relaxation techniques are recommended. If sleep does not initiate within 15-30 minutes, it is recommended that they rest in a different environment.
- *Sleep Restriction Therapy:* Sleep restriction therapy aims to optimize the time spent in bed only for sleep to improve sleep quality. This therapy increases the time spent in bed by 20 minutes when the individual's sleep efficiency is above 90%, and decreases it by 20 minutes when it falls below 80%; however, it should not be below 5 hours (Yılmaz et al., 2014). Gradually reducing the time spent awake in bed using Spielman's method has shown positive results in mild insomnia cases (Spielman et al., 1987). Family physicians and primary healthcare services play a critical role in implementing these approaches.
- *Relaxation Techniques:* Various therapy methods are used in the treatment of insomnia. The method of relaxing muscles enables to relax the body and calm the mind of the individual, within this scope, imagery training aims to clear the mind of negative thoughts (Debellemaniere et al., 2018). Consulting for professional help is recommended to reduce the high arousal and anxiety that occur during wakefulness.
- *Cognitive Therapy:* Individuals experiencing insomnia often have anxiety and fear during the process of falling asleep, which can impair the problem further. Cognitive therapy focuses on correcting misleading beliefs and expectations about sleep in these individuals, and recent studies show a 54% improvement in sleep initiation with this method (Edinger et al., 2001). Therefore, the effectiveness rates of relaxation therapy and placebo treatment are 16% and 12%, respectively (Edinger et al., 2001). Especially in elderly individuals, cognitive therapy has been observed to have positive results

parallel to the pharmacological treatment applied by family physicians and in primary care.

- *Paradoxical Intention:* Paradoxical intention therapy enables patients to consciously stay awake, helping them to cope with the fear of insomnia (Jansson-Fröjmark et al., 2022). This method relieves concerns about the possible consequences of inadequate sleep and reduces performance anxiety during the transition to sleep.

The meta-analysis of 48 studies on behavioral therapy indicates the effectiveness of stimulus control therapy and shows its superiority over other methods (Smith et al., 2002). Progressive muscle relaxation has been found to be more effective compared to placebo (Smith et al., 2002). However, a recent meta-analysis comparing pharmacotherapy with behavioral therapy found no significant difference between the two methods except that behavioral therapy was more successful in reducing the sleep initiation period (Smith et al., 2002).

Non-pharmacological methods provide effective strategies in the management of sleep problems. Especially approaches such as sleep hygiene education, sleep restriction therapy, and cognitive therapy are used to improve an individual's sleep quality.

Pharmacological Treatments

In selecting pharmacological methods for insomnia treatment, the primary goal is to resolve nighttime sleep problems and eliminate the negative effects they produce during the day (Lou & Oks, 2021). First, before initiating treatment, physicians should identify potential causes of insomnia such as respiratory disorders, restless leg syndrome, or psychiatric disorders, and consider these issues as a priority (Janette D Lie et al., 2015). Parallel to pharmacological treatment, priority should be given to non-pharmacological methods in the treatment of insomnia, especially those that focus on the biological and psychological rhythms of sleep (Matheson & Hainer, 2017).

Antihistamines

Antihistamines, especially hydroxyzine and diphenhydramine, are commonly preferred in the treatment of insomnia due to their moderate sedative effects (Culpepper & Wingertzahn, 2015). The duration of action of these medications typically ranges from 6 to 8 hours, with hydroxyzine lasting up to 6 to 24 hours. When taken late at night, these medications can lead to side effects, such as morning grogginess due to their long half-lives (Li et al., 2010). On the other hand, tolerance to the sedative effects of these medications can develop over time. However, it should be noted that some antihistamines can cause anticholinergic side effects; therefore, they should be used with caution, especially in the elderly and those taking other medications with anticholinergic effects.

Benzodiazepines

Benzodiazepines are commonly used pharmacological agents in the treatment of insomnia. These compounds are rapidly absorbed from the gastrointestinal system, reaching maximum plasma concentration within 1-3 hours after ingestion. However, it has been observed that the absorption of these compounds is slowed by food and antacids. The effectiveness of medications, especially in the treatment of insomnia, depends on their distribution rates (Karadag, 2016). Some benzodiazepines such as diazepam affect rapidly, while lipophobic medications such as oxazepam and lorazepam have a long-acting. The half-lives of medications are directly related to their elimination processes, and medications with longer half-lives can accumulate, causing the risk of increased sedation (Yılmaz et al., 2014).

Elderly individuals metabolize benzodiazepines differently. It is known that metabolism slows down and increased neurological sensitivity is observed in this population. These medications shorten the time it takes to fall asleep, while also reducing total sleep time. However, the tendency of benzodiazepines to reduce REM sleep indicates that short-acting types (for instance, triazolam) can lead to REM rebound in the later hours of the night (Pagel & Parnes, 2001).

Benzodiazepines are classified based on their duration of action. They are grouped into three main categories: long-acting (e.g., Diazepam, Flurazepam), intermediate-acting (e.g., Oxazepam, Lorazepam), and short-acting (e.g., Triazolam, Temazepam) (Griffin et al., 2013). While short-acting benzodiazepines are recommended for patients experiencing difficulty initiating sleep, intermediate-acting agents are more suitable for those with sleep maintenance problems (Chen et al., 2016). While long-acting benzodiazepines can provide benefits for patients with daytime anxiety and early awakening, their potential to negatively affect daytime performance should be considered, especially in elderly patients (Chen et al., 2016). Additionally, the use of benzodiazepines is not recommended during pregnancy and breastfeeding. There is also a risk of tolerance and dependence with long-term use.

In the treatment of chronic insomnia, the choice of medication and dosage adjustment are of great importance. During the treatment process, selecting the lowest effective dose or choosing medications with a short half-life is essential. The medication treatment should not exceed four weeks and, if necessary, should be used intermittently (Janette D Lie et al., 2015). At the end of the treatment process, the medications should be gradually reduced.

In summary, benzodiazepines play a significant role in the treatment of insomnia. However, it is essential to use them correctly, considering their effects and side effects. The ideal treatment should be personalized according to the individual's needs and risk factors.

Non-Benzodiazepine Benzodiazepine Receptor Agonists

Hypnotic medications such as zolpidem, zopiclone, and zaleplon have a safer profile compared to classical benzodiazepines and disrupt the sleep architecture less. These medications have fewer side effects, such as psychomotor and memory issues, because they have a more selective effect on the α-1 subtype of the GABA-A receptor complex. In the case where short-acting benzodiazepines are preferred, medications such as zolpidem and zaleplon provide a safer alternative for patients with respiratory disorders (Sys et al., 2020).

Benzodiazepine receptor agonists are generally well tolerated and are particularly recommended for short-term use (Wagner & Wagner, 2000). They have side effects such as drowsiness and headache; however, excessive use can lead to serious side effects.

Zopiclone, different from benzodiazepines, is from the cyclopyrrolone class and reaches its peak plasma level within 2 hours; its duration of action lasts 6-8 hours, with a short half-life of 4-6 hours (Terzano et al., 2003). Its impact on sleep architecture differs from benzodiazepines; it does not affect REM sleep, reduces Stage 1 sleep, but does not significantly alter Stages 3-4 sleep duration (Terzano et al., 2003). This medication is typically used in a dosage range of 7.5-15 mg, but should be reduced to 3.75 mg in elderly individuals and those with liver disease. Its anxiolytic, muscle relaxant, and anticonvulsant effects are similar to benzodiazepines, with less occurrence of rebound insomnia and tolerance development (Terzano et al., 2003).

Eszopiclone is the I-enantiomer of zopiclone and is particularly preferred for patients experiencing difficulty in initiating sleep and for elderly individuals who do not desire daytime sedation. It is an FDA-approved cyclopyrrolone class medication for the long-term pharmacological treatment of chronic primary insomnia (Rösner et al., 2018).

Zolpidem, different from benzodiazepines, has a minimal impact on sleep architecture, reduces the number of awakenings, and prolongs total sleep duration. It shows features such as delayed REM sleep and increased Stage 3-4 sleep, and it does not exhibit anxiolytic, muscle relaxant, or anticonvulsant effects. It is a medication that can be preferred, especially for patients who have difficulty falling asleep and for elderly patients, due to its short-acting and rare occurrence of the daytime sedation effect (Greenblatt & Roth, 2012).

Zaleplon shortens the sleep initiation period depending on the dose with minimal effect on sleep architecture, but due to its short-acting, it does not prolong the total sleep time. Especially, it is recommended for patients experiencing difficulty initiating sleep and has anxiolytic, muscle relaxant, and anticonvulsant effects (Ebbens & Verster, 2010).

Antidepressants

Antidepressants and other psychotropic medications are commonly used in the treatment of insomnia symptoms (Wichniak et al., 2012). Particularly, quetiapine from antipsychotic; gabapentin, pregabalin, and tiagabine from antiepileptics are used for this purpose (Matheson & Hainer, 2017). However, the lack of evidence on the use of these medications in the treatment of patients with insomnia causes difficulties in guiding healthcare professionals. It is observed that sedative antidepressants, especially those from the tricyclic group, are advantageous for insomnia patients with depression experiencing (Wichniak et al., 2012). Nevertheless, the risks and benefits of using these medications as a first-line treatment for chronic insomnia should be carefully evaluated.

Trazodone is the most commonly prescribed medication among sedating antidepressants, known for its low cost, long-term usability, and lower risk of misuse compared to benzodiazepines. This medication increases slow-wave sleep in patients and does not decrease REM sleep (Yi et al., 2018). However, it should be considered that trazodone can cause orthostatic hypotension and can pose a risk to elderly patients. The selective histamine receptor antagonist doxepin, approved by the FDA for the treatment of insomnia, is effective in low doses for the treatment of insomnia (Matheson & Hainer, 2017). Mirtazapine, in patients with major depression and insomnia, leads to improvements in sleep duration and efficacy (Kamphuis et al., 2015). However, this medication can cause weight gain and daytime sedation in some patients. It is essential to consider the potential side effects of all these antidepressants during their use in the treatment of insomnia.

Antipsychotics

Quetiapine, an atypical antipsychotic, increases total sleep time, sleep efficiency, and Stage 2 sleep in healthy individuals; however, it does not have an official indication for this use, although it is used as a sleep aid in patients with psychiatric disorders (Doroudgar et al., 2013).

Melatonin

Melatonin is considered a weak hypnotic and is used as a rhythm regulator in patients with disrupted circadian rhythms. It is known that the night secretion of this neurohormone from the pituitary gland, and its suppression in bright light, regulation of sleep and circadian rhythm (Lemoine & Zisapel, 2012). Irregularities in melatonin secretion can lead to sleep disorders, and this secretion decreases with age (Cardinali et al., 2012). Melatonin is typically used in doses ranging from 0.3 to 5 mg, with a half-life ranging from 30 to 50 minutes. Ramelteon, approved by the FDA, is a melatonin receptor agonist and is preferred for insomnia with difficulty initiating sleep (Kuriyama et al., 2014). However, it should be considered that incorrect use of melatonin can cause sleep disorders, and ramelteon has a very short duration, lasting approximately one hour.

Conclusion

Insomnia has serious negative effects on individuals and society, being quite prevalent in the community, and this condition is significantly associated with morbidity, mortality, and economic costs. Nevertheless, these costs can be significantly reduced with appropriate diagnosis and treatment methods. In light of this data, insomnia needs to be considered as a significant public health issue. Family physicians, the primary source of health for patients, play a critical role in actively questioning patients about their sleep habits and concerns to prevent the negative effects of insomnia. In this context, family physicians listening to their patients with an empathetic approach and asking relevant questions about their sleep patterns help diagnose individuals experiencing insomnia problems. Especially considering patients' lifestyles and habits, a patient-centered treatment planning increases the effectiveness of insomnia therapy. Moreover, as the 'gatekeepers' of primary care, family physicians refer patients to advanced levels or specialists when necessary allow diagnosis and treatment to continue with a more specific and focused approach.

References

Agargun, M. (1996). Validity and reliability of the Pittsburgh sleep quality index. *Turk Psikiyatri Dergisi*, *7*, 107-115.

Aikens, J. E., & Rouse, M. E. (2005). Help-seeking for insomnia among adult patients in primary care. *The Journal of the American Board of Family Practice*, *18*(4), 257-261. https://doi.org/10.3122/jabfm.18.4.257.

Akerstedt, T., Fredlund, P., Gillberg, M., & Jansson, B. (2002). A prospective study of fatal occupational accidents–relationship to sleeping difficulties and occupational factors. *Journal of sleep research*, *11*(1), 69-71. https://doi.org/10.1046/j.1365-2869.2002.00287.x.

Ancoli-Israel, S. (2000). Insomnia in the elderly: a review for the primary care practitioner. *Sleep*, *23*, S23-30; discussion S36.

Aslan, S., Gulcat, Z., Selda Albayrak, F., Maral, I., Yetkin, S., Sutcigil, L., Aycan, S., Isik, E., & Aydin, H. (2006). Prevalence of insomnia symptoms: results from an urban district in Ankara, Turkey. *International journal of psychiatry in clinical practice*, *10*(1), 52-58. https://doi.org/10.1080/13651500500410364

Aydın, R., Ünal, E., Uzuner, G., Erdinç, O., & Metintaş, S. (2014). Turkish Adaptation of the Pittsburgh Insomnia Rating Scale: A Validity and Reliability Study. 15th National Sleep Medicine Congress. *J Turk Sleep Med*, *1*(Suppl 1), 103.

Aysan, E., Karaköse, S., Zaybak, A., & İsmailoğlu, E. G. (2014). Sleep quality in university students and affecting factors. *Dokuz Eylül Üniversitesi Hemşirelik Fakültesi Elektronik Dergisi*, *7*(3), 193-198.

Baldwin Jr, D. C., & Daugherty, S. R. (2004). Sleep deprivation and fatigue in residency training: results of a national survey of first-and second-year residents. *Sleep*, *27*(2), 217-223. https://doi.org/10.1093/sleep/27.2.217.

Basner, M., & McGuire, S. (2018). WHO environmental noise guidelines for the European region: a systematic review on environmental noise and effects on sleep. *International journal of environmental research and public health*, *15*(3), 519. https://doi.org/10.3390/ijerph15030519.

Bastien, C. H., & Morin, C. M. (2000). Familial incidence of insomnia. *Journal of sleep research*, *9*(1), 49-54. https://doi.org/10.1046/j.1365-2869.2000.00182.x.

Bastien, C. H., Vallières, A., & Morin, C. M. (2001). Validation of the Insomnia Severity Index as an outcome measure for insomnia research. *Sleep Med*, *2*(4), 297-307. https://doi.org/10.1016/s1389-9457(00)00065-4.

Bjorvatn, B., Sagen, I. M., Oyane, N., Waage, S., Fetveit, A., Pallesen, S., & Ursin, R. (2007). The association between sleep duration, body mass index and metabolic measures in the Hordaland Health Study. *Journal of sleep research*, *16*(1), 66-76. https://doi.org/10.1111/j.1365-2869.2007.00569.x.

Bluestein, D., Rutledge, C. M., & Healey, A. C. (2010). Psychosocial correlates of insomnia severity in primary care. *The Journal of the American Board of Family Medicine*, *23*(2), 204-211. https://doi.org/10.3122/jabfm.2010.02.090179.

Boysan, M., Gulec, M., Besiroglu, L., & Kalafat, T. (2010). Psychometric properties of the Insomnia Severity Index in Turkish sample. *Anadolu Psikiyatri Dergisi-Anatolian Journal of Psychiatry*, *11*(3).

Buysse, D. J., Reynolds III, C. F., Kupfer, D. J., Thorpy, M. J., Bixler, E., Manfredi, R., Kales, A., Vgontzas, A., Stepanski, E., & Roth, T. (1994). Clinical diagnoses in 216 insomnia patients using the International Classification of Sleep Disorders (ICSD), DSM-IV and ICD-10 categories: a report from the APA/NIMH DSM-IV Field Trial. *Sleep*, *17*(7), 630-637. https://doi.org/10.1093/sleep/17.7.630.

Buysse, D. J., Reynolds III, C. F., Monk, T. H., Berman, S. R., & Kupfer, D. J. (1989). The Pittsburgh Sleep Quality Index: a new instrument for psychiatric practice and research. *Psychiatry research*, *28*(2), 193-213. https://doi.org/10.1016/0165-1781(89)90047-4.

Buysse, D. J., Soehner, A., Abbott, S., Kapur, V. K., Mahowald, M. W., Parker, K. P., Honeycutt, E. F., Redline, S., Schenck, C. H., & Zee, P. C. (2015). Sleep and Sleep–Wake Disorders. *Psychiatry*, 1264-1310. https://doi.org/10.1002/9781118753378.ch66.

Cappuccio, F. P., Taggart, F. M., Kandala, N.-B., Currie, A., Peile, E., Stranges, S., & Miller, M. A. (2008). Meta-analysis of short sleep duration and obesity in children and adults. *Sleep*, *31*(5), 619-626. https://doi.org/10.1093/sleep/31.5.619.

Cardinali, D. P., Srinivasan, V., Brzezinski, A., & Brown, G. M. (2012). Melatonin and its analogs in insomnia and depression. *Journal of pineal research, 52*(4), 365-375. https://doi.org/10.1111/j.1600-079X.2011.00962.x.

Chehri, A., Kiamanesh, A., Ahadi, H., & Khazaie, H. (2016). Psychometric Properties of the Persian Version of Sleep Hygiene Index in the General Population. *Iran J Psychiatry Behav Sci, 10*(3), e5268. https://doi.org/10.17795/ijpbs-5268.

Chen, L., Bell, J. S., Visvanathan, R., Hilmer, S. N., Emery, T., Robson, L., Hughes, J. M., & Tan, E. C. (2016). The association between benzodiazepine use and sleep quality in residential aged care facilities: a cross-sectional study. *BMC Geriatr, 16*(1), 196. https://doi.org/10.1186/s12877-016-0363-6.

Chung, K. F., Lee, C. T., Yeung, W. F., Chan, M. S., Chung, E. W. Y., & Lin, W. L. (2018). Sleep hygiene education as a treatment of insomnia: a systematic review and meta-analysis. *Family practice, 35*(4), 365-375. https://doi.org/10.1093/fampra/cmx122 .

Culpepper, L., & Wingertzahn, M. A. (2015). Over-the-counter agents for the treatment of occasional disturbed sleep or transient insomnia: a systematic review of efficacy and safety. *The Primary Care Companion for CNS Disorders, 17*(6), 26162. https://doi.org/10.4088/PCC.15r01798.

Daley, M., Morin, C. M., LeBlanc, M., Grégoire, J. P., & Savard, J. (2009). The economic burden of insomnia: direct and indirect costs for individuals with insomnia syndrome, insomnia symptoms, and good sleepers. *Sleep, 32*(1), 55-64.

Debellemaniere, E., Gomez-Merino, D., Erblang, M., Dorey, R., Genot, M., Perreaut-Pierre, E., Pisani, A., Rocco, L., Sauvet, F., & Leger, D. (2018). Using relaxation techniques to improve sleep during naps. *Industrial health, 56*(3), 220-227. https://doi.org/10.2486/indhealth.2017-0092.

Demir, A. U., Ardic, S., Firat, H., Karadeniz, D., Aksu, M., Ucar, Z. Z., Sevim, S., Ozgen, F., Yilmaz, H., & Itil, O. (2015). Prevalence of sleep disorders in the Turkish adult population epidemiology of sleep study. *Sleep and Biological Rhythms, 13*, 298-308. https://doi.org/10.1111/sbr.12118.

Diagnostic and Statistical Manual of Mental Disorders, (DSM 5). . (2013). (fifth ed.). American Psychiatric Association.

Doroudgar, S., Tony, I., Chou, F., Yu, J., Trinh, K., Pal, J., & Perry, P. J. (2013). Evaluation of trazodone and quetiapine for insomnia: an observational study in psychiatric inpatients. *The Primary Care Companion for CNS Disorders, 15*(6), 26342. https://doi.org/10.4088/PCC.13m01558.

Drake, C., Roehrs, T., Shambroom, J., & Roth, T. (2013). Caffeine effects on sleep taken 0, 3, or 6 hours before going to bed. *J Clin Sleep Med, 9*(11), 1195-1200. https://doi.org/10.5664/jcsm.3170.

Ebbens, M. M., & Verster, J. C. (2010). Clinical evaluation of zaleplon in the treatment of insomnia. *Nature and science of sleep*, 115-126. https://doi.org/10.2147/NSS.S6853.

Edinger, J. D., & Morin, C. M. (2012). *Sleep disorders classification and diagnosis*. Oxford Library of Psychology. https://doi.org/10.1093/oxfordhb/9780195376203.013.0019.

Edinger, J. D., & Sampson, W. S. (2003). A primary care 'friendly' cognitive behavioral insomnia therapy. *Sleep, 26*(2), 177-182. https://doi.org/10.1093/sleep/26.2.177.

Edinger, J. D., Wohlgemuth, W. K., Radtke, R. A., Marsh, G. R., & Quillian, R. E. (2001). Cognitive behavioral therapy for treatment of chronic primary insomnia: a randomized controlled trial. *Jama, 285*(14), 1856-1864. https://doi.org/10.1001/jama.285.14.1856.

Fujieda, M., Uchida, K., Ikebe, S., Kimura, A., Kimura, M., Watanabe, T., Sakamoto, H., Matsumoto, T., & Uchimura, N. (2017). Inquiring about insomnia may facilitate diagnosis of depression in the primary care setting. *Psychiatry and clinical neurosciences, 71*(6), 383-394. https://doi.org/10.1111/pcn.12507.

Gagnon, C., Bélanger, L., Ivers, H., & Morin, C. M. (2013). Validation of the Insomnia Severity Index in primary care. *The Journal of the American Board of Family Medicine, 26*(6), 701-710. https://doi.org/10.3122/jabfm.2013.06.130064.

Gamsızkan, Z. (2017). Insomnia; Definition, Classification and Insomnia Management in Primary Care. *Duzce Medical Journal, 19*(2), 48-50.

Gamsızkan, Z., & Aslan, S. (2014). Evaluation of Insomnia Frequency and Related Beliefs and Attitudes in Primary Care. *Journal of Cognitive Behavioral Psychotherapy and Research, 3*, 156-161. https://doi.org/10.5455/JCBPR.38154.

Garbarino, S., Magnavita, N., Guglielmi, O., Maestri, M., Dini, G., Bersi, F. M., Toletone, A., Chiorri, C., & Durando, P. (2017). Insomnia is associated with road accidents. Further evidence from a study on truck drivers. *PLoS One*, *12*(10), e0187256. https://doi.org/10.1371/journal.pone.0187256.

Genç, S., & Dikmen, N. (2017). New Classification of Sleep Disorders (Icsd-3): Changes in the Classification of Sleep Breathing Disorders with Icsd-3. *Mustafa Kemal Üniversitesi Tıp Dergisi*, *8*(31), 23-31. https://doi.org/10.17944/mkutfd.376521.

Greenblatt, D. J., & Roth, T. (2012). Zolpidem for insomnia. *Expert opinion on pharmacotherapy*, *13*(6), 879-893. https://doi.org/10.1517/14656566.2012.667074.

Griffin, C. E., 3rd, Kaye, A. M., Bueno, F. R., & Kaye, A. D. (2013). Benzodiazepine pharmacology and central nervous system-mediated effects. *Ochsner J*, *13*(2), 214-223.

Hajak, G. o., & Group, S. S. (2001). Epidemiology of severe insomnia and its consequences in Germany. *European Archives of Psychiatry and Clinical Neuroscience*, *251*, 49-56. https://doi.org/10.1007/s004060170052.

Holliday, E. G., Magee, C. A., Kritharides, L., Banks, E., & Attia, J. (2013). Short sleep duration is associated with risk of future diabetes but not cardiovascular disease: a prospective study and meta-analysis. *PLoS One*, *8*(11), e82305. https://doi.org/10.1371/journal.pone.0082305.

Im, E., & Kim, G.-S. (2017). Relationship between sleep duration and Framingham cardiovascular risk score and prevalence of cardiovascular disease in Koreans. *Medicine*, *96*(37). https://doi.org/10.1097/MD.0000000000007744.

Irish, L. A., Kline, C. E., Gunn, H. E., Buysse, D. J., & Hall, M. H. (2015). The role of sleep hygiene in promoting public health: A review of empirical evidence. *Sleep medicine reviews*, *22*, 23-36. https://doi.org/10.1016/j.smrv.2014.10.001.

Jansson-Fröjmark, M., Alfonsson, S., Bohman, B., Rozental, A., & Norell-Clarke, A. (2022). Paradoxical intention for insomnia: A systematic review and meta-analysis. *J Sleep Res*, *31*(2), e13464. https://doi.org/10.1111/jsr.13464.

Kahraman, M. (2006). Clinical update on epidemiology, pathogenesis and nonpharmacological treatment of insomnia. *Turk Noroloji Dergisi*, *12*, 87-97.

Kamphuis, J., Taxis, K., Schuiling-Veninga, C. C., Bruggeman, R., & Lancel, M. (2015). Off-label prescriptions of low-dose quetiapine and mirtazapine for insomnia in the Netherlands. *Journal of clinical psychopharmacology*, *35*(4), 468-470. https://doi.org/10.1097/JCP.0000000000000338.

Kapur, V. K., Redline, S., Nieto, F. J., Young, T. B., Newman, A. B., & Henderson, J. A. (2002). The relationship between chronically disrupted sleep and healthcare use. *Sleep*, *25*(3), 289-296.

Karadag, H. (2016). Cognitive and Pharmacological Treatments for Insomnia. *Journal of Turkish Sleep Medicine*, *3*(1), 11.

Keskin, N., & Tamam, L. (2018). Sleep disorders: Classification and treatment. *Arşiv Kaynak Tarama Dergisi*, *27*(2), 241-260. https://doi.org/10.17827/aktd.346010.

Krystal, A. D., Prather, A. A., & Ashbrook, L. H. (2019). The assessment and management of insomnia: an update. *World Psychiatry*, *18*(3), 337-352. https://doi.org/10.1002/wps.20674.

Kuriyama, A., Honda, M., & Hayashino, Y. (2014). Ramelteon for the treatment of insomnia in adults: a systematic review and meta-analysis. *Sleep medicine*, *15*(4), 385-392. https://doi.org/10.1016/j.sleep.2013.11.788.

Lemoine, P., & Zisapel, N. (2012). Prolonged-release formulation of melatonin (Circadin) for the treatment of insomnia. *Expert opinion on pharmacotherapy*, *13*(6), 895-905. https://doi.org/10.1517/14656566.2012.667076.

Li, B.-F., Moree, W. J., Yu, J., Coon, T., Zamani-Kord, S., Malany, S., Jalali, K., Wen, J., Wang, H., & Yang, C. (2010). Selectivity profiling of novel indene H1-antihistamines for the treatment of insomnia. *Bioorganic & Medicinal Chemistry Letters*, *20*(8), 2629-2633. https://doi.org/10.1016/j.bmcl.2010.02.055.

Lie, J. D., Tu, K. N., Shen, D. D., & Wong, B. M. (2015). Pharmacological treatment of insomnia. *Pharmacy and Therapeutics*, *40*(11), 759.

Lie, J. D., Tu, K. N., Shen, D. D., & Wong, B. M. (2015). Pharmacological Treatment of Insomnia. *P t*, *40*(11), 759-771.

Lou, B. X., & Oks, M. (2021). Insomnia: pharmacologic treatment. *Clinics in Geriatric Medicine*, *37*(3), 401-415. https://doi.org/10.1016/j.cger.2021.04.003.

Mastin, D. F., Bryson, J., & Corwyn, R. (2006). Assessment of sleep hygiene using the Sleep Hygiene Index. *Journal of behavioral medicine*, *29*, 223-227. https://doi.org/10.1007/s10865-006-9047-6.

Matheson, E., & Hainer, B. L. (2017). Insomnia: pharmacologic therapy. *American family physician*, *96*(1), 29-35.

Meyer, T. J. (1998). Evaluation and management of insomnia. *Hosp Pract (1995)*, *33*(12), 75-78, 83-76. https://doi.org/10.3810/hp.1998.12.122.

Morin, C. M., Belleville, G., Bélanger, L., & Ivers, H. (2011). The Insomnia Severity Index: psychometric indicators to detect insomnia cases and evaluate treatment response. *Sleep*, *34*(5), 601-608. https://doi.org/10.1093/sleep/34.5.601.

Morin, C. M., Mimeault, V., & Gagné, A. (1999). Nonpharmacological treatment of late-life insomnia. *Journal of psychosomatic research*, *46*(2), 103-116. https://doi.org/10.1016/S0022-3999(98)00077-4.

Oğuz, S., Keskin Dilbay, N., Çeliktaş, E., Balcılar, R., & Polat, M. G. (2019). Effect of progressive relaxation exercises on stress level, sleep quality and exercise capacity in young adults. *Sağlık Bilimleri ve Meslekleri Dergisi*, *6*(3), 534-544.

Ozdemir, P. G., Boysan, M., Selvi, Y., Yildirim, A., & Yilmaz, E. (2015). Psychometric properties of the Turkish version of the Sleep Hygiene Index in clinical and non-clinical samples. *Compr Psychiatry*, *59*, 135-140. https://doi.org/10.1016/j.comppsych.2015.02.001.

Pagel, J. F., & Parnes, B. L. (2001). Medications for the Treatment of Sleep Disorders: An Overview. *Prim Care Companion J Clin Psychiatry*, *3*(3), 118-125. https://doi.org/10.4088/PCC.v03n0303.

Radecki, S. E., & Brunton, S. A. (1993). Management of insomnia in office-based practice: national prevalence and therapeutic patterns. *Archives of Family Medicine*, *2*(11), 1129. https://doi.org/10.1001/archfami.2.11.1129.

Rakel, R. E. (1993). Insomnia: concerns of the family physician. *Journal of family practice*, *36*, 551-551.

Ram, S., Seirawan, H., Kumar, S. K., & Clark, G. T. (2010). Prevalence and impact of sleep disorders and sleep habits in the United States. *Sleep Breath*, *14*(1), 63-70. https://doi.org/10.1007/s11325-009-0281-3.

Ringdahl, E. N., Pereira, S. L., & Delzell, J. E. (2004a). Treatment of primary insomnia. *The Journal of the American Board of Family Practice*, *17*(3), 212-219. https://doi.org/10.3122/jabfm.17.3.212.

Ringdahl, E. N., Pereira, S. L., & Delzell, J. E. J. (2004b). Treatment of primary insomnia. *J Am Board Fam Pract*, *17*(3), 212-219. https://doi.org/10.3122/jabfm.17.3.212.

Rösner, S., Englbrecht, C., Wehrle, R., Hajak, G., & Soyka, M. (2018). Eszopiclone for insomnia. *Cochrane Database of Systematic Reviews*(10). https://doi.org/10.1002/14651858.CD010703.pub2.

Sabanayagam, C., & Shankar, A. (2010). Sleep duration and cardiovascular disease: results from the National Health Interview Survey. *Sleep*, *33*(8), 1037-1042. https://doi.org/10.1093/sleep/33.8.1037.

Safer, V. B. (2017). Factors Affecting the Sleep Quality of Children and Mothers with Cerebral Palsy and Depression in Mothers. *Zeynep Kamil Tıp Bülteni*, *48*(2), 53-59.

Sarısaltık, A., & Topuzoğlu, A. (2019). Screening and Evaluation of Sleep Disorders in Primary Health Care Services. *ESTÜDAM Halk Sağlığı Dergisi*, *4*(2), 232-243. https://doi.org/10.35232/estudamhsd.526007.

Sateia, M. J. (2014). International classification of sleep disorders. *Chest*, *146*(5), 1387-1394. https://doi.org/10.1378/chest.14-0970.

Savard, M. H., Savard, J., Simard, S., & Ivers, H. (2005). Empirical validation of the Insomnia Severity Index in cancer patients. *Psycho-Oncology: Journal of the Psychological, Social and Behavioral Dimensions of Cancer*, *14*(6), 429-441. https://doi.org/10.1002/pon.860.

Saygın, M., Öztürk, Ö., Şenel, F. A., & Yalçın, A. (2021). Family physicians' awareness levels about sleep disorders. *Uyku Bülteni*, *2*(2), 26-31.

Shochat, T., Umphress, J., Israel, A. G., & Ancoli-Israel, S. (1999). Insomnia in primary care patients. *Sleep*, *22*, S359-365.

Siebern, A. T., Suh, S., & Nowakowski, S. (2012). Non-pharmacological treatment of insomnia. *Neurotherapeutics*, *9*(4), 717-727. https://doi.org/10.1007/s13311-012-0142-9.

Smith, M. T., Perlis, M. L., Park, A., Smith, M. S., Pennington, J., Giles, D. E., & Buysse, D. J. (2002). Comparative meta-analysis of pharmacotherapy and behavior therapy for persistent insomnia. *Am J Psychiatry*, *159*(1), 5-11. https://doi.org/10.1176/appi.ajp.159.1.5.

Spicuzza, L., Caruso, D., & Di Maria, G. (2015). Obstructive sleep apnoea syndrome and its management. *Therapeutic advances in chronic disease*, *6*(5), 273-285. https://doi.org/10.1177/2040622315590318.

Spielman, A. J., Saskin, P., & Thorpy, M. J. (1987). Treatment of chronic insomnia by restriction of time in bed. *Sleep*, *10*(1), 45-56.

Sys, J., Van Cleynenbreugel, S., Deschodt, M., Van der Linden, L., & Tournoy, J. (2020). Efficacy and safety of non-benzodiazepine and non-Z-drug hypnotic medication for insomnia in older people: a systematic literature review. *European Journal of Clinical Pharmacology*, *76*, 363-381. https://doi.org/10.1007/s00228-019-02812-z.

Terzano, M. G., Rossi, M., Palomba, V., Smerieri, A., & Parrino, L. (2003). New drugs for insomnia: comparative tolerability of zopiclone, zolpidem and zaleplon. *Drug safety*, *26*, 261-282. https://doi.org/10.2165/00002018-200326040-00004.

Tjepkema, M. (2005). Insomnia. *Health Rep*, *17*(1), 9-25.

Tümer, A., İlhan, B., & Kartal, A. (2017). Prevelance of insomnia in young people. *OPUS International Journal of Society Researches*, *7*(13), 426-439. https://doi.org/10.26466/opus.337353.

Wagner, J., & Wagner, M. L. (2000). Non-benzodiazepines for the treatment of insomnia. *Sleep medicine reviews*, *4*(6), 551-581. https://doi.org/10.1053/smrv.2000.0126.

Wagner, J., Wagner, M. L., & Hening, W. A. (1998). Beyond benzodiazepines: alternative pharmacologic agents for the treatment of insomnia. *Annals of Pharmacotherapy*, *32*(6), 680-691. https://doi.org/10.1345/aph.17111.

Wichniak, A., Wierzbicka, A., & Jernajczyk, W. (2012). Sleep and antidepressant treatment. *Current Pharmaceutical Design*, *18*(36), 5802-5817. https://doi.org/10.2174/138161212803523608.

Yi, X.-y., Ni, S.-f., Ghadami, M. R., Meng, H.-q., Chen, M.-y., Kuang, L., Zhang, Y.-q., Zhang, L., & Zhou, X.-y. (2018). Trazodone for the treatment of insomnia: a meta-analysis of randomized placebo-controlled trials. *Sleep medicine*, *45*, 25-32. https://doi.org/10.1016/j.sleep.2018.01.010.

Yılmaz, H., Tuncel, D., Aksu, M., Akyıldız, U. O., Alp, R., Arslan, K., Baklan, B., Bakar, E. E., Benbir, G., & Demir, C. F. (2014). Treatment Guide for Sleep Disorders.

Chapter 26

Periodic Health Examination

Aydan Çevik Varol[*]**, MD**
Department of Family Medicine, Namık Kemal University, Tekirdag, Turkiye

Abstract

Periodic health examination underscores the pivotal role of regular health assessments in family medicine, particularly within the realm of respiratory system diseases. Periodic health examinations, commonly known as check-ups, have immense value in identifying potential health concerns before they escalate. The chapter emphasizes the significance of early detection and prevention through these examinations. By delving into patient history, conducting comprehensive physical examinations, and employing diagnostic tools such as pulmonary function tests and chest X-rays, practitioners can effectively address respiratory ailments. The chapter also stresses the importance of patient education in matters of respiratory health, including advising on habits such as smoking cessation and strategies for minimizing exposure to pollutants. This holistic approach empowers healthcare professionals in family medicine to proactively enhance patient care and contribute significantly to the management of respiratory conditions. In conclusion, periodic health examinations performed are critical for respiratory health in society within family medicine practice in terms of early diagnosis, early management of the disease, and prevention of some complications.

Keywords: periodic health examination

Introduction

In the realm of contemporary medical practice, the significance of periodic health assessments in the identification and management of respiratory system ailments cannot be overstated. For family physicians, a proficient comprehension of the intricacies surrounding regular health evaluations for respiratory diseases is essential. This chapter attemps to elucidate the pivotal role that periodic health examinations play in discerning and mitigating respiratory system afflictions (Wodwaski, & Webber, 2023; Riobó et al., 1992; Simpson, 2006).

The human respiratory system, a dynamic nexus of anatomical structures and physiological mechanisms, stands as a cornerstone of vitality. It is imperative that family physicians

[*] Corresponding Author's Email: dracevik@gmail.com.

In: Common Diseases According to Family Medicine Practice Guidelines
Editors: Esra Meltem Koç and Hilal Aksoy
ISBN: 979-8-89530-302-3

understand the nuances of this intricate system to effectively safeguard the well-being of their patients. Within the context of respiratory system diseases, early detection, and timely intervention wield a formidable influence on prognosis and therapeutic efficacy (Riobó et al., 1992; Simpson, 2006; Moore, 2007; Tokman, & Huang, 2013).

The ensuing sections of this chapter shall delve into the anatomical foundations of the respiratory system, elucidate prevalent respiratory diseases, expound on the indispensability of periodic health assessments, and elaborate upon the multifaceted components therein. By navigating this compilation, family physicians will be equipped not only to comprehend the nuances of respiratory health examinations, but also to utilize this knowledge to optimize patient care. Through this exploration, the chapter aspires to empower family physicians with the tools requisite for informed decision-making and superior patient outcomes in the domain of respiratory health.

The Importance of Periodic Health Examination (PHE)

In the intricate tapestry of modern medical practice, periodic health examinations emerge as a paramount strategy in the preservation of respiratory wellness. For family practitioners, a deep appreciation of the crucial role these assessments play in the early detection and management of respiratory diseases is imperative (Wodwaski, & Webber, 2023; Riobó et al., 1992; Sharp, & Rozanski, 2013; Hinchcliff, & Byrne, 1991).

Respiratory system diseases, ranging from the insidious progression of chronic conditions such as chronic obstructive pulmonary disease (COPD) to the potentially aggressive manifestation of lung malignancies, underscore the gravity of the matter. Periodic health examinations serve as the vanguard in this battle, acting as a potent conduit for the identification of subtle deviations from physiological norms (Simpson, 2006, Moore, 2007, Tokman, & Huang, 2013). Early detection of respiratory irregularities through these examinations provides a dual advantage. Firstly, it affords clinicians the opportunity to initiate interventions in the nascent stages of disease progression, thereby thwarting its potential exacerbation. Secondly, it paves the way for a more precise assessment of treatment modalities, thereby amplifying therapeutic efficacy (Sharp, & Rozanski, 2013; Hinchcliff, & Byrne, 1991; Benbassat, & Baumal, 2010).

The ramifications of a comprehensive respiratory health assessment cascade in multiple domains. Family physicians, as the primary custodians of patient well-being, are sentinels in averting the downstream consequences of undiagnosed and unmanaged respiratory diseases. Using the insights gleaned from these examinations, healthcare providers can orchestrate personalized care plans, thus minimizing morbidity, mortality, and the attendant burden of healthcare. It is incumbent on family physicians to foster an environment of proactive engagement with patients, highlighting the value of periodic health examinations as an investment in sustained respiratory health. Through this collaborative effort, patients are empowered to take charge of their well-being, engendering a harmonious synergy between medical expertise and patient agency (Bowman et al., 2023; Teixeira et al., 2020; Woodruff, 2021; Lemire, & Mang, 2020).

PHEs can help detect respiratory system diseases early when they are most treatable. They can also help identify risk factors for respiratory system diseases, such as smoking and exposure to environmental pollutants. PHEs typically include a physical examination, a review of the patient's medical history, and laboratory tests. The physical examination may include listening to the lungs for abnormal sounds, such as wheezing or crackles. The review of the medical history can focus on the patient's risk factors for respiratory system diseases. Laboratory tests may include a chest X-ray, a blood test, or a sputum culture (Wodwaski, & Webber, 2023; Riobó et al., 1992; Simpson, 2006; Moore, 2007; Benbassat, & Baumal, 2010).

Here are some of the benefits of periodic health examinations for respiratory system diseases (Riobó et al., 1992; Simpson, 2006; Moore, 2007; Tokman, & Huang, 2013; Sharp, & Rozanski, 2013):

- Early detection and diagnosis of respiratory system diseases can lead to earlier and more effective treatment.
- PHEs can help identify risk factors for respiratory system diseases, such as smoking and exposure to environmental pollutants.
- PHEs can help educate patients about respiratory system diseases and how to prevent them.
- PHEs can help improve the quality of life of people with respiratory system diseases.

Family physicians play an important role in promoting periodic health examinations for respiratory system diseases. They can educate patients about the importance of PHEs and help to make sure that they receive the recommended screenings. In the ensuing segments of this chapter, the intricacies of the creation of a comprehensive respiratory health examination are elucidated. By mastering this discipline, family physicians assume a pivotal role in the pursuit of holistic patient care, steering the course toward optimal respiratory well-being and improved quality of life (Riobó et al., 1992; Hinchcliff, & Byrne, 1991; Bowman et al., 2023; Teixeira et al., 2020).

Components of a Periodic Health Examination for Respiratory System Diseases

The meticulous orchestration of a comprehensive respiratory health examination requires a systematic approach, enabling family physicians to unravel potential anomalies within the intricate domain of the respiratory system. This section unveils the multifaceted components integral to such assessments, fostering a nuanced understanding vital for accurate detection and adept management of respiratory ailments (Hinchcliff, & Byrne, 1991; Benbassat, & Baumal, 2010; Donn & Sinha, 2017).

An exhaustive inquiry into the patient's medical history unveils invaluable insight. Scrutinizing familial predispositions, previous respiratory conditions, and occupational exposures provides a foundational framework for further evaluation. The meticulous auscultation of lung sounds, assessment of respiratory rate and evaluation of chest expansion form the bedrock of physical evaluations. Subtle signs such as wheezing, crackles, or diminished breath sounds are indicative of underlying respiratory aberrations (Benbassat, & Baumal, 2010; Donn & Sinha, 2017; Bertrand et al., 2020).

The inclusion of spirometry and peak flow measurements provides quantitative data on lung capacity and airway obstruction. These metrics provide essential information for the diagnosis of conditions such as asthma and COPD. Radiological modalities, including chest X-rays and computed tomography (CT), scans provide anatomical insight. Interpretation of these images detects structural abnormalities, infiltrates, and masses that may denote underlying respiratory pathologies (Bertrand et al., 2020; Puente Maestú, & García de Pedro, 2012; Nagewo et al., 2015).

Blood tests facilitating the analysis of biomarkers such as C-reactive protein (CRP) and arterial blood gases elucidate systemic inflammation and gas exchange derangements, respectively. Sputum analysis aids in diagnosing infections and determining optimal treatment strategies. In cases suggestive of allergic etiologies, allergy testing assists in identifying specific triggers. This knowledge guides therapeutic decisions, mitigating allergen-induced respiratory distress (Donn & Sinha, 2017; Bourouiba, 2021; Wise et al., 2018).

Cognizant integration of these components culminates in a panoramic assessment, enabling precise diagnosis and tailored interventions. Recognition of abnormal findings demands meticulous interpretation, thus necessitating a synthesis of clinical experience and scientific data. The subsequent steps involve personalized patient engagement. Articulating findings to patients, outlining the significance of detected anomalies, and elucidating the proposed course of action establishes a collaborative dynamic. Should the need arise, judicious referrals to respiratory specialists ensure specialized care, thereby enhancing patient outcomes. The cardinal principle herein resides in the holistic comprehension of the respiratory system's intricacies. Family physicians, as custodians of comprehensive patient care, use these components to orchestrate interventions that resonate across the spectrum of respiratory health (Moore, 2007; Tokman, & Huang, 2013; Donn & Sinha, 2017).

Assessment of Lung Function

The evaluation of lung function is an integral aspect of periodic health examinations, especially in the context of respiratory health. This section delves into the various techniques and tools used to assess lung function, elucidating how these assessments provide invaluable insights into respiratory well-being and aid in the early detection of lung-related issues (Donn & Sinha, 2017; Bertrand et al., 2020; Puente Maestú, & García de Pedro, 2012).

Spirometry is a cornerstone in the evaluation of lung function. This non-invasive test measures the volume of air an individual can inhale and exhale and the rate at which these exchanges occur. By quantifying metrics such as forced vital capacity (FVC) and forced expiratory volume in one second (FEV1), spirometry aids in diagnose conditions such as asthma, COPD, and restrictive lung diseases (Zhao et al., 2022; Serifoglu & Ulubay, 2019).

Peak expiratory flow monitoring gauges the maximum speed at which an individual can forcefully exhale. This technique is particularly valuable for individuals with asthma, as it provides insights into the narrowing of the airways and the efficacy of bronchodilator medications. Regular PEF measurements facilitate the early detection of worsening symptoms and prompt adjustments to treatment plans (Hanon et al., 2021; Ruffin, 2004).

Pulmonary function testing encompasses a suite of evaluations that delve deeper into lung mechanics. These tests include measurements of lung volumes, diffusion capacity, and airway resistance. PFTs provide a comprehensive picture of lung health, aiding in the diagnosis and monitoring of a range of respiratory conditions, including interstitial lung disease and lung fibrosis (Ruppel, & Enright, 2012; Bernstein., 2012).

Arterial blood gas (ABG) analysis assesses the levels of oxygen and carbon dioxide in the blood. This evaluation offers insights into respiratory efficiency, acid-base balance, and overall oxygenation. ABG analysis is particularly useful in critical care settings and for individuals with severe respiratory illnesses, guiding treatment decisions and ventilator management (Carlino et al., 2020; Larkin, & Zimmanck, 2015).

Exercise testing evaluates lung function under exertion, shedding light on an individual's respiratory capacity during physical activity. These tests not only aid diagnose exercise-induced bronchoconstriction and other exertional respiratory issues but also guide the development of personalized exercise regimens that optimize respiratory health (Tran, 2018; DeCato et al., 2020).

Radiological imaging, including chest X-rays and computed tomography scans, provides a visual representation of lung structures. These images assist in identifying structural abnormalities, such as tumors, infections, and pneumothorax. Radiological assessments contribute to a comprehensive understanding of respiratory health and inform subsequent diagnostic steps (Ley., 2015; San José Estépar., 2022).

Risk Factor Considerations

In the nuanced landscape of respiratory health evaluations, family physicians are tasked with a judicious amalgamation of age-related dynamics and intricate risk factor assessments. This section explores the vital interaction between age and risk factors, providing family physicians with a compass to navigate the tailored landscape of periodic health examinations for respiratory system diseases (Hogea et al., 2020; Almirall et al., 2017).

The continuum of age significantly impacts respiratory health trajectories. From the dynamic developmental nuances in pediatric patients to the age-associated vulnerabilities in geriatric individuals, the astute consideration of age guides examination parameters. Pediatric assessments emphasize developmental milestones, whereas geriatric evaluations encompass the discernment of physiological decline (Hogea et al., 2020; Almirall et al., 2017; Akhter et al., 2021).

The pervasive influence of tobacco use requires meticulous inquiry. From adolescents experimenting with nicotine to long-term smokers, a detailed exploration of smoking history unveils potential risks for respiratory ailments such as COPD and lung cancer. Occupational exposures to airborne irritants or toxins further amplify risk profiles. Geographic location and environmental exposure garner prominence. Urban environments laden with pollutants, allergens, and particulate matter contrast with rural settings characterized by allergenic triggers. Awareness of these contextual factors increases the precision of assessments (Hogea et al., 2020; Almirall et al., 2017; Akhter et al., 2021; Masarweh et al., 2021; Povoa et al., 2021).

Genetic predispositions underscore the familial clustering of respiratory disorders. A comprehensive investigation of family history unravels hereditary tendencies, making it an invaluable dimension for early detection and preventive strategies. Coexisting medical conditions such as cardiovascular diseases and diabetes interweave with respiratory health. Family physicians must unravel these intricacies, recognizing how intertwined ailments increase susceptibility to respiratory diseases (Almirall et al., 2017; Akhter et al., 2021; Masarweh et al., 2021).

Vaccination status, particularly against influenza and pneumococcal infections, significantly mitigates the burdens of respiratory diseases. Tracking immunization records and advocating for vaccinations are integral to preventive measures. The burgeoning obesity epidemic reverberates within respiratory health. Family physicians assess metabolic parameters and body composition, recognizing the propensity of obesity to exacerbate respiratory conditions. Allergic predispositions often serve as precursors to respiratory disorders such as asthma. The examination of allergies and atopic tendencies equips family physicians with anticipatory strategies (Hogea et al., 2020; Almirall et al., 2017; Akhter et al., 2021; Masarweh et al., 2021).

By adeptly marrying age-specific considerations with the intricate tapestry of risk factors, family physicians chart personalized courses of action. The art herein rests in an adept blend of clinical acumen and scientific insight, transcending simple identification into the realm of tailored interventions. As this chapter unfolds, the case illustrations will further illuminate the fusion of age and risk factors, nurturing a comprehensive mastery of respiratory health evaluations (Hogea et al., 2020; Almirall et al., 2017; Akhter et al., 2021).

Pediatric Respiratory Health Assessments

Children's respiratory health is of paramount importance, laying the foundation for a lifetime of well-being. This section delves into the significance of pediatric respiratory health assessments in the context of periodic health examinations, highlighting the unique considerations, assessment methods, and interventions that contribute to optimal lung function in young individuals (Masarweh et al., 2021; Shah et al., 2017).

Pediatric respiratory health assessments require a specialized approach due to the distinct physiological characteristics of growing bodies. Children have smaller airways, making them more susceptible to respiratory infections and obstructions. Their respiratory systems are still developing, which influences the way illnesses manifest and the potential long-term effects of respiratory issues. Periodic health examinations for pediatric respiratory health encompass a range of assessment techniques tailored to children's needs. Objective measures such as lung function tests, including peak expiratory flow measurements, can provide insight into lung capacity and potential restrictions. Healthcare practitioners also rely on thorough medical history reviews, assessing symptoms, and observing breathing patterns to detect early signs of respiratory disorders (Masarweh et al., 2021; Shah et al., 2017; Ventre et al., 2011; Goetz & Singh, 2016).

Pediatric respiratory assessments are intricately related to developmental milestones. Monitoring the attainment of these milestones, such as proper breathing patterns, chest expansion, and normal speech development, provides healthcare professionals with information on potential deviations that might indicate underlying respiratory issues. Periodic health examinations serve as essential opportunities to identify and address common pediatric respiratory issues. Asthma, wheezing, bronchiolitis, and upper respiratory infections are prevalent in children. Through vigilant assessments, healthcare providers can offer timely interventions, treatments, and education to parents and caregivers, thus ensuring optimal respiratory health as children grow (Shah et al., 2017; Ventre et al., 2011; Goetz & Singh, 2016; Camargos, & Watts, 2021).

Pediatric respiratory health assessments offer a platform to educate parents and caregivers about preventive measures. Educating families about reducing exposure to environmental triggers, ensuring proper vaccination, and fostering healthy lifestyle habits can significantly contribute to minimizing respiratory risks in children. As children transition into adolescence and adulthood, their respiratory health needs evolve. Periodic health examinations play a vital role in monitoring this transition, assessing lung function changes, and addressing any ongoing respiratory concerns. This continuity of care ensures a seamless shift from pediatric to adult healthcare settings (Ventre et al., 2011; Goetz & Singh, 2016; Camargos, & Watts, 2021).

Pediatric respiratory health assessments lay the foundation for a lifetime of optimal lung function and overall well-being. By promoting early detection, prevention, and parental education, healthcare professionals prepare the way for children to grow into adults with a heightened awareness of the importance of respiratory health and the tools to maintain it (Masarweh et al., 2021; Shah et al., 2017; Camargos, & Watts, 2021).

Interpreting Examination Results

The culmination of a meticulous respiratory health examination unveils a tapestry of clinical data, necessitating astute interpretation to unearth diagnostic insights. This section explores the realm of deciphering examination results, arming family physicians with the ability to navigate the intricacies of respiratory health assessment. Synthesizing the patient's medical history with the examination findings enriches contextual comprehension. Family physicians correlate symptoms, exposures, and familial tendencies, thus fostering a holistic diagnostic framework (Hinchcliff, & Byrne, 1991; Benbassat, & Baumal, 2010; Donn & Sinha, 2017).

The auscultation of lung sounds, detection of wheezing, or the presence of accessory muscle usage serve as corroborative evidence. The correlation between clinical observations and examination outcomes improves diagnostic accuracy. Spirometry and peak flow measurements reveal quantitative lung capacity and airway obstruction. These figures, juxtaposed with established norms, illuminate conditions such as asthma or COPD (Bertrand et al., 2020; Puente Maestú, & García de Pedro, 2012; Nagewo et al., 2015).

Radiological images obtained from chest X-rays and computed tomography (CT) scans require skilled interpretation. Recognition of infiltrates, masses, and anatomical anomalies underpins diagnosis, enriching the diagnostic tableau. Blood tests provide biochemical information. Elevation of biomarkers such as CRP signals inflammation, guiding diagnostic trajectories. Arterial blood gases unravel aberrations of gas exchange, guiding interventions for respiratory failure (Donn & Sinha, 2017; Ley., 2015; San José Estépar., 2022).

Identification of allergens or pathogens through tests such as sputum analysis or allergy panels substantiates etiological attributions. These findings, linked to clinical presentation, aid in the design of therapeutic strategies. The convergence of various data streams fortifies diagnostic precision. Integration of history, physical findings, laboratory results, and imaging studies creates a comprehensive diagnostic mosaic (Wise et al., 2018; Goetz & Singh, 2016; Zhang et al., 2022).

Deciphering the delineation between normal and aberrant findings underscores clinical acumen. Distinctive alterations from baseline norms serve as sentinel markers, directing clinical focus. Precision in interpretation fuels personalized patient management. Family physicians, through skillful analysis, delineate the diagnostic trajectory, paving the path for customized interventions. The strategic interplay of scientific rigor and clinical intuition navigates the intricate waters of respiratory health (1; Simpson, 2006; Donn & Sinha, 2017).

Preventive Measures and Lifestyle Recommendations

Within the realm of respiratory health assessments, family physicians have the imperative responsibility of not only to identify afflictions but also to instill preventive paradigms that mitigate disease progression. This section embarks on an exploration of preventive measures and lifestyle advice, equipping family physicians to guide patients toward optimal respiratory well-being. Tobacco's insidious impact necessitates an unwavering focus on smoking cessation. Family physicians employ evidence-based techniques, guiding patients through nicotine dependence management to curtail the precipitous progression of chronic respiratory ailments (Hogea et al., 2020; Almirall et al., 2017; Akhter et al., 2021).

Regular physical activity bestows multi-faceted respiratory benefits. Family physicians advocate for exercise regimens tailored to patient capacities, increasing lung capacity, and fortifying overall respiratory vigor. The intricate nexus between obesity and respiratory diseases demands vigilance in weight management. Family physicians orchestrate customized dietary interventions, fostering weight modulation that is harmonized with optimal respiratory function (Teixeira et al., 2020; Woodruff, 2021; Lemire, & Mang, 2020).

Education in indoor air quality optimization reduces allergen and irritant exposures. Family physicians guide patients in minimizing triggers such as mold, dust mites, and pet dander, resulting in notable alleviation of respiratory symptoms. The advocacy for influenza and pneumococcal vaccinations is integral to respiratory wellness. Family physicians elucidate the protective mantle conferred by immunization, significantly reducing susceptibility to respiratory infections (Hogea et al., 2020; Alderson et al., 2020; Martin et al., 2018).

Allergy-prone patients benefit from targeted allergen avoidance strategies. Family physicians decipher allergen sources, facilitating personalized precautions that reduce the burden of allergic respiratory manifestations. Patients grappling with asthma gain empowerment through personalized action plans. Family physicians define proactive steps for symptom exacerbations, ensuring timely intervention and reducing disease exacerbations (Wise et al., 2018; D'Amato et al., 2020; Principi et al., 2018).

Awareness of occupational exposures is paramount in preventive efforts. Family physicians inform patients of potential workplace irritants or toxins, making informed decisions that safeguard respiratory health. The interaction of medical expertise with patient education propels preventive paradigms, forging a potent alliance against respiratory diseases. Family physicians illuminate the trajectory of wellness through lifestyle modifications, reducing the encroachment of respiratory diseases (Principi et al., 2018; Emamian et al., 2013; Seele & Spallek, 2015).

Follow-Up and Referrals

The continuum of care in respiratory health examinations extends beyond a simple assessment, encompassing vigilant follow-up and judicious referrals. This section navigates the intricate tapestry of post-examination management, equipping family physicians with the discernment to steer patient trajectories toward optimal respiratory well-being. Family physicians chart meticulous follow-up protocols, tailoring the frequency of subsequent evaluations based on examination findings and patient characteristics. A nuanced approach ensures the timely detection of evolving respiratory dynamics (Riobó et al., 1992; Woodruff, 2021; Lemire, & Mang, 2020; Donn & Sinha, 2017).

The legacy of the assessment is gauged through the efficacy of the instituted interventions. Family physicians use objective metrics and patient-reported outcomes to track treatment effectiveness, adapting strategies as needed. The continuum of care thrives on patient empowerment. Family physicians improve patient education by elucidating the importance of adherence to prescribed medications, lifestyle adjustments, and self-monitoring regimens. The recognition of complex or refractory cases prompts judicious referrals to respiratory specialists. Family physicians leverage interdisciplinary collaboration to ensure that patients have access to specialized insights and interventions. Periodic respiratory health assessments are sentinel markers of disease progression. Family physicians monitor trends in examination findings, facilitating timely escalation of interventions in response to evolving respiratory dynamics (Woodruff, 2021; Lemire, & Mang, 2020; Donn & Sinha, 2017; Kim et al., 2016).

Complex cases demand a multidisciplinary approach. Family physicians coordinate seamless collaboration with pulmonologists, allergists, and other specialists to obtain comprehensive information for holistic patient management. The thread that binds follow-up and referrals lies in patient-centric communication. Family physicians communicate the significance of follow-up evaluations and referrals, educating patients about their integral role in their respiratory health journey. Chronic respiratory conditions warrant long-term vigilance. Family physicians design continuous monitoring to ensure the timely detection of relapses, exacerbations, or emerging comorbidities. Through meticulous orchestration of follow-up and judicious referrals, family physicians guide patient trajectories toward sustained respiratory wellness. The artistry herein emerges through a fusion of medical expertise, patient engagement, and interdisciplinary collaboration (Woodruff, 2021; Lemire, & Mang, 2020; Donn & Sinha, 2017; Kim et al., 2016; Zurbano & Zurbano, 2017).

Patient Education and Empowerment

In the realm of respiratory health evaluations, family physicians serve as torchbearers of patient education, igniting a paradigm of informed decision-making and proactive engagement. This section embarks on an exploration of patient education and empowerment, endowing family physicians with the tools to foster a symbiotic partnership with patients for optimal respiratory well-being. Family physicians reveal the intricacies of respiratory diseases, elucidating the underlying pathophysiological mechanisms. By imparting this knowledge, patients gain a profound comprehension of their conditions, promoting adherence to therapeutic regimens (Ouksel et al., 2022; Price et al., 2011; Hammoud et al., 2020).

The interpretation of examination outcomes forms the basis for patient education. Family physicians demystify the findings, illustrating their relevance and guiding patients in comprehending the implications for their respiratory health. Armed with medical insights, family physicians prescribe personalized lifestyle adjustments. Patients are enlightened on tailored strategies, such as smoking cessation, exercise routines, and dietary modifications that increase respiratory vitality. The nuances of prescribed medications are expounded upon. Family physicians underline the significance of adherence, ensuring patients grasp the pivotal role that pharmacotherapy plays in curbing disease progression. Patients susceptible to allergens and irritants gain empowerment through allergen avoidance education. Family physicians meticulously detail avoidance strategies, enabling patients to navigate environments conducive to respiratory well-being (Ouksel et al., 2022; Price et al., 2011; Hammoud et al., 2020; Cano-De La Cuerda et al., 2010).

The cultivation of vigilant self-monitoring habits arms patients with the ability to recognize subtle symptom fluctuations. Family physicians impart the skills to discern potential exacerbations, thus promoting timely intervention. Patients grappling with respiratory conditions receive comprehensive action plans. Family physicians outline steps to undertake during exacerbations and emergencies, instilling a sense of preparedness and confidence. Family physicians promote a long-term perspective on disease management. Patients are educated on the evolving nature of respiratory diseases, nurturing a proactive attitude that transcends periodic assessments. The nexus between patient education and empowerment is a bedrock of enduring wellness. Family physicians, as educators and advocates, infuse patients with the tools to steer their respiratory health journeys (Price et al., 2011; Hammoud et al., 2020; Cano-De La Cuerda et al., 2010; Boise, 2014; Laporte & Bellocq, 2021).

Conclusion

In the intricate domain of periodic health examinations for respiratory system diseases, family physicians assume an indelible role as custodians of comprehensive patient care. This journey through the nuances of assessment, interpretation, prevention, and patient engagement illuminates the multifaceted nature of respiratory well-being. The significance of these examinations as sentinel markers cannot be overstated. The interplay of medical knowledge, scientific insights, and patient collaboration unveils a panorama wherein early detection and personalized interventions culminate in improved patient outcomes.

Family physicians are poised at the confluence of medical expertise and patient advocacy. The knowledge obtained from this exploration equips us to navigate the intricate contours of respiratory health assessments with precision, compassion, and dedication. By embracing the principles expounded within this chapter, we chart a course toward enhanced respiratory vitality for our patients, fostering not only disease detection but also its prevention, mitigation, and management.

The continuum of respiratory wellness is perpetuated through an unwavering commitment to knowledge application and patient empowerment. This chapter serves as a compass, guiding family physicians toward excellence in the realm of respiratory health evaluations. With this comprehension, we journey forward, kindling a beacon of respiratory well-being that illuminates the path to optimal health for our patients. Sources that support the information presented in the chapter.

References

Akhter, Z., Razzaq, S., Rabbani, U., Irfan, M., Burney, P., & Nafees, A. A. (2021). Prevalence of and risk factors for respiratory symptoms in an adult urban population. *The international journal of tuberculosis and lung disease : the official journal of the International Union against Tuberculosis and Lung Disease*, 25(1), 16–22. https://doi.org/10.5588/ijtld.20.0057.

Alderson, M. R., Murphy, T., Pelton, S. I., Novotny, L. A., Hammitt, L. L., Kurabi, A., Li, J. D., Thornton, R. B., & Kirkham, L. S. (2020). Panel 8: Vaccines and immunology. *International journal of pediatric otorhinolaryngology*, 130 Suppl 1(Suppl 1), 109839. https://doi.org/10.1016/j.ijporl.2019.109839.

Almirall, J., Serra-Prat, M., Bolíbar, I., & Balasso, V. (2017). Risk Factors for Community-Acquired Pneumonia in Adults: A Systematic Review of Observational Studies. *Respiration; international review of thoracic diseases*, 94(3), 299–311. https://doi.org/10.1159/000479089.

Benbassat, J., & Baumal, R. (2010). Narrative review: should teaching of the respiratory physical examination be restricted only to signs with proven reliability and validity?. *Journal of general internal medicine*, 25(8), 865–872. https://doi.org/10.1007/s11606-010-1327-8.

Bernstein, W. K. (2012). Pulmonary function testing. *Current opinion in anaesthesiology*, 25(1), 11–16. https://doi.org/10.1097/ACO.0b013e32834e7ad2.

Bertrand Z, F., Segall K, D., Sánchez D, I., & Bertrand N, P. (2020). La auscultación pulmonar en el siglo 21 [Lung auscultation in the 21th century]. *Revista chilena de pediatria*, 91(4), 500–506. https://doi.org/10.32641/rchped.v91i4.1465.

Boise, E. (2014). Patient education and designing an asthma action plan. *Otolaryngologic clinics of North America*, 47(1), 127–134. https://doi.org/10.1016/j.otc.2013.09.008.

Bourouiba, L. (2021). Fluid Dynamics of Respiratory Infectious Diseases. *Annual review of biomedical engineering*, 23, 547–577. https://doi.org/10.1146/annurev-bioeng-111820-025044.

Bowman, M. A., Seehusen, D. A., & Ledford, C. J. W. (2023). Family Physicians Can/Should Do: What? Where? And How?. *Journal of the American Board of Family Medicine: JABFM*, 36(1), 1–3. https://doi.org/10.3122/jabfm.2022.220413R0.

Camargos, P., & Watts, K. D. (2021). Inequalities and Inequities in Pediatric Respiratory Diseases. *Pediatric clinics of North America*, 68(1), 293–304. https://doi.org/10.1016/j.pcl.2020.09.017.

Cano-De La Cuerda, R., Useros-Olmo, A. I., & Muñoz-Hellín, E. (2010). Eficacia de los programas de educación terapéutica y de rehabilitación respiratoria en el paciente con asma [Effectiveness of therapeutic education and respiratory rehabilitation programs for the patient with asthma]. *Archivos de bronconeumologia*, 46(11), 600–606. https://doi.org/10.1016/j.arbres.2010.07.003.

Carlino, M. V., Guarino, M., Izzo, A., Carbone, D., Arnone, M. I., Mancusi, C., & Sforza, A. (2020). Arterial blood gas analysis utility in predicting lung injury in blunt chest trauma. *Respiratory physiology & neurobiology*, 274, 103363. https://doi.org/10.1016/j.resp.2019.103363.

D'Amato, G., Chong-Neto, H. J., Monge Ortega, O. P., Vitale, C., Ansotegui, I., Rosario, N., Haahtela, T., Galan, C., Pawankar, R., Murrieta-Aguttes, M., Cecchi, L., Bergmann, C., Ridolo, E., Ramon, G., Gonzalez Diaz, S., D'Amato, M., & Annesi-Maesano, I. (2020). The effects of climate change on respiratory allergy and asthma induced by pollen and mold allergens. *Allergy*, 75(9), 2219–2228. https://doi.org/10.1111/all.14476.

DeCato, T. W., Haverkamp, H., & Hegewald, M. J. (2020). Cardiopulmonary Exercise Testing (CPET). *American journal of respiratory and critical care medicine*, 201(1), P1–P2. https://doi.org/10.1164/rccm.2011P1.

Donn, S. M., & Sinha, S. K. (2017). Pulmonary diagnostics. *Seminars in fetal & neonatal medicine*, 22(4), 200–205. https://doi.org/10.1016/j.siny.2017.03.006.

Emamian, M. H., Hassani, A. M., & Fateh, M. (2013). Respiratory Tract Infections and its Preventive Measures among Hajj Pilgrims, 2010: A Nested Case Control Study. International journal of preventive medicine, 4(9), 1030–1035.

Goetz, D. M., & Singh, S. (2016). Respiratory System Disease. *Pediatric clinics of North America*, 63(4), 637–659. https://doi.org/10.1016/j.pcl.2016.04.007.

Hammoud, S., Amer, F., Lohner, S., & Kocsis, B. (2020). Patient education on infection control: A systematic review. *American journal of infection control*, 48(12), 1506–1515. https://doi.org/10.1016/j.ajic.2020.05.039.

Hanon, S., Vanderhelst, E., Vincken, W., Schuermans, D., & Verbanck, S. (2021). Peak In- and Expiratory Flow Revisited: Reliability and Reference Values in Adults. *Respiration; international review of thoracic diseases*, 100(1), 11–18. https://doi.org/10.1159/000511694.

Hinchcliff, K. W., & Byrne, B. A. (1991). Clinical examination of the respiratory system. The Veterinary clinics of North America. *Equine practice, 7(1)*, 1–26. https://doi.org/10.1016/s0749-0739(17)30513-8.

Hogea, S. P., Tudorache, E., Fildan, A. P., Fira-Mladinescu, O., Marc, M., & Oancea, C. (2020). Risk factors of chronic obstructive pulmonary disease exacerbations. *The clinical respiratory journal*, 14(3), 183–197. https://doi.org/10.1111/crj.13129.

Kim, W., Lee, K. S., Kim, H. S., Koh, W. J., Jeong, B. H., Chung, M. J., & Jang, H. W. (2016). CT and microbiologic follow-up in primary multidrug-resistant pulmonary tuberculosis. *Acta radiologica (Stockholm, Sweden : 1987)*, 57(2), 197–204. https://doi.org/10.1177/0284185115575196.

Laporte, J. C., & Bellocq, A. (2021). Éducation thérapeutique des personnes atteintes de maladie respiratoire chronique [Therapeutic education for people with chronic respiratory disease]. *Revue de l'infirmiere*, 70(269), 20–23. https://doi.org/10.1016/j.revinf.2021.01.007.

Larkin, B. G., & Zimmanck, R. J. (2015). Interpreting Arterial Blood Gases Successfully. *AORN journal*, 102(4), 343–357. https://doi.org/10.1016/j.aorn.2015.08.002.

Lemire, F., & Mang, E. J. (2020). Advancing family medicine, improving lives: 2020 in review. *Canadian family physician Medecin de famille canadien*, 66(12), 940. https://doi.org/10.46747/cfp.6612940.

Ley, S. (2015). Lung imaging. *European respiratory review : an official journal of the European Respiratory Society*, 24(136), 240–245. https://doi.org/10.1183/16000617.00011214.

Martin, C., Aguilo, N., & Gonzalo-Asensio, J. (2018). Vaccination against tuberculosis. Vacunación frente a tuberculosis. *Enfermedades infecciosas y microbiologia clinica (English ed.)*, 36(10), 648–656. https://doi.org/10.1016/j.eimc.2018.02.006.

Masarweh, K., Gur, M., Toukan, Y., Bar-Yoseph, R., Kassis, I., Gut, G., Hakim, F., Nir, V., & Bentur, L. (2021). Factors associated with complicated pneumonia in children. *Pediatric pulmonology*, 56(8), 2700–2706. https://doi.org/10.1002/ppul.2Boise, 201468.

Moore T. (2007). Respiratory assessment in adults. *Nursing standard (Royal College of Nursing (Great Britain) : 1987)*, 21(49), 48–58. https://doi.org/10.7748/ns2007.08.21.49.48.c4605.

Negewo, N. A., Gibson, P. G., & McDonald, V. M. (2015). COPD and its comorbidities: Impact, measurement and mechanisms. *Respirology (Carlton, Vic.)*, 20(8), 1160–1171. https://doi.org/10.1111/resp.12642.

Ouksel, H., Chambouleyron, M., Grosbois, J. M., Surpas, P., Lino, A., Kermelly, S. B., & Bourbeau, J. (2022). Éducation thérapeutique du patient au cours de la réadaptation respiratoire [Therapeutic patient education in respiratory rehabilitation]. *Revue des maladies respiratoires*, 39(2), 152–169. https://doi.org/10.1016/j.rmr.2021.11.007.

Povoa, P., Martin-Loeches, I., & Nseir, S. (2021). Secondary pneumonias in critically ill patients with COVID-19: risk factors and outcomes. *Current opinion in critical care*, 27(5), 468–473. https://doi.org/10.1097/MCC.0000000000000860.

Price, E. L., Mackenzie, T. D., Metlay, J. P., Camargo, C. A., Jr, & Gonzales, R. (2011). A computerized education module improves patient knowledge and attitudes about appropriate antibiotic use for acute respiratory tract infections. *Patient education and counseling*, 85(3), 493–498. https://doi.org/10.1016/j.pec.2011.02.005.

Principi, N., Di Pietro, G. M., & Esposito, S. (2018). Bronchopulmonary dysplasia: clinical aspects and preventive and therapeutic strategies. *Journal of translational medicine*, 16(1), 36. https://doi.org/10.1186/s12967-018-1417-7.

Puente Maestú, L., & García de Pedro, J. (2012). Lung function tests in clinical decision-making. *Archivos de bronconeumologia*, 48(5), 161–169. https://doi.org/10.1016/j.arbres.2011.12.012.

Riobó, P., Walker, R., Sanz, T., Plaza, P., Olalla, T., Gómez, P., Muñoz, F., & Monge, V. (1992). El examen periódico de slaud [Periodic health examination]. *Revista clinica espanola*, 190(7), 361–366.

Ruffin, R. (2004). Peak expiratory flow (PEF) monitoring. Thorax, 59(11), 913–914. https://doi.org/10.1136/thx.2004.027029.

Ruppel, G. L., & Enright, P. L. (2012). Pulmonary function testing. *Respiratory care*, 57(1), 165–175. https://doi.org/10.4187/respcare.01640.

San José Estépar, R. (2022). Artificial intelligence in functional imaging of the lung. *The British journal of radiology*, 95(1132), 20210Hammoud et al., 20107. https://doi.org/10.1259/bjr.20210Hammoud et al., 20107.

Seele, S., & Spallek, M. (2015). Occupational preventive measures. *Deutsches Arzteblatt international*, 112(33-34), 561–562. https://doi.org/10.3238/arztebl.2015.0561b.

Şerifoğlu, İ., & Ulubay, G. (2019). The methods other than spirometry in the early diagnosis of COPD. KOAH erken tanısında spirometri dışındaki yöntemler. *Tuberkuloz ve toraks*, 67(1), 63–70. https://doi.org/10.5578/tt.68162.

Shah, S. N., Bachur, R. G., Simel, D. L., & Neuman, M. I. (2017). Does This Child Have Pneumonia?: The Rational Clinical Examination Systematic Review. *JAMA*, 318(5), 462–471. https://doi.org/10.1001/jama.2017.9039.

Sharp, C. R., & Rozanski, E. A. (2013). Physical examination of the respiratory system. *Topics in companion animal medicine*, 28(3), 79–85. https://doi.org/10.10Cano-De La Cuerda et al., 2010/j.tcam.2013.06.005.

Simpson, H. (2006). Respiratory assessment. *British journal of nursing (Mark Allen Publishing)*, 15(9), 484–488. https://doi.org/10.12968/bjon.2006.15.9.484.

Teixeira, P. M., Lemos, F., Yaphe, J., Alves, L., & de Sousa, J. C. (2020). Respiratory medicine curriculum in Portuguese family medicine training: A Delphi study. *Pulmonology*, S2531-0437(20)30251-8. Advance online publication. https://doi.org/10.1016/j.pulmoe.2020.10.014.

Tran, D. (2018). Cardiopulmonary Exercise Testing. *Methods in molecular biology (Clifton, N.J.)*, 1735, 285–295. https://doi.org/10.1007/978-1-4939-7614-0_18.

Tsang, H. F., Chan, L. W. C., Cho, W. C. S., Yu, A. C. S., Yim, A. K. Y., Chan, A. K. C., Ng, L. P. W., Wong, Y. K. E., Pei, X. M., Li, M. J. W., & Wong, S. C. (2021). An update on COVID-19 pandemic: the epidemiology, pathogenesis, prevention and treatment strategies. *Expert review of anti-infective therapy*, 19(7), 877–888. https://doi.org/10.1080/14787210.2021.1863146.

v). Evaluation of respiratory disease. *Clinics in chest medicine*, 34(2), 191–204. https://doi.org/10.1016/j.ccm.2013.02.005.

Ventre, K. M., Wolf, G. K., & Arnold, J. H. (2011). Pediatric respiratory diseases: 2011 update for the Rogers' Textbook of Pediatric Intensive Care. *Pediatric critical care medicine : a journal of the Society of Critical Care Medicine and the World Federation of Pediatric Intensive and Critical Care Societies*, 12(3), 325–338. https://doi.org/10.1097/PCC.0b013e31821Hammoud et al., 2010661.

Wise, S. K., Lin, S. Y., Toskala, E., Orlandi, R. R., Akdis, C. A., Alt, J. A., Azar, A., Baroody, F. M., Bachert, C., Canonica, G. W., Chacko, T., Cingi, C., Ciprandi, G., Corey, J., Cox, L. S., Creticos, P. S., Custovic, A., Damask, C., DeConde, A., DelGaudio, J. M., ... Zacharek, M. (2018). International Consensus Statement on Allergy and Rhinology: Allergic Rhinitis. *International forum of allergy & rhinology*, 8(2), 108–352. https://doi.org/10.1002/alr.22073.

Wodwaski, N., & Webber, E. (2023). Respiratory Assessment. *Home healthcare now*, 41(4), 182–189. https://doi.org/10.1097/NHH.0000000000001184.

Woodruff, A. (2021). Keeping the Family in Family Medicine. *The American journal of hospice & palliative care*, 38(3), 313–314. https://doi.org/10.1177/1049909120933273.

Zhang, R., Wu, Y., Deng, G., & Deng, J. (2022). Value of sputum Gram stain, sputum culture, and bronchoalveolar lavage fluid Gram stain in predicting single bacterial pathogen among children with community-acquired pneumonia. *BMC pulmonary medicine*, 22(1), 427. https://doi.org/10.1186/s12890-022-02234-1.

Zhao, N., Wu, F., Peng, J., Zheng, Y., Tian, H., Yang, H., Deng, Z., Wang, Z., Li, H., Wen, X., Xiao, S., Huang, P., Dai, C., Lu, L., Zhou, K., Chen, S., Zhou, Y., & Ran, P. (2022). Preserved ratio impaired spirometry is associated with small airway dysfunction and reduced total lung capacity. *Respiratory research*, 23(1), 298. https://doi.org/10.1186/s12931-022-02216-1.

Zurbano, L., & Zurbano, F. (2017). Qué debe saber el médico de familia sobre el trasplante pulmonar. Complicaciones, promoción de la salud y supervivencia (Parte 2) [What the family doctor must know about lung transplantation. Complications, health promotion, and outcomes (Part 2)]. *Semergen*, 43(7), 511–518. https://doi.org/10.1016/j.semerg.2016.11.001.

Chapter 27

Cancer Screening

Meryem Cakir*, **MD**
Department of Family Medicine, Izmir Katip Celebi University, Atatürk Training and Research Hospital, Izmir, Turkey

Abstract

Cancer is a global public health issue, and its increasing incidence day by day has adverse effects on the social, economic, and healthcare systems. Early detection and screenings play a crucial role in cancer prevention, and there are specific screening strategies and international recommendations for different types of cancer. Three commonly screened cancer types worldwide are breast, colon, and cervical cancers.

While developing screening strategies, the World Health Organization suggests shaping these strategies based on a country's healthcare infrastructure, the acceptance of the test by the public, and the budget allocated for screening services. The general recommendation for breast cancer screenings is mammography for women aged 40 to 74 years. For colorectal cancer screenings, the use of fecal occult blood tests in individuals aged 50-75 is recommended, and in the presence of abnormal results, further examination through colonoscopy is advised. For cervical cancer screenings, human papillomavirus testing, Pap smear tests, or co-testing using both are recommended. Although not widely accepted globally, lung cancer screenings, particularly emphasized in guidelines in the United States, suggest annual low-dose computed tomography for individuals at high risk.

Cancer screenings are among the secondary preventive methods widely attempted worldwide to reduce healthcare expenses, prolong individuals' lifespans, and improve their quality of life. As developed countries have better healthcare infrastructure and budgets allocated for healthcare expenditures, the implementation rate of screening strategies is higher compared to developing nations. Strategies should continue to be developed globally to increase the prevalence of cancer screenings worldwide.

Keywords: breast cancer, cervical cancer, colon cancer, lung neoplasms, cancer screening

Introduction

Cancer is a significantly important public health concern worldwide. With the increasing and aging global population, there is greater exposure to variables involved in cancer etiology.

* Corresponding Author's Email: obgndrmeryem@hotmail.com.

In: Common Diseases According to Family Medicine Practice Guidelines
Editors: Esra Meltem Koç and Hilal Aksoy
ISBN: 979-8-89530-302-3

Consequently, the incidence of cancer and its associated social and economic burden is increasing (WHO, Cancer Key facts, 2022). This rapid increase in the burden of cancer constitutes a significant crisis for healthcare systems worldwide. In the future, for many countries, including those with ample resources, allocating funds for the treatment of numerous diagnosed cancer patients and providing palliative and supportive care could become a serious issue (WHO, Cancer Today, 2020). However, regardless of resource levels, all countries have the potential to achieve success in cancer prevention. Presently, approximately 30-50% of cancers can be prevented by avoiding risk factors and implementing evidence-based prevention strategies. Additionally, if diagnosed early and adequately treated, many cancers have a high probability of recovery (WHO, Guide to cancer early diagnosis, 2017).

Health screenings are programs applied at regular intervals to healthy individuals with the aim of early disease recognition, consequently reducing disease and mortality (WHO, Guide to cancer early diagnosis, 2017). The goal of screening tests is to identify conditions that can be confirmed using advanced methods before symptoms occur in individuals at risk. Individuals diagnosed through screening programs generally receive early-stage diagnoses, making their treatments both easier and more cost-effective (Ratushnyak et al., 2019).

The appropriateness of screening in communities was first introduced by Wilson and Jungner in 1968 (WHO, Cancer Key facts, 2022). According to the World Health Organization's (WHO) Wilson-Jungner criteria, diseases to be included in national screening programs should have the following characteristics:

- The disease should be a significant health problem prevalent in the community.
- The natural history of the disease should be well understood, with symptoms potentially appearing in the early or latent stage.
- The screening test should have a procedure that ensures continuity.
- The disease to be screened should have a safe, practical, and socially accepted test and examination.
- A clear timing for the repetition of screening tests should be known.
- There should be an appropriate treatment method available for the disease diagnosed through screening.
- The screening test should have high selectivity and sensitivity.
- The screening test should be economically balanced in terms of cost-effectiveness.

Each type of cancer has its own etiology, risk factors, diagnostic, and treatment methods. Therefore, early diagnosis and screening strategies vary depending on the type of cancer. Cancer screenings constitute a complex public health strategy that requires additional resources, infrastructure, and coordination. Screening programs should only be implemented when their effectiveness is proven, when resources are adequate to cover almost the entire target group, when healthcare facilities are available to confirm diagnoses and provide treatment for those with abnormal results, and when the prevalence of the disease justifies screening efforts and costs (WHO, Cancer Key facts, 2022). When effectively planned, adequately financed, and implemented, screening can reduce deaths from cancer and, in some types of cancer, can reduce the risk of developing cancer (Shulman et al., 2010; WHO, Guide to cancer early diagnosis, 2017).

Breast Cancer Screening

According to WHO data, in 2020, there were 2,261,419 newly diagnosed breast cancer patients worldwide, making breast cancer the most commonly occurring cancer globally (WHO, Cancer Today, 2020). The reasons behind this increase in breast cancer diagnoses include population growth and aging, changes in patient lifestyles such as obesity, sedentary behavior, late childbirth, higher levels of education and awareness among women, and policies promoting breast cancer awareness, leading to a tendency among women to undergo irregular mammography.

Many international guidelines recommend mammography screening every one to two years for average-risk populations aged 40 to 74 years. For high-risk populations, they suggest annual mammography or magnetic resonance imaging (MRI) from a younger age (Ren et al., 2022). The World Health Organization suggests mammography screenings every two years for women aged 50-69. For women aged 40-49 and 70-75 years, mammography screenings could be considered in the presence of a strong and widespread healthcare system based on economic conditions (WHO, WHO position paper on mammography screening, 2014).

In the United States, the Centers for Disease Control and Prevention (CDC) supports the cancer screening recommendations of the U.S. Preventive Services Task Force (USPSTF). USPSTF recommends a biennial mammography for women aged 50-74 with an average risk of breast cancer. For women aged 40-49, they advise discussing with their doctors when to start mammography and how often. Women are recommended to consider the benefits and risks of mammography before starting screening before the age of 50. For women over 75 years old, there is insufficient evidence supporting breast cancer screening; hence, it is not recommended (Siu, 2016).

The National Cancer Institute (NCI) in the United States states that mammography is the most commonly used screening method for detecting breast cancer and reduces breast cancer mortality in women aged 50-69. However, its benefit for women aged 40-49 remains debated (NCI, Breast Cancer Screening, 2023; Sickles, 1998). Some randomized controlled trials suggest that clinical breast examinations (CBE) as a screening test might be effective in detecting advanced-stage breast cancer but lack sufficient evidence to reduce mortality. Self-breast examination has not shown a mortality benefit (NCI, Breast Cancer Screening, 2023; Jatoi and Pinsky, 2021). Women with BRCA1/2 mutations, a family history of breast cancer, or various genetic syndromes such as Li-Fraumeni or Cowden syndrome are considered at high risk and could undergo breast MRI as a screening test (Warner et al., 2011). While breast MRI is more sensitive, it is less specific and significantly more expensive, up to 35 times, compared to mammography (NCI, Breast Cancer Screening, 2023).

The National Comprehensive Cancer Network (NCCN) suggests breast cancer screening for women at average risk, recommending breast awareness and clinical encounters every 1-3 years for women aged 25-39. For women aged 40 years and older, the NCCN recommends breast awareness, annual clinical encounters, annual mammography, and additional screening methods such as MRI for heterogeneous or extremely dense breasts. Individuals with a history of thoracic radiation, genetic predisposition, or a family history of breast cancer between ages 10-30 are considered at high risk, where clinical encounters are recommended every 6-12 months and initiating screenings ten years before the age of the affected family member diagnosed with breast cancer. For these individuals, an annual MRI in addition to mammography is advised (NCCN, Breast Cancer Screening and Diagnosis, 2023).

In December 2022, the European Health Union published new decisions aiming to provide screenings to 90% of the EU population eligible for breast, cervical, and colorectal cancer screenings by 2025. They also called for expanding screenings gradually to include prostate, lung, and, under specific conditions, stomach cancer. The recommendation for breast cancer screening involves biennial mammography for women aged 50-69, setting the lower age limit at 45 and the upper age limit at 74. Digital breast tomosynthesis or digital mammography is recommended for screening, with consideration for MRI when medically appropriate (European Health Union, 2022).

As per the European Society for Medical Oncology (ESMO) recommendations, women aged 50-69 are suggested to undergo annual or biennial mammography screenings. The evidence supporting mammography for women aged 40-49 and 70-74 is less conclusive. Women with or without BRCA mutations but with a strong family history of breast cancer are recommended to have annual MRI and mammography (concurrently or alternately) (Cardoso et al., 2019). The United Kingdom National Screening (NHS) Committee released a revision in 2023 for the Breast Screening Program, recommending inviting all eligible women aged 50-71 years for mammography screenings every three years. Additionally, women identified as at very high risk for breast cancer should be invited annually for screenings (NHS, Breast screening programme, 2023).

In Turkiye, due to the fact that a significant proportion of women diagnosed with breast cancer are younger than 50 years old, screening starts at the age of 40, inviting women aged 40-69 to mammography screenings every two years. Additionally, women are encouraged to gain breast awareness, conduct monthly self-examinations, and have yearly clinical breast examinations (Turkey Cancer Control Programme, 2021).

Colorectal Cancer Screening

Colorectal cancer (CRC) is the third most prevalent cancer globally, and various methods are recommended by health authorities for its screening and early detection (WHO, Cancer Today, 2020). Screening by fecal occult blood tests for individuals aged 50-75 years and subsequent advanced diagnostic procedures such as colonoscopy after detecting abnormal findings constitute the most common screening scenario, as recommended by WHO (IARC, 2019).

In the United States, the CDC and USPSTF recommend the screening for colorectal cancer for adults aged 45-75 years. For adults aged 76-85, screening is selectively suggested based on overall health status, previous screening history, and preferences. Various tests are proposed for screening, emphasizing shared decision-making between clinicians and patients based on individual conditions and preferences (CDC, Colorectal Cancer Screening Tests, 2021; USPSTF, Screening for Colorectal Cancer, 2021). The screening strategies recommended by the CDC and USPSTF are as follows:

- Annual high-sensitivity guaiac-based fecal occult blood test (HSgFOBT) or fecal immunochemical test (FIT) screening
- Screening every 1-3 years using the fecal DNA-FIT test
- Screening every 5 years using computed tomography and colonography
- Screening every 5 years with flexible sigmoidoscopy

- Screening every 10 years with flexible sigmoidoscopy + annual FIT
- Screening every 10 years with a colonoscopy.

According to the NCCN, individuals aged 45 and over with a history of adenoma or sessile serrated polyp/adenoma in the colon, history of inflammatory bowel disease, personal history of high-risk colorectal cancer genetic syndromes, cystic fibrosis, childhood cancer history, or a family history of advanced adenoma (high-grade dysplasia, ≥1 cm, villous or tubulovillous histology) without a first-, second-, or third-degree relative's history of colorectal cancer are considered at moderate risk. The recommendation for these individuals involves annual evaluation of HSgFOBT and FIT, Multitargeted stool DNA (mt-sDNA) test every 3 years, computed tomography (CT) colonography every 5 years, flexible sigmoidoscopy every 5-10 years, and colonoscopy every 10 years. The presence of any a mentioned risk factor calls for an increased screening frequency (NCCN, Colorectal Cancer Screening, 2023).

The American Cancer Society (ACS) advises regular screening for individuals at average colorectal cancer risk starting at 45. It is recommended for individuals in good health with a life expectancy of more than 10 years to continue regular colorectal cancer screening until 75. Between ages 76-85, screening decisions should consider personal preferences, life expectancy, overall health, and past screening history. Screening for individuals over 85 for colorectal cancer is not recommended. The ACS suggests stool-based tests and visual examination of the colon and rectum. For stool-based tests, options include annual HSgFOBT, annual FIT, or mt-sDNA every 3 years. Structural examination involves colonoscopy every 10 years, CT colonography every 5 years, or flexible sigmoidoscopy every 5 years (ACS, Colorectal Cancer Early Detection, Diagnosis, and Staging, 2020).

The European Union's cancer consensus report proposes screening using FIT before referring individuals aged 50-74 for colonoscopy. FIT screenings are anticipated to provide quantitative information, enabling risk-specific strategies, and potentially requiring further investigation based on gender, age, and previous test results. Endoscopy could be adopted as the primary tool for implementing combined strategies (European Health Union, 2022). In Turkey, individuals aged 50-70 are recommended to undergo biennial fecal occult blood tests and a colonoscopy every 10 years (Turkey Cancer Control Programme, 2021).

Cervical Cancer Screening

Cervical cancer ranks as the fourth most common cancer in women worldwide (WHO, Cancer Today, 2020). The ability to detect precursor lesions before cancer develops and ensure early diagnosis enhances the success of cervical cancer screening. For years, successful cervical cancer screening programs have been implemented globally, resulting in a decrease in the morbidity and mortality associated with cervical cancer. According to the ACS, the significant reduction of approximately 65% in cervical cancer burden from 2012 to 2019 is partly attributed to the widespread administration of human papillomavirus (HPV) vaccines. In developed countries, screening programs are applied more extensively, thereby reducing the burden of cervical cancer. Conversely, in developing nations, the lack of widespread cervical cancer screening and vaccination programs maintains cervical cancer as a significant public health issue (Siegel et al., 2023).

Cervical intraepithelial neoplasia (CIN) is a premalignant lesion found in three stages: CIN1, CIN2, or CIN3 (referred to as CIN2+). If left untreated, CIN2 or CIN2+ can progress to cervical cancer. It is estimated that approximately 1-2% of women are affected by CIN2+. This rate is reported to be around 10% in HIV-positive women. Cervical cancer screening can be conducted using HPV testing, Pap smear tests, or a co-test combining HPV and Pap smears. The WHO emphasizes the regular screening of women aged 30-49 and recommends initiating screening for HIV-diagnosed women at age 25. After turning 50, cessation of screening is suggested if two consecutive screenings yield negative results. Priority in screening is recommended for women aged 50-65 who have never been screened (WHO, WHO guideline for screening and treatment of cervical pre-cancer lesions for cervical cancer prevention, 2021).

In the United States, the USPSTF recommends cervical cancer screening for women aged 21-29 years using cervical cytology every three years. For women aged 30-65, screening options include cervical cytology alone every three years, high-risk human papillomavirus (hrHPV) testing alone every five years, or co-testing with cytology and hrHPV testing every five years (USPSTF, Screening for Cervical Cancer, 2018).

The NCI provides screening recommendations based on age and health history. Considering that the HPV vaccine does not prevent infections caused by all high-risk HPV types, individuals who have received the vaccine are also advised to undergo a cervical cancer screening. They suggest Pap smear testing every three years for individuals aged 21-29, emphasizing that there is no need for Pap smear testing before 21, even if sexually active. For individuals aged 30-65 years, they recommend screening every five years using HPV testing, HPV/Pap smear co-testing, or Pap smear alone every three years. Women over 65 years of age with regular screenings and normal results may discontinue screening. It is highlighted that those who are HIV-positive, have a weakened immune system, were exposed to diethylstilbestrol (DES) before birth, had recent abnormal cervical screening test results or biopsy, or previously had cervical cancer might require more frequent screenings (NCI, Cervical Cancer Screening, 2023).

According to the updated cervical cancer screening guidelines by the ACS, screening should commence at age 25 with HPV testing and continue every five years until age 65. Nevertheless, it is emphasized that co-testing with HPV/Pap smear every five years or Pap smear every three years could still be considered valid (Fontham et al., 2020).

The European Union's cancer consensus report recommends HPV testing every five years for women aged 30-65 years for cervical cancer screening. The report also suggests adapting the age and interval of HPV testing based on individuals' HPV vaccination histories and providing self-sampling kits to allow women to collect their own samples, particularly for non-responsive screening invitations (European Health Union, 2022). In Turkiye, asymptomatic women 30-65 years of age are recommended to undergo cervical smears every five years (Turkey Cancer Control Programme, 2021).

Lung Cancer Screening

According to WHO data from 2020, lung cancer is the second most prevalent cancer worldwide after breast cancer and ranks the first in cancer-related fatalities (WHO, Cancer Today, 2020). While there is not a universally agreed-upon approach to lung cancer screening, it is noted that screening can be conducted for individuals at higher risk (USPTSF, Screening for Lung Cancer, 2021).

The USPSTF recommends annual lung cancer screening using low-dose computed tomography (LDCT) for adults aged 50 to 80 years with a 20-pack-year smoking history and who are current smokers or who have quit smoking within the past 15 years. It is suggested that screening should be discontinued if a person hasn't smoked for 15 years or if a significant health issue arises that substantially limits life expectancy or the ability or desire for curative lung surgery (USPSTSF, Screening for Lung Cancer, 2021).

The NCI indicates that they examine LDCT, chest X-rays, and sputum cytology to determine whether they reduce the risk of dying from lung cancer. The National Lung Screening Trial investigated individuals aged 55 to 74 who had smoked at least 1 pack per day for 30 years or longer (either current smokers or former smokers who quit within the last 15 years) and showed that LDCT screenings reduced the risk of dying from lung cancer in heavy smokers. However, it is emphasized that lung cancer screening tests entail certain risks. These risks include the possibility that the detection of lung cancer may not necessarily improve health or prolong life, potential false-negative and false-positive test results, and exposure to radiation by chest X-rays and CT scans. NCI notes ongoing research on lung cancer screening tests in clinical trials (NCI, Lung Cancer Screening, 2023).

NCCN states that in the United States, most professional organizations, including the American College of Radiology, American Cancer Society, American Lung Association, and American College of Chest Physicians, indicate that lung cancer risk is determined based on age and smoking history. They mention that other potential risk factors for lung cancer, such as personal cancer or lung disease history, family history of lung cancer, exposure to radon, and occupational exposure to lung carcinogens, could also be factored into calculations. The NCCN recommends that individuals at high risk for lung cancer, who have participated in shared decision-making or were offered this decision-making process, undergo screening using LDCT. It is not recommended to screen low-risk individuals or those with functional status or comorbidities that would prevent them from receiving lung cancer treatment. Chest X-rays are not recommended for lung cancer screening (NCCN, Lung cancer screening, 2023).

The European Union's Cancer Consensus report suggests that member countries investigate the feasibility and effectiveness of LDCT screening programs, considering preliminary evidence for screening and the need for a stepwise approach. The report emphasizes the importance of developing primary and secondary preventive strategies, starting with identifying high-risk profiles, particularly heavy and former heavy smokers, and highlights the necessity for further research on how to reach and invite the target group due to the lack of systematic data on smoking habits (European Health Union, 2022).

Conclusion

The most widely accepted and implemented cancer screenings worldwide are for breast, cervical, and colorectal cancers. For a screening program to be deemed successful, it is necessary to reach 70% of the target population, a rate that can be achieved in developed countries but requires improvement in the screening infrastructure and efforts in developing nations. While ongoing efforts persist for lung cancer screening, notably in the United States, guidelines there primarily recommend screening with LDCT. Prostate and stomach cancer screenings are still under study, and based on future evidence, screening programs for these cancers are hoped to commence in the coming years.

References

Breast cancer screening (PDQ). *National Cancer Institute (NCI).* (2023). https://www.cancer.gov/types/breast/hp/breast-screening-pdq. Accessed: 20/10/2023.

Breast cancer screening and diagnosis. *National Comprehensive Cancer Network (NCCN).* (2023). https://www.nccn.org/professionals/physician_gls/pdf/breast-screening.pdf. Accessed: 20/10/2023.

Breast screening programme: Standards. *National Health Service (NHS).* (2023). https://www.gov.uk/government/publications/breast-screening-consolidated-programme-standards/breast-screening-supporting-information. Accessed: 20/10/2023.

Cardoso, F., Kyriakides, S., Ohno, S., Penault-Llorca, F., Poortmans, P., Rubio, I. T., Zackrisson, S., & Senkus, E. (2019). Early breast cancer: ESMO Clinical Practice Guidelines for diagnosis, treatment and follow-up. *Annals of Oncology, 30*(8), 1194–1220. https://doi.org/10.1093/annonc/mdz173.

Cervical cancer screening. *National Cancer Institute (NCI).* (2023). https://www.cancer.gov/types/cervical/screening. Accessed: 20/10/2023.

Colorectal cancer early detection, diagnosis, and staging. *American Cancer Society (ACS).* (2020). https://www.cancer.org/content/dam/CRC/PDF/Public/8606.00.pdf. Accessed: 20/10/2023.

Colorectal cancer screening tests. *Centers for Disease Control and Prevention (CDC*). (2021). https://www.cdc.gov/cancer/colorectal/basic_info/screening/tests.htm. Accessed: 20/10/2023.

Colorectal cancer screening. *National Comprehensive Cancer Network (NCCN*). (2023). https://www.nccn.org/professionals/physician_gls/pdf/colorectal_screening.pdf. Accessed: 20/10/2023.

European Health Union: Commission welcomes adoption of new EU cancer screening recommendations. *European Commission.* (2022). https://ec.europa.eu/commission/presscorner/detail/en/ip_22_7548. Accessed: 20/10/2023.

Fontham, E. T. H., Wolf, A. M. D., Church, T. R., Etzioni, R., Flowers, C. R., Herzig, A., Guerra, C. E., Oeffinger, K. C., Shih, Y. C. T., Walter, L. C., Kim, J. J., Andrews, K. S., DeSantis, C. E., Fedewa, S. A., Manassaram-Baptiste, D., Saslow, D., Wender, R. C., & Smith, R. A. (2020). Cervical cancer screening for individuals at average risk: 2020 guideline update from the American Cancer Society. *CA: A Cancer Journal for Clinicians, 70*(5), 321-346. https://doi.org/10.3322/caac.21628.

International Agency for Research on Cancer (IARC). (2019). *Colorectal cancer screening. In IARC Handbooks of Cancer Prevention* (Vol. 17, p. 300). Lyon, France: International Agency for Research on Cancer.

Jatoi, I., & Pinsky, P. F. (2021). Breast cancer screening trials: Endpoints and overdiagnosis. *Journal of the National Cancer Institute, 113*(9), 1131-1135. https://doi.org/10.1093/jnci/djaa140.

Lung cancer screening (PDQ®)–Health Professional Version. *National Cancer Institute (NCI).* (2023). https://www.cancer.gov/types/lung/hp/lung-screening-pdq. Accessed: 20/10/2023.

Lung cancer screening. *National Comprehensive Cancer Network (NCCN).* (2023). https://www.nccn.org/professionals/physician_gls/pdf/lung_screening.pdf. Accessed: 20/10/2023.

Ratushnyak, S., Hoogendoorn, M., & Baal, P. H. M. (2019). Cost-effectiveness of cancer screening: Health and costs in life years gained. *American Journal of Preventive Medicine, 57*(6), 792-799. https://doi.org/10.1016/j.amepre.2019.07.027.

Ren, W., Chen, M., Qiao, Y., & Zhao, F. (2022). Global guidelines for breast cancer screening: A systematic review. *Breast, 64*, 85-99. https://doi.org/10.1016/j.breast.2022.04.003.

Shulman, L. N., Willett, W., Sievers, A., & Knaul, F. M. (2010). Breast cancer in developing countries: Opportunities for improved survival. *Journal of Oncology, 2010*, 595167. https://doi.org/10.1155/2010/595167.

Sickles, E. A. (1998). Findings at mammographic screening on only one standard projection: Outcomes analysis. *Radiology, 208*(2), 471-475. https://doi.org/10.1148/radiology.208.2.9680578.

Siegel, R. L., Miller, K. D., Wagle, N. S., & Jemal, A. (2023). Cancer statistics, 2023. *CA: A Cancer Journal for Clinicians, 73*(1), 17-48. https://doi.org/10.3322/caac.21763.

Siu, A. L. (2016). Screening for breast cancer: U.S. Preventive Services Task Force Recommendation Statement. *Annals of Internal Medicine, 164*(4), 279-296. https://doi.org/10.7326/M15-2886.

Turkiye Cancer Control Programme. T.R. *Ministry of Health General Directorate of Public Health.* (2021). https://hsgm.saglik.gov.tr/depo/birimler/kanser-db/Dokumanlar/Raporlar/Turkey_NCCP_18_April_2022.pdf. Accessed: 20/10/2023.

U.S. Preventive Services Task Force (USPSTF). (2018). Screening for cervical cancer: U.S. Preventive Services Task Force Recommendation Statement. *JAMA, 320*(7), 674-686. https://doi.org/10.1001/jama.2018.10897.

U.S. Preventive Services Task Force (USPSTF). (2021). Screening for colorectal cancer: U.S. Preventive Services Task Force Recommendation Statement. *JAMA, 325*(19), 1965-1977. https://doi.org/10.1001/jama.2021.6238.

U.S. Preventive Services Task Force (USPSTF). (2021). Screening for lung cancer: U.S. Preventive Services Task Force Recommendation Statement. *JAMA, 325*(10), 962-970. https://doi.org/10.1001/jama.2021.1117.

Warner, E., Hill, K., Causer, P., Plewes, D., Jong, R., Yaffe, R., Foulkes, W. D., Ghadirian, P., Lynch, H., Couch, F., Wong, J., Wright, F., Sun, P., & Narod, S. A. (2011). Prospective study of breast cancer incidence in women with a BRCA1 or BRCA2 mutation under surveillance with and without magnetic resonance imaging. *Journal of Clinical Oncology, 29*(13), 1664-1669. https://doi.org/10.1200/JCO.2009.27.0835.

World Health Organization. (2014). *WHO position paper on mammography screening.* https://www.who.int/publications/i/item/who-position-paper-on-mammography-screening. Accessed: 20/10/2023.

World Health Organization. (2017). *Guide to cancer early diagnosis.* https://www.who.int/publications/i/item/9789241511940. Accessed: 20/10/2023.

World Health Organization. (2020). *Cancer today.* https://gco.iarc.fr/today/home. Accessed: 20/10/2023.

World Health Organization. (2021). *WHO guideline for screening and treatment of cervical pre-cancer lesions for cervical cancer prevention.* https://iris.who.int/bitstream/handle/10665/342365/9789240030824-eng.pdf?sequence=1. Accessed: 20/10/2023.

World Health Organization. (2022). *Cancer key facts.* https://www.who.int/en/news-room/fact-sheets/detail. Accessed: 20/10/2023.

Chapter 28

Contraception

Gökçe Işcan[1,*], MD
and Serhan Can Işcan[2], MD
[1]Department of Family Medicine, Süleyman Demirel University, Isparta, Turkey
[2]Department of Gynecologic Oncology, Isparta City Hospital, Isparta, Turkey

Abstract

The utilization of contraception is of utmost significance in the realm of family planning since it grants women the ability to make well-informed decisions regarding their reproductive well-being. The field of contraception has had notable advancements, encompassing both conventional approaches like hormonal contraceptives and barrier methods, as well as state-of-the-art breakthroughs like long-acting reversible contraceptives (LARCs) and new non-hormonal alternatives. There has been a significant increase in the focus on tailored ways of contraception, which incorporate individual preferences and health factors.

Prominent aspects encompass the growing accessibility of non-prescription contraceptives, heightened recognition of fertility awareness-based approaches, and the continuous investigation into male contraceptive alternatives. Notwithstanding the progress made, there are still persistent difficulties that need to be addressed, such as the need to tackle discrepancies in access to contraceptives and to overcome cultural obstacles.

This summary provides a comprehensive overview of the evolving field of contraception, highlighting the various approaches used to improve the effectiveness, availability, and inclusiveness of family planning techniques. The ongoing development of contraceptive technology highlights the dedication to offering women a wide range of options to address their distinct reproductive health requirements.

Keywords: contraception, emergency contraception, contraception behavior

Introduction

Contraceptive methods refer to the various techniques and devices employed to prevent pregnancy. These approaches are designed to inhibit or interfere with the different contemporary contraceptive methods used globally, including barrier methods such as

* Corresponding Author's Email: dr_gokcedilek@yahoo.com.

In: Common Diseases According to Family Medicine Practice Guidelines
Editors: Esra Meltem Koç and Hilal Aksoy
ISBN: 979-8-89530-302-3

spermicide applications, diaphragms, and condoms, as well as intrauterine devices, oral contraceptives, patches, implants, injectables, intrauterine devices, and sterilization. According to the Turkish Society of Gynecology and Obstetrics (TJOD), the guideline of Faculty Health Sexual and Reproductive Healthcare (FSRH) contraception methods are examined under 8 major headings (Royal College of Obstetrician and Gynaecologists, 2016; Turkish Society of Gynecology and Obstetrics, 2012).

Intrauterin Contraception (IUC)

As we mentioned in Figure 1 this is one of the popular type of contraception. The intrauterine device (IUD) bears resemblance to the intrauterine system (IUS), however with a distinction in the release of copper into the uterus, as opposed to the progestogen hormone released by the IUS. IUD usage is the most prevalent form of reversible contraception on a global scale, with an average of 23% of female contraceptive consumers employing it (K. J. Buhling et al., 2014). The percentage varies from 2% to over 40%, contingent upon the country (K. J. Buhling et al., 2014). Also among contraceptive-using women in the United States, IUD usage increased from 2% to 14% between 2002 and 2014 (Kimberly Daniels et al., 2015; Lawrence B Finer et al., 2012; Megan L Kavanaugh & Jenna Jerman, 2018).

IUC methods are long-acting reversible contraceptives (LARCs) and are authorized for use for periods varying from three to ten years. IUC may be more convenient and cost-effective than shorter-acting methods such as oral contraceptives due to its substantially lower typical use failure rate and the reduced frequency with which users must visit contraceptive services (Royal College of Obstetricians and Gynaecologists, 2023b).

Copper Intrauterine Device (Cu-IUD)

Cu-IUDs differ in size and morphology and are non-hormonal. In addition to copper and plastic, they might also incorporate barium to impart radio-opacity. Certain varieties include a core of silver or another inert metal, which aids in wire integrity. Cu-IUD insertion is permissible whenever there is reasonable certainty that the woman is not carrying a pregnancy. Also, it can be used for Emergency contraception. Inserted no later than five days after the initial instance of unprotected sexual intercourse (UPSI) during that particular cycle or five days before the earliest anticipated date of ovulation (Royal College of Obstetricians and Gynaecologists, 2023b).

There are some side effects of Cu-IUD such as unscheduled spotting or light bleeding, as well as severe or protracted bleeding. Usually, these are frequent in the first 3–6 months of Cu-IUD treatment, harmless, and reduced with use. Can consider an underlying gynecological problem, such as Cu-IUD displacement, an sexually transmitted diseases (STD), pregnancy, or new pathological uterine conditions (e.g., polyps or fibroids), if clinically indicated, especially in women who have used the Cu-IUD for a few months and developed heavy or prolonged bleeding. During the menstrual period, in cases where no gynecological abnormalities have been identified and the lady seeks medical intervention, the following therapeutic modalities can be taken into consideration: The administration of nonsteroidal anti-inflammatory drugs

(NSAIDs) for five days is suggested as a therapeutic option. Alternatively, in cases where bleeding persists and the woman expresses dissatisfaction with this approach, it is advisable to explore alternative contraceptive techniques (M. Bofill Rodriguez et al., 2019).

Levonorgestrel Intrauterine Device (LNG-IUS)

The LNG-IUS is a contraceptive intrauterine device (IUD) characterized by its T-shaped structure that contains the progestogen hormone levonorgestrel within an elastomer core. The insertion of the object in question is deemed appropriate when an acceptable level of certainty exists regarding the absence of pregnancy in the woman. The LNG-IUS does not necessitate supplementary contraceptive measures during the initial seven days after insertion, coinciding with the commencement of menstrual menstruation. In the event that the LNG-IUS is inserted beyond a period of seven days subsequent to the initiation of monthly flow, it is advised that the woman abstains from engaging in sexual activity for the subsequent week or employ an extra form of contraception (Centers for Disease Control and Prevention, 2016).

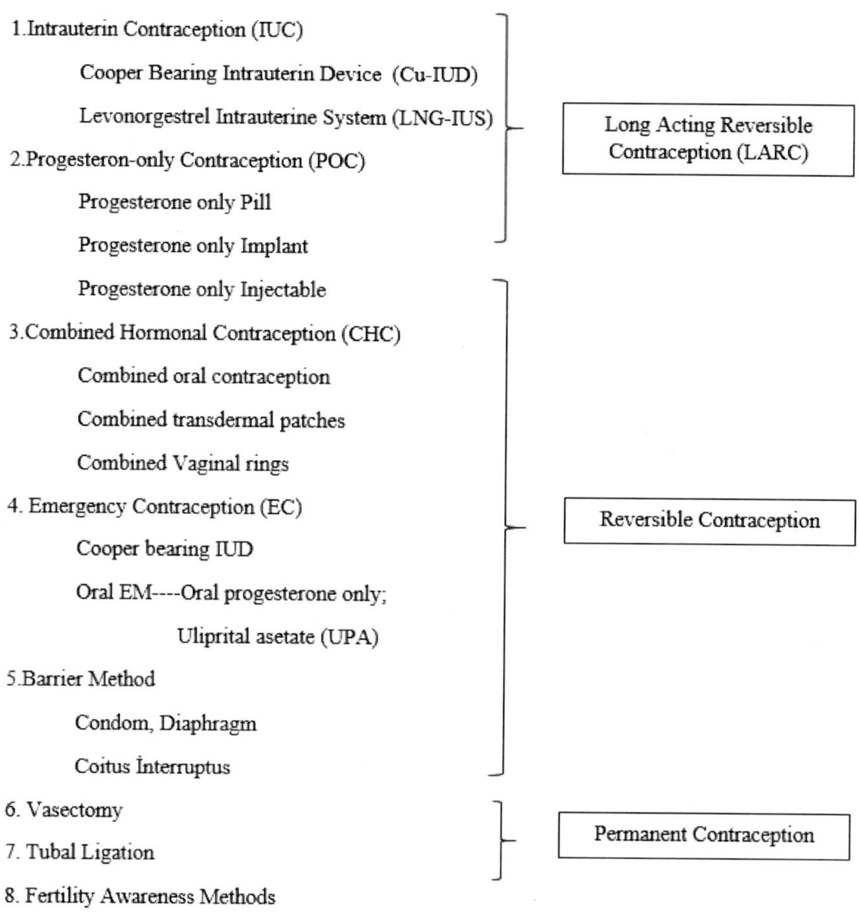

Figure 1. Types of contraception.

The anticipated contraceptive failure rate for a Copper Intrauterine Device (Cu-IUD) during the initial year of usage has been reported as 0.8% under usual use conditions and 0.6% under perfect use conditions. The projected contraceptive failure rate for a 52 mg LNG-IUD during the initial year of usage is 0.2%, regardless of whether it is used typically or ideally. According to research findings, the rate of contraceptive failure during authorized usage is estimated to be approximately 0.3% for both the 19.5 mg and 13.5 mg LNG intrauterine devices (IUDs) (Evidence Level C) (Royal College of Obstetricians and Gynaecologists, 2023b). Although most IUD insertions can be performed in primary care and community settings without complications, the process of inserting an intrauterine device (IUD) has the potential to facilitate the dissemination of bacteria, hence increasing the risk of developing complications such as pelvic inflammatory disease (PID) (D. A. Grimes & K. F. Schulz, 1999). While the likelihood of pelvic inflammatory disease (PID) was shown to be elevated within the initial 20 days following IUD insertion, the overall occurrence of PID among women who underwent IUD insertion remained very low (T. M. Farley et al., 1992).

Progesterone Only Contraception (POC)

Progesterone-Only Pills (POPs)

Progesterone-only pills (POPs) only consist of a progestin compound and do not contain any estrogen. The data suggests that, on average, around 9% of women experience pregnancy during the initial year of using progestin-only pills (POPs) under usual circumstances (J. Trussell, 2011), and POPs have an effectiveness rate of over 99% when used correctly (Royal College of Obstetricians and Gynaecologists, 2023b). POPs possess the potential for utilization among women across all age groups but do not protect against sexually transmitted diseases (STDs). The existing body of evidence is insufficient to determine if there exists a substantial disparity in contraceptive efficacy between standard progestin-only pills (POPs) and drospirenone-containing desogestrel (DSG/DRSP) POPs (James Trussell, 2004).

Progestin-only pills (POPs)(POPs) can be administered at any given time, supplied that there exists a reasonable degree of certainty that the female individual in issue is not presently pregnant. The initiation of POPs is feasible within a five-day window following the onset of menstrual bleeding without the need for additional contraceptive measures. Women who initiate POPs after experiencing five days of menstruation need to either abstain from sexual activity or use additional contraception for two days.

In the case of healthy women, there is no requirement for any examinations or tests before the commencement of progestogen-only pills (POPs). However, getting baseline weight and BMI measurements may be beneficial to monitor POP users longitudinally. Women who have pre-existing medical illnesses or unique circumstances may require supplementary examinations or tests to assess their suitability as candidates for a specific contraceptive method. When faced with uncertainty regarding a woman's pregnancy status, healthcare providers should initiate progestin-only pills (POPs) due to the likelihood of their advantages outweighing potential risks. Consequently, the initiation of POPs should be contemplated at any given moment, accompanied by a subsequent pregnancy test within a timeframe of 2 to 4 weeks (Centers for Disease Control and Prevention, 2016). A dose is considered missed if it has been more than three hours (or less than 12 hours late for a desogestrel pill) since it should have been administered.

Missed Use

- Immediately consume a single tablet.
- Use backup contraception (such as condoms) or refrain from sexual activity until the pills have been taken accurately and on time for two consecutive days.
- Continue taking one medication daily at the same time every day, even if it means taking two pills on the same day.
- If a woman has had unprotected sexual activity, she should consider emergency contraception (except UPA).

Situations to Watch Out For

- The guideline development group (GDG) recommends measuring urea, electrolytes, and blood pressure before prescribing the DRSP POP for anyone over 50 with high-risk factors for chronic renal disease.
- According to the manufacturer, patients with severe renal insufficiency or acute renal failure should not use the DRSP POP.
- The GDG advises avoiding DRSP POP for those with hyperkalemia or untreated hypoaldosteronism, such as Addison's illness.
- Women who are on potassium-sparing diuretics, aldosterone antagonists, or potassium supplements should exercise caution when utilizing these medications.
- DRSP POP should be used cautiously by people with mild/moderate renal impairment or treated hypoaldosteronism (e.g., Addison's illness) (Royal College of Obstetricians and Gynaecologists, 2023a).

Progesterone-Only Implant

Single-rod etonogestrel implants (ENG-IMP) of 68 mg are available in the US, UK, and Turkey. Only 1 in 100 women with standard etonogestrel implant use got pregnant in the first year (Royal College of Obstetricians and Gynaecologists, 2023a; Ministry of Health General Directorate of Maternal and Child Health and Family Planning, 2019; James Trussell, 2011). When there is uncertainty regarding the potential pregnancy status of a woman, it is advisable to weigh the potential risks against the benefits of initiating the implant. Consequently, it is recommended to consider commencing the implantation process at any given moment while also ensuring a subsequent pregnancy test is conducted within a timeframe of 2-4 weeks.

If a woman transitions from one contraceptive technique to an implant, it is advisable to contemplate the implementation of supplementary contraceptive measures. Specifically, it is recommended to maintain the use of the previous contraceptive method for seven days after the placement of the implant. There is a lack of direct empirical evidence about the potential consequences of initiating the etonogestrel implant at various points within the menstrual cycle (Centers for Disease Control and Prevention, 2016). The ENG-IMP is a widely recognized and productive kind of long-acting reversible contraception, authorized for three years for contraceptive purposes. The current recommendation is to avoid prolonged usage of the ENG-IMP for a duration exceeding three years. Based on the existing body of knowledge, it may be inferred that the contraceptive efficacy of the ENG-IMP is unaffected by variations in body weight or body mass index (Evidence Level C) (Royal College of Obstetricians and Gynaecologists, 2023a).

Side Effects of Progesteron-Only Implants

According to a study, hormonal contraception, particularly progestogen-only implants, may increase the risk of breast cancer. Ectopic pregnancy is rare using ENG-IMP contraception. Despite limited data, the ENG-IMP does not appear to enhance the venous or arterial thromboembolic events risk. Irregular bleeding and headaches are often reported symptoms associated with the use of ENG-IMP. Conversely, new onset acne, depression, and weight gain are infrequently observed in women utilizing this medication. For those who are medically eligible, it may be worth considering a 3-month trial of an extra combination oral contraceptive (COC) or a 5-day course of mefenamic acid as potential interventions to address troublesome bleeding. In contrast to combination oral contraceptives containing both estrogen and progestin, progestin-only pills do not pose an elevated risk of developing hypertension or cardiovascular ailments. Moreover, women with specific medical issues, such as a prior occurrence of deep vein thrombosis (DVT) or unregulated hypertension, might still opt for progestin-only pills (American College of Obstetricians and Gynecologists, 2023a).

The ENG-IMP contraceptive method can be administered at any point throughout a natural menstrual cycle within a timeframe of 1 to 5 days. It can also be issued on the 21st day after childbirth or the 5th day following a medical or surgical abortion without requiring supplementary contraception. According to the instructions provided by the Faculty of Sexual and Reproductive Healthcare (FSRH), following the implementation of ENG-IMP, it is advised to utilize condoms for seven days and, if deemed suitable, to have a subsequent pregnancy test. After administering levonorgestrel emergency contraception (LNG-EC) promptly or ulipristal acetate emergency contraception (UPA-EC) within a 5-day window, the initiation of ENG-IMP can be expedited. It is advised to employ condoms for seven days and undergo a subsequent pregnancy test as part of the follow-up procedure (Royal College of Obstetricians and Gynaecologists, 2023a).

Progesterone-Only Injectables

The primary mechanism of action of progestogen-only injectable contraception is the inhibition of ovulation. Additionally, there is an observed impact on cervical mucus, leading to suboptimal cervical mucus scores and restricted sperm penetration. Most women experience an effect on cervical mucus within the initial few days, as supported by studies (Nathalie Kapp & Mary E Gaffield, 2013; Carlos A Petta et al., 1998). Because of the endometrium, implantation can not happen. When progestogen-only injectable contraception is administered according to the recommended dose interval, the failure rate is estimated to be around 0.2% within the initial year of usage. The failure rate under regular usage conditions is calculated to be about 6% (Evidence Level A).

The birth control injection is composed of the hormone depot medroxyprogesterone acetate (DMPA) and norethisterone enanthate (NET-EN). DMPA is formulated for deep intramuscular (IM) injection as Depo-Provera® (150 mg medroxyprogesterone acetate in 1 ml) (Health Products Regulatory Authority, 2021) and subcutaneous (SC) injection as Sayana Press® (104 mg MPA in 0.65 ml) (Health Products Regulatory Authority, 2020). Sayana Press® (Royal College of Obstetrician and Gynaecologists, 2013) is a subcutaneous injection formulation of DMPA (depot medroxyprogesterone acetate) with a concentration of 104 mg in 0.65 ml. It was initially granted a license in the United Kingdom in 2011. The substance in question is considered bioequivalent to Depo-Provera®, a pharmaceutical product. Utilizing Depo-Provera® may be more advantageous for women who use anticoagulants or have a bleeding condition. It is available as Noristerat® (200 mg in 1 ml), administered by IM injection (Electronic Medicines Compendium Bayer Schering, 2019; Arthi Thirumalai & John K Amory, 2021). Methods that lack estrogen are suitable for use during breastfeeding, commencing six weeks postpartum, and are appropriate for women who cannot utilize estrogen-containing techniques. The progesterone-only injection functions by suppressing the process of ovulation. Progesterone induces an elevation in viscosity and a decrease in the volume of cervical mucus. This occurrence presents a problem for sperm in terms of their capacity to navigate the uterine cavity and effectively accomplish the fertilization of an egg. It induces a decrease in the thickness of the endometrial lining.

Essential Instructions

- If the client and their healthcare provider are confident that there is no pregnancy, the injection can be given anytime during the menstrual cycle.
- If the first dose of contraception is given within seven days of menstruation, no additional steps are needed.
- If the contraceptive injection is given more than seven days after menstruation, use a different birth control method or abstain from sexual activity for seven days.
- It is recommended to discontinue the use of the previous contraceptive technique while initiating the administration of the injection. In cases where the duration of menstruation exceeds seven days, it is advisable to consider employing supplementary contraceptive methods or refraining from engaging in sexual intercourse.
- Many options exist for switching from an intrauterine device (IUD). After the injection, the IUD can be removed after seven days. Before removing the intrauterine device (IUD) and giving the initial infusion, people can use condoms or abstain from sexual activity for seven days (Royal College of Obstetricians and Gynaecologists, 2023b).

Contraindications (Health Products Regulatory Authority, 2020, 2021; Electronic Medicines Compendium Bayer Schering, 2019; Royal College of Obstetrician and Gynaecologists, 2016)

- Breast cancer was diagnosed within the past five years.
- Aberrant human chorionic gonadotrophin (hCG) levels are present in gestational trophoblastic neoplasia.
- Women who are currently experiencing significant liver dysfunction or have a medical history of hepatic adenoma or cholestatic jaundice induced by steroid use.
- Women with a documented history of severe arterial disease or those who possess a multitude of high-risk variables are more susceptible to an elevated risk of thrombosis and arterial disease.
- The presence of acute porphyria, especially without a documented history of active disease.
- Before administering the injection, it is imperative to exclude the possibility of pregnancy. A sufficient indicator for this exclusion is a recent history of regular menstruation.
- The administration of Noristerat® is contraindicated in nursing newborns who have severe or persistent jaundice.
- The occurrence of vaginal bleeding without a clear or identifiable cause.

Combined Hormonal Contraception (CHC)

Combined hormonal contraception options include birth control pills, the birth control patch, and the vaginal birth control ring. These substances consist of two hormones, namely estrogen and progestin (American College of Obstetricians and Gynecologists, 2023a). When CHC contraceptives are utilized with optimal adherence, the likelihood of failure is minimal, amounting to less than 1%. However, when considering typical usage patterns, it has been predicted that approximately 9% of women experience unintended pregnancies within the initial year of CHC utilization. The efficacy of contraceptive techniques may also be influenced by drug interactions (in all combined hormonal contraceptive methods) and malabsorption (in combined oral contraceptives only). Additionally, the contraceptive transdermal patch may have reduced effectiveness in women with a body weight above 90 kg (Royal College of Obstetricians and Gynaecologists, 2023c).

The primary mode of operation of combined hormonal contraceptives (CHC) is the inhibition of ovulation. The contraceptive hormone combination (CHC) exerts its effects on the hypothalami pituitary-ovarian axis by suppressing the secretion of luteinizing hormone (LH) and follicle-stimulating hormone (FSH), thus inhibiting the process of ovulation. The contraceptive function may be influenced by alterations in cervical mucus, endometrium, and tubal motility caused by exposure to progestogens (P. G. Crosignani et al., 1996; T. M. Mulders & T. O. Dieben, 2001).

Combined Oral Contraceptives (COC)

Combined oral contraceptives (COCs) consist of a combination of estrogen and progesterone compounds and were initially launched in the 1960s. Combined oral contraceptives (COCs) are commonly referred to by various names, including "the Pill," low-dose combined pills, OCPs, and OCs. The primary mechanism of action involves the inhibition of ovulation, hence preventing the release of ova from the ovaries. The efficacy of contraceptive pills is contingent upon the user's adherence to the prescribed regimen. The likelihood of conception is significantly heightened if a woman commences taking a new pack of pills three or more days beyond the recommended start date or neglects to consume three or more tablets near the commencement or conclusion of a pill pack. Typically, the utilization of combined oral contraceptives (COCs) results in approximately seven births per 100 women within the initial year of usage. This implies that the contraceptive effectiveness rate of combined oral contraceptives (COCs) is 93% among women, indicating that the likelihood of pregnancy is low for the majority of users ((Johns Hopkins Bloomberg School of Public Health World Health Organization Department of Sexual and Reproductive Health and Research & United States Agency for International Development Bureau for Global Health Office of Population and Reproductive Health Center for Communication Programs Knowledge for Health Project, 2022).

When adhered to without any errors, the use of combined oral contraceptives (COCs) results in a pregnancy rate of less than 1 per 100 women during the initial year of usage. There is no delay in the resumption of fertility following the discontinuation of combined oral contraceptives (COCs). There is a lack of protection against sexually transmitted diseases (STIs) (Johns Hopkins Bloomberg School of Public Health World Health Organization Department of Sexual and Reproductive Health and Research & United States Agency for International Development Bureau for Global Health Office of Population and Reproductive Health Center for Communication Programs Knowledge for Health Project, 2022).

The implications of different contraceptive methods should be considered, and it may be necessary to select the proper contraceptive method for each woman. Certain combined oral contraceptives (COCs) are prescribed to be taken for 21 consecutive days, followed by a subsequent 7-day interval without medication.

Women may opt to utilize a hormone-free placebo or tablets providing iron preparations without interruption as an alternative during a specified duration. It is advised to refrain from consuming pharmaceuticals that include active hormones.

Withdrawal bleeding is a phenomenon that takes place during the menstrual period, contributing to the occurrence of cyclic bleeding. The regimen consists of 28 tablets, 24 tablets containing hormone, and four tablets containing placebo. These tablets are taken continuously without any interruption. In addition, progesterone-only pills (POPs) raise concerns when used for extended periods without interruption. Extended-cycle oral contraceptives, which consist of 84 days of combined low-dose placebo or ethynyl on day seven after contraceptive use, are now unavailable in our nation. In certain countries, estradiol-containing pills are utilized to induce withdrawal bleeding every quarter. This approach involves the administration of mixed preparations (S. Krishnan & J. Kiley, 2010).

Oral contraceptives usually contain ethinyl estradiol, or they contain estradiol valerate. Over time, the doses of estrogen used in oral contraceptives have been reduced, and estrogenic side effects have decreased accordingly. COCs contain different synthetic progesterones with various efficacy and spectrum of action at different doses. Synthetic progesterones can produce estrogenic, anti-estrogenic, and anti-androgenic effects. Synthetic progesterones are derived from the chemical structures of strains (norethindrone, etinodiol diacetate) and gonan (levonorgestrel, desogestrel, norgestimat). These compounds can be categorized as pregnane, precisely medroxyprogesterone acetate (A. Black et al., 2004).

The progestogens used in combined hormonal contraceptives (CHC) are occasionally categorized into "generations" based on the chronological order in which they were initially introduced as elements of combined oral contraceptives (COCs). The classification is noteworthy. The first group was norethisterone (NET), and the second was levonorgestrel (LNG). The third group includes desogestrel, gestodene, and norgestimate. Additionally, there are newer or alternative options such as drospirenone (DRSP), dienogest, and nomegestrol acetate (A. E. Schindler et al., 2008; Regine Sitruk-Ware, 2002).

Indications for Combined Oral Contraceptives

For all women who are healthy and want contraception (nulliparous or multiparous), combined oral contraceptives at any age, from menarche to menopause, can be used.

The Absolute Contraindications Associated with The Use of Combination Oral Contraceptives (Royal College of Obstetricians and Gynaecologists, 2023c; World Health Organization, 2015)

- Postpartum period: 6 weeks in breastfeeding, three weeks in non-breastfeeding
- Smoking at least 15 cigarettes a day over the age of 35
- Hypertension (≥160 mmHg systolic or ≥100 mmHg diastolic)
- History of venous thromboembolism (VTE)/pulmonary embolism (PE)
- Ischemic heart disease
- History of cerebrovascular events
- Complicated valvular heart disease (pulmonary hypertension, atrial fibrillation, history of subacute bacterial endocarditis
- Migraine with aura (regardless of age)
- Active breast cancer
- Diabetes with retinopathy/nephropathy/neuropathy
- Diabetes for >20 years
- Severe cirrhosis
- Liver tumor (adenoma or hepatoma)
- Major surgical procedures that cause prolonged immobilization
- Thrombogenic mutations (Factor V Leiden, prothrombin mutation, Protein S, C, and antithrombin deficiency)
- Viral hepatitis
- A combination of multiple risks for arterial heart disease (diabetes, obesity, hypertension, smoking, advanced age)
- Antiphospholipid antibody positivity.

The Utilization of Contraceptive Methods in Women Who Have a Coexisting Medical Condition

The utilization of benign breast diseases and a family history of breast cancer is not deemed to be prohibited.

For females presenting with mild lupus and lacking positive antiphospholipid antibodies, the utilization of Combined Oral Contraceptives (COCs) is permissible.

The incidence of cardiovascular disease exhibits an upward trend beyond the age of forty. Women who are in good health and do not smoke may consider taking progestogen-only pills (POPs) until they reach menopause, as long as the potential risks and benefits are carefully evaluated.

Caution should be exercised by hypertensive women who are over the age of 35 and maintain controlled blood pressure levels.

Women who are in their younger years, devoid of any further health complications such as end-organ damage, and do not engage in smoking have the option to utilize POPs.

Women with diabetes who are below the age of 35 and also have hypertension, nephropathy, retinopathy, and other vascular disorders may be eligible to take combined oral contraceptives (COCs), provided that their diabetes diagnosis does not exceed 20 years.

There is currently insufficient evidence to establish a causal relationship between the usage of progestogen-only pills (POP) and the exacerbation of depression in women.

The majority of women who have well-managed dyslipidemia at dosages of 35 mcg or lower can utilize combined oral contraceptives (COCs) that contain estrogen. However, suppose their LDL levels are equal to or greater than 160 mg/dl. In that case, if their triglyceride levels are similar to or greater than 250 mg/dl, and they have risk factors for coronary artery disease, alternate approaches should be considered.

Women over 40 years of age who are healthy and have no risk factors to interfere can use COCs. COCs have an additional benefit in the presence of perimenopausal symptoms may provide. The lowest possible dose of ethinyl estrogen in this age group. It is preferable to use POPs. Before starting to use POPs, a full assessment should be made, and people with obesity, smoking, hypertension, or women with diabetes should not be offered COCs.

Combined Oral Contraceptives and Associated Side Effects and Consultancies

Unscheduled Bleeding: This side effect has been observed in clinical trials involving combined oral contraceptives (COCs). These trials have revealed diverse rates of irregular bleeding, often exhibiting a decreasing trend as time progresses (M. C. Audet et al., 2001; M. J. Rosenberg et al., 1999; L. H. Schilling et al., 1989). It would be appropriate to inform patients that this adverse effect is predominantly transient, as opposed to altering the course of contraceptive oral combination (COC) therapy. If the duration of bleeding exceeds three months or if bleeding commences after the initiation of combined oral contraceptive (COC) use, it is advisable to explore alternative factors that may be contributing to the bleeding. One possible factor contributing to COC (combined oral contraceptive) failure may be attributed to the irregular usage and concurrent administration of medications such as anticonvulsants and rifampin (A. Black et al., 2004; J. E. Krettek et al., 1993). In the context of prolonged use of combined oral contraceptives (COCs) among women, it has been shown that Chlamydia infection was detected in a considerable proportion, specifically up to 29%, of cases presenting with breakthrough bleeding.

Consequently, it is advisable to consider Chlamydia testing in such instances (J. E. Krettek et al., 1993). When encountering breakthrough bleeding, it is advisable to exclude alternative etiologies before proceeding. Subsequently, it is recommended to provide the patient with more education regarding the utilization of combined oral contraceptives (COCs), with a particular emphasis on consistent and timely administration. If the patient engages in smoking behavior, it is advisable to recommend smoking cessation due to the potential association between breakthrough bleeding and smoking. Short-term oral estrogen therapy may be considered as a viable option in cases of recent or persistent bleeding (precisely, 1.25 mg of conjugated estrogen or 2 mg of 17beta estradiol for seven days) (J. E. Krettek et al., 1993).

Amenorrhea, The condition of amenorrhea is observed in approximately 2-3% of women who utilize combined oral contraceptives (COCs). In this particular scenario, it is crucial to ascertain the absence of pregnancy. In cases where pregnancy is absent, and the patient is presenting with amenorrhea, it may be deemed suitable to administer supplementary estrogen for 10 days. The desired outcome can be attained by administering a dosage of 0.625-1.25 mg of conjugated estrogen or 1-2 mg of 17beta estradiol (I. H. Thorneycroft, 1999).

Pregnancy: In the event that a woman who is using combination oral contraceptives (COCs) becomes pregnant, it is crucial to discontinue the use of COCs immediately. It is imperative to communicate to the woman that the utilization of combination oral contraceptives (COCs) throughout the initial stages of pregnancy does not present an increased likelihood of congenital defects (Michael B Bracken, 1990; I. H. Thorneycroft, 1999).

Mastalgia commonly exhibits a decrease and final cessation within a few months of commencing the use of combination oral contraceptives (COCs). The adoption of strategies such as decreasing caffeine use and utilizing combined oral contraceptives (COCs) with reduced estrogen levels can yield advantageous outcomes (Robert A Hatcher & John Guillebaud, 1998).

Nausea is a commonly observed side effect that tends to decrease during combined oral contraceptive (COC) usage. The administration of COCs in conjunction with meals or before sleep has been observed to diminish the occurrence of nausea. The utilization of contraceptive oral contraceptives (COCs) that possess a low concentration of estrogen is advantageous (Robert A Hatcher & John Guillebaud, 1998; Michael J Rosenberg et al., 1999).

Combined Transdermal Patches

The transdermal contraceptive patch, which combines estrogen and progestin, has been observed to improve persistence in comparison to oral contraceptives because to its effectiveness and comfort (David F Archer et al., 2002; Rosanna M Galzote et al., 2017). The norelgestromin (NGMN) and ethinyl estradiol (EE) transdermal contraceptive patch, commonly called the NGMN-EE patch, are now distributed in 60 countries globally. This contraceptive patch comprises 6 mg of NGMN and 600 mg of EE. According to the study, the patch with a surface area of 20 cm2 is applied once a week for three weeks, followed by a week without the patch. The average daily release rates for NGMN and EE are around 203 mg/day and 33.9 mg/day, respectively. The concentrations of NGMN and EE reached steady-state levels of approximately 0.8 ng/mL and 50 pg/mL, respectively, within 48 hours after a single application. These concentrations were then maintained consistently during the suggested duration of wear.

Combined Vaginal Ring

The Combined Contraceptive Vaginal Ring (CVR) is a pliable device composed of ethylene acetate that releases a daily dosage of 15 mcg of ethinylestradiol and 120 mcg of etonogestrel (Devorah R Wieder & Lynn Pattimakiel, 2010).

These methods are under the user's control and are safe and very effective when consistently and correctly employed. Both vaginal rings and other combined treatments have similar benefits and hazards, but one advantage of vaginal rings is their extended duration of effect. The market offers several fused hormonal contraceptive rings that are readily accessible. These include the etonogestrel/ethinyl estradiol ring (ENG/EE), designed for monthly use and available under brand names such as NuvaRing and EluRyng. Additionally, there is the progesterone acetate/ethinyl estradiol ring (SA/EE), intended for annual use and marketed under Annovera. The utilization of hormonal contraceptive vaginal rings offers the benefit of circumventing challenges associated with daily or weekly administration (MD Jennifer Kerns, Philip D Darney, MD, MSc, 2023).

The Etonogestrel and Ethinyl Estradiol Ring: The etonogestrel/ethinyl estradiol (ENG/EE) ring, which is commonly referred to as NuvaRing, EluRyng, Haloette, and EnilloRing, is a flexible contraceptive device that measures 54 mm in diameter and has a cross-section of 4 mm. The previously mentioned ring is specifically intended for vaginal insertion and is intended to be used continuously for three weeks. Following this period, the ring is subsequently removed and discarded, allowing for a one-week break before a new ring is installed. The outer ring comprises a combination of ethinyl estradiol (EE) and an ethylene vinyl acetate copolymer, which incorporates crystals of ENG, specifically the 3-keto-metabolite of desogestrel. According to the cited sources, the device can release an average of 120 mcg/day of ENG and 15 mcg/day of EE during 21 days (MD Jennifer Kerns, Philip D Darney, MD, MSc, 2023).

Progesterone Acetate and Ethinyl Estradiol Ring: The reusable Annovera contraceptive ring contains progesterone acetate and ethinyl estradiol. The ring diameter is 56 mm, and the cross-sectional diameter is 8.4 mm. The ring is used for three weeks, removed for one week, and repeated 13 times. The observed use pattern causes withdrawal bleeding and a 2.98 per 100 woman-year Pearl index for unwanted pregnancies. The ring has two internal channels: one with SA and EE, the other with SA. The device delivers 150 micrograms of SA and 13 micrograms of EE daily for 21 days. Inactive ingredients include silicone elastomers, titanium dioxide, dibutyltin dilaurate, and silicone medical glue. The median Tmax of both hormones is 2 hours after vaginal implantation, and concentrations stabilize about 96 hours. The drug may be stored without refrigeration and has no oral activity, making it appealing to breastfeeding mothers who want to avoid progestin exposure. The one-year ring is FDA-approved and available (MD Jennifer Kerns, Philip D Darney, MD, MSc, 2023).

COCs and vaginal rings have similar systemic adverse effects. Ring users experience vaginitis, dampness, and leukorrhea more than COC users. These symptoms seldom cause ring withdrawal and do not require treatment. The contraceptive ring may be subject to unplanned removal or expulsion. In the event of an unintentional displacement, the object can be cleansed using cool or warm water (avoiding hot water) and subsequently reintroduced into the vaginal cavity. The subsequent actions, such as the requirement for additional contraception, are contingent upon the duration of time without the ring and the specific week of the menstrual cycle (about the ENG/EE ring exclusively). The resumption of fertility often occurs within approximately one month following the cessation of ring usage (MD Jennifer Kerns, Philip D Darney, MD, MSc, 2023).

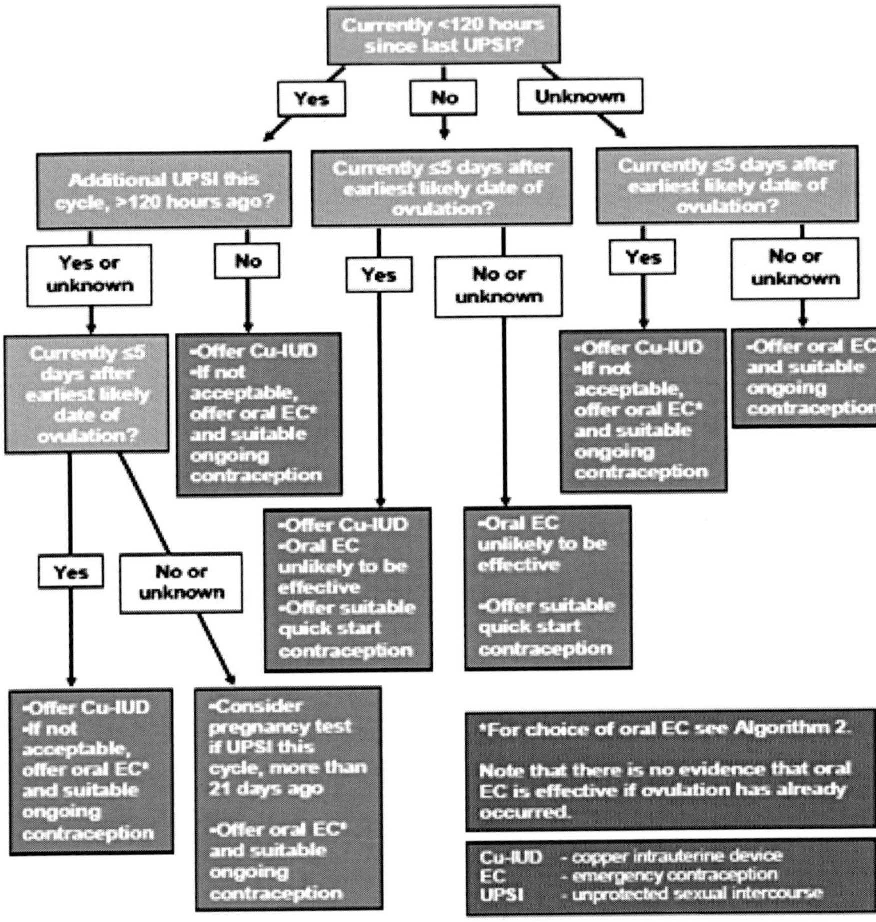

Figure 2. Decision-making algorithms for emergency contraception (Faculty of Sexual & Reproductive Healthcare Clinical Guidance, 2023).

The contraceptive ring has the potential to disrupt the efficacy of certain female barrier contraceptives, such as the diaphragm, cervical cap, and female condom. However, it generally does not interfere with the effectiveness of most vaginal drugs. An important caveat to consider is that the utilization of the SA/EE ring is contraindicated in conjunction with oil-based vaginal treatments or pharmaceuticals. During the menstrual period, tampons can be utilized without affecting the absorption of hormones from the ring (MD Jennifer Kerns, Philip D Darney, MD, MSc, 2023).

Emergency Contraception (EC)

Emergency contraception (EC) encompasses a range of contraceptive methods that are intended to be utilized within a limited timeframe following instances of unprotected or inadequately protected sexual activity or sexual assault to mitigate the likelihood of pregnancy. Emergency contraceptive pills (ECPs) should be promptly administered within a maximum timeframe of five days following instances of unprotected sexual intercourse. The existing emergency contraception (EC) methods offered in the United States comprise the copper intrauterine device (IUD), the levonorgestrel (LNG) 52 mg IUD, oral LNG choices like My Way, and Take Action, as well as oral ulipristal acetate (UPA) in the form of Ella (K. Cleland et al., 2012; A. Glasier, 2014). As you see in Figure 2 there is an algorithm to choose the true way of EC.

Emergency contraception (EC) encompasses a range of contraceptive methods that are administered within a short timeframe following instances of unprotected or inadequately protected sexual intercourse or sexual assault to mitigate the likelihood of pregnancy. The existing emergency contraception (EC) methods offered in the United States comprise the copper intrauterine device (IUD), the levonorgestrel (LNG) 52 mg IUD, oral levonorgestrel and oral ulipristal acetate (Ella). All available approaches for emergency contraception have demonstrated (Figure 1) efficacy, safety, and typically high levels of tolerability. Oral methods can be obtained without the need for a visit to a clinic (Faculty of Sexual & Reproductive Healthcare Clinical Guidance, 2023). Emergency contraception (EC) is distinct from pharmaceutical abortion in that it is specifically employed to prevent conception in the early stages rather than terminating an already established pregnancy.

Cooper Bearing IUD

Cu-IUDs utilized as emergency contraception (EC) demonstrate a notably higher level of efficacy compared to emergency contraceptive pills (ECPs), as evidenced by a pregnancy rate of 0.09% (K. Cleland et al., 2012). The LNG 52 mg intrauterine device (LNG-IUD) is recommended as a first choice for emergency contraception (EC), in addition to other available EC options (GRADE 1B). Patients seeking emergency contraception (EC) through the use of an intrauterine device (IUD) should get appropriate counseling regarding the potential risks associated with this method. Specifically, they should be informed about the possibility of ectopic pregnancy in the event of IUD failure, as well as the risk of pregnancy while an IUD is in place, including miscarriage and intrauterine infection (K. M. Curtis et al., 2016).

According to the available evidence (GRADE 1A), the copper intrauterine device (Cu-IUD) demonstrates a higher level of effectiveness compared to emergency contraceptive pills (ECPs). Also, it has been determined that UPA emergency contraceptive pills (ECPs) exhibit greater efficacy than LNG ECPs, as indicated by a GRADE 1A recommendation. The efficacy of the LNG 52 mg intrauterine device (IUD) is comparable to that of the copper IUD for emergency contraception (EC) when used within five days following unprotected intercourse, based on evidence of high quality (GRADE 1B) (Faculty of Sexual & Reproductive Healthcare Clinical Guidance, 2023).

Oral Emergency Contraception

Ulipritral Asetate (UPA) and LNG-EC

The drug UPA 30 mg, classified as a selective progesterone receptor modulator, postpones ovulation for a minimum duration of 5 days. This delay ensures that any sperm resulting from unprotected sexual intercourse (UPSI) in which emergency contraception (EC) was administered becomes nonviable. The use of ulipristal acetate emergency contraception (UPA-EC) has been found to cause a delay in ovulation, even after the onset of the luteinizing hormone (LH) surge. In contrast, levonorgestrel emergency contraception (LNG-EC) is no longer efficacious once the LH surge has commenced. The UPA-EC medication does not possess the ability to impede ovulation either during or after the LH peak (V. Brache et al., 2013).

The effectiveness of UPA and levonorgestrel emergency contraceptive pills (ECPs) is comparable when administered within three days following unprotected sexual intercourse. Nonetheless, studies have demonstrated that UPA exhibits greater efficacy compared to the levonorgestrel formulation when taken between 3 and 5 days after unprotected sexual intercourse (A. F. Glasier et al., 2010). The effectiveness of UPA and levonorgestrel emergency contraceptive pills (ECPs) is comparable when administered within three days following unprotected sexual intercourse. Nevertheless, research indicates that UPA demonstrates superior efficacy compared to the levonorgestrel formulation when taken between 3 and 5 days after unprotected sexual intercourse (Faculty of Sexual & Reproductive Healthcare Clinical Guidance, 2023; Elizabeth Raymond et al., 2004).

Barrier Methods

The category of on-demand contraception encompasses several methods, such as barrier methods like male and female condoms, vaginal sponges, diaphragms, and cervical caps. Additionally, chemical barriers in the form of spermicides can be utilized either independently or in combination with other contraceptive approaches. The methods above possess characteristics of safety, accessibility, affordability, and reversibility (C. C. Baker & M. J. Chen, 2022).

A *diaphragm or cervical* cap may be implanted before sexual intercourse, accompanied by the use of spermicide (Evidence Level C). It is recommended to reapply spermicide in situations when sexual activity is planned, and the diaphragm or cap has been in place for three hours or longer, or if sexual activity is repeated while the contraceptive device remains on site (Evidence Level C). It is recommended to retain a diaphragm or cervical cap for a minimum of 6 hours following the most recent instance of sexual intercourse (Evidence Level C). It is essential for women utilizing a diaphragm or cervical cap to be aware of the little empirical support on the efficacy of these approaches in mitigating the risk of HIV/STI transmission or the occurrence of cervical intraepithelial neoplasia (Evidence Level C).

Male *condoms* have been found to exhibit a 98% efficacy rate in preventing pregnancy, while female condoms have demonstrated a 95% efficacy rate. However, it is essential to note that these rates are contingent upon regular and correct usage of the respective contraceptive methods (Evidence Level B).

The pregnancy rates for both latex and non-latex condoms exhibit comparable outcomes. When employed constantly and accurately, alongside the use of spermicide, diaphragms and cervical caps are predicted to show a contraceptive efficacy ranging from 92% to 96% in preventing conception (Evidence Level C).

It is strongly advised to consistently and accurately employ male latex condoms to mitigate the likelihood of HIV transmission (Evidence Level A). It is recommended to utilize male condoms during oral sexual activity to minimize the potential for HIV transmission (Evidence Level C). It is recommended that those who are living with HIV be counseled on the need to use condoms as a preventive measure against the transmission of HIV to others, the possibility of superinfection with distinct strains of HIV, and the acquisition of additional STIs. (Evidence Level B) (C. C. Baker & M. J. Chen, 2022).

Coitus Interruptus

Coitus interruptus, often referred to as withdrawal, is a conventional form of family planning wherein the male partner withdraws his penis entirely from the vaginal canal and external genitalia of the female partner before ejaculation. The practice of coitus interruptus involves the withdrawal of the penis from the woman's vagina before ejaculation, effectively obstructing the entry of sperm into the vaginal canal. Consequently, this method impedes the interaction between spermatozoa and the ovum.

This approach may be suitable for;

- Women who possess a strong drive and can efficiently utilize this approach.
- Due to religious or philosophical convictions, women may choose not to employ alternative means of contraception.
- Women who require rapid access to contraception and find themselves engaged in a sexual encounter without access to alternate techniques.
- Women who engage in sexual activity on a less frequent basis.

There are several advantages associated with the practice of coitus interruptus. Firstly, when employed correctly, this approach does not interfere with breastfeeding. Additionally, it can be consistently utilized as a primary contraceptive method or as a supplementary option. Furthermore, coitus interruptus is characterized by the absence of economic expenses or the utilization of chemical substances, and it lacks any immediate health hazards. The practice of coitus interruptus does not protect against sexually transmitted diseases (STDs), such as human immunodeficiency virus (HIV). It is important to advise women who choose this approach that the consistent and correct use of male latex condoms significantly decreases the risk of transmitting HIV and other STDs. The utilization of female condoms has the potential to offer protection against the transmission of sexually transmitted diseases (STDs), although the available data on this matter are currently limited.

The method of coitus interruptus is susceptible to improper use, and its efficacy is contingent upon the couple's commitment and capability to employ withdrawal during each instance of sexual intercourse consistently. Women who have medical disorders that pose a significant danger during pregnancy should be informed that the adoption of the withdrawal method may not be suitable for them due to its comparatively higher rates of failure in real-world scenarios (K. M. Curtis et al., 2016).

Abstinence

If a woman does not want to get pregnant, she should avoid sexual activity or utilize contraception like condoms. Women may choose to employ barrier measures or abstain from intercourse based on personal preferences, religious or cultural norms, and partner preferences.

Using spermicides or barrier techniques with lubricants can hinder the detection of cervical secretion alterations. Using cervical secretions in conjunction with other fertility markers reduces the problem. Using a diaphragm may help women monitor changes in their cervix. Barrier methods can be used as an alternative to sexual abstinence during the fertile window. Still, couples must be appropriately taught and accept a greater failure rate during peak ovulation (Faculty of Sexual & Reproductive Healthcare Clinical Guidance, 2015).

Permanent Contraception

Vasectomy

The vas deferensces are a pair of tubular structures responsible for transporting spermatozoa from the testes. Spermatozoa are incorporated into the seminal fluid of males. During a vasectomy procedure, the vas deferens tubes are subjected to various methods such as ligation, incision, clipping, or sealing, with the intention of impeding the passage of sperm into the seminal fluid. This mechanism inhibits the fusion of a female gamete (egg) with a male gamete (sperm). Following a vasectomy, there is no discernible alteration in a man's sexual function. Due to the typical composition of semen, wherein sperm constitute a mere 5 percent, the volume of fluid expelled after ejaculation is not expected to undergo significant alterations. The efficacy of vasectomy in contraceptive effectiveness over one year surpasses that of female sterilization by a little margin. Similar to female sterilization, vasectomy does not provide protection against STIs (American College of Obstetricians and Gynecologists, 2023b).

A vasectomy is a surgical technique that is characterized by its efficiency and relatively low level of pain. In the majority of instances, women are typically permitted to return to their place of residence on the same day. It is recommended to abstain from engaging in sexual activity for a minimum duration of 7 days subsequent to undergoing a vasectomy procedure. During the initial 8 to 12 weeks following the procedure, it is advisable to employ an alternative contraceptive method, since the process of eliminating residual sperm from the fallopian tubes may require this duration.

Approximately 12 weeks post-procedure, it will be necessary to provide a semen sample for the purpose of assessing sperm presence. Upon the completion of tests that have verified the absence of sperm in your semen, the vasectomy procedure can be deemed efficacious, hence obviating the need for supplementary contraceptive measures. It is possible that certain women of the male gender may require two separate tests. However, it is imperative to employ an alternative method of contraception until the absence of sperm in your semen has been definitively established. Some women may have persistently low levels of sperm in their reproductive system, characterized by reduced motility and diminished fertility potential. Consequently, the likelihood of impregnating one's spouse is significantly reduced in such cases. If an individual belongs to this demographic, their healthcare provider will engage in a discussion regarding the available choices. The duration of this process varies among women. There remains a potential for conception during this period (NHS, 2023).

Tubal Sterilization

Tubal sterilization involves the occlusion or excision of the fallopian tubes. The aforementioned mechanism hinders the downward movement of the egg within the fallopian tube, hence impeding the sperm's ability to reach and fertilize the egg. This is a widely recognized and efficacious method for preventing pregnancy. The incidence of pregnancy within one year following the surgical procedure is less than 1% among women. In the event of an infrequent occurrence of pregnancy following tubal sterilization, there is an elevated likelihood that the pregnancy may manifest as an ectopic pregnancy. However, the incidence of ectopic pregnancy in women who have undergone tubal sterilization is reduced compared to those who do not utilize any contraception. There exist additional dangers that are contingent upon the particular nature of the process (American College of Obstetricians and Gynecologists, 2023b).

Fertility Awareness Methods

Calendar-Based Methods

Standard Day Method

Fertility awareness-based (FAB) approaches of family planning encompass the identification of fertile days within the menstrual cycle. This can be achieved through the observation of fertility markers, such as cervical secretions and basal body temperature, or by tracking cycle days. The utilization of Fertility Awareness-Based (FAB) approaches in conjunction with abstinence or barrier strategies is a viable approach during the fertile period.

The Standard Days technique (SDM) is a simpler variant of the calendar technique that employs a consistent mathematical equation. The Standard Days Method (SDM) entails the practice of refraining from engaging in unprotected sexual intercourse (UPSI) throughout the period between Day 8 and Day 19 of a woman's menstrual cycle. The rule was formulated by evaluating the chance of pregnancy on various cycle days using a comprehensive existing dataset. The researchers demonstrated that among women whose menstrual cycles ranged from 26 to 32 days in length, the period of highest fertility was observed to be between Days 8 and 19.

The use of the Standard Days Method (SDM) is not recommended for women who have menstrual cycle durations that are shorter than 26 days, greater than 32 days, or those who experience irregular periods. The utilization of this approach is not recommended in cases when two or more cycles have occurred outside of this specified range throughout the preceding 12-month period (American College of Obstetricians and Gynecologists, 2023b).

Calendar Rhythm Method

A comprehensive study of eight research examining the effectiveness of calendar techniques revealed an aggregate failure rate of roughly 20% (with a range of 5-47%) after 12 months of observation. Inconsistencies between self-reported cycle days and hormonal data have been observed, indicating that relying just on cycle days to compute risk may not always accurately represent the actual risk.

Prospective multicenter research was conducted to evaluate the efficacy of the Symptothermal Method (SDM) in a cohort of 478 women aged 18-39 years. A total of 218 female participants completed 13 cycles of method use, accounting for 46% of the total sample. However, 28% of the participants were excluded from the study because two cycles fell outside the predetermined range. The one-year pregnancy rate, encompassing all cycles and pregnancies, was 12%, with a 95% confidence interval ranging from 8.47% to 15.3% (Marcos Arévalo et al., 2002).

Symptom-Based Methods

Cervical Secretion Method

Observing variations in cervical secretions is utilized to monitor the initiation and conclusion of the fertile window. Women can discern the existence of secretions by examining mucus indications on their undergarments' toilet paper and/or by tactile assessment of their genital region. Once the vaginal secretions are no longer dry and become noticeable, it indicates the beginning of their fertile period. The final day on which women know the significantly fecund and lubricating secretions is commonly referred to as the peak day, typically occurring close to ovulation. The identification of the peak day can only be determined in hindsight, as the secretions will return to a thicker consistency or cease altogether (Faculty of Sexual & Reproductive Healthcare Clinical Guidance, 2015).

The period of highest fertility occurs on the peak day and the two days leading up to it. However, it is important to note that conception can still occur from unprotected sexual intercourse (UPSI) that takes place at any point within the fertile window. The period of fertility commences upon the initial detection of any secretions and lasts for a duration of three complete days following the occurrence of the peak. The period of fertility concludes on the fourth day following the occurrence of the peak day. Women may require a minimum of three menstrual cycles to develop a sufficient level of confidence in accurately identifying and interpreting changes in their vaginal discharges. While cervical secretions are present, sexual activity increases the risk of conception, so women who want to avoid pregnancy should abstain or use an extra contraceptive until three days of dryness are seen (Evidence Level B) (Faculty of Sexual & Reproductive Healthcare Clinical Guidance, 2015).

Basal Body Temperature Method (BBT)

To use this indication, women must monitor their BBT daily with a digital thermometer. Women should take their temperature daily at the same time. Take the temperature before rising after a minimum of 3 hours of rest. Additional contraceptive precautions are not needed for intercourse occurring three days following a fever rise until menstruation begins. To avoid pregnancy, women should avoid sex or use extra contraceptive measures until higher temperatures are reported on three consecutive days in the next cycle (Evidence Level B) (Faculty of Sexual & Reproductive Healthcare Clinical Guidance, 2015).

Conclusion

Several contraceptive methods have been previously mentioned. Nevertheless, it is imperative to speak with family physicians, obstetricians, gynecologists, or allied health professionals who possess expertise in this domain, in order to select the most suitable contraceptive method. Additionally, it is crucial to reassess the condition during subsequent follow-up appointments.

References

Archer, D. F., Bigrigg, A., Smallwood, G. H., Shangold, G. A., Creasy, G. W., & Fisher, A. C. (2002). Assessment of compliance with a weekly contraceptive patch (Ortho Evra™/Evra™) among North American women. *Fertility and Sterility, 77*, 27-31.

Arévalo, M., Jennings, V., & Sinai, I. (2002). Efficacy of a new method of family planning: The Standard Days Method. *Contraception, 65*(5), 333-338.

Baker, C. C., & Chen, M. J. (2022). New contraception update - Annovera, Phexxi, Slynd, and Twirla. *Current Obstetrics and Gynecology Reports, 11*(1), 21-27. https://doi.org/10.1007/s13669-021-00321-4.

Bayer Schering. (2019). *Summary of Product Characteristics (SPC) - Noristerat® 200 mg, solution for intramuscular injection.* Retrieved 24/10/2023 from https://www.bayer.com/sites/default/files/NUR-ISTERATE_EN_PI.pdf.

Black, A., Francoeur, D., Rowe, T., Collins, J., Miller, D., Brown, T., David, M., Dunn, S., Fisher, W. A., Fleming, N., Fortin, C. A., Guilbert, E., Hanvey, L., Lalonde, A., Miller, R., Morris, M., O'Grady, T., Pymar, H., Smith, T., & Henneberg, E. (2004). SOGC clinical practice guidelines: Canadian contraception consensus. *Journal of Obstetrics and Gynaecology Canada, 26*(3), 219-296.

Bofill Rodriguez, M., Lethaby, A., & Farquhar, C. (2019). Non-steroidal anti-inflammatory drugs for heavy menstrual bleeding. *Cochrane Database of Systematic Reviews, 9*(9), CD000400. https://doi.org/10.1002/14651858.CD000400.pub4.

Brache, V., Cochon, L., Deniaud, M., & Croxatto, H. B. (2013). Ulipristal acetate prevents ovulation more effectively than levonorgestrel: Analysis of pooled data from three randomized trials of emergency contraception regimens. *Contraception, 88*(5), 611-618. https://doi.org/10.1016/j.contraception.2013.05.010.

Bracken, M. B. (1990). Oral contraception and congenital malformations in offspring: A review and meta-analysis of the prospective studies. *Obstetrics & Gynecology, 76*(3 Part 2), 552-557.

Buhling, K. J., Zite, N. B., Lotke, P., & Black, K. (2014). Worldwide use of intrauterine contraception: A review. *Contraception, 89*(3), 162-173. https://doi.org/10.1016/j.contraception.2013.11.011.

Cleland, K., Zhu, H., Goldstuck, N., Cheng, L., & Trussell, J. (2012). The efficacy of intrauterine devices for emergency contraception: A systematic review of 35 years of experience. *Human Reproduction, 27*(7), 1994-2000. https://doi.org/10.1093/humrep/des140.

Crosignani, P. G., Testa, G., Vegetti, W., & Parazzini, F. (1996). Ovarian activity during regular oral contraceptive use. *Contraception, 54*(5), 271-273. https://doi.org/10.1016/s0010-7824(96)00178-3.

Curtis, K. M., Jatlaoui, T. C., Tepper, N. K., Zapata, L. B., Horton, L. G., Jamieson, D. J., & Whiteman, M. K. (2016). U.S. selected practice recommendations for contraceptive use, 2016. *MMWR Recommendations and Reports, 65*(4), 1-66. https://doi.org/10.15585/mmwr.rr6504a1.

Daniels, K., Daugherty, J., & Mosher, W. D. (2015). *Current contraceptive use and variation by selected characteristics among women aged 15-44: United States, 2011-2013.*

Health Products Regulatory Authority. (2020). *SAYANA PRESS®104 mg/0.65 ml suspension for injection single-dose container Medroxyprogesterone acetate.* Retrieved 23/10/2023 from http://www.hpra.ie/img/uploaded/swedocuments/2153241.PA0019_054_002.af1c8e9c-ea4d-477f-a4a2-808f536a06f4.000001PIL.150824.pdf.

Health Products Regulatory Authority. (2021). *Depo-Provera Summary of Product Characteristics.* Retrieved 23/10/2023 from http://www.hpra.ie/img/uploaded/swedocuments/Licence_PA0822-124-001_21062021164149.pdf.

American College of Obstetricians and Gynecologists. (2023a). *Progestin-Only Hormonal Birth Control: Pill and Injection.* https://www.acog.org/womens-health/faqs/progestin-only-hormonal-birth-control-pill-and-injection.

American College of Obstetricians and Gynecologists. (2023b). *Sterilization for Women and Men.* https://www.acog.org/womens-health/faqs/sterilization-for-women-and-men.

Centers for Disease Control and Prevention. (2016). *US Selected Practice Recommendations for Contraceptive Use.* Retrieved from https://www.cdc.gov/reproductivehealth/contraception/mmwr/spr/references.html.

Faculty of Sexual & Reproductive Healthcare Clinical Guidance. (2015). *Fertility Awareness Methods Clinical Effectiveness Unit.* https://www.fsrh.org/standards-and-guidance/documents/ceuguidancefertilityawarenessmethods/.

Faculty of Sexual & Reproductive Healthcare Clinical Guidance. (2023). *Emergency Contraception.* https://www.fsrh.org/standards-and-guidance/documents/ceu-clinical-guidance-emergency-contraception-march-2017/.

Farley, T. M., Rosenberg, M. J., Rowe, P. J., Chen, J. H., & Meirik, O. (1992). Intrauterine devices and pelvic inflammatory disease: An international perspective. *Lancet, 339*(8796), 785-788. https://doi.org/10.1016/0140-6736(92)91904-m.

Finer, L. B., Jerman, J., & Kavanaugh, M. L. (2012). Changes in use of long-acting contraceptive methods in the United States, 2007–2009. *Fertility and Sterility, 98*(4), 893-897.

Galzote, R. M., Rafie, S., Teal, R., & Mody, S. K. (2017). Transdermal delivery of combined hormonal contraception: A review of the current literature. *International Journal of Women's Health*, 315-321.

Glasier, A. (2014). The rationale for use of Ulipristal Acetate as first-line in emergency contraception: Biological and clinical evidence. *Gynecological Endocrinology, 30*(10), 688-690. https://doi.org/10.3109/09513590.2014.950645.

Glasier, A. F., Cameron, S. T., Fine, P. M., Logan, S. J., Casale, W., Van Horn, J., Sogor, L., Blithe, D. L., Scherrer, B., Mathe, H., Jaspart, A., Ulmann, A., & Gainer, E. (2010). Ulipristal acetate versus levonorgestrel for emergency contraception: A randomised non-inferiority trial and meta-analysis. *Lancet, 375*(9714), 555-562. https://doi.org/10.1016/s0140-6736(10)60101-8.

Grimes, D. A., & Schulz, K. F. (1999). Prophylactic antibiotics for intrauterine device insertion: A meta-analysis of the randomized controlled trials. *Contraception, 60*(2), 57-63. https://doi.org/10.1016/s0010-7824(99)00071-2.

Hatcher, R. A., & Guillebaud, J. (1998). The pill: Combined oral contraceptives. *Contraceptive Technology, 17*, 405-466.

Kapp, N., & Gaffield, M. E. (2013). Initiation of progestogen-only injectables on different days of the menstrual cycle and its effect on contraceptive effectiveness and compliance: A systematic review. *Contraception, 87*(5), 576-582.

Kavanaugh, M. L., & Jerman, J. (2018). Contraceptive method use in the United States: Trends and characteristics between 2008, 2012, and 2014. *Contraception, 97*(1), 14-21.

Kerns, J., & Darney, P. D. (2023). *Contraception: Hormonal contraceptive vaginal rings.* Retrieved 14/11/2023 from https://www.uptodate.com/contents/contraception-hormonal-contraceptive-vaginal-rings.

Krettek, J. E., Arkin, S. I., Chaisilwattana, P., & Monif, G. R. (1993). *Chlamydia trachomatis* in patients who used oral contraceptives and had intermenstrual spotting. *Obstetrics & Gynecology, 81*(5 Pt 1), 728-731.

Krishnan, S., & Kiley, J. (2010). The lowest-dose, extended-cycle combined oral contraceptive pill with continuous ethinyl estradiol in the United States: A review of the literature on ethinyl estradiol 20 μg/levonorgestrel 100 μg + ethinyl estradiol 10 μg. *International Journal of Women's Health, 2*, 235-239. https://doi.org/10.2147/ijwh.s6437.

Ministry of Health General Directorate of Maternal and Child Health and Family Planning. (2019). *Family Planning Method Implementation Guide.* Retrieved 24/10/2023 from https://uremesagligi.org/wp-content/uploads/2019/03/aile-planlamasi-yontemi-uygulama-rehberi.pdf.

Mulders, T. M., & Dieben, T. O. (2001). Use of the novel combined contraceptive vaginal ring NuvaRing for ovulation inhibition. *Fertility and Sterility, 75*(5), 865-870. https://doi.org/10.1016/s0015-0282(01)01689-2.

NHS. (2023). *Vasectomy (Male Sterilisation).* https://www.nhs.uk/conditions/contraception/vasectomy-male-sterilisation/.

Petta, C. A., Faundes, A., Dunson, T. R., Ramos, M., Delucio, M., Faundes, D., & Bahamondes, L. (1998). Timing of onset of contraceptive effectiveness in Depo-Provera users: Part I. Changes in cervical mucus. *Fertility and Sterility, 69*(2), 252-257.

Rosenberg, M. J., Meyers, A., & Roy, V. (1999). Efficacy, cycle control, and side effects of low- and lower-dose oral contraceptives: A randomized trial of 20 μg and 35 μg estrogen preparations. *Contraception, 60*(6), 321-329.

Royal College of Obstetricians and Gynaecologists. (2013). *New Product Review: Sayana Press®.* Retrieved 24/10/2023 from https://www.fsrh.org/standards-and-guidance/documents/cec-ceu-newproductreview-sayana-press-jun-2013/.

Royal College of Obstetricians and Gynaecologists. (2016). *UK Medical Eligibility Criteria for Contraceptive Use (UKMEC).* Retrieved October 17, 2023, from http://ukmec.pagelizard.com/2016#sectiona/effectiveness_of_contraceptive_method.

Royal College of Obstetricians and Gynaecologists. (2023a). *Faculty of Sexual & Reproductive Healthcare Clinical Guideline: Progestogen-only Implant.* https://www.fsrh.org/standards-and-guidance/documents/cec-ceu-guidance-implants-feb-2014/.

Royal College of Obstetricians and Gynaecologists. (2023b). *Faculty of Sexual & Reproductive Healthcare Intrauterine Contraception.* Retrieved 18/10/2023 from https://www.fsrh.org/standards-and-guidance/documents/ceuguidanceintrauterinecontraception/.

Royal College of Obstetricians and Gynecologists. (2023c). *Faculty of Sexual & Reproductive Healthcare Combined Hormonal Contraception.* Retrieved 23/10/2023 from https://www.rcog.org.uk/guidance/browse-all-guidance/green-top-guidelines/venous-thromboembolism-and-hormonal-contraception-green-top-guideline-no-40/.

Schindler, A. E., Campagnoli, C., Druckmann, R., Huber, J., Pasqualini, J. R., Schweppe, K. W., & Thijssen, J. H. (2008). Classification and pharmacology of progestins. *Maturitas, 61*(1-2), 171-180. https://doi.org/10.1016/j.maturitas.2008.11.013.

Sitruk-Ware, R. (2002). Hormonal replacement therapy. *Reviews in Endocrine and Metabolic Disorders, 3*(3), 243-256. https://doi.org/10.1023/A:1020028510797.

Thirumalai, A., & Amory, J. K. (2021). Emerging approaches to male contraception. *Fertility and Sterility, 115*(6), 1369-1376.

Thorneycroft, I. H. (1999). Cycle control with oral contraceptives: A review of the literature. *American Journal of Obstetrics and Gynecology, 180*(2 Pt 2), 280-287. https://doi.org/10.1016/s0002-9378(99)70719-2.

Trussell, J. (2004). Contraceptive failure in the United States. *Contraception, 70*(2), 89-96.

Trussell, J. (2011). Contraceptive failure in the United States. *Contraception, 83*(5), 397-404. https://doi.org/10.1016/j.contraception.2011.01.021.

Turkish Society of Gynecology and Obstetrics. (2012). *Oral Contraception Guide.* https://www.tjod.org/wp-content/uploads/2012/12/Demir-C-ve-ark.-Ed-I%CC%87til-I%CC%87M.-Oral-Kontrasepsiyon-K%C4%B1lavuzu-TJOD-2012.pdf.

Wieder, D. R., & Pattimakiel, L. (2010). Examining the efficacy, safety, and patient acceptability of the combined contraceptive vaginal ring (NuvaRing®). *International Journal of Women's Health*, 401-409.

World Health Organization Department of Sexual and Reproductive Health and Research, Johns Hopkins Bloomberg School of Public Health, & Center for Communication Programs Knowledge for Health Project, United States Agency for International Development Bureau for Global Health Office of Population and Reproductive Health. (2022). Chapter 1 - Combined oral contraceptives. In *Family Planning: A Global Handbook for Providers.* https://fphandbook.org/sites/default/files/WHO-JHU-FPHandbook-2022Ed-v221115a.pdf.

World Health Organization. (2015). *Medical eligibility criteria for contraceptive use — 5th ed.* https://iris.who.int/bitstream/handle/10665/181468/9789241549158_eng.pdf?sequence=9.

Chapter 29

Menopause

Enver Ciftel*, MD

Department of Endocrinology and Metabolism, Sivas State Hospital, Sivas, Turkey

Abstract

Menopause is a physiological period in the reproductive lifespan of women, marked by the loss of ovarian function and the discontinuation of menstrual cycles. Menopause is the cessation of a woman's reproductive potential, which typically occurs between the ages of 45 and 55. During this phase, hormonal fluctuations and a noticeable decrease in estrogen levels occur. The physiological, psychological, and sociological implications of menopause can significantly impact the overall well-being of numerous women. The initiation of menopause, its symptoms, and physiological alterations during this phase are significant factors in the well-being of women. Furthermore, the substantial impact of hormonal changes induced by the menopausal transition on cardiovascular health, bone density, and metabolic alterations cannot be overstated. Menopause exhibits psychological effects, including mood changes, increased vulnerability to depression, and noticeable impacts on quality of life. Menopause, a natural event in the life of a woman, is complex and requires a range of treatment options for management. These alternatives include hormone replacement medications, lifestyle modifications, and alternative treatments. This page aims to serve as a complete guide for healthcare professionals, researchers, and general readers seeking to understand the complex and diverse aspects of menopause and its wide-ranging impact on women's health.

Keywords: menopause, hormone therapy, estrogen, progesterone

Introduction

Definition and Process of Menopause

The STRAW (Stages of Reproductive Aging Workshop) staging system, regarded as the benchmark, defines the reproductive aging process from the reproductive years to menopause (Harlow et al., 2012). It was built using data from multiple longitudinal cohort studies. Based on this classification, the lives of adult women can be divided into three main stages: the

* Corresponding Author's Email: enver-ciftel@hotmail.com.

In: Common Diseases According to Family Medicine Practice Guidelines
Editors: Esra Meltem Koç and Hilal Aksoy
ISBN: 979-8-89530-302-3

reproductive period, the phase of transitioning to menopause/perimenopause, and postmenopause (Harlow et al., 2012). The menopausal transition and the postmenopausal era can be further categorized into "early" and "late" stages. The provided information is displayed in Table 1.

Menopause is the cessation of ovarian activity and menstrual cycles, which occurs permanently after 12 consecutive months of amenorrhea (Talaulikar, 2022). The onset typically happens around the age of 51.4 years. It is characterized by depletion of the ovarian follicles, leading to low estrogen levels and high follicle-stimulating hormone (FSH) (Jayasinghe et al., 2018). The perimenopausal period is the transitional phase after the reproductive years and encompasses the pre-menopausal period. It is characterized by symptoms such as irregular menstrual cycles, significant hormonal fluctuations, and the onset of hot flashes, typically starting around four years before the last menstrual period (LMP) (Nagy & Dolenc, 2021). Early menopause refers to the cessation of ovarian functions between the ages of 40 and 45 without any identifiable secondary reason (Sochocka et al., 2023). The occurrence of menopause characterizes premature ovarian failure (POF) before the age of 40 (C. Pillay & Manyonda, 2022). The hormonal changes that occur during the menopausal transition and menopause lead to the development of bothersome vasomotor symptoms (VMS), mood problems, temporary cognitive dysfunction, genitourinary complaints, and other disease processes that negatively impact the quality of life (Jayasinghe et al., 2018).

The menopausal transition is a protracted and distressing process that can last beyond ten years and induces symptoms in the majority of women. Clinicians must have the ability to identify initial indications and manifestations of transition and be ready to provide treatment to reduce these symptoms. Menopause treatment encompasses a variety of secure and efficacious treatments, such as hormone replacement therapy (HRT) (Kingsberg et al., 2023).

Table 1. Premenopausal-postmenopausal period characteristics

	Premenopausal Period		Postmenopausal Period	
Parameters	Early	Late	Early	Late
FSH	High/Variable	High (>25ıu)	High/Variable	High/Stable
AMH	Low	Low	Low	Very Low
INHIBIN	Low	Low	Low	Very Low
AFC	Low	Low	Low	Very Low
E2	Normal	Low	Low	Very Low
VMS	There İs No	Mostly	Very Likely	İncreasing Symptoms of Urogenitoal Atrofi
Diagnosis	40-45 Age Menstrual irregularities VMS Differential diagnosis; BHCG, PRL, TSH >45 Age The diagnosis is clinical. Based on the presence of irregular menstrual periods and/or menopausal symptoms. Laboratory evaluation is not required.		Permanent cessation of ovarian activity and menstrual periods following >12 months of amenorrhea	

Abbreviations: AMH (Anti Mullerian Hormone), AFC (Antral folicule count), E2 (Estradiol), VMS (Vasomotor Symptoms), PRL (Prolactın), LMP (Last menstrual period).

Physiology of Menopause

The onset of the menopausal transition, also known as perimenopause, typically occurs four years before the final menstrual period and encompasses many physiological changes (Verdonk et al., 2022). The condition is distinguished by unpredictable menstrual cycles and notable hormonal variations, frequently accompanied by menopausal indications, including sudden episodes of intense heat, disruptions in sleep patterns, changes in mood, and dryness in the vaginal area (Woods & Mitchell, 2005). Furthermore, alterations in lipids and the onset of bone loss commence, leading to enduring health consequences (Marlatt et al., 2022).

The early transition is characterized by a shift in the intermenstrual interval of at least seven days. The typical duration between menstrual cycles during the reproductive phase is 25 to 35 days. However, during the menopausal transition, this duration can extend to 40–50 days, or there may be a reduction in the length of intermenstrual intervals, particularly in the later reproductive years. During the initial stage of the menstrual cycle, known as the early follicular phase, follicle-stimulating hormone (FSH) levels exhibit variability, but often remain elevated. The levels of AMH (Antimullerian Hormone), inhibin B, and antral follicle count (AFC) are below average. No clinical signs are present (Jayasinghe et al., 2018; Sochocka et al., 2023). During the late transition stage, there is a progression toward more pronounced changes in the menstrual cycle. These changes include longer intervals between periods, skipped periods, episodes of amenorrhea, and an increase in cycles where ovulation does not occur (Harlow et al., 2012). Irregular menstrual cycles are commonly accompanied by variations in the levels of follicle-stimulating hormone (FSH) and estradiol in the blood. According to a study, serum FSH levels greater than 25 IU/L were indicative of a late menopausal transition (Freeman et al., 2005). Nevertheless, because of the fluctuation in blood FSH levels during the later stages of the menopausal transition, it is not advisable to regularly evaluate them. During the menopausal transition, there are further hormonal changes that occur. These include a gradual decline in the levels of serum inhibin B as well as a drop in the levels of anti-Mullerian hormone (AMH), which is also produced by the cells in the ovaries known as granulosa cells (Jayasinghe et al., 2018). Furthermore, the antral follicle count (AFC), which refers to the number of follicles measuring between 2 and 10 mm in diameter on transvaginal ultrasound, consistently diminishes. Studies have examined AMH, AFC, FSH, and estradiol levels to evaluate menopausal status; however, none of these measures have been confirmed for practical use (Harlow et al., 2012).

Menopause is the term used to describe the permanent cessation of ovarian activity and menstrual cycles after 12 consecutive months of amenorrhea, after years irregularity in the monthly calendar (Shifren, 2019). In the STRAW staging system, the period ranging from the first two to six years after the last menstrual period is designated as "early postmenopause," while the period following that is referred to as "late postmenopause (Harlow et al., 2012)." The mean age of onset of spontaneous menopause is 51.4 years, and the occurrence of menopause is influenced by various factors such as genetic predisposition, tobacco use, and reproductive background (Dunneram et al., 2019). The elevation in serum FSH levels continues near the last menstrual period. Subsequently, over multiple years, follicle-stimulating hormone (FSH) gradually increases to levels ranging from 70 to 100 IU/L and then decreases as one age (Hall, 2004).

Clinic

Menopause Signs and Symptoms

Following menopause, there is a decline in the production and release of estradiol by the ovaries. Nevertheless, the ovaries persist in releasing testosterone. Estrogen insufficiency leads to several chronic consequences, such as osteoporosis, cardiovascular disease (CVD), dementia, osteoarthritis, balance difficulties, and skin alterations. While vasomotor symptoms (VMS) are the primary symptom throughout the menopausal transition and the early postmenopausal years, there are many additional symptoms, such as sleep difficulties, depression, genitourinary complaints, and, less frequently, joint disorders (Johnston et al., 2021; Lee et al., 2022; Williams et al., 2009; Woods & Mitchell, 2005).

Vasomotor Symptoms

While some women who have reached menopause may not experience any symptoms, up to 85% of cases are characterized by vasomotor symptoms (such as hot flashes and sweating) (Talaulikar, 2022). The prevalence of symptoms during the early menopausal transition is around 40%, but this percentage increases to 60% to 80% during the late menopausal transition and early postmenopausal periods (Sochocka et al., 2023). Hot flashes often commence as an abrupt sensation of warmth localized in the upper chest and face and swiftly spread (Talaulikar, 2022). The sensation of warmth typically endures for two to four minutes, frequently accompanied by profuse perspiration and intermittent palpitations, and occasionally followed by sensations of coldness, tremors, and unease. VMS exhibits fluctuating frequency throughout the day. It typically happens multiple times within a day, with the frequency varying from 1-2 times daily to once every hour. Nocturnal hot flashes, sometimes known as "night sweats," are particularly prevalent (Flores et al., 2021).

While the exact causes of the variations in geographical distribution remain uncertain, research has demonstrated notable disparities in vasomotor symptoms (VMS) among different geographic regions and ethnic groups. Despite the varied and conflicting prevalence data, the highest prevalence is observed in black women, while the lowest prevalence is found in East Asian women (Kingsberg et al., 2023).

Several variables influence the intensity and length of the VMS. Menopausal status, hormone therapy, age, high body mass index (BMI), depression, anxiety, poor physical health, high perceived stress, smoking, and low education level are factors that are linked to a prolonged duration of vasomotor symptoms (VMS) (Harlow et al., 2022). The US-based Survey of Women's Health Nationwide (SWAN) reports that the duration of symptoms averages 7.4 years (Kingsberg et al., 2023). Nevertheless, it has the potential to persist for a duration of up to 20 years after the last menopause period.

Women experiencing vasomotor symptoms (VMS) commonly encounter sleep difficulties (94%), concentration (84%), mood (85%), energy (77%), and sexual activity (61%). However, the degree and frequency of VMS may differ (12). The greater the severity of VMSs, the more they impair daily activities and work performance. This can lead to adverse consequences such as absences, layoffs, and job transitions (Williams et al., 2009).

Genitourinary Syndrome of Menopause (GSM)

Vulvar vaginal atrophy (VVA) is a condition that occurs in menopausal women due to a decrease in estrogen levels. It is characterized by a combination of symptoms and findings that affect the labia, clitoris, vagina, urethra, and bladder. These changes result in hypoestrogenic symptoms and urinary dysfunction. While there is less information on the impact of androgens in the hypoestrogenic state, they are similarly believed to have a role in safeguarding the structure and function of genitourinary tissue (Flores et al., 2021). Estrogen is responsible for preserving a well-lined vaginal cavity throughout the reproductive period. Estrogen acts on receptors in specific areas of the female reproductive system, including the trigone of the vagina, vulva, urethra, and bladder. This action promotes optimal blood flow to the genitals, maintains a healthy balance of microorganisms in the vagina, thickens the stratified non-keratinized squamous epithelium of the vagina, and protects the urogenital region against infections (Rahn et al., 2014). Vaginal atrophy is mainly caused by a substantial decrease in estrogen levels (Scavello et al., 2019).

The structures of the urinary tract share the same embryological genesis as the genital system and have estrogen receptors. The hypoestrogenic state has an impact on the bladder, urethra, pelvic floor musculature, and endopelvic fascia. Possible ramifications of urinary tract atrophy include sensations of discomfort in the urethra, an increased frequency of urination, urinary incontinence, blood in the urine, painful urination, and an increased incidence of urinary tract infections (Yenice et al., 2020). The length of time that hypoestrogenism persists is a crucial determinant in the onset and intensity of MGS. Additional factors, in addition to reduced estrogen and androgen levels, such as having never given birth vaginally, previous vaginal surgery, abstaining from sexual activity, smoking, depression, and urine incontinence, can intensify the symptoms of vaginal atrophy or increase the probability of experiencing these symptoms (Harlow et al., 2022). Approximately 70% of women experiencing signs of vaginal atrophy refrain from disclosing their problem to a healthcare provider (Johnston et al., 2021; Scavello et al., 2019). These symptoms are often seen as an anticipated and important aspect of the aging process. Patients may have discomfort addressing genitourinary issues due to factors such as embarrassment, cultural norms, religious beliefs, and social conventions. Moreover, many patients lack knowledge regarding the many therapy alternatives available. Patients frequently use lifestyle modifications to manage their symptoms instead of actively pursuing medical intervention. Without therapy, the condition will often advance in the majority of women, leading to long-lasting alterations in the structure and function of the urogenital tissue that may prove challenging to reverse, even with medical intervention. The manifestations of GSM encompass the following (Johnston et al., 2021; Lee et al., 2022).

- Vulvovaginal dryness and pain
- Lack of lubrication
- Impairment in sexual functions (Decreased arousal, orgasm, or sexual desire)
- Vulvar or vaginal bleeding, burning, irritation, or itching
- Vaginal discharge (leucorrhea or yellow and foul smelling)
- Urinary tract symptoms (e.g., urinary frequency, urgency, dysuria, urethral discomfort, hematuria, recurrent urinary tract infections).
- Urethral prolapse.

Regular screening for symptoms and signs of genitourinary syndrome of menopause (GSM) is recommended for menopausal women due to the potential for symptoms to develop gradually and become unpleasant even after the menopausal transition. The evaluation for GSM typically encompasses a comprehensive medical history assessment and a thorough pelvic examination. Laboratory testing is typically unnecessary. During clinic appointments, it is important to inquire about symptoms of urogenital atrophy in patients in the perimenopausal or postmenopausal period or those who have other causes of hypoestrogenism. Assessments of quality of life matters should also be conducted. These factors encompass the level of discomfort, behavioral reactions to symptoms, and the influence of symptoms on everyday activities and partner relationships (Avis et al., 2015; Scavello et al., 2019).

Effects of Menopause on Women's Health

Menopause and Diabetes Mellitus (DM)

Women have phenotypic, metabolic, and biochemical changes during the menopausal transition, which increase the likelihood of developing type 2 diabetes mellitus (T2DM). Whether these alterations are unrelated to age and if menopause raises the risk of T2DM remains a subject of discussion (18). Menopause is associated with an adverse metabolic profile that increases susceptibility to diabetes. During the menopausal transition, several changes can increase the risk of developing type 2 diabetes mellitus (T2DM). These changes include an increase in fat tissue, a decline in the ability of the body to produce and respond to insulin, and weight gain (Opoku et al., 2023). Elevated production of proinflammatory cytokines, circulating free fatty acids, and reactive oxygen species resulting from visceral adiposity, hyperandrogenic state, and reduced estrogen receptor-α (ERα) activity, as demonstrated in experimental research, could potentially contribute to the increased insulin resistance observed during menopause (19,20). Research has indicated that experiencing menopause during the menopausal transition is associated with a 47% higher likelihood of developing Type 2 Diabetes Mellitus (T2DM). Similarly, undergoing menopause before the age of 45 is associated with a 20% increased risk of T2DM compared to the average age of menopause. Furthermore, experiencing menopause before the age of 40 is associated with a 32% higher risk of T2DM. Research on the impact of diabetes mellitus (DM) on the onset of menopause yields diverse and conflicting findings (Slopien et al., 2018).

Menopause and Dyslipidemia

The onset of menopause is accompanied by an elevation in levels of total cholesterol (TK), low-density lipoprotein cholesterol (LDL-C), triglycerides (TG), apolipoprotein B (apoB), and perhaps lipoprotein (a). Conversely, there is a reduction in the concentration of high-density lipoprotein cholesterol (HDL-C). The atherogenic lipid profile is related to it, and these alterations seem to be unrelated to age, BMI, and the duration since the last menopausal period (Marlatt et al., 2022). Table 2 demonstrates the impact of menopause on lipid levels.

Table 2. Effects of menopause on lipid profile

Parameters	Effects Of Menopause
LDL-C	Increases
TriglycerideTotal-C	Increases
HDL-C	Increases
Lipoprotein (a)	Decreases
Apolipoprotein A-1	Increases/Stable
Apolipoprotein B	Increases

Menopause and Sexual Health

Sexual dysfunctions in menopausal women can be categorized as disorders encompassing diminished sexual desire, arousal, discomfort, and orgasmic difficulties. A concise sexual screening history and physical examination are essential when assessing menopausal women (Scavello et al., 2019; Shifren, 2019).

Menopause and Sleep Disorders

Sleep quality is frequently compromised during the perimenopausal and postmenopausal phases, as indicated by subjective and objective measurements. Sleep disturbances are primarily related to nocturnal hot flashes, which exhibit a higher frequency the nighttime (Sochocka et al., 2023). The estimated prevalence during the early menopausal transition is between 32-40%, and this percentage increases to 38-46% during the late transition. White women exhibited a higher prevalence of sleep problems compared to East Asian women (Kingsberg et al., 2023).

Menopause and Depression

The perimenopausal phase is a critical period for the emergence of depressive symptoms and major depressive episodes. The incidence of developing depression for the first time is approximately 30%, and this risk doubles to 60% in individuals with a previous history of depression (Sochocka et al., 2023). The incidence of depression diminishes during the postmenopausal phase.

Menopause and Cognitive Changes

During the perimenopause and menopause stages, individuals can have cognitive symptoms, including transient amnesia, reduced focus, cognitive processing deceleration, and other cognitive manifestations (Sochocka et al., 2023).

Menopause and Bone Health

Osteoporosis initiation commences during the perimenopausal phase. The most significant decrease in bone mineral density occurs over one year before and two years following the final menstrual period. During perimenopause and menopause, joint problems are more prevalent compared to the reproductive phase (Massé et al., 2010).

Menopause and Cardiovascular Health

A correlation between the onset of menopause and a higher likelihood of cardiovascular events has been observed. However, it remains uncertain whether this is due to the natural aging process or is specifically attributable to menopause. The cardiovascular risk related to menopause seems to arise from the confluence of various risk factors, including abdominal obesity, insulin resistance, hyperglycemia, and atherogenic dyslipidemia (Opoku et al., 2023; Slopien et al., 2018).

Menopause and Migraine

Fluctuations in estrogen levels can precipitate headaches, including migraines. Estrogen has the most significant impact on migraines, which are a specific type of headache. The incidence of migraine in females starts to increase throughout early adolescence, reaches its highest point in the 20s and 30s, and decreases after menopause (Sochocka et al., 2023).

Diagnosis and Evaluation in Menopause

Initially, it is necessary to assess whether the patient is experiencing menopause. The assessment is contingent upon the patient's age, categorized as either under 40 years, between 40 and 45 years, or over 45 years. A comprehensive method involves conducting a monthly cycle analysis for all patients, conducting a thorough investigation of menopausal symptoms, and performing pelvic examinations to assess vaginal atrophy in women experiencing symptoms such as vaginal dryness, dyspareunia, or sexual dysfunction (Jayasinghe et al., 2018).

For women aged 45 and older, additional tests are unnecessary if menopausal symptoms accompany irregular menstruation. Nevertheless, a follicle-stimulating hormone (FSH) level beyond 30-40 mIU/mL and an estradiol level lower than 20 pg/mL could potentially signify the onset of menopause (Talaulikar, 2022). A low AMH level can suggest the onset of menopause within the following five years, although it is inconclusive (Davis SR, Pinkerton J, Santoro N, 2023). During the menopausal transition, it is advisable to review women's bone health, smoking habits, alcohol use, cardiovascular risk, and cancer screening and prevention (Lobo RA, 2022). Women between the ages of 40 and 45 who experience irregular menstruation should undergo an evaluation similar to individuals with oligomenorrhea/amenorrhea. In cases when pregnancy is a potential concern, it is advisable to test for serum HCG, TSH, and prolactin

(PRL) levels to investigate any suspicions. Women of all age groups experiencing unusual hot flashes or night sweats should have a thorough evaluation to consider the possibility of other conditions, such as carcinoid syndrome, pheochromocytoma, or underlying cancer (Avis et al., 2015). Women less than 40 years old should undergo a comprehensive evaluation to determine the cause of their irregular or absent menstrual periods. Subsequently, we will thoroughly examine health factors relevant to individuals in their middle years of life. The topics addressed encompass VMS (Vasomotor Symptoms), MGS (Musculoskeletal Symptoms), mood assessment and management, sleep issues, cognition, bone health, cardiovascular risk assessment and management, cancer screening and prevention, and optimization of lifestyle factors (Lobo R. A., 2022).

Premenopausal/Menopausal Patient Management and the Treatment of Symptoms

Treatment of Vasomotor Symptoms

Menopausal hormone therapy (MHT) is considered the most effective treatment for vasomotor symptoms (VMS) (Flores et al., 2021). It is recommended to regularly assess the necessity for MHT and tailor the treatment according to symptoms, concurrent medical conditions, potential dangers, treatment objectives, and personal preferences (Society, 2023).

Menopausal Hormone Therapy

Hormone therapy (HT) is the optimal therapeutic modality for addressing vasomotor symptoms (VMS) and the genitourinary syndrome of menopause (GSM). Additional symptoms related to estrogen sensitivity during perimenopause and menopause encompass sleep disruptions, depression/anxiety, and joint discomfort. Research indicates that hormone therapy (HT) is comparatively safer during the early stages of menopause as opposed to later stages, and it has a more significant number of beneficial impacts on coronary heart disease and overall mortality. Hormone therapy (HT) is advised for women who experience moderate to severe vasomotor symptoms (VMS), are under the age of 60 or within ten years of menopause onset, have no medical conditions that make HT unsafe, and have a low risk of cardiovascular disease and breast cancer. The impact of hormone therapy (HT) differs based on factors such as age, duration since menopause, presence of other medical conditions, type of therapy, dosage, and method of administration (Flores et al., 2021; SR & RJ, 2022).

When a woman goes through early menopause or premature ovarian insufficiency (POI), hormone therapy (HT) can help with both the symptoms of low estrogen levels and the long-term health problems that can come with estrogen deficiency, such as osteoporosis, fractures, cardiovascular disease (CVD), memory loss, mood disorders, and a higher risk of death (Davis SR, Pinkerton J, Santoro N, 2023). For these women, hormone therapy is seen as a form of hormone replacement (Lobo RA, 2022).

Women who undergo surgical menopause also undergo a sudden and significant decrease in the levels of ovarian androgens in their bloodstream. Systemic estrogen therapy effectively alleviates symptoms caused by low estrogen levels and can even prevent the early-onset genitourinary syndrome of menopause (GSM). However, women who undergo surgical menopause and subsequently suffer reduced sexual desire may find it beneficial to supplement estrogen therapy with androgens (Flores et al., 2021). Nevertheless, the potential long-term usage hazards remain uncertain, and there are currently no authorized formulations specifically designed for women.

Before deciding on menopausal hormone therapy, it is important to take into account the patient's age, the severity of their symptoms, their risk of cardiovascular disease and breast cancer, and the available evidence-based data on the risks and benefits related explicitly to their hormone therapy. The dangers associated with hormone therapy (HT) are contingent upon factors such as the specific medication, dosage, duration of usage, method of administration, timing of the beginning, and the inclusion of progestogen. Women who have previously had breast cancer, coronary heart disease (CHD), a past venous thromboembolic (VTE) incident or stroke, current liver disease, or are at high risk for these issues are susceptible to MHT.

Women under 60 years old or within ten years of starting menopause and who do not have any medical reasons to avoid it will find that the advantages outweigh the disadvantages when it comes to treating uncomfortable vasomotor symptoms (VMS) and preventing bone loss. Women who initiate hormone therapy ten years after the start of menopause or who are over the age of 60 experience a less advantageous benefit-risk ratio. This is primarily due to the increased absolute risks of coronary heart disease, stroke, venous thromboembolism (VTE), and dementia. Insufficient research has been conducted on the potential hazards of prolonged hormone therapy. Consequently, choosing to proceed with treatment in specific, well-informed women aged 60 or 65 and above is a personal decision. There is insufficient evidence to justify the regular cessation of the medication in females aged 65 and above (Flores et al., 2021). According to analyses, the duration of exposure affects the risk of cardiovascular disease (CVD), and there is no appreciable increase in risk among women younger than 60 years old and who have gone through menopause. Furthermore, it seems that mortality rates are reduced among young postmenopausal individuals who use hormone therapy compared to those who do not utilize it.

Postmenopausal women with hypertriglyceridemia, active gallbladder disease, known thrombophilias such as factor V Leiden, a history of VTE, migraine headaches with aura, risk factors for cardiovascular disease, or obesity should refrain from using oral estrogens. Transdermal estrogen is the recommended choice for these women. Transdermal estrogens bypass the initial metabolic processing of the liver, and research conducted so far has not identified a higher likelihood of developing venous thrombosis (AE & S., 2023; Lobo R. A., 2022; S. R. & R. J., 2022).

Situations in which HT should not be used are as follows (AJ et al., 2021).

- Breast cancer (known, suspected, or previous)
- Estrogen-sensitive malignant disease (ovary, cervix, and endometrium)
- Coronary heart disease, stroke
- Previous thromboembolic event (deep vein thrombosis, pulmonary embolism)
- Untreated hypertension

- Furthermore, HT is not recommended in women with high-risk factors for these diseases, as well as in undiagnosed genital bleeding and untreated endometrial hyperplasia.

Drugs

Table 3. Drugs used in menopausal hormone therapy

MENAPOUSAL HORMONE THERAPY

Progesterone Therapy

Oral synthetic	Bioidentical	İntrauterin
MPA Norethindrone Megestrol acetate Didrogesterone Medrogestone Nomegestrol asetat Promegestone	Mikronize Progesterone	Levonorgestrel

Estrogen Therapy

Oral	Transdermal	Vaginal
Micronized E CEE	E2 Patch E2 Gel E2 Nasal Spray	E2 Cream E2 Ring

Other
Tibolone Bazedoxifen-CEE

Combined Treatments
Oral MPA+CEE NETA+E2 CyproteroneAsetat+E2 Norgestimate+E2 Drosperinone+E2 Didrogesterone+E2
Transdermal E2+NETA E2+Norethindrone E2+Levonorgestrel

Estrogen Therapy

Estrogen is offered in many formulations, including oral, transdermal, and subcutaneous implants, each with distinct potencies and dosages, as indicated in Table 3. When selecting estrogen, it is advisable to prioritize oral or transdermal estradiol as the initial option. Due to its similar structure to the estrogen that ovaries naturally produce, 17-beta estradiol is the preferred option (Johnston et al., 2021). When used to treat vasomotor symptoms, vaginal rings, and creams in high doses have a systemic effect. On the other hand, vaginal estrogen in medium and low doses has a localized effect and is used for managing genitourinary syndrome of menopause (GSM) (Scavello et al., 2019). To alleviate menopausal symptoms in the majority of women, a minimal dosage of estrogen (17β-estradiol 0.5–1 mg/day oral, 0.05 mg transdermal) is adequate. Young women with bilateral oophorectomies are rare (C. Pillay & Manyonda, 2022). Typically, greater doses (such as 2 mg of oral estradiol, 0.1 mg of transdermal estradiol, or a comparable dosage) are commonly needed within the initial two to three years following surgery (C. Pillay & Manyonda, 2022). Nevertheless, the present method involves initiating treatment with smaller quantities, such as transdermal estradiol at a dosage of 0.025 mg or oral estradiol at a daily dosage of 0.5 mg, and adjusting the dosage based on symptom observation (Kingsberg et al., 2023).

Progesterone Therapy

Progestogens, such as medroxyprogesterone acetate (MPA), norethindrone acetate (NETA), and micronized progesterone (MP), are frequently prescribed alongside estrogen. These progestogens are included in Table 3. While MP has the same structure as the corpus luteum's progesterone naturally produces, MPA, levonorgestrel, and NETA are artificial progestins (Flores et al., 2021; Johnston et al., 2021).

The purpose of using progestogen during estrogen therapy (ET) is to prevent excessive development of the endometrium and reduce the chance of developing endometrial cancer (32,36,37). Progestins are unnecessary for women who have undergone a hysterectomy or who use modest amounts of vaginal estrogen. The dosage and duration of progestogen use play a crucial role in the protection of the endometrium. The choice of a progestogen dosage regimen to ensure endometrial safety is dependent on the potency of the progestogen and is subject to variation based on the estrogen dose (Journal et al., 2007). The preferred initial option for progestin is oral natural micronized progesterone, administered at a dosage of 200 mg/day or 100 mg/day as a continuous regimen for 10-14 days every month. Recent investigations have demonstrated the adverse impact of continuous progesterone use of on the breast, thus making this treatment not advisable (Johnston et al., 2021). Monthly administration of progestins is necessary for women who receive conventional levels of estrogen. Progesterone treatment for 14 days every three months may be indicated to minimize breast exposure to progesterone in individuals taking lower levels of estrogen. However, the effectiveness of this treatment has not been thoroughly assessed (Lobo RA, 2022). Administering progestin every three months is not considered adequately effective and cannot be advised for women who are on regular dosages of estrogen. Occasionally, vaginal progesterone insertions are attempted, but there is a lack of comprehensive evidence on the safety of these insertions in the endometrium (Dunneram et al., 2019). It is advisable to prioritize the occasional use of natural progesterone or norethindrone above MPA as a form of progesterone. Oral progestational agents shown to protect the endometrium include:

- Medroksiprogesteron acetate (MPA) (2,5 mg/day or 5 mg 10-12 days/month)
- Progesterone (100 mg/day or 200 mg 10-12 days/month)
- Norethindrone acetate (combined preparation 0.35 mg/day, or 5 mg 10-12 days/month)
- Drospirenon (2-3 mg/day),
- Levonorgestrel (0,075 mg/day).

The Use of Combined Oral Contraceptives (COCs) During the Menopausal Transition

Perimenopausal women who desire relief from menopausal symptoms while also requiring contraception or management of heavy bleeding may consider using low-estrogen combined oral contraceptives (COCs) (Harlow et al., 2022). The transition from combined oral contraceptives (COCs) to hormone therapy (HT) often occurs around the average age of menopause, which is roughly 52 years. Alternatively, switching might be based on an individual's family reproductive history and personal profile (Flores et al., 2021).

Other Hormonal Agents Used in VMS Treatment

Tibolon

Tibolone is a synthetic steroid that produces metabolites with estrogenic, androgenic, and progestogenic characteristics. It exhibits estrogenic and progestogenic actions that are specific to certain tissues. It does not have any estrogenic effects on the uterus or breast. It decreases vasomotor symptoms (VMS) but is not as efficacious as estrogen therapy (Am, 2016; SR & RJ, 2022). It is not used together with other MHTs.

Conjugated Estrogens with Bazedoxifene

A choice involves the utilization of bazedoxifene (BZA), which is a selective estrogen receptor modulator (SERM), in conjunction with conjugated estrogen (CCE). Research conducted over 2 years has indicated that the combination of BZA with CEE offers endometrial protection (Parth M. Raina, 2024). Bazedoxifene, in this combination, serves to inhibit estrogen-induced endometrial hyperplasia, obviating the necessity of progestin administration. Similar to other Selective Estrogen Receptor Modulators (SERMs), bazedoxifene carries an elevated risk of venous thromboembolism (VTE).

Follow-Up and Treatment Duration of Women Receiving Hormonal Therapy

Women undergoing hormone therapy (HT) should undergo assessment for both the effects and side effects of the treatment during the initial three months and subsequently at intervals of 6–12 months. According to many menopause guidelines, it is advised to assess patients every year to determine if medication should be continued and to strive for the shortest possible length of treatment. The recommended length for the usage of MHT is five years, and it should not be continued beyond the age of 60 (Carolyn J Crandall, Jaya M Mehta, 2023). Nevertheless, the majority of women experience persistent hot flashes for a duration of 10 to 20 years following their final menstrual period. As a result, several professional organizations believe that continued hormone therapy (HT) is a sensible choice for generally healthy women experiencing ongoing vasomotor symptoms (VMS) as long as counseling and collaborative decision-making are taken into account (Lobo R. A., 2022).

The duration of treatment and the cessation of hormone therapy (HT) should be determined by considering the patient's specific preferences and their personalized risk-benefit assessment. The potential dangers associated with the prolonged use of hormone therapy (HT) in women who initiated treatment at an early age but now have over 60 years old remain uncertain. It is unclear whether these risks are comparable to those of initiating HT in women over 60 years or more than ten years after the onset of menopause. Some important things to think about are how bad the symptoms are, whether non-hormonal and lifestyle therapies can help, and the underlying risk of osteoporosis, cardiovascular disease (CVD), cerebrovascular disease (CVD), venous thromboembolism (VTE), and breast cancer (Marlatt et al., 2022). Patients should be educated about the potential to develop breast cancer and advised to have appropriate breast cancer screenings for their age. If there is abnormal vaginal bleeding, it is necessary to assess the endometrium for hyperplasia and malignancy (Freeman et al., 2005).

Termination of Hormone Therapy

The majority of associations concur that the utilization of MHT should be tailored to each individual and should not be terminated purely based on the patient's age. There are a limited number of studies that assess the optimal method to cease hormone therapy (HT), and vasomotor symptoms (VMS) will reoccur in around 50% of women following the end of the medication. There is a dearth of data that directly compare the consequences of suddenly stopping hormone therapy versus gradually reducing the dosage. However, it is typically recommended to reduce the dosage gradually. Consider providing alternative therapeutic choices upon discontinuation of systemic hormone therapy.

Clinicians should consider risk reduction techniques, such as implementing risk stratification, transitioning from oral to transdermal E, and minimizing dose regimens. Hormone therapy (HT) can be explored for women over the age of 65 years who are at high risk for osteoporosis and also exhibit permanent vasomotor symptoms (VMS). Additionally, HT may be considered for selected women who are at low risk of cardiovascular disease (CVD) despite their advancing age. Opting for transdermal estrogen, with or without medroxyprogesterone (MP), helps mitigate certain dangers, such as venous thromboembolism (VTE) while providing advantages such as symptom management and decreased long-term fracture risk. Therefore, it is a safer option for long-term HT (Flores et al., 2021; Jayasinghe et al., 2018).

Future Directions

Ongoing research is focused on developing more accurate and non-hormonal remedies to treat VMS. The neurokinin-3 receptor antagonist fezolinant, which has demonstrated favorable outcomes in clinical studies for vasomotor symptoms (VMS), has recently obtained approval in the United States for the management of moderate to severe VMS resulting from menopause (Depypere et al., 2021). An additional field of research to consider is the assessment of the conservation of ovarian function through cryopreservation and subsequent reimplantation of ovarian tissue. The discovery of ovarian stem cells has facilitated the exploration of regenerative medicine, particularly in women with premature ovarian insufficiency (POI).

Hormone Therapy and Long-Term Health

Quality of Life

The impact of estrogen on the quality of life in postmenopausal women varies based on factors such as age, the presence of symptoms, and any additional medical issues. Estrogen has been found to enhance the overall well-being in postmenopausal women experiencing vasomotor symptoms (VMS).

Bone Health

Menopause is related to increased bone resorption, while ET decreases bone resorption and the likelihood of fractures (Yong Eu-Leong & Logan Susan, 2021). Hormone therapy (HT) has received approval from the FDA to prevent bone loss. However, it does not have approval for the treatment of osteoporosis. Hormone therapy is a viable choice for women who have a high likelihood of experiencing osteoporotic fractures and for whom other treatments for osteoporosis are not appropriate or result in adverse consequences (Flores et al., 2021; Massé et al., 2010).

Joint Pain

Estrogen provides a safeguard for biomechanical integrity, functionality, and overall joint well-being. Nevertheless, the impact of estrogen on osteoarthritis remains a subject of debate (Geraci et al., 2021; Jayasinghe et al., 2018).

Sarcopenia

Preclinical investigations of hormone therapy (HT) in postmenopausal women have shown some indication that combining estrogen therapy (ET) with exercise may help prevent the decline of muscle mass, strength, and performance. However, this potential advantage has not been confirmed in clinical research (Geraci et al., 2021).

Gallbladder and Liver

Oral estrogen medication is strongly associated with a notable increase in the likelihood of developing biliary tract disease [44]. The use of estrogen after menopause is linked to a higher likelihood of developing gallstones and cholecystitis. Nevertheless, there is no evidence indicating any risk linked to biliary tract cancer. Observational studies have shown that the use of the transdermal route of administration, which avoids the liver's first-pass metabolism, is related to a reduced incidence of gallbladder disease. Preclinical and observational studies indicate the potential advantages of hormone therapy in addressing liver fibrosis and fatty liver disease (Randolph et al., 2005; Selli et al., 2016). However, further investigation is required to establish conclusive recommendations.

Metabolic Syndrome and Diabetes

Menopausal hormone therapy positively impacts various metabolic parameters, such as diminishing the buildup of belly fat, augmenting lipid oxidation, and increasing energy expenditure (Carr, 2003; Opoku et al., 2023). Research indicates that estrogens enhance insulin sensitivity by directly influencing estrogen receptors (ERs) in the liver, muscle, and adipose tissue. Additionally, estrogens can potentially boost insulin production in pancreatic beta cells (Slopien et al., 2018). Significant randomized controlled trials demonstrate that hormone therapy (MHT) effectively reduces the risk of type 2 diabetes mellitus (T2DM). Moreover, women who use MHT experience a 25% reduction in the occurrence of T2DM (Slopien et al., 2018). For women diagnosed with type 2 diabetes, the administration of menopausal hormone therapy (MHT) should be based on their risk of cardiovascular disease (CVD). In women with type 2 diabetes mellitus (T2DM) and a low risk of cardiovascular disease (CVD), it may be preferable to use oral estrogens. However, in women with T2DM and other risk factors for CVD such as obesity, it is recommended to use transdermal 17β-estradiol. Progestins exert a neutral impact on glucose metabolism.

Dyslipidemia

A customized strategy is necessary for menopausal hormone therapy (MHT) for women with dyslipidemia due to the varied effects of hormones on lipids (Table 4). This approach should consider parameters such as dosage, method of administration, and other relevant considerations.

Progestogens have a minimal impact on the estrogen-induced decrease in TC and LDL-C levels. Micronized progesterone or dydrogesterone are the chosen progestogens since they neutrally impact the lipid profile. Tibolone has the ability to decrease total cholesterol (TC), low-density lipoprotein cholesterol (LDL-C), triglycerides (TG), and lipoprotein(a) (Lp(a)) levels while also reducing high-density lipoprotein cholesterol (HDL-C) concentrations. The use of low-dose vaginal estrogen has been found to have a beneficial impact on the lipid profile. However, there is currently inadequate data to determine the effects of dehydroepiandrosterone (DHEA) on this profile (Carr, 2003).

CVD and All-Cause Mortality

The impact of hormone therapy on cardiovascular disease (CVD) can differ based on factors such as a woman's age, the duration since the start of menopause, and the timing of hormone therapy initiation (Marlatt et al., 2022). Observational data and meta-analyses indicate that women who initiate hormone therapy before the age of 60 or within ten years of the onset of menopause have a lower risk of coronary heart disease (CHD) (Lee et al., 2022). Initiating hormone therapy in postmenopausal older women purely to prevent cardiovascular disease is not recommended, as there are insufficient data to support this indication.

Women with a high risk of cardiovascular disease (CVD) should start using nonhormonal treatments instead of menopausal hormone therapy (MHT) to relieve vasomotor symptoms (VMS). On the other hand, women with an intermediate risk of CVD should use transdermal therapy to reduce VMS (Society, 2023).

Cerebrovascular Disease

Evidence demonstrates that there is no elevated risk of cerebrovascular accident among women below the age of 60 years or those who initiate hormone therapy within 10 years after the onset of menopause. However, the risk escalates with age (Selli et al., 2016).

Venous Thromboembolism

The likelihood of developing venous thromboembolism (VTE) when undergoing menopausal hormone therapy (MHT) is higher in those who are older, obese, have the factor V Leiden mutation, and have a history of deep vein thrombosis (DVT). Transdermal therapy has a reduced risk of deep vein thrombosis (DVT) compared to oral medication. It should be chosen only when the advantages outweigh the potential drawbacks (Depypere et al., 2021; Johnston et al., 2021).

Endometrial Hyperplasia and Cancer

The likelihood of developing endometrial hyperplasia and cancer increases with systemic administration of unopposed estrogen therapy, with the risk depending on the dosage and length of treatment. While the use of low-dose vaginal estrogen therapy (ET) does not seem to increase the likelihood of developing endometrial cancer, the available research on endometrial biopsy findings is restricted to a one-year timeframe (Rahn et al., 2014).

Table 4. Effect of mht on lipid profile

Parameters	Effect Of MHT
TC	Decreases
LDL-C	Decreases
Lipoprotein (a)	Decreases
TG	Increases
HDL-C	Increases
Apolipoprotein B	Stable
Apolipoprotein A–I	Increases

Breast Cancer

The association between hormone use and breast cancer is a major concern for women considering MHT. It is crucial to comprehend the potential influence of HT on the chance of developing breast cancer. The impact of this phenomenon is contingent upon the specific hormone therapy used, the length of time it is administered, the prescribed regimen, prior exposure, the timing of the beginning, and individual characteristics. Given the correlation between the duration of use and the risk of developing breast cancer, it is advisable to regularly assess the advantages and disadvantages of hormone therapy (HT). Multiple observational studies have demonstrated a positive correlation between the duration of hormone therapy use, namely over five years, and an elevated risk of developing breast cancer. This includes both unopposed estrogen therapy and combined estrogen-progestin therapy (Dunneram et al., 2019).

The choice of progestin can impact the chance of developing breast cancer. Initial observations indicate that natural micronized progesterone may not carry any additional risk. Most studies have found that the risk of breast cancer is greater in individuals who receive combination therapy as opposed to those who just receive estrogen (Dunneram et al., 2019). Additionally, there is a hypothesis that continuous administration of progestin can be related to a greater risk compared to cyclic regimens. However, it is important to note that not all studies have documented this association.

Observational studies have shown that hormone therapy generally decreases the likelihood of dying from breast cancer, although not all research has reached the same conclusion (Pocobelli G, Newcomb PA, Li CI, Cook LS, Barlow WE, 2014). This can be attributed to the observation that breast tumors in hormone therapy (HT) users have a higher prevalence of benign histological characteristics compared to non-HT users in the majority of studies. HT users may undergo more regular mammograms and diagnostic exams, particularly in the presence of signs or symptoms, which could result in early detection and reduced mortality.

Ovarian Cancer

The use of oral contraceptives is related to a substantial decrease in the likelihood of developing ovarian cancer. The risk decreases as the duration of usage increases. A drop in risk is observed after 1 to 4 years of use and persists for up to 30 years after stopping the oral contraceptive (Dunneram et al., 2019).

Colorectal Cancer

Observational studies have indicated that the occurrence of colorectal cancer declined among women aged 50–59 who currently use hormone therapy (HT); however, this finding did not reach statistical significance (Society, 2023).

Lung Cancer

HT exhibits a generally neutral impact on both the occurrence and survival rates of lung cancer (Maki P. M., Kornstein S. G., Joffe H., Bromberger J. T., Freeman E. W., Athappilly G., Bobo W. V., Rubin L. H., Koleva H. K., Cohen L. S., 2018).

Falls

Estrogen therapy has the potential to enhance balance and decrease the propensity to fall, which may lead to a decrease in the likelihood of fractures. Several studies suggest that estrogen therapy can enhance balance, but there are conflicting findings (Sochocka et al., 2023).

Skin Health

Estrogen is believed to contribute to the preservation of skin thickness and collagen levels in women after menopause (Kamp et al., 2022).

Eye Health

Long-term estrogen medication seems to reduce the likelihood of developing dry eyes and cataracts. MHT may decrease intraocular pressure and mitigate the likelihood of primary open-angle glaucoma (Vajaranant T. S., Maki P. M., Pasquale L. R., Lee A., Kim H., 2016).

Systemic Lupus Erythematosus (SLE)

Estrogen is associated with an elevated likelihood of acquiring Systemic Lupus Erythematosus (SLE) and experiencing illness exacerbations in women diagnosed with SLE (A. Gompel, 2020).

Epilepsy

A study including 42 menopausal women with epilepsy found that hormone therapy (HT) was related to a higher frequency of seizures (Vanessa Carvalho, Isabella Colonna, Giulia Curia, Maria Teresa Ferretti, Gennarina Arabia, Maria Judit Molnar, Elena R Lebedeva, Elena Moro, Marianne de Visser, 2023).

Alzheimer's Disease

Research provides evidence that the timing of hormone therapy's (HT) beginning has a crucial role in determining the likelihood of developing Alzheimer's disease. Initiating HT early decreases the risk, while initiating it late is related to an increased risk (Imtiaz B, Tuppurainen M, Rikkonen T, Kivipelto M, Soininen H, Kröger H, 2017; Sochocka et al., 2023).

Non-Hormonal Therapies to Control VMS

Almost all randomized research indicates that a placebo decreases vasomotor symptoms (VMS) in approximately one-third of women. Based on randomized research, soy, isoflavones, and phytoestrogens have demonstrated inconclusive outcomes in alleviating symptoms. Weight loss, mindfulness, hypnosis, cognitive behavioral therapy, and stress reduction have been found to be advantageous, although the benefits of yoga, exercise, and acupuncture vary and are not consistently positive (AJ et al., 2021; Society, 2023).

Lifestyle Changes

For individuals experiencing mild vasomotor symptoms (VMS), lifestyle modifications such as maintaining a cool environment and wearing breathable cotton clothing can provide relief. Abstaining from smoking, alcohol, caffeine, and spicy meals, as well as minimizing weight and stress, can have advantageous effects (AE & S., 2023; Xu et al., 2014).

Antidepressants

SSRI and SNRI antidepressants are advised for women looking for a pharmacological intervention for moderate to severe vasomotor symptoms (VMS) in cases where hormone therapy (HT) is not prescribed or desired. Among this group, venlafaxine appears to be the most efficacious preparation. The FDA has exclusively approved Paroxetine at a dosage of 7.5 mg per day for this specific purpose (Kingsberg et al., 2023).

Gabapentin and Pregabalin

An individual administration of gabapentin in a dosage range of 300-1200 mg is a potent remedy. A dosage of 75-150 mg of pregabalin can be used twice a day (Flores et al., 2021).

Clonidine

Women who do not have a positive response to or cannot handle nonhormonal prescription medications, selective serotonin reuptake inhibitors (SSRIs), serotonin-norepinephrine reuptake inhibitors (SNRIs), or gabapentin and pregabalin should consider the use of clonidine as a potential treatment option (Nguyen et al., 2017).

Complementary Herbal and Natural Products

The available evidence supporting the efficacy of most complementary and alternative treatments in treating vasomotor symptoms (VMS) is limited. Due to the lack of substantial evidence regarding their efficiency and little information on their safety, it is not advisable to advocate these approaches (Elizabeth A. Casiano Evans, Deslyn T. G. Hobson, Sarit O. Aschkenazi, Alexandriah N. Alas, Sunil Balgobin, Ethan M. Balk, Alexis A. Dieter, Gregory Kanter, Francisco J. Orejuela, Tatiana V. D. Sanses, 2023; Lobo R. A., 2022). Phytoestrogens are compounds obtained from plants that can mimic the effects of estrogen on the body. Genistein and daidzein are two types of phytoestrogens derived from isoflavones. Soy isoflavones are abundant in soybeans, soy products, and red clover. The findings of studies examining the impact of these drugs on VMS are inconclusive. Specifically, the impact of red clover was determined to be comparable to that of a placebo (S. R. & R. J., 2022).

Cognitive Behavioral Therapy (CBT)

The latest draft guidance from NICE asserts that Cognitive Behavioral Therapy (CBT) can effectively alleviate menopausal symptoms, including hot flashes, night sweats, depressive symptoms, and sleep disturbances. The draft guideline asserts that Cognitive Behavioral Therapy (CBT) diminishes the occurrence and intensity of hot flashes and night sweats. It recommends that CBT be considered alongside or instead of Hormone Replacement Therapy (HRT) (Sochocka et al., 2023).

Sleeping Disorders

Hormone therapy (HT) enhances sleep quality by diminishing instances of nighttime awakenings in women experiencing troublesome nocturnal vasomotor symptoms (VMS). Estrogen may exert certain sleep influences unrelated to vasomotor symptoms (Nagy & Dolenc, 2021). The administration of hormone therapy in the form of low dosages of estrogen or progesterone can improve the condition of persistent insomnia in women experiencing menopause. Certain data, regardless of vasomotor symptoms (VMS), suggest that transdermal estrogen therapy (ET) may improve sleep quality in perimenopausal women (Kingsberg et al., 2023).

Treatment of Genitourinary Symptoms

Long-term treatment is essential for many patients because of the wide range of negative consequences, which include not only symptom alleviation but also the management of more problematic issues such as sexual dysfunction, post-coital bleeding, and recurring urinary tract infections. Multiple vaginal estrogen formulations for menopausal genitourinary syndrome (GSM) are accessible, including creams, pills, and rings. Recently, a synthetic form of DHEA called prasterone has been introduced as a vaginal suppository to treat GSM (Courtney R Cameron, Stacey Cohen, Keri Sewell, 2023). According to a comprehensive study on the treatment of GSM, vaginal estrogen preparations were shown to be the most effective treatment for genitourinary symptoms. They were found to be superior to vaginal lubricants and moisturizers (Colton Biehl, Olivia Plotsker, 2019).

The recommended treatment for symptoms of vaginal dryness, discomfort, or painful sexual intercourse associated with vaginal atrophy typically involves the use of non-hormonal vaginal moisturizers and lubricants to be applied at least twice a week (Rahn et al., 2014). Vaginal preparations of estrogen therapy (ET) at low doses are both effective and typically safe for treating genitourinary symptoms associated with menopausal genital syndrome (Johnston et al., 2021). These preparations have minimal absorption into the bloodstream and are preferred over systemic treatments in cases where ET is solely used to address genitourinary symptoms (Journal et al., 2007). If initial therapies do not sufficiently alleviate symptoms, individuals without any contraindications can consider using low-dose vaginal estrogen therapy or other hormonal drugs (Scavello et al., 2019). All existing vaginal estrogen treatments are effective in alleviating symptoms of vaginal atrophy. Conjugated estrogen cream, intravaginal sustained-release estradiol rings, and low-dose estradiol vaginal tablets are all suggested as effective therapies for vaginal atrophy. There is no evidence to indicate any variation in safety or effectiveness between different vaginal estrogen therapy preparations (Colton Biehl, Olivia Plotsker, 2019).

Vaginal dehydroepiandrosterone (DHEA), also known as prastrone, is a therapeutic choice for dyspareunia associated with the genitourinary syndrome of menopause. Vaginal DHEA can be considered a treatment option for people with symptomatic VVA who do not experience improvement with vaginal lubricants and moisturizers and who are eligible for hormonal therapy. This approach is suitable for patients who do not have significant reasons to avoid estrogen medication but prioritize avoiding its use (Colton Biehl, Olivia Plotsker, 2019).

Ospemifene is a selective estrogen receptor modulator (SERM) that functions as an estrogen agonist, specifically in the vagina. It does not appear to have any noteworthy estrogenic effects on the endometrium or breast that are of therapeutic significance. Ospemifene has received FDA approval for addressing moderate to severe dyspareunia and/or vaginal dryness in menopausal individuals (Johnston et al., 2021).

Existing studies offer limited evidence to suggest that vaginal testosterone has the potential to activate the vaginal mucosa and alleviate symptoms associated with vaginal atrophy. Nevertheless, the FDA has not approved the use of these products in women (Colton Biehl, Olivia Plotsker, 2019).

Treatment of Sexual Dysfunctions

Addressing sexual dysfunction requires a comprehensive strategy that includes medical, psychological, and relational aspects. To streamline treatment, it is necessary to categorize the patient's issue as either desire-related, arousal-related, pain-related, or orgasm-related (Scavello et al., 2019). Postmenopausal women with hypoactive sexual desire disorder have several effective choices to consider, including pain medication, psychotherapy, and the use of transdermal testosterone (off-label) or flibanserin. Studies have demonstrated that flibanserin can enhance women's desire, but transdermal testosterone has been proven to improve desire, arousal, and the occurrence of gratifying sexual experiences while also reducing personal distress (Reed et al., 2022). According to current guidelines, testosterone therapy is recommended for postmenopausal women who have been diagnosed with hypoactive sexual desire disorder or dysfunction using internationally recognized diagnostic criteria (Scavello et al., 2019). Psychological interventions such as cognitive behavioral therapy, mindfulness-based therapy, couple therapy, and sexual therapy are effective in addressing sexual dysfunctions. Vaginal estrogens, lubricants, moisturizers, vaginal DHEAS, and ospemifene are viable options for treating vaginal atrophy associated with menopause (Journal et al., 2007; Scavello et al., 2019).

Depression Treatment

This is necessary to establish awareness of depressive symptoms, early identification, standardized diagnostic processes, tailored treatment, and a suitable follow-up program (Williams et al., 2009). The impact of estrogen therapy varies based on the specific phase of menopause. There is evidence that hormone therapy has antidepressant effects that are similar to those seen with traditional antidepressants in perimenopausal women who are depressed, with or without symptoms of vasomotor syndrome (Talaulikar, 2022). However, this is not true for women who have reached menopause, particularly those with vasomotor symptoms (VMS). Both MHT (Menopausal Hormone Therapy) and SSRIs (Selective Serotonin Reuptake Inhibitors) have been found to be effective in the treatment of mood disorders that significantly hinder the ability to perform (Maki PM, Kornstein SG, Joffe H, Bromberger JT, Freeman EW, Athappilly G, Bobo WV, Rubin LH, Koleva HK, Cohen LS, 2018). Choosing the initial treatment based on the most prominent symptom is advisable. If the primary issue is depression and the hot flashes are not severe, it is advisable to receive treatment with a selective serotonin reuptake inhibitor (SSRI). On the other hand, if the major symptom is vasomotor symptoms (VMS) and depression or mood symptoms are mild, it is recommended to undergo treatment with menopausal hormone therapy (MHT). Both medications are advised concomitantly for women experiencing severe depression and vasomotor symptoms (VMS) (Maki P. M., Kornstein S. G., Joffe H., Bromberger J. T., Freeman E. W., Athappilly G., Bobo W. V., Rubin L. H., Koleva H. K., Cohen L. S., 2018).

Conclusion

This episode delves into the intricate and diverse aspects of menopause and its impact on women's well-being. Menopause is a phase characterized by substantial physiological and psychological transformations experienced by several women. Hormonal fluctuations in the body can result in physiological manifestations such as hot flashes, sleep disturbances, vaginal dryness, and various other symptoms. In addition to the aforementioned physical alterations, menopause can also present psychological difficulties. Women at this stage may frequently encounter issues such as mood fluctuations, anxiety, and despair.

Customizing menopause treatment to suit individual requirements and personal choices is essential. Although hormonal medications can be successful for certain women, others may find lifestyle modifications, herbal remedies, or other therapies to be more suitable. It is crucial to understand that each woman's experience of menopause is distinct, and treatment methods should be tailored to the person.

It is crucial to acknowledge and address the social and cultural aspects of menopause. Societal expectations and standards can have an impact on how women perceive and express their menopausal experiences. Hence, providing menopausal education and boosting awareness could help women manage the difficulties associated with this phase.

Further investigations of different aspects of menopause with greater scrutiny can enhance the provision of improved assistance to women throughout this phase. Moreover, incorporating extensive and varied populations in studies on menopause and women's health will enable us to acquire more thorough and all-encompassing data. To adequately support women during the significant life stage of menopause, it is essential to adopt a multidisciplinary strategy that comprehends the intricate nature and effects of this process.

References

Am, M. (2016). *Short-term and long-term effects of tibolone in postmenopausal women* [Review]. https://doi.org/10.1002/14651858.CD008536.pub3.

Avis, N. E., Crawford, S. L., Greendale, G., Bromberger, J. T., Everson-Rose, S. A., Gold, E. B., Hess, R., Joffe, H., Kravitz, H. M., Tepper, P. G., & Thurston, R. C. (2015). Duration of menopausal vasomotor symptoms over the menopause transition. *JAMA Internal Medicine, 175*(4), 531–539. https://doi.org/10.1001/jamainternmed.2014.8063.

Biehl, C., Plotsker, O., & Stuenkel, C. A. (2019). A systematic review of the efficacy and safety of vaginal estrogen products for the treatment of genitourinary syndrome of menopause. *Menopause, 26*(4), 431–453. https://doi.org/10.1097/GME.0000000000001221.

Cameron, C. R., Cohen, S., Sewell, K., & Lachance, L. M. (2023). The art of hormone replacement therapy (HRT) in menopause management. *Journal of Pharmacy Practice*. https://doi.org/10.1177/08971900231167925.

Carr, M. C. (2003). The emergence of the metabolic syndrome with menopause. *Journal of Clinical Endocrinology & Metabolism, 88*(6), 2404–2411. https://doi.org/10.1210/jc.2003-030242.

Carter, A. E., & Merriam, S. (2023). Menopause. *Medical Clinics of North America, 107*(2), 199–212. https://doi.org/10.1016/j.mcna.2022.10.003.

Carvalho, V., Colonna, I., Curia, G., Ferretti, M. T., Arabia, G., Molnar, M. J., Lebedeva, E. R., Moro, E., de Visser, M., & Gaitatzis, A. (2023). Sex steroid hormones and epilepsy: Effects of hormonal replacement therapy on seizure frequency of postmenopausal women with epilepsy—A systematic review. *European Journal of Neurology, 30*(9), 2884–2898. https://doi.org/10.1111/ene.15916.

Crandall, C. J., Mehta, J. M., & Manson, J. E. (2023). Management of menopausal symptoms: A review. *JAMA, 329*(7), 405–420. https://doi.org/10.1001/jama.2022.24140.

Davis, S. R., & Brinton, R. D. (2022). Treating menopause—MHT and beyond. *Nature Reviews Endocrinology, 18*(8), 490–502. https://doi.org/10.1038/s41574-022-00685-4.

Davis, S. R., Pinkerton, J., Santoro, N., & Teten, T. (2023). Menopause—Biology, consequences, supportive care, and therapeutic options. *Cell, 186*(19), 4038–4058. https://doi.org/10.1016/j.cell.2023.08.016.

Depypere, H., Lademacher, C., Siddiqui, E., & Fraser, G. L. (2021). Fezolinetant in the treatment of vasomotor symptoms associated with menopause. *Expert Opinion on Investigational Drugs, 30*(7), 681–694. https://doi.org/10.1080/13543784.2021.1893305.

Dunneram, Y., Greenwood, D. C., & Cade, J. E. (2019). Diet, menopause, and the risk of ovarian, endometrial, and breast cancer. *Proceedings of the Nutrition Society, 78*(3), 438–448. https://doi.org/10.1017/S0029665118002884.

Evans, E. A. C., Hobson, D. T. G., Aschkenazi, S. O., Alas, A. N., Balgobin, S., Balk, E. M., Dieter, A. A., Kanter, G., Orejuela, F. J., Sanses, T. V. D., & Rahn, D. D. (2023). Nonestrogen therapies for treatment of genitourinary syndrome of menopause: A systematic review. *Obstetrics & Gynecology, 142*(1), 555–570. https://doi.org/10.1097/AOG.0000000000005288.

Flores, V. A., Pal, L., & Manson, J. E. (2021). Hormone therapy in menopause: Concepts, controversies, and approach to treatment. *Endocrine Reviews, 42*(6). https://doi.org/10.1210/endrev/bnab011.

Freeman, E. W., Sammel, M. D., Gracia, C. R., Kapoor, S., Lin, H., Liu, L., & Nelson, D. B. (2005). Follicular phase hormone levels and menstrual bleeding status in the approach to menopause. *Fertility and Sterility, 83*(2), 383–392. https://doi.org/10.1016/j.fertnstert.2004.06.066.

Geraci, A., Calvani, R., Ferri, E., Marzetti, E., Arosio, B., & Cesari, M. (2021). Sarcopenia and menopause: The role of estradiol. *Frontiers in Endocrinology, 12*, 1–5. https://doi.org/10.3389/fendo.2021.682012.

Gompel, A. (2020). Systemic lupus erythematosus and menopause. *Climacteric, 23*(2), 109–115. https://doi.org/10.1080/13697137.2019.1679113.

Hall, J. E. (2004). Neuroendocrine physiology of the early and late menopause. *Endocrinology & Metabolism Clinics of North America, 33*(4), 637–659. https://doi.org/10.1016/j.ecl.2004.08.002.

Harlow, S. D., Burnett-Bowie, S.-A. M., Greendale, G. A., Avis, N. E., Reeves, A. N., Richards, T. R., & Lewis, T. T. (2022). Disparities in reproductive aging and midlife health between Black and White women: The study of women's health across the nation (SWAN). *Women's Midlife Health, 8*(1), 1–17. https://doi.org/10.1186/s40695-022-00073-y.

Harlow, S. D., Gass, M., Hall, J. E., Lobo, R., Maki, P., Rebar, R. W., Sherman, S., Sluss, P. M., & De Villiers, T. J. (2012). Executive summary of the stages of reproductive aging workshop +10: Addressing the unfinished agenda of staging reproductive aging. *Journal of Clinical Endocrinology and Metabolism, 97*(4), 1159–1168. https://doi.org/10.1210/jc.2011-3362.

Imtiaz, B., Tuppurainen, M., Rikkonen, T., Kivipelto, M., Soininen, H., & Kröger, T. A. (2017). Postmenopausal hormone therapy and Alzheimer disease: A prospective cohort study. *Neurology, 88*(14), 1062–1088. https://doi.org/10.1212/WNL.0000000000003696.

Jayasinghe, Y. L., Wallace, W. H. B., & Anderson, R. A. (2018). Ovarian function, fertility, and reproductive lifespan in cancer patients. *Expert Review of Endocrinology & Metabolism, 13*(3), 125–136. https://doi.org/10.1080/17446651.2018.1455498.

Johnston, S., Bouchard, C., Fortier, M., & Wolfman, W. (2021). Guideline No. 422b: Menopause and genitourinary health. *Journal of Obstetrics and Gynaecology Canada, 43*(11), 1301-1307.e1. https://doi.org/10.1016/j.jogc.2021.09.001.

Kamp, E., Ashraf, M., Musbahi, E., & DeGiovanni, C. (2022). Menopause, skin, and common dermatoses. Part 1: Hair disorders. *Clinical and Experimental Dermatology, 47*(12), 2110–2116. https://doi.org/10.1111/ced.15327.

Kingsberg, S. A., Schulze-Rath, R., Mulligan, C., Moeller, C., Caetano, C., & Bitzer, J. (2023). Global view of vasomotor symptoms and sleep disturbance in menopause: A systematic review. *Climacteric, 26*(6), 537–549. https://doi.org/10.1080/13697137.2023.2256658.

Lee, E., Anselmo, M., Tahsin, C. T., Vanden Noven, M., Stokes, W., Carter, J. R., & Keller-Ross, M. L. (2022). Vasomotor symptoms of menopause, autonomic dysfunction, and cardiovascular disease. *American Journal of Physiology - Heart and Circulatory Physiology, 323*(6), H1270–H1280. https://doi.org/10.1152/ajpheart.00477.2022.

Lobo, R. A., & Greendale, G. A. (2022). Management of menopause: A view toward prevention. *The Lancet Diabetes & Endocrinology, 10*(6), 457–470. https://doi.org/10.1016/S2213-8587(21)00269-2.

Maki, P. M., Kornstein, S. G., Joffe, H., Bromberger, J. T., Freeman, E. W., Athappilly, G., Bobo, W. V., Rubin, L. H., Koleva, H. K., Cohen, L. S., & Society for the North American Menopause (NAMS). (2018). Guidelines for the evaluation and treatment of perimenopausal depression: Summary and recommendations. *Menopause, 25*(10), 1069–1085. https://doi.org/10.1097/GME.0000000000001174.

Marlatt, K. L., Pitynski-Miller, D. R., Gavin, K. M., Moreau, K. L., Melanson, E. L., Santoro, N., & Kohrt, W. M. (2022). Body composition and cardiometabolic health across the menopause transition. *Obesity, 30*(1), 14–27. https://doi.org/10.1002/oby.23289.

Massé, P. G., Pacifique, M. B., Tranchant, C. C., Arjmandi, B. H., Ericson, K. L., Donovan, S. M., Delvin, E., & Caissie, M. (2010). Bone metabolic abnormalities associated with well-controlled type 1 diabetes (IDDM) in young adult women: A disease complication often ignored or neglected. *Journal of the American College of Nutrition, 29*(4), 419–429. https://doi.org/10.1080/07315724.2010.10719859.

Nagy, M., & Dolenc, M. S. (2021). Disorders. *Clinical Obstetrics and Gynecology, 1*(1), 1–20.

Nguyen, V., Tiemann, D., Park, E., & Salehi, A. (2017). Alpha-2 agonists. *Anesthesiology Clinics, 35*(2), 233–245. https://doi.org/10.1016/j.anclin.2017.01.009.

North, T., Menopause, A., & Vol, S. (2007). The role of local vaginal estrogen for treatment of vaginal atrophy in postmenopausal women. *Menopause, 14*(3), 357–369. https://doi.org/10.1097/gme.0b013e31805170eb.

Opoku, A. A., Abushama, M., & Konje, J. C. (2023). Obesity and menopause. *Best Practice & Research Clinical Obstetrics & Gynaecology, 88*, 102348. https://doi.org/10.1016/j.bpobgyn.2023.102348.

Pillay, C. O., & Manyonda, I. (2022). The surgical menopause. *Best Practice & Research: Clinical Obstetrics & Gynaecology, 81*, 111–118. https://doi.org/10.1016/j.bpobgyn.2022.03.001.

Pocobelli, G., Newcomb, P. A., Li, C. I., Cook, L. S., & Barlow, W. E. (2014). Fatal breast cancer risk in relation to use of unopposed estrogen and combined hormone therapy. *Breast Cancer Research and Treatment, 145*(2), 439–447. https://doi.org/10.1007/s10549-014-2911-0.

Rahn, D. D., Carberry, C., Sanses, T. V., Mamik, M. M., Ward, R. M., Meriwether, K. V., Olivera, C. K., Abed, H., Balk, E. M., & Murphy, M. (2014). Vaginal estrogen for genitourinary syndrome of menopause. *Obstetrics and Gynecology, 124*(6), 1147–1156. https://doi.org/10.1097/AOG.0000000000000526.

Raina, P. M. (2024). Bazedoxifene. In *StatPearls* [Internet]. StatPearls Publishing. https://www.statpearls.com.

Randolph, J. F., Sowers, M. F., Bondarenko, I., Gold, E. B., Greendale, G. A., Bromberger, J. T., Brockwell, S. E., & Matthews, K. A. (2005). The relationship of longitudinal change in reproductive hormones and vasomotor symptoms during the menopausal transition. *Journal of Clinical Endocrinology & Metabolism, 90*(11), 6106–6112. https://doi.org/10.1210/jc.2005-1374.

Reed, S. D., Carpenter, J. S., Larson, J., Mitchell, C. M., Shifren, J., Heiman, J., Woods, N. F., Lindau, S. T., Lacroix, A. Z., & Guthrie, K. A. (2022). Toward a better measure of midlife sexual function: Pooled analyses in nearly 1,000 women participating in MsFLASH randomized trials. *Menopause, 29*(4), 397–407. https://doi.org/10.1097/GME.0000000000001940.

Scavello, I., Maseroli, E., Di Stasi, V., & Vignozzi, L. (2019). Sexual health in menopause. *Medicina (Lithuania), 55*(9). https://doi.org/10.3390/medicina55090559.

Selli, J., Unal, D., Mercantepe, F., Akaras, N., Kabayel, R., Unal, B., & Atilay, H. (2016). Protective effects of beta-glucan in brain tissues of post-menopausal rats: A histochemical and ultra-structural study. *Gynecological Endocrinology, 32*(3), 1–8. https://doi.org/10.3109/09513590.2015.1110139.

Shifren, J. L. (2019). Midlife sexuality in women's words. *Menopause, 26*(10), 1088–1089. https://doi.org/10.1097/GME.0000000000001408.

Slopien, R., Wender-Ozegowska, E., Rogowicz-Frontczak, A., Meczekalski, B., Zozulinska-Ziolkiewicz, D., Jaremek, J. D., Cano, A., Chedraui, P., Goulis, D. G., Lopes, P., Mishra, G., Mueck, A., Rees, M., Senturk, L. M., Simoncini, T., Stevenson, J. C., Stute, P., Tuomikoski, P., Paschou, S. A., … Lambrinoudaki, I. (2018). Menopause and diabetes: EMAS clinical guide. *Maturitas, 117*, 6–10. https://doi.org/10.1016/j.maturitas.2018.08.009.

Sochocka, M., Karska, J., Pszczołowska, M., Ochnik, M., Fułek, M., Fułek, K., Kurpas, D., Chojdak-Łukasiewicz, J., Rosner-Tenerowicz, A., & Leszek, J. (2023). Cognitive decline in early and premature menopause. *International Journal of Molecular Sciences, 24*(7), 1–16. https://doi.org/10.3390/ » ijms24076566.

Society, T. N. A. M. (2023). The 2023 nonhormone therapy position statement of The North American Menopause Society. *Menopause, 30*(69), 573–590. https://doi.org/10.1097/GME.0000000000002200.

Talaulikar, V. (2022). Menopause transition: Physiology and symptoms. *Best Practice & Research Clinical Obstetrics & Gynaecology, 81*, 3–7. https://doi.org/10.1016/j.bpobgyn.2022.03.003.

Vajaranant, T. S., Maki, P. M., Pasquale, L. R., Lee, A., Kim, H., & Hwang, M. (2016). Effects of hormone therapy on intraocular pressure: The Women's Health Initiative-Sight Exam Study. *American Journal of Ophthalmology, 165*, 115–124. https://doi.org/10.1016/j.ajo.2016.02.025.

Verdonk, P., Bendien, E., & Appelman, Y. (2022). Menopause and work: A narrative literature review about menopause, work, and health. *Work, 72*(2), 483–496. https://doi.org/10.3233/WOR-205214.

Voedisch, A. J., Dunsmoor-Su, R., & Kasirsky, J. (2021). Menopause: A global perspective and clinical guide for practice. *Clinical Obstetrics and Gynecology, 64*(3), 528–554. https://doi.org/10.1097/GRF.0000000000000639.

Williams, R. E., Levine, K. B., Kalilani, L., Lewis, J., & Clark, R. V. (2009). Menopause-specific questionnaire assessment in a U.S. population-based study shows negative impact on health-related quality of life. *Maturitas, 62*(2), 153–159. https://doi.org/10.1016/j.maturitas.2008.12.006.

Woods, N. F., & Mitchell, E. S. (2005). Symptoms during the perimenopause: Prevalence, severity, trajectory, and significance in women's lives. *American Journal of Medicine, 118*(12 Suppl 2), 14–24. https://doi.org/10.1016/j.amjmed.2005.09.031.

Xu, Y., Ding, J., Ma, X. P., Ma, Y. H., Liu, Z. Q., & Lin, N. (2014). Treatment with Panax ginseng antagonizes the estrogen decline in ovariectomized mice. *International Journal of Molecular Sciences, 15*(5), 7827–7840. https://doi.org/10.3390/ijms15057827.

Yenice, M. G., Danacıoğlu, Y. O., Mert, M., Karakaya, P., Seker, K. G., Akkaş, F., Şimşek, A., Şahin, S., & Taşçı, A. I. (2020). Evaluation of factors affecting sexual dysfunction in female patients with diabetes mellitus. *Archives of Endocrinology and Metabolism, 64*(3), 319–325. https://doi.org/10.20945/2359-3997000000238.

Yong, E. L., & Logan, S. (2021). SMJ-62-159. *Singapore Medical Journal, 62*(4), 156–166.

Chapter 30

Burns

Ezgi Gün Soytürk[1], MD
and Ümmühan Kiliç[2], PhD
[1]Department of Pediatric Surgery, Samsun Training and Research Hospital, Samsun, Turkey
[2]R&D and Projects Specialist, Samsun Provincial Health Directorate, Samsun, Turkey

Abstract

Burns are common traumatic injuries that cause tissue damage and can lead to serious medical and social problems. Such injuries can occur as a result of exposure to a variety of factors, and proper management is of great importance. This book chapter examines the prevalence, causes, risk factors, and management of burns by reviewing the literature and analyzing the data obtained. The study of burns helps us to understand the impact of such injuries on individuals and society. Accurate identification of the risk factors and management of burns allows the development of an effective treatment and rehabilitation strategy. A better understanding of the significance of burns can significantly improve the quality of life of those affected by such injuries through correct diagnosis and treatment.

Keywords: burns, burn incidence, burn risk factors, burn treatment, burn rehabilitation

Introduction

Burn injuries encompass tissue damage resulting from exposure to diverse stimuli such as heat, chemicals, electricity, or radiation. The severity of burns, ranging from minor medical issues to life-threatening emergencies, depends on the extent and depth of tissue involvement (Pratama and Lewa, 2022).

Burns represent a traumatic event with substantial implications at both individual and societal levels, characterized not only by physical and biological consequences but also by pronounced psychosocial effects (Liang et al., 2022). The comprehensive management of burn trauma, ranging from initial first aid interventions to long-term rehabilitation strategies, significantly influences treatment outcomes. Strategies informed by scientific and clinical insights into burns are pivotal in equipping both individuals and communities with effective coping mechanisms (Hafizurrachman et al., 2023).

In: Common Diseases According to Family Medicine Practice Guidelines
Editors: Esra Meltem Koç and Hilal Aksoy
ISBN: 979-8-89530-302-3

Incidence

The incidence of burn injuries exhibits regional, age-specific, and socioeconomic variability. Globally, pediatric populations constitute approximately half of all burn cases, with the majority falling below the age of 5 years (Brusselaers et al., 2010). The global mortality rate attributable to burns ranges from 1.3 to 1.6 per 100,000 individuals annually (Wolf et al., 2018). It is estimated that pediatric burn-related fatalities reach approximately 180,000 annually worldwide (Jordan KC et al., 2022). Enhanced survival rates among burn patients can be attributed to advancements in surgical techniques, sophisticated intensive care capabilities, and the introduction of novel antimicrobial agents (Özlü et al., 2022; Kazanasmaz and Dinç , 2019).

Causes and Risk Factors of Burns

Burn injuries of varying severity can arise from excessive exposure to various stimuli, including hot liquids and surfaces, fire, chemicals, electrical current, sunlight, and cold. The vulnerability to burns is increased among children and the elderly. Skin type constitutes a prevalent risk factor, particularly in sun-exposed settings, with individuals possessing fair and sensitive skin exhibiting increased susceptibility. Occupations involving chemical contact and elevated temperatures, inadequate fire safety measures within domestic environments, personal neglect, inadvertence, specific health conditions (such as diabetes, neuropathy, immune dysfunction, and dermatological disorders), as well as certain sporting activities, contribute to the increased risk of burn injuries. Emphasizing fundamental safety measures and exercising caution is imperative in mitigating burn risks.

Accurate assessing burn severity is crucial for effective treatment. Common methods include:

Wallace Rule of Nines: This method determines the percentage of the total body surface area affected by burns. It involves dividing the body into approximately nine distinct areas or regions and estimating the surface area of each (Moore et al., 2023). While the rule of nines (Figure 1) is more accurate for adults, a modified Lund-Browder diagram is used for children (Figure 2) (Murari and Singh, 2019).

Burn Depth: Burn depth assessment: Visual examination of the physical characteristics present on the burning surface represents the predominant method to determine burn depth, although histological and advanced imaging modalities are also available. In clinical settings, burns are classified into four categories based on depth, according to burn treatment guidelines: (Table 1) superficial (first degree), superficial partial thickness (second degree), deep partial thickness (second degree), indeterminate depth burn, and full thickness (third degree) (Jackson, 1970). The depth classification plays a crucial role in determining the treatment approach and evaluating the severity of the burn. Superficial burns exhibit minimal or no skin damage and typically heal within 3 weeks without complications. Conversely, deep burns involve partial or complete dermal damage, with a classification based on the extent of the damage to the deep tissues. These burns typically require longer than 3 weeks to heal and may necessitate surgical intervention (Karim et al., 2020).

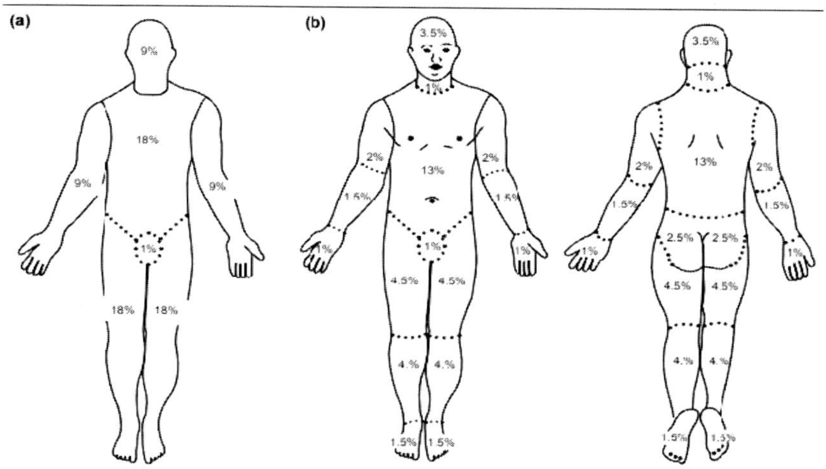

Figure 1. Yastı et al., Guideline and Treatment Algorithm for Burn Injuries. (a) The rule of nines diagram. (b) Schema for estimation of body surface area in adults.

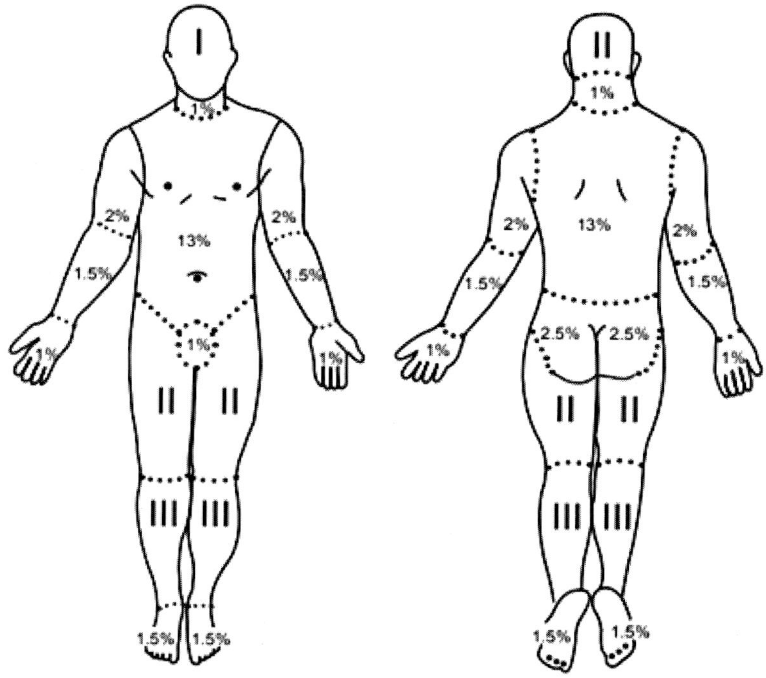

Age		0	1	5	10	15	Adult
Front or back half		(%)	(%)	(%)	(%)	(%)	(%)
I	(Head)	9½	8½	6½	5½	4½	3½
II	(Thigh)	2¾	3¼	4	4¼	4½	4¾
III	(Leg)	2½	2½	2¾	3	3¼	3½

Figure 2. Lund-Browder chart for estimating the extent of burns in children (Lund & Browder, 1994; Murari, 2017).

Table 1. Visual assessment of burn depth (Karim et al., 2020)

Visual Assessment of Burn Depth	Clinical Depth	Layer Affected	Visual Characteristics	Tactile Characteristics	Prognosis
	Superficial (First Degree)	Epidermis only	Erythema, dry	Painful	Heals within a few days
	Superficial Partial Thickness (Second Degree)	Epidermis and superficial dermis	Erythema, blisters, moist, weeping	Painful, blanchable with applied pressure	Heals within 3–15 days
	Deep Partial Thickness (Second Degree)	Epidermis and deep dermis	Erythema or pale, +/– blisters, moist or dry	Painful or anesthetic, non-blanchable with applied pressure	May heal within 2–3 weeks
	Indeterminate Depth Burn	Epidermis and deep dermis or full dermis	Erythema or pale, +/– blisters, moist or dry	Painful or anesthetic, non-blanchable with applied pressure	Healing time unknown but likely longer than 2–3 weeks
	Full Thickness (Third Degree)	Complete destruction of the epidermis and dermis in the subcutaneous layer.	Dry, leathery, white/brown/black in color	Non-painful, non-blanchable with applied pressure	Healing slowly from edges only, requires autograft for normal orderly healing

Table 2. Classification of burn severity (Yasti et al., 2015)

Minor Burns	Moderate Burns	Major Burns	
• Second degree adult burns less than 15% TBSA • Second degree child burns less than 10% TBSA • Third degree child or adult burns less than 2% TBSA.	• Second degree adult burns involving 15 to 25% TBSA • Second degree child burns involving 10 to 20% TBSA • Third degree child or adult burns involving 2 to 10% TBSA	• In adults, second degree burns greater than 25% TBSA • In children, second degree burns greater than 20% TBSA • hird degree burns greater than 10% in an adult or a child • Inhalation injury • Electrical burns	• Burns with concomitant additional trauma (such as head trauma, intra-abdominal injury, fractures) • Burns during pregnancy • Co-morbidities adding significant risk to burns (such as Diabetes Mellitus, corticosteroid use, immune suppression) • Burns of the eye, ear, face, hand, foot, major joint and genitalia.

Burn Surface Area: Calculated by multiplying the length and width of the burn area by square centimeters.

Burns can be thermal, chemical, electrical, or radiation-related. First-degree burns affect the epidermis, causing sunburn-like symptoms. Second-degree burns involve damage to the epidermal and sometimes upper dermal layers, characterized by blisters and fluid-filled lesions. Third-degree burns affect all dermal layers, resulting in hard, dark, and painless skin with necrosis. Fourth-degree burns extend to deeper tissues, requiring specialized treatment (Yasti et al., 2015). Classification of burn severity is depicted in Table 2.

Mild burns can be managed in outpatient settings or burn units, while moderate to severe burns require hospitalization for specialized care.

Medical Intervention for Burn Patients

Burn injuries are significant traumas where the primary concern, similar to any trauma, is the assessment of the airway, breathing, and circulation. In the cases of multiple traumas, prioritizing life-threatening injuries is crucial, following the principle of addressing immediate threats before focusing on burns. The information presented in this section is based on burn treatment guidelines established by the International Society for Burn Injuries in collaboration with the World Health Organization, as well as the Burn Injuries Treatment Algorithm endorsed by the Turkish Ministry of Health (WHO, 2023; ISBI Practice Guidelines for Burn Care, 2016; Smolle et al., 2016; Yasti, 2015).

Interventions to be implemented at the scene include safe evacuation of the victim from the site of the fire and the cessation of the fire itself. For minor burns, immediate application of cold running water to the burn area for 15-20 minutes is recommended. In cases of scald injuries, removing all damp clothing is advised. In instances of electrical burns, deactivating the power source and moving the patient to a secure environment is essential. The necessity of cardiopulmonary resuscitation must be promptly assessed. In situations involving chemical burns, the initial step involves the removal of dry chemicals, followed by thorough irrigation with running water. The use of neutralizing agents is not recommended. In the event of substantial burns, establishing intravenous access and administering lactate Ringer solution for fluid resuscitation within the first 24 hours are crucial. Considering the anticipated edema, removal of jewelry is advised. Burn injuries should not be covered with medication or substances but should be dressed with a clean cloth and transported to the nearest emergency department. If available, medical coolants can be applied to the affected area. Areas of the body unaffected by burns should be shielded to maintain body temperature.

Following the initial medical intervention for burn patients, pertinent information including the patient's demographic details (age, gender), injury specifics (cause, location, time), burn severity (extent, depth), associated injuries, comorbidities, overall health status, and administered medical interventions should be conveyed to the receiving medical facility prior to transfer.

The emergency department management of burn patients is summarized as follows:

1. *The assessment of airway and breathing:* Airway patency must be ensured, respiratory support should be provided to patients with respiratory distress, and endotracheal

intubation should be performed promptly when necessary, with the patient placed on ventilator support. Assessment of inhalation burns is crucial.

2. *The assessment of circulation and establishment of intravenous access:* Peripheral venous access should be quickly established, considering central catheterization in extensive burns. In children with large burns requiring close monitoring, central catheterization is preferred. In children under 6 years old, if peripheral venous access fails after two attempts, intraosseous access should be utilized promptly. Using a 16-18 G needle (or spinal needle) under local anesthesia, systemic fluids can be administered into the bone marrow at a rate of over 100 mL/hour from the distal femur or proximal tibia (care should be taken to avoid growth plate damage). Due to the risk of systemic hypothermia development, the temperature of administered fluids should be close to the body temperature.
3. *The assessment of associated injuries:* Identification and appropriate management of associated injuries are crucial. In patients with multiple traumas and burns, the section related to life-threatening injuries should follow up on the patient.
4. *The evaluation of body surface area:* Assessing the patient's body surface area is fundamental for fluid resuscitation. While the "Rule of Nines" may be used for adults, the Lund and Browder charts are more suitable for children.
   *Estimating body surface area in children: Body surface (m2) = [4 x body weight (kg) + 7]/[90 + body weight (kg)].
5. *Forensic examination:* Each burn case should be evaluated forensically, and in suspicious cases, the police or forensic institution should be notified.
6. *Wound care:* Wounds should be covered with a clean dressing during the pre-hospital period. In extensive burns, edema is expected, so jewelry should be removed. Silver sulfadiazine may be an option for wound care (except for the face).
7. *Fluid resuscitation:* Intravenous fluid resuscitation should be initiated if the burn body surface area is over 10% in children or over 20% in adults. The fluid regimen in burn treatment requires adjustments based on the clinical condition.

For adults in the first 24 hours: Parkland Formula: 4 mL/kg of lactated Ringer's solution per % of the total body surface area burned Modified Brooke Formula: 2 mL/kg per % total body surface area burned
For children in the first 24 hours: Galveston Formula: 2000 mL/m² of body surface area + 5000 mL/m² per % of the total body surface area burned, lactated Ringer's solution
Half of the calculated amount is administered within the first eight hours, and the remaining half is given over the next 16 hours.

The presence of associated additional trauma, alcohol intake, inhalation injury, delayed onset or inadequate fluid resuscitation, dehydration, and electrical burns, among other conditions, can necessitate administering more fluid than calculated.

In cases of extensive burns and/or perineal burns requiring close monitoring, a urinary catheterization should be performed. The targeted urinary output in adults is 30-50 mL per hour, while in children, it is 1-2 mL/kg per hour. The targeted urine specific gravity is 1.015. In electrical burns and inhalation injuries, the targeted urinary output should be double the mentioned amount.

The use of topical creams or ointments containing local anesthetics to relieve pain is not recommended. The patient's pain will subside after the wound has been dressed.

Chemical burns can occur in the form of acid and alkali burns, with alkali burns having the ability to progress into deeper tissues through liquefaction necrosis. The burning continues as long as the active substance remains in contact with the skin. After the patient has been completely removed, they should shower with water at body temperature, but should not be in a bathtub to avoid prolonged exposure that can lead to hypothermia. Patients with electrical burns, chemical burns, and large and/or deep burns should be hospitalized. Serum electrolytes and arterial blood gas should be monitored, and EKG monitoring should be performed as needed. In high-voltage electrical burns, intravenous (IV) fluids should be administered until the urine clears and becomes alkaline. In cases of edema and/or eschar formation, escharotomy or fasciotomy of the chest, abdomen, limbs, and neck should be considered. Unconscious patients and/or patients with burned TBSA > 30% are at risk of gastro-paralysis and ileus, and nasogastric decompression should be performed as needed.

In patients with moderate or large burns and those with high-risk accompanying illnesses and/or injuries, basic blood and urine tests should be performed (crossmatching, Rh testing, serum electrolytes, blood glucose, complete blood count, myoglobinuria/hemoglobinuria at minimum). Patients with large burns receive prophylaxis according to general tetanus prophylaxis protocols.

Patients Requiring Hospitalization (Yastı et al., 2015):

- All ages, TBSA >%20, second and third degree burns
- All ages, TBSA ≥%5-10, third degree burns
- Patients younger than 10 or older than 50 years, TBSA ≥%10, second and third degree burns
- Burns to the face, ears, hands, and feet
- Burns involving major joints
- Genital and perineal burns
- Chemical burns
- Electrical burns
- Lightning strikes
- Respiratory injuries
- Associated multiple traumas
- Chronic comorbidities (diabetes, hypertension, cardiac pathologies, immune deficiency, neurological disorders)
- Pregnancy
- Presence or suspicion of child abuse

Treatment Options, New Research, and Developments in Burn Care

In burn care, various treatment options are available depending on whether the patient is managed as an outpatient or hospitalized. Initially, cleansing the wound and removing debris is of paramount importance; therefore, wounds are cleansed by washing with warm tap water or saline at room temperature, followed by dressing application. However, non-neutral pH antiseptic solutions and brushes should not be used during this process (Canadian Association of Wound Care, 2021). The risk of infection is a major concern in burn care, and minimizing this risk is crucial. Sterile wound care, debridement, and topical antimicrobial agents should be meticulously addressed as appropriate prevention and treatment methods. In addition to traditional methods, alternatives such as silver sulfadiazine, mafenide acetate, and silver nanoparticles play a significant role in antimicrobial efficacy in burn treatment (Slaviero et al., 2018).

In minor burns, the use of topical antimicrobial creams or ointments is not mandatory, and pain during dressing changes can be reduced by using paraffin-impregnated dressings. Polyurethane film layers may be preferred in cosmetically visible areas. If these materials are not available, dressings with paraffin or oily ointments (e.g., 0.2% Nitrofurazone ointment) are suitable. The dressing materials should be separate and single-use for each patient. In the presence of infection or eschar, 1% silver sulfadiazine is used in extensive burns. Due to its potential to delay wound healing, the use of silver preparations should be discontinued once epithelialization is observed. Small, controlled blisters can be left intact, while large blisters need to be drained or removed for dressing follow-up (Cambiaso-Daniel et al., 2019).

During outpatient treatment of burn wounds, signs of infection should be carefully monitored; any signs such as redness, swelling, pain, pus, or fever should prompt immediate medical attention. The strict adherence to hygiene rules is essential, with hands kept constantly clean, and hygienic measures carefully applied during wound care. Infection of burn wounds can lead to serious complications; therefore, appropriate prevention and treatment methods are of paramount importance. Delayed wound healing exceeding three weeks can lead to discoloration, hypertrophic scarring, keloid formation, and/or contracture development, necessitating prompt referral of patients to burn units/centers (Yasti, 2015).

The Common Topical Antimicrobial Agents

1. Silver-based agents

The antimicrobial properties of silver have been recognized for centuries, and there are many silver-based products used in situations with infection risk such as burn wounds. Silver ions (Ag^+) are highly effective against bacteria, yeasts, and fungi at low concentrations, disrupting the survival capabilities of microorganisms and causing their death (Landsdown A, 2002). Silver can exist in different oxidation states, such as Ag^+, Ag^{++}, and Ag^{+++}, which provide different mechanisms of action against microorganisms. These mechanisms include enzyme inhibition, damage to cell membranes or cell walls, and inhibition of DNA and RNA replication (Marx & Barillo, 2014) (Fong & Woods F, 2006).

Silver-based products are used in the treatment of wound infections such as burn wounds and come in forms such as silver sulfite, silver sulfadiazine, and silver nitrate. They are commonly used for wound cleansing and bacterial control, accelerating the healing process.

However, ionic silver may delay the healing of second-degree burns by adversely affecting keratinocytes and fibroblasts, so this potential slowing effect should be considered before using silver-based agents (Cartotto, 2017).

1a. Silver Nitrate: A 0.5% silver nitrate (AgNO3) solution is used as a topical antimicrobial agent for wounds. However, AgNO3 can easily precipitate free silver ions, rendering the silver ineffective (Paddock et al., 2007).

1b. Silver Sulfadiazine (SSD): SSD is a topical antimicrobial cream commonly used for burns. It is effective due to the continuous release and accumulation of silver ions, but it has cytotoxic effects on keratinocytes and fibroblasts (Robert Cartotto, 2017).

1c. Silver-Impregnated Dressings: There are various silver-impregnated dressings available, such as nanocrystalline dressings, hydrocolloid and hydrofiber silver dressings, and silver dressings containing activated charcoal. These dressings provide continuous release of silver ions and may require fewer painful dressing changes (Brown et al., 2016; Malic et al., 2014).

2. Mafenide Acetate

Mafenide acetate is a sulfonamide antibiotic used for deep burns. It is effective against bacteria but does not show antifungal activity and can cause skin irritation (Cartotto, 2017).

3. Antibiotic Ointments

Antibiotic ointments such as Bacitracin, Polymyxin B sulfate, Neomycin, and Mupirocin are used to treat burn wounds and generally provide a moist wound environment. After applying a thick layer of one of these ointments, the wound is covered with a non-adherent dressing (e.g., paraffin gauze, Xeroform®, or Adaptic®), followed by a bulky gauze dressing (Cartotto, 2017).

4. Antiseptic Solutions.

The use of hypochlorous solutions (Dakin's solution), acetic acid, chlorhexidine, and cerium nitrate is available (Scholten-Jaegers et al., 2017; Barsoumian et al., 2013; Halstead et al., 2015; Peterson et al., 1990).

Burn Debridement

Debridement plays a critical role in the burn treatment process, involving the removal of dead tissue, eschar, and foreign materials from the burn wound. This function of debridement can expedite the healing process, reduce the risk of infection, and support tissue regeneration (Novak et al., 2022). Debridement is performed through various methods:

1. *Physical Debridement:* Dead tissue and eschar are physically removed using surgical instruments or various medical devices (Butts et al., 2020).
2. *Mechanical Debridement:* Dead tissue and foreign objects are cleared from the wound area using pressurized water or specialized devices (Butts et al., 2020).
3. *Enzymatic Debridement:* Products such as gels or creams containing specific enzymes are used to dissolve dead tissue and eschar (Singer, 2010; Hirche et al., 2020).

4. *Bioactive Debridement:* A special gel or tissue applied to the wound area contains natural components and helps remove dead tissue and foreign objects, supporting healing (Fernández-Guarino et al., 2023).
5. *Larval Debridement:* Sterile fly larvae are placed in the wound area; these larvae feed on dead tissue and clean the wound surface (Gaffari, 2023).

Debridement is typically performed by surgeons, wound care specialists, or plastic surgery specialists. The appropriate debridement method is selected based on the severity and type of burn. Proper cleansing and care of burn wounds can expedite the healing process and minimize scarring. Therefore, debridement plays a vital role in effectively treating burns.

Graft Applications in Burn Wound Treatment

The management of burn injuries necessitates surgical graft procedures designed to address substantial tissue loss and expedite the healing process. Grafting emerges as a pivotal area within the tissue engineering and surgical disciplines, offering efficacious strategies for reconstructing burn wounds. Burn wound grafts are broadly categorized into autografts (tissue sourced from the patient's own skin) and allografts (tissue obtained from a donor individual). Moreover, grafting is one of the predominant and efficacious modalities to address tissue loss (Wang et al., 2020).

The application of grafts in burn wounds typically encompasses the following methodologies to address tissue deficits:

1. *Full-Thickness Autografts:* This technique involves the direct placement of a full-thickness skin segment harvested from the burn area on the wound bed. Primarily used in the management of deep burns, this approach encompasses the entirety of the skin layer and facilitates more enduring outcomes (Keenan et al., 2023).
2. *Split-Thickness Autografts:* In this approach, a portion of the upper skin layer (epidermis) and a segment of the underlying layer (dermis) are harvested and utilized. These grafts find extensive application in the treatment of superficial burns (Leon et al., 2023).
3. *Mesh Grafts:* Mesh grafts are made by cutting and stretching the harvested skin segment at specific intervals. This method is instrumental in covering larger wound areas with a smaller graft size, leading to expedited healing times (Dahmardehei et al., 2020).
4. *Allografts:* Allografts entail the use of skin grafts obtained from a donor individual. Designed as a rapid intervention in extensive burn wounds, these grafts serve as a temporary measure, particularly preferred in cases where the patient lacks adequate autologous tissue for grafting (Hermans, 2014).

The selection of grafts to address tissue loss in burn injuries relies on factors such as patient suitability, burn severity, and the extent of tissue replacement needed. Surgical specialists and plastic surgeons perform graft applications, which are pivotal in facilitating the patient's healing process.

Progress in tissue engineering has led to the development of skin substitutes that aid wound healing. These substitutes, comprising synthetic and biological dermal matrices, address the challenge of limited availability of autologous skin grafts to treat extensive burn injuries (Concannon, 2023). While promoting skin regeneration and restoring primary skin functions, these substitutes may exhibit mechanical fragility and lack durability. Skin substitutes are categorized by their composition, including amnion, cultured epithelial autografts, acellular allografts, cellular allografts, xenografts, composites, and synthetics (Davis et al., 2023). Innovative techniques such as 3D tissue printing aim to create more complex skin substitutes for clinical use (Fu et al., 2023). Additionally, utilizing tissue-engineered skin substitutes enriched with stem cells shows promise in expediting wound healing and improving recovery outcomes (Kumar, 2023). Overall, advancements in tissue engineering have expanded the range of options for wound treatment and offer potential for further advancements in skin tissue biomaterials through the integration of nanotechnology.

Management of Burn Scars

The formation of scars as a result of burn wound healing can present both aesthetic and functional challenges. Recent advancements in scar treatment and management have introduced novel techniques and products. These encompass laser therapies, corrective surgical procedures for scars, and advanced technological solutions for scar treatment. The approach to scar treatment is tailored to each individual, taking into account their specific characteristics and the severity of the burn injury (Obaidi et al., 2023).

Pain Management

Burn injuries commonly elicit intense pain, making effective pain management a pivotal aspect of burn care. Recent efforts have focused on enhancing pain control through the integration of non-pharmacological interventions, such as virtual reality therapy and meditation, alongside pharmacological treatments (Kilic et al., 2024).

Pharmacological management of burn pain often involves the use of opioids in severe cases, although their potential for addiction necessitates caution. Non-opioid analgesics are generally preferred for managing mild to moderate pain. Additionally, topical analgesics administered directly to the wound site and adjuvant medications targeting neuropathic pain are viable treatment options. Local anesthetics such as Anestol are not recommended for pediatric burn patients due to the risk of methemoglobinemia. Non-pharmacological approaches, including cold therapy, cognitive-behavioral therapy, and physical rehabilitation techniques, have proven to be effective in alleviating burn pain and facilitating the healing process. These comprehensive strategies are used to promote both physical and psychological recovery in individuals with burn injuries (Romanovski et al., 2020).

Complications and Long-Term Effects of Burns

Burn injuries, initially associated with an elevated risk of infection due to a compromised skin barrier, can have significant health implications over time. During the reparative phase of deep tissue damage, the development of scar tissue and contractures can profoundly impact the patient's mobility and overall aesthetic appearance. Burns, especially those affecting the face, neck, and chest regions, can induce respiratory challenges, psychological distress, and enduring metabolic perturbations (Zang, 2023). Furthermore, deep burns often necessitate recurrent surgical interventions, while extensive burns can precipitate profound blood loss and complications such as anemia. Concurrently, the loss of protein during therapeutic interventions can exacerbate hypoalbuminemia and bodily edema, thereby complicating the recovery process. Addressing these complications requires a multidisciplinary therapeutic approach, aimed not only at mitigating adverse outcomes but also at augmenting the patient's health status and quality of life (Li, 2023).

Prevention Strategies

The primary prevention strategies center around the regulation of hot water and ensuring child safety. It is imperative to adjust the temperature of hot water, particularly during bathing and showering for children and the elderly, ensuring that it does not exceed 49°C. Essential measures include restricting children's access to flammable materials, safeguarding hot surfaces, and preventing children from engaging in fire-related activities (Hicks & Komar, 2023).

Moreover, practicing careful cooking methods to prevent hot pots and pans from overflowing and positioning large pots used on stovetops in safer locations are crucial. Vigilance is necessary in smoking-permitted areas, especially considering the risk of children being affected by forgotten cigarettes while asleep in bed or on furniture.

Routine maintenance of electrical appliances is essential to prevent overheating, and they should be used correctly. Lighters and matches should be stored out of children's reach. When exposed to the sun for extended periods, appropriate sunscreen with adequate sun protection factor (SPF) and protective clothing should be used. Caution should be exercised when serving hot beverages to children, and cooling accelerators should be used. Hazardous substances such as household chemical cleaning products must be stored safely away from children. Organizing educational programs aimed at both children and adults to raise awareness of burn risks and promote safe behaviors is paramount (Burgess & Jacqueline, 2019).

These strategies are applicable for burn prevention and establishing a safe environment. Enhancing awareness among individuals regarding burn prevention can lead to a notable reduction in burn occurrences.

Rehabilitation and Recovery

Physical therapy and rehabilitation play a pivotal role in the prevention and management of physical complications arising from burns, particularly contractures. These interventions focus on preserving range of motion, rebuilding muscle strength, and enhancing functional independence. Post-burn psychosocial support is essential to address the emotional distress experienced by both patients and their families, aiding in the management of depression, anxiety, and stress. Furthermore, burns can lead to increased metabolic demands and physiological strain, underscoring the critical importance of proper nutrition and sufficient fluid intake.

The management of burn scars encompasses aesthetic surgical procedures and laser treatments designed to mitigate the prominence of long-term scarring. Active participation in long-term monitoring and rehabilitation programs is vital to the early detection and management of potential complications, thereby promoting optimal recovery and successful reintegration into daily life. This multidisciplinary approach underscores the collaborative efforts among healthcare professionals to ensure comprehensive burn treatment and rehabilitation (Daniel et al., 2018).

Conclusion

This chapter provides crucial information on the treatment, rehabilitation, and prevention of burn injuries. By offering guidance to both burn survivors and healthcare practitioners, this information aims to contribute to the reduction of future burn occurrences by fostering burn awareness within the community. With a shared commitment to building a knowledgeable, compassionate, and empathetic society in combating burn injuries, we extend our wishes for continued health and safety.

References

Barsoumian, A., Sanchez, C. J., Mende, K., Tully, C. C., Beckius, M. L., & Akers, K. S., et al., (2013). In vitro toxicity and activity of Dakin's solution, mafenide acetate, and amphotericin B on filamentous fungi and human cells. *Journal of Orthopaedic Trauma, 27*(8), 428–436.

Brown, M., Dalziel, S. R., Herd, E., Johnson, K., Wong, S. R., & Shepherd, M. (2016). A randomized controlled study of silver-based burns dressing in a pediatric emergency department. *Journal of Burn Care & Research, 37*, e340–e347.

Brusselaers, N., Monstrey, S., Vogelaers, D., Hoste, E., & Blot, S. (2010). Severe burn injury in Europe: A systematic review of the incidence, etiology, morbidity, and mortality. *Critical Care, 14*(5), R188. https://doi.org/10.1186/cc9300.

Burgess, J. (2019). *Prevention of paediatric hot beverage scalds* (PhD Thesis). Faculty of Medicine, The University of Queensland. https://doi.org/10.14264/uql.2019.182.

Butts, C. C., Holmes, J. H., & Carter, J. E. (2020). Surgical escharotomy and decompressive therapies in burns. *Journal of Burn Care & Research, 41*(2), 263–269. https://doi.org/10.1093/jbcr/irz152.

Cambiaso-Daniel, J., Boukovalas, S., Bitz, G. H., Branski, L. K., Herndon, D. N., & Culnan, D. M. (2019). Topical antimicrobials in burn care: Part I – Topical antiseptics. *Annals of Plastic Surgery*, PMC. https://doi.org/10.1097/SAP.0000000000001297.

Canadian Association of Wound Care. (2021). *Best practice recommendations for the prevention and management of burns*. Retrieved from https://www.woundscanada.ca.

Concannon, E., Damkat-Thomas, L., Coghlan, P., & Greenwood, J. E. (2023). Wound healing - Recent advances and future opportunities. In Puri, P., & Höllwarth, M. E. (Eds.), *Pediatric Surgery* (pp. 1–16). Springer. https://doi.org/10.5772/intechopen.105179.

Dahmardehei, M., Vaghardoost, R., Saboury, M., Zarei, H., Saboury, S., Molaei, M., Seyyedi, J., & Maleknejad, A. (2020). Comparison of modified Meek technique with standard mesh method in patients with third-degree burns. *World Journal of Plastic Surgery, 9*(3), 267–273. https://doi.org/10.29252/wjps.9.3.267.

Daniel, J. C., Suman, O. E., Jaco, M., & Benjamin, D. A., Herndon, D. N. (2018). Teamwork for total burn care: Burn centers and multidisciplinary burn teams. In *Total Burn Care* (5th ed., pp. 8-13.e1). Elsevier. https://doi.org/10.1016/B978-0-323-47661-4.00002-2.

Davis, M., Dugan, K., Neill, B. C., et al., (2023). The role of skin substitutes in dermatologic surgery: A practical review. *Journal of Drugs in Dermatology, 22*(5), 475–480. https://doi.org/10.36849/JDD.7132.

Fernández-Guarino, M., Bacci, S., González, L. A. P., Bermejo-Martínez, M., & Cecilia-Matilla, A. (2023). The role of physical therapies in wound healing and assisted scarring. *International Journal of Molecular Sciences, 24*, 7487. https://doi.org/10.3390/ijms24087487.

Fong, J., & Woods, F. (2006). Nanocrystalline silver dressings in wound management: A review. *International Journal of Nanomedicine, 1*(4), 441–449.

Fu, H., Zhang, D., & Zeng, J. (2023). Application of 3D-printed tissue-engineered skin substitute using innovative biomaterial loaded with human adipose-derived stem cells in wound healing. *International Journal of Bioprinting, 9*(2), 674. https://doi.org/10.18063/ijb.v9i2.674.

Gaffari, J., Akbarzadeh, K., Baniardalani, M., Hosseini, R., Masoumi, S., Amiri, Z. S., Kordshouli, R. S., Rafinejad, J., & Dahmardehei, M. (2023). Larval therapy vs conventional silver dressings for full-thickness burns: A randomized controlled trial. *BMC Medicine, 21*(1), 361. https://doi.org/10.1186/s12916-023-03063-7.

Hafizurrachman, M., Menna, C., & Lesmana, E. (2023). Review of traditional first aid for burn injuries in the 21st century. *Annals of Plastic Surgery, 91*(3), 337-347. https://doi.org/10.1097/SAP.0000000000003584.

Halstead, F. D., Rauf, M., Moiemen, N. S., Bamford, A., Wearn, C. M., & Fraise, A. P. (2015). The antibacterial activity of acetic acid against biofilm-producing pathogens of relevance to burns patients. *PLoS One.* https://doi.org/10.1371/journal.pone.0136190.

Hermans, M. H. E. (2014). Porcine xenografts vs. (cryopreserved) allografts in the management of partial thickness burns: Is there a clinical difference? *Burns, 40*(3), 408–415. https://doi.org/10.1016/j.burns.2013.08.020.

Hicks, A., & Komar, L. (2023). Too hot! Preventing, recognizing and managing heat injury in children. *Paediatrics & Child Health, 28*(2), 72–74. https://doi.org/10.1093/pch/pxac092.

Hirche, C., Almeland, S. K., Dheansa, B., Fuchs, P., Governa, M., Hoeksema, H., Korzeniowski, T., Lumenta, D. B., Marinescu, S., Martinez-Mendez, J. R., Plock, J. A., Sander, F., Ziegler, B., & Kneser, U. (2020). Eschar removal by bromelain-based enzymatic debridement (Nexobrid®) in burns: European consensus guidelines update. *Burns, 46*(4), 782–796. https://doi.org/10.1016/j.burns.2020.03.002.

ISBI Practice Guidelines Committee. (2016). ISBI practice guidelines for burn care. *Burns, 42*(5), 953–1021. https://doi.org/10.1016/j.burns.2016.05.013.

Jackson, D. M. (1970). A historical review of the use of local physical signs in burns. *British Journal of Plastic Surgery, 23*(3), 211–218.

Jackson, D. M. (1970). In search of an acceptable burn classification. *British Journal of Plastic Surgery, 23*(3), 219–226.

Jordan, K. C., Di Gennaro, J. L., von Saint André-von Arnim, A., & Stewart, B. T. (2022). Global trends in pediatric burn injuries and care capacity from the World Health Organization Global Burn Registry. *Frontiers in Pediatrics, 10*, 954995. https://doi.org/10.3389/fped.2022.954995.

Karim, A. S., Shaum, K., & Gibson, A. L. F. (2020). Indeterminate depth burn injury: Exploring the uncertainty. *Journal of Surgical Research, 245*, 183–197. https://doi.org/10.1016/j.jss.2019.07.063.

Kazanasmaz, Ö., & Dinç, N. (2019). Yanık ünitesinde takip edilen pediatrik yaş grubu olguların klinik değerlendirmesi [Clinical evaluation of pediatric cases followed in the burn unit]. *Harran Üniversitesi Tıp Fakültesi Dergisi, 16*(3), 535-539.

Keenan, C. S., Cooper, L., Nuutila, K., Chapa, J., Christy, S., Chan, R. K., & Carlsson, A. H. (2023). Full-thickness skin columns: A method to reduce healing time and donor site morbidity in deep partial-thickness burns. *Wound Repair and Regeneration, 31*(5), 586–596. https://doi.org/10.1111/wrr.13114.

Kilic, Ü., Tural, E. B., Oruc, M. A., & Avci, İ. A. (2024). The effect of VR headsets used during burn dressing in children on satisfaction and anxiety level of their parents. *Journal of Pediatric Nursing*. https://doi.org/10.1016/j.pedn.2024.01.006.

Kumar, V. S., Diksha, A. D., & Kumar, V. R. (2023). Recent advancements in skin tissue engineering in the application of nanotechnology. *Research Journal of Biotechnology, 18*(2), 127–136. https://doi.org/10.25303/1802rjbt1270136.

Lansdown, A. (2002). Silver 1: Its antibacterial properties and mechanism of action. *Journal of Wound Care, 11*, 125–133.

Leon, J. L. A., Rivero, C. R., Guerrero, L., Alviar, J. D., Rodríguez, M. A., Arocha, A. M., & Pineda, G. G. (2023). Immediate results of the use of split-thickness skin autografts with and without acellular dermal matrix in patients with burns: A comparative study in a Colombian population. *Journal of Burn Care & Research*. https://doi.org/10.1093/jbcr/irad131.

Li, X. J., & Tang, W. B. (2023). Pay attention to persistent inflammation-immunosuppression-catabolism syndrome in the late stage of severe burns. *Zhonghua Shao Shang Za Zhi, 39*(5), 407–410. https://doi.org/10.3760/cma.j.cn501225-20230131-00030.

Liang, J., Li, R., Wang, C., Zhang, R., Yue, K., Li, W., & Li, Y. (2022). A spiking neural network based on retinal ganglion cells for automatic burn image segmentation. *Entropy, 24*, 1526. https://doi.org/10.3390/e24111526.

Lund, C. C., & Browder, N. C. (1994). The estimation of areas of burns. *Surgery, Gynecology & Obstetrics, 79*, 352–358.

Malic, C., Verchere, C., & Arneja, S. N. (2014). Inpatient silver sulphadiazine versus outpatient nanocrystalline silver models of care for pediatric scald burns: A value analysis. *Plastic Surgery, 22*(2), 99–102.

Marx, D. E., & Barillo, D. J. (2014). Silver in medicine: The basic science. *Burns, 40*(S), S9–S18.

Miller, L. M., Loder, J. S., Hansborough, J. F., Peterson, H. D., Monafo, W. W., & Jordan, M. H. (1990). Patient tolerance of topical chlorhexidine diphosphanilate: A new topical agent for burns. *Burns, 16*(3), 217–220.

Moore, R. A., Waheed, A., & Burns, B. (2022). Rules of nines. In *StatPearls* [Internet]. StatPearls Publishing.

Murari, A. (2017). A modified Lund and Browder chart. *Indian Journal of Plastic Surgery, 50*(2), 220–221. https://doi.org/10.4103/ijps.IJPS_77_17.

Murari, A., & Singh, K. N. (2019). Lund and Browder chart-modified versus original: A comparative study. *Acute Critical Care, 34*(4), 276-281. https://doi.org/10.4266/acc.2019.00647.

Nowak, M., Mehrholz, D., Barańska-Rybak, W., & Nowicki, R. J. (2022). Wound debridement products and techniques: Clinical examples and literature review. *Advances in Dermatology and Allergology, 39*(3), 479–490. https://doi.org/10.5114/ada.2022.117572.

Obaidi, N., Keenan, C., & Chan, R. K. (2023). Burn scar management and reconstructive surgery. *Surgical Clinics of North America, 103*(3), 515–527. https://doi.org/10.1016/j.suc.2023.01.012.

Özlü, Ö., & Başaran, A. (2022). Majör yanığı olan çocuk hastalarda yanıkla ilişkili enfeksiyonlar [Burn-related infections in pediatric patients with major burns]. *J Pediatr Emerg Intensive Care Med, 9*(1), 31-36.

Paddock, H. N., Fabia, R., Giles, S., Hayes, J., Lowell, W., & Besner, G. E. (2007). A silver impregnated antimicrobial dressing reduces hospital length of stay for pediatric patients with burns. *Journal of Burn Care & Research, 28*, 409–411.

Pratama, A. M. O., & Lewa, A. (2022). The protective role of strong antioxidant astaxanthin on burn wound and burn-induced early acute kidney injury through abilities to relieve oxidative stress and inhibit apoptosis by modulating mitochondrial apoptotic pathways. *International Journal of Medical Science and Clinical Research Studies, 12*(2), 1591-1595. https://doi.org/10.47191/ijmscrs/v2-i12-37.

Rogers, A. D., & Rode, H. (2023). Burns. In *Pediatric Surgery*. Springer. https://doi.org/10.1007/978-3-030-81488-5_24.

Romanowski, K. S., Carson, J., Pape, K., Bernal, E., Sharar, S., Wiechman, S., Carter, D., Liu, Y. M., Nitzschke, S., Bahalla, P., Litt, J., Przkora, R., Friedman, B., Popiak, S., Jeng, J., Ryan, C. M., & Joe, V. (2020). American Burn Association guidelines on the management of acute pain in the adult burn patient: A review of the literature, a compilation of expert opinion, and next steps. *Journal of Burn Care & Research, 41*(6), 1129–1151. https://doi.org/10.1093/jbcr/iraa119.

Scholten-Jaegers, S. M. H. J., Niewenhuis, M. K., van Baar, M. E., Niemeijer, A. S., Hiddingh, J., & Beerthuizen, G. I. J. M. (2017). Epidemiology and outcome of patients with burns treated with cerium nitrate silversulfadiazine. *Journal of Burn Care & Research, 38*, e432–e442.

Singer, A. J., Taira, B. R., Anderson, R., McClain, S. A., & Rosenberg, L. (2010). The effects of rapid enzymatic debridement of deep partial-thickness burns with Debrase on wound reepithelialization in swine. *Journal of Burn Care & Research, 31*(5), 795–802. https://doi.org/10.1097/BCR.0b013e3181eed48e.

Slaviero, L., Avruscio, G., Vindigni, V., & Tocco-Tusardi, I. (2018). Antiseptics for burns: A review of the evidence. *Annals of Burns and Fire Disasters, 31*(3), 198–203.

Smolle, C., Janos Cambiaso-Daniel, Abigail A Forbes, Paul Wurzer et al., (2016). Recent trends in burn epidemiology worldwide: A systematic review. *Burns*. https://doi.org/10.1016/j.burns.2016.08.013.

Wang, C., Zhang, F., & Lineaweaver, W. C. (2020). Clinical applications of allograft skin in burn care. *Annals of Plastic Surgery, 84*(3S Suppl 2), S158–S160. https://doi.org/10.1097/SAP.0000000000002282.

Wolf, S. E., Cancio, L. C., & Pruitt, B. A. (2018). Epidemiological, demographic, and outcome characteristics of burns. In *Total Burn Care: Fifth Edition* (pp. 14-27.e2). Elsevier Inc. https://doi.org/10.1016/B978-0-323-47661-4.00003-4.

World Health Organization. (n.d.). Burns. Retrieved from https://www.who.int/news-room/fact-sheets/detail/burns.

Yastı, A. Ç., Şenel, E., Saydam, M., Özok, G., Çoruh, A., & Yorgancı, K. (2015). Guideline and treatment algorithm for burn injuries. *Ulus Travma Acil Cerrahi Derg, 21*(2), 95-107.

Zhang, W., Zhang, W. D., Chen, L., Luan, X. G., Yang, F., Li, Z., Liu, F., & Wang, D. Y. (2023). Clinical effects of expanded flaps in reconstructing scar contracture deformities in the face and neck after extensive burns. *Zhonghua Shao Shang Za Zhi, 39*(9), 826–834. https://doi.org/10.3760/cma.j.cn501225-20230706-00248.

Chapter 31

Pressure Ulcers

Demet Kelleci Demir*, MD, PhD
Department of Family Medicine, Çamoluk District State Hospital, Giresun, Turkey

Abstract

Pressure ulcers are one of the most common adverse events in hospitalized patients worldwide. It prolongs hospital stays, increases medical expenses, reduces the quality of life, and causes nosocomial infections, disability, morbidity, and mortality. The risk factors for the formation of pressure ulcers are divided into two main groups: extrinsic risk factors and internal risk factors. Extrinsic risk factors can be listed as pressure, friction, tear, and moisture. Internal risk factors can be listed as nutritional deficiency, advanced age, activity and movement limitation, deterioration of sensory and motor functions, a disorder of body temperature regulation, urinary incontinence, anemia, widespread use of anesthetic-sedative-analgesic and muscle relaxant drugs, metabolic disorders, circulatory disorders, and ventilation disorders. Pressure ulcers are classified according to the International NPUAP/EPUAP Pressure Ulcer Classification System. In 2016, NPUAP collected the things that need to be done to prevent the formation of pressure ulcers in 5 main articles. These are risk management, the provision of skin care, the provision and maintenance of nutrition, patient positioning, and education. Despite the precautions taken, it is not always possible to prevent the formation of pressure sores. Different treatment methods can be used to prevent infection, eliminate it if present, and accelerate wound healing.

Keywords: pressure ulcers, bed sores, risk factors, prevention, treatment

Introduction

Many terms are used to describe pressure-induced deterioration in tissue integrity. Bed sore, decubitus ulcer, decubitus, pressure sore, pressure necrosis, ischemic ulcer, and pressure ulcers are the most commonly used terms (Mervis and Phillips, 2019). The National Pressure Sore Advisory Panel (NPUAP) in America and the European Pressure Sore Advisory Panel (EPUAP) define decubitus ulcer as skin and/or tissue damage that usually occurs on bone protrusions as a result of pressure, compression, or both. Although pressure ulcers mostly occur

* Corresponding Author's Email: dr.demet.kelleci@gmail.com.

In: Common Diseases According to Family Medicine Practice Guidelines
Editors: Esra Meltem Koç and Hilal Aksoy
ISBN: 979-8-89530-302-3

on a bone protrusion, there may be a connection with a medical device or object (Korkut Kurtoğlu &Yılmaz, 2023).

Pressure ulcers are one of the most frequently occurring adverse events in hospitalized patients worldwide. It prolongs hospital stays, increases medical expenses, reduces the quality of life, and causes nosocomial infections, disability, morbidity, and mortality. It causes depression, pain, muscle and bone inflation in the patient, and even threatens the lives of elderly individuals, those with multiple chronic diseases, and patients with limited mobility (Jaul et al., 2018).

Pressure ulcers are caused by pressure that completely or partially blocks blood flow to soft tissue. The possibility of developing pressure ulcers is very high, especially in patients with limited mobility who are confined to a wheelchair or bed for long periods. Areas of the body, especially those where bony or cartilaginous protrusions are covered only by thin, soft tissue, are high-risk areas for pressure ulcers. Therefore, the areas where ulcers are most commonly seen are the cutaneous surfaces on the coccyx, spinous processes, heels, ankles, and elbows, and in side-lying patients, the iliac crest, trochanters, and, less commonly, the ear areas (Anders et al., 2010). Nearly 70% of all pressure ulcers occur in the hip and sacral regions, troenteric and ischial regions. Furthermore, pressure ulcers occur in the pretibial regions, patellar, and heel regions, which constitute approximately 15%-25% of all pressure ulcers (Fatima et al., 2023; Black et al., 2015). The most common stages are Stage I (43.5%) and Stage II (28.0%) (Li et al., 2020).

It is estimated that there are approximately one million patients in the United States who develop pressure ulcers. According to research on the prevalence of pressure ulcers in Europe, the prevalence was found to be between 5.7% and 28.2%, and in the USA, it was between 9.2% and 17% (Clark et al., 2017). A study conducted in France reported a 7.8% prevalence of pressure ulcers at admission and a 12.3% prevalence of pressure ulcers at discharge (Dugaret et al., 2014). In studies conducted in our country, the prevalence of pressure ulcers was found to be 2.5-12.7% and 10.5-26.2% in patients in intensive care (Kısacık and Sönmez, 2020). However, the incidence and prevalence of pressure ulcers cannot be determined exactly due to the insufficient number of studies conducted in our country and the differences in data received from healthcare areas.

Main Body

Risk Factors

The risk factors in the formation of pressure ulcers are divided into two main groups: extrinsic risk factors (not belonging to the patient) and intrinsic risk factors (belonging to the patient).

Extrinsic Risk Factors

They can be listed as pressure, friction, tear, and humidity. The most important factor in pressure sore development is pressure. Long-term pressure blocks blood flow in the capillaries of that area. Pressure ulcers occur when the delivery of oxygen and nutrients to the tissue stops.

The blood pressure in the capillaries is between 10 and 30 mmHg, and when the pressure in the area exceeds this range, there is a risk of ulcer (Tayyib et al., 2013). The effect created by the pressure is related to the intensity of the pressure, the tolerance of the exposed area, and the exposure time.

The force created by two objects moving in opposite directions is the friction force. In particular, friction occurs between the skin and the patient's clothes or bed surface. Friction is caused by patients sliding up or down on the bed and by caregivers holding the patient and pulling them up without using the sheets that are under the patient and used for positioning while positioning the patient. The friction factor is the beginning of skin deterioration. Repeated friction creates deeper ulcers (Agrawal and Chauhan, 2012).

It is the downward sliding of the patient's structure on a surface by the effect of gravity, while the skin and subcutaneous tissue remain fixed and the underlying soft tissue, such as muscle and fascia, moves in opposite directions. This shear is an important pathomechanical factor. The force generated between tissues causes stretching and tearing of blood vessels, interruption of blood flow, and ischemic tissue necrosis in that area. Especially in healthcare areas, shearing is seen to occur when the gravity distribution of patients lying semi-reclined for a long time is shifted or when caregivers position the patient without lifting the beds to ensure the continuation of their sections. For this reason, it is especially important to pay attention to the explanations of the processes of the authorities who provide 24-hour service to the patient, and information and topics on the subject are important (Agrawal and Chauhan, 2012).

Humidity causes increased sensitivity of the epidermis layer and a disruption of tissue integrity. Conditions such as urinary and fecal incontinence, excessive sweating, and wound drainage are conditions that cause a moist environment in the body. In patients who are bedridden for a long time, moist skin, especially in contact with clothes or bedspreads for a long time, causes shearing and facilitates the development of pressure sores (Coleman et al., 2013).

Internal Risk Factors

They can be listed as nutritional deficiency, advanced age, activity and movement limitation, deterioration in sensory and motor diseases, dysregulation of the body system, incontinence, anemia, widespread use of anesthetic-sedative-analgesic and muscle relaxant systems, metabolism-circulation-ventilation disorders, and mechanical ventilation application.

Insufficient intake of protein, vitamins, and minerals causes malnutrition. Malnutrition is one of the most important risk factors for the development and healing of pressure ulcers in the care of elderly patients. As people age, the fat tissue decreases, and the skin loses its elasticity. As a result, the decrease in resistance to pressure and friction increases the risk of pressure ulcers (Cooper 2013).

Among the problems that limit physical activity and movement in people, the most common features are; brain hemorrhage, spinal cord injury, and femur fracture. The risk of pressure values that encounter the system of this system and remain motionless remains in areas such as the gluteal region, sacrum, and heel.

Many diseases such as burns, diabetes, damage to peripheral nerves, and spinal cord injury cause patients to experience loss of sensation and sensation in tissues. Since the pain in the tissue of the patient with sensory loss is not felt, the risk of damage in the area where the pressure is applied is quite high. In patients with motor dysfunction, lymphedema occurs in the lymphatic system. This lymphedema also increases the risk of pressure ulcers (Bhattacharya and Mishra 2015).

It is thought that antibiotics, analgesics, and hormone drugs used especially in the treatment process of patients with chronic diseases affect the structural properties of the skin, increasing the risk of pressure ulcers. Ersoy et al., (2013) found in their study that all patients with pressure ulcers received sedation and steroid treatment.

Table 1. International NPUAP/EPUAP pressure ulcer classification system (2009, 2014)

Category/Stage I: Nonblanchable Erythema	It is an erythema of intact skin that does not fade with pressure. It is intact skin with localized, non-blanchable redness, usually over a bony prominence. It may be painful, hard, soft, warmer, or colder than the adjacent tissue. It may be difficult to detect in individuals with a dark skin color.
Category/Stage II: Partial Thickness Skin Loss	It is a partial thickness loss of skin. Partial-thickness dermis loss presenting as a shallow open ulcer with a red-pink wound bed, without fibrinous scar tissue (slough). It may also present as an intact or open/ruptured serum-filled blister.
Category/Stage III: Full Thickness Skin Loss	It is the loss of the full thickness of the skin. Fibrinous scar tissue (slough) may be present but does not mask the depth of tissue loss. It may include cavitation (undermining) and tunneling under the edges of the wound. Subcutaneous tissue is absent in the bridge of the nose, ear, occiput, and malleolus, and Category/Stage III ulcers can be shallow. Conversely, certain areas of fat can develop extremely deep Category/Stage III pressure ulcers. The bone/tendon is not visible or directly palpable.
Category/Stage IV: Full Thickness Tissue Loss	It is a full-thickness tissue loss with exposed bone, tendon, or muscle. Fibrinous scar tissue (slough) or crusted dead skin (eschar) may be present in some parts of the wound bed. It often involves cavitation (undermining) and tunneling under the edges of the wound. There is no subcutaneous tissue on the bridge of the nose, ear, occiput, and malleolus, and these ulcers can be shallow. Category/Stage IV ulcers can extend into muscle and/or supporting structures (e.g., fascia, tendon, or joint capsule), allowing osteomyelitis. Exposed bone/tendon is visible or can be directly palpated.
Unstageable: Depth Unknown	Its depth is unknown. It is the exact tissue loss where the base of the ulcer is covered with fibrinous scar tissue (scab) and/or crusted dead skin (eschar) in wound formation, the depth of which is unknown. The actual depth and therefore the Category/Stage cannot be determined until sufficient fibrinous scar tissue (scab) and/or crusted dead skin (eschar) have been removed to expose the wound base. Stable eschar on the heels should act as a biological cover and should not be removed.
Suspected Deep Tissue Injury: Depth Unknown	A purple or maroon localized area containing discolored intact skin or a blood-filled blister due to mild underlying air temperatures and/or shear damage. It may be painful, hard, soft, mud-like, hotter, or colder than the adjacent tissue. Identifying deep tissue injury can be difficult in individuals with a darker skin color. During its development, a thin blister may be visible on a dark wound bed. The wound can progress further and become covered with thin crusted dead skin (eschar). Although it is an optimal treatment, it can progress rapidly, exposing other tissue layers of the wound.

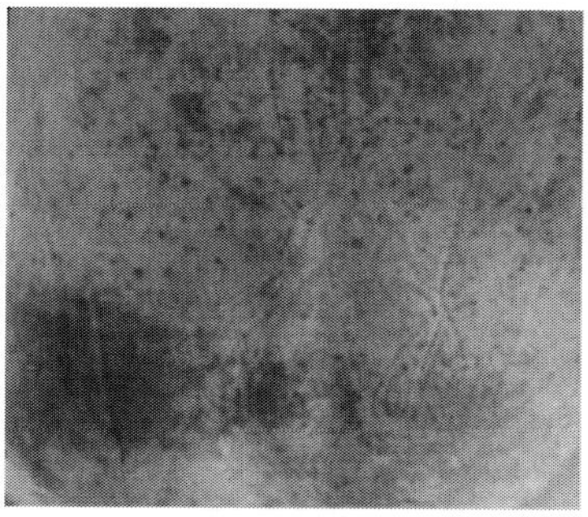

Stage I

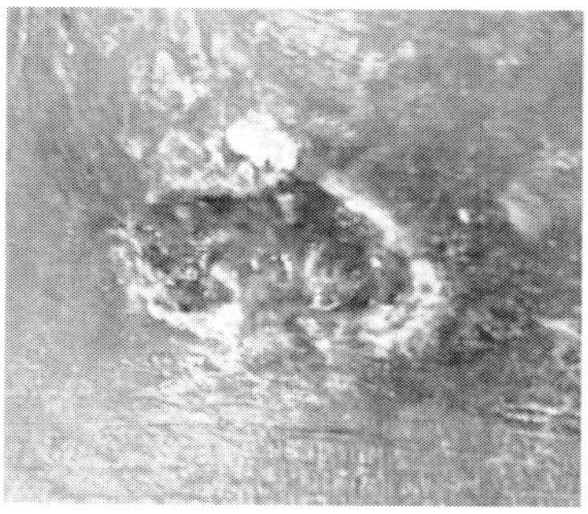

Stage II

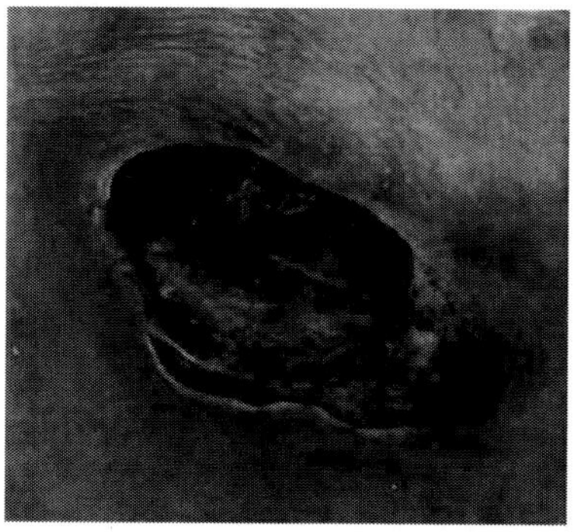

Stage III

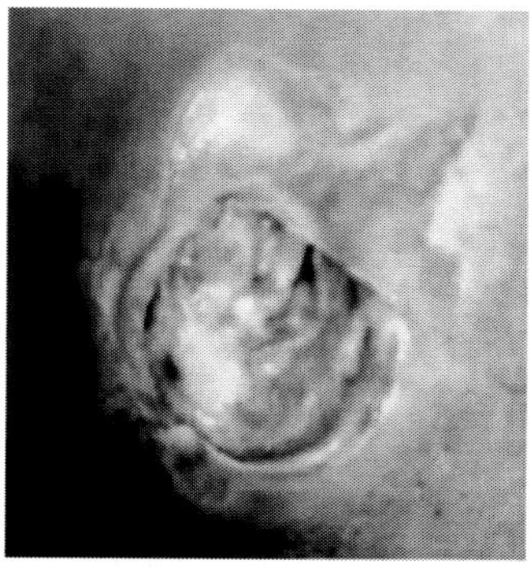

Stage IV

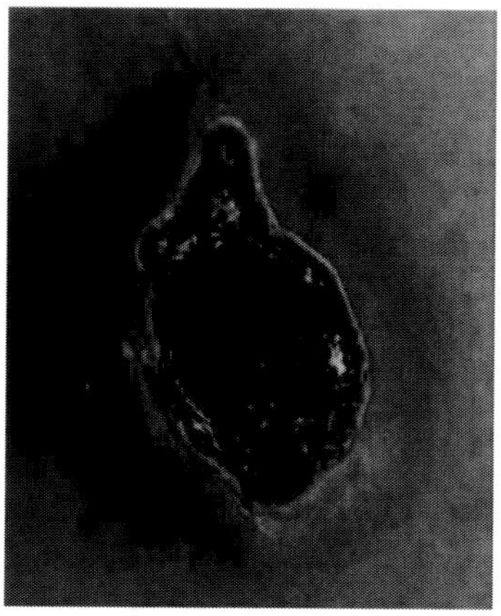

Unstageable Ulcer

Figure 1. Photos of pressure ulcers according to their stages (Photos belong to the author's archive).

Classification

The International NPUAP/EPUAP Pressure Ulcer Classification System (2009, 2014) is generally used for decubitus ulcer classification (Table 1). Other classification systems are the WHO ICD-11 (2018) and the NPUAP Classification System (April 2016). Photos of the stages of pressure ulcers are presented in Figure 1.

Table 2. Braden risk assessment scale (Braden, 2012)

Braden Risk Assessment Scale					
Sensory/Mental	Moisture	Activity	Mobility	Nutrition	Friction/Shear
1. Totally limited	1. Constantly moist	1. Bedfast	1. %100 immobile	1. Very poor	1. Frequent sliding
2. Very limited	2. Very moist	2. Chairfast	2. Very limited	2. <½ daily portion	2. Feeble corrections
3. Slightly limited	3. Occasionally moist	3. Walks w/assistance	3. Slightly limited	3. Most of portion	3. Independent corrections
4. No impairment	4. Dry	4. Walks w/out assistance	4. Full mobility	4. Eats everything	

Total Braden Score
15-16 Mild Risk 12-14 Moderate Risk <12 High Risk
15-18 is considered Mild Risk for those > 75 years.

Prevention

In 2016, NPUAP collected the things that need to be done to prevent the formation of pressure ulcers in 5 main articles.

Risk Management

Scales developed for the risk assessment of decubitus ulcer formation are used to implement appropriate preventive measures by analyzing the scores that determine the individual risk level. The scales also include factors that cannot be controlled and therefore cannot be completely prevented for critically ill patients. Various risk assessment tools have been developed for risk identification since the early 1960s, with more than 50 scales such as the Norton Scale, Waterlow Scale, and Braden Scale (Shi et al., 2019). The Braden scale is the most common worldwide due to its ease of use by including more risk factors (Huang et al., 2021). By focusing on the duration of pressure, the Braden scale addresses the intensity of external pressure (sensory function, activity, mobility) and the skin's tolerance to potentially harmful factors (moisture, nutritional status, friction, shear forces) (Anders, 2010). The scale consists of 6 items in total. These substances are sensory perception, moisture, activity, mobility, nutrition, and friction/shear (Table 2).

Providing Skin Care

In patients, a whole skin evaluation should be performed at short intervals, and in hospitalized patients, the whole skin should be evaluated within eight hours at most. Especially for stage 1 pressure ulcers, pressure points under the sacrum, coccyx, hip, heel, thoracanter, elbows, and medical instruments should be observed at least once a day. Immediately after contact with urine, the skin should be cleaned with pH-balanced skin cleansers. In addition to protecting the skin from moisture, dry skin should also be moisturized daily. It is necessary to avoid routine massage and rubbing in the area at risk of pressure ulcers. Bed linens should always be clean, dry, wrinkle-free and stretched, and foreign objects such as treatment materials, cables, etc. should not be kept in the bed (Duncan, 2007).

Providing and Maintaining Nutrition

Individuals at risk for pressure sores should be supported for adequate and balanced nutrition, and if necessary, the individual should be assisted in their nutrition. A protein-rich diet should be provided according to weight, calorie needs, and medical diagnosis. Weight loss should be determined early. It should be evaluated whether oral, enteral, or parenteral intake is sufficient. If possible, nutritional supplements should be provided. Making the patient gain weight by overfeeding them increases the pressure and reduces mobility, making positioning difficult and accelerating the development of pressure ulcers (Wilborn, 2015).

Positioning the Patient

Position changes should be made every two hours at most, taking into account the condition of the individual and the resistance of the skin to pressure, in the order of left lateral, back, and right lateral, avoiding repetitions. The frequency of positioning should be determined by considering the sleep pattern throughout the night. When giving the individual a side-lying position, it should be checked whether the sacrum touches the bed. Positioning should not be performed in the area with a pressure injury. A mattress pad that allows the skin to ventilate should be used. For individuals sitting in a wheelchair, a chair cushion that distributes pressure evenly should be preferred. Sedentary or weak chair-bound individuals should be positioned hourly. If the individual is motionless or in a head elevation position, a polyurethane sacrum support cushion should be used. Polyurethane support should be used for the heels of individuals at high risk for heel sores. A thin breathable barrier should be used under medical devices (Duncan, 2007).

Education

Patients and their relatives should be informed about pressure injuries. The patient and the patient's family should be involved in care (Anders, 2010).

Treatment

Despite the precautions taken, it is not always possible to prevent the formation of pressure sores. The aim of the treatment of decubitus ulcer is to prevent infection, eliminate it if present, and accelerate wound healing. It is also important to assess and treat pain. To relieve pain, analgesic wound dressings and analgesic medications (topical or oral) should be used (Yoshikawa et al., 2002). Another important step in decubitus ulcer treatment is wound cleaning. The wound can be cleaned with physiological saline or antiseptic solutions. Wounds that are infected or contain necrotic debris can be cleaned with surfactants and/or antimicrobial agents. Debridement is necessary for wounds with dead and necrotic residues and an adequate blood supply. Debridement can also be applied to wounds with suspected biofilm formation. Debridement can be performed surgically, autolytically, enzymatically, larvally or mechanically. It is recommended not to debride stable, hard, and dry scar tissues unless there are signs of infection. It is important to evaluate signs of infection and treat them, if present, to ensure wound healing. Appropriate strength, and non-toxic topical antiseptics can be used for a limited time to control the bacterial load. The use of topical antibiotics should be restricted except in special cases due to side effects and the risk of resistance development. Systemic antibiotics should be used in the presence of signs of a systemic infection. Osteomyelitis should be suspected if there are signs of delayed wound healing or visible bone. Moisture must be controlled to ensure proper wound healing. It is important to dry the skin after getting wet due to sweating, wound drainage, urinary incontinence, and other reasons. Barrier creams can be used when necessary. Various wound dressings are available to accelerate wound healing. When choosing a wound dressing, care should be taken to ensure that the wound bed does not remain moist, meets the patient's expectations, prevents the formation of a bacterial load, and is appropriate for the amount of wound exudate, the size and depth of the ulcer, and the surrounding tissue. Therefore, hydrocolloid dressings, clear film dressings, hydrogel dressings, alginate dressings, foam dressings, silver or honey-impregnated dressings, silicone dressings, collagen matrix dressings, or gauze can be used. Platelet-derived growth factors can be used in decubitus wounds where wound healing is delayed. Apart from these, there are also methods such as electromagnetic wave-based electrical stimulation method, pulsed radio frequency energy, phototherapy, high- or low-frequency ultrasound, negative pressure therapy, kinetic energy-based methods, and hyperbaric and topical oxygen therapy. Negative pressure therapy can be applied to pressure ulcers that are free of necrotic tissues. In addition to these, reconstructive surgical methods can also be applied when necessary, in the treatment of pressure ulcers (Reddy et al., 2008).

Conclusion

With the increase in the elderly population and chronic diseases worldwide, the incidence of pressure ulcers has also increased and has become an important health problem, especially in the patient group requiring palliative care. It causes patients to prolong hospital stays, increase medical expenses, decrease quality of life, and increase hospital infection, disability, morbidity, and mortality. Its treatment is also quite difficult and costly. Therefore, preventing pressure sores is important for both the patient and the healthcare system. Knowing the factors that cause the development or progression of pressure ulcers and making plans to prevent them by considering their effects on morbidity and mortality are necessary for good management of resource expenditures.

References

Agrawal, K., & Chauhan, N. (2012). Pressure ulcers: Back to the basics. *Indian Journal of Plastic Surgery*, 45(02), 244-254. https://doi.org/10.4103/0970-0358.101287.

Anders, J., Heinemann, A., Leffmann, C., Leutenegger, M., Pröfener, F., & Renteln-Kruse, W. (2010). Decubitus ulcers: pathophysiology and primary prevention. *Deutsches Ärzteblatt International*, 107(21), 371–382. https://doi.org/10.3238/arztebl.2010.0371.

Bhattacharya, S., & Mishra, R. K. (2015). Pressure ulcers: current understanding and newer modalities of treatment. *Indian Journal of Plastic Surgery*, 48(01), 004-016. https://doi.org/10.4103/0970-0358.155260.

Black, J., Alves, P., Brindle, C. T., Dealey, C., Santamaria, N., Call, E., & Clark, M. (2015). Use of wound dressings to enhance prevention of pressure ulcers caused by medical devices. *International Wound Journal*, 12(3), 322-327. https://doi.org/10.1111/iwj.12111.

Braden, B. J. (2012). The Braden scale for predicting pressure sore risk: reflections after 25 years. *Advances in Skin & Wound Care*, 25(2), 61. https://doi.org/10.1097/01.ASW.0000411403.11392.10.

Clark, M., Semple, M. J., Ivins, N., Mahoney, K., & Harding, K. (2017). National audit of pressure ulcers and incontinence-associated dermatitis in hospitals across Wales: a cross-sectional study. *BMJ Open*, 7(8), e015616. https://doi.org/10.1136/bmjopen-2016-015616.

Coleman, S., Gorecki, C., Nelson, E. A., Closs, S. J., Defloor, T., Halfens, R., & Nixon, J. (2013). Patient risk factors for pressure ulcer development: systematic review. *International Journal of Nursing Studies*, 50(7), 974-1003. https://doi.org/10.1016/j.ijnurstu.2012.11.019.

Cooper, K. L. (2013). Evidence-based prevention of pressure ulcers in the intensive care unit. *Critical Care Nurse*, 33(6), 57-66. https://doi.org/10.4037/ccn2013985.

Dugaret, E., Videau, M. N., Faure, I., Gabinski, C., Bourdel-Marchasson, I., & Salles, N. (2014). Prevalence and incidence rates of pressure ulcers in an emergency department. *International Wound Journal*, 11(4), 386-391. https://doi.org/10.1111/j.1742-481X.2012.01103.x.

Duncan, K. D. (2007). Preventing pressure ulcers: the goal is zero. *The Joint Commission Journal on Quality and Patient Safety*, 33(10), 605-610. https://doi.org/10.1016/S1553-7250(07)33069-9.

Ersoy, E. O., Öcal, S., Öz, A., Yılmaz, P., Arsava, B., & Topeli, A. (2013). Evaluation of risk factors for decubitus ulcers in intensive care unit patients. *Intensive Care Journal*, 4(1), 9-12. https://doi.org/10.5152/dcbybd.2013.03.

Fatima, A., Altaf, F., Hassan, M. A., Ali, H., Manzoor, U., Hayat, M. D., & Fatima, A. (2023). Prevalence of pressure ulcers among patients in Ibn e Sina Hospital. *Pakistan Journal of Medical & Health Sciences*, 17(02), 265-265. https://doi.org/10.53350/pjmhs2023172265.

Huang, C., Ma, Y., Wang, C., Jiang, M., Yuet, L., Lv, L., & Han, L. (2021). Predictive validity of the Braden scale for pressure injury risk assessment in adults: A systematic review and meta-analysis. *Nursing Open*, 8(5), 2194–2207. https://doi.org/10.1002/nop2.792.

Jaul, E., Barron, J., Rosenzweig, J. P., & Menczel, J. (2018). An overview of co-morbidities and the development of pressure ulcers among older adults. *BMC Geriatrics*, 18(1), 1-11. https://doi.org/10.1186/s12877-018-0997-7.

Kısacık, Ö. G., & Sönmez, M. (2020). Pressure ulcers prevention: Turkish nursing students' knowledge and attitudes and influencing factors. *Journal of Tissue Viability*, 29(1), 24-31. https://doi.org/10.1016/j.jtv.2019.11.003.

Korkut Kurtoğlu, Y., & Yılmaz, M. T. (2023). Research of the change of CRP/Albumin ratio according to wound stage in patients with decubitus ulcer. *Journal of Health Sciences of Adıyaman University*, 9(2), 111-118. https://doi.org/10.30569/adiyamansaglik.1246302.

Li, Z., Lin, F., Thalib, L., & Chaboyer, W. (2020). Global prevalence and incidence of pressure injuries in hospitalised adult patients: A systematic review and meta-analysis. *International Journal of Nursing Studies*, 105, 103546. https://doi.org/10.1016/j.ijnurstu.2020.103546.

Mervis, J. S., & Phillips, T. J. (2019). Pressure ulcers: Pathophysiology, epidemiology, risk factors, and presentation. *Journal of the American Academy of Dermatology*, 81(4), 881-890. https://doi.org/10.1016/j.jaad.2018.12.069.

Reddy, M., Gill, S. S., Kalkar, S. R., Wu, W., Anderson, P. J., & Rochon, P. A. (2008). Treatment of pressure ulcers: A systematic review. *JAMA*, 300(22), 2647-2662. https://doi.org/10.1001/jama.2008.778.

Shi, C., Dumville, J. C., & Cullum, N. (2019). Evaluating the development and validation of empirically-derived prognostic models for pressure ulcer risk assessment: A systematic review. *International Journal of Nursing Studies*, 89, 88–103. https://doi.org/10.1016/j.ijnurstu.2018.08.005.

Tayyib, N. A. H., Coyer, F., & Lewis, P. (2013). Pressure ulcers in the adult intensive care unit: A literature review of patient risk factors and risk assessment scales. *Journal of Nursing Education and Practice*, 3(11), 28-42. https://doi.org/10.5430/jnep.v3n11p28.

Wilborn, W. (2015). Pressure ulcer prevention strategies. *Nursing Made Incredibly Easy!*, 13(6), 10-12. https://doi.org/10.1097/01.NME.0000471848.53131.8c.

Yoshikawa, T. T., Livesley, N. J., & Chow, A. W. (2002). Infected pressure ulcers in elderly individuals. *Clinical Infectious Diseases*, 35(11), 1390-1396. https://doi.org/10.1086/344059.

Index

A

B

C

D

J

L

M

N

O

P